Advanced Manufacturing Technologies in Biomedical Science

As healthcare challenges such as human aging and traffic accidents continue to increase exponentially, the biomedical sector faces a significant obstacle in arranging patient-specific biomedical products. Over the past two decades, additive manufacturing's printing quality and ease of production have gained global attention, particularly in the development of scaffolds and implants.

This book explores additive manufacturing technologies and their categorization, materials, processing factors, output responses, advantages, challenges, and biomedical applications. It provides a critical analysis of past biomedical applications of additive manufacturing technology, explores recent advancements, and examines the design, applications, and characterizations of biomedical components using additive manufacturing techniques. Moreover, it discusses notable applications of additive fabrication in aerospace, education, and medicine, as it showcases the medical applications of rapid prototyping, addressing computational and experimental aspects of 3D-printed biomedical devices. Also, it provides future human implications and developments.

Advanced Manufacturing Technologies in Biomedical Science: Practical Applications, Case Studies, and Future Trends offers a unique framework for understanding and evaluating the latest advancements in biomedical additive manufacturing. This book targets individuals interested in conducting research, providing valuable insights, and can serve as an authoritative source of information for manufacturers and academic researchers in the business sector.

Sustainable Manufacturing Technologies: Additive, Subtractive, and Hybrid

Series Editors: Chander Prakash, Sunpreet Singh, Seeram Ramakrishna, and Linda Yongling Wu

This book series offers the reader comprehensive insights of recent research breakthroughs in additive, subtractive, and hybrid technologies while emphasizing their sustainability aspects. Sustainability has become an integral part of all manufacturing enterprises to provide various techno-social pathways toward developing environmental friendly manufacturing practices. It has also been found that numerous manufacturing firms are still reluctant to upgrade their conventional practices to sophisticated sustainable approaches. Therefore this new book series is aimed to provide a globalized platform to share innovative manufacturing mythologies and technologies. The books will encourage the eminent issues of the conventional and non-conventual manufacturing technologies and cover recent innovations.

Modern Hybrid Machining and Super Finishing Processes
Technology and Applications
Edited by Ankit Sharma, Amrinder S. Uppal, Bhargav P. Prajwal, Atul Babbar and Chander Prakesh

Green Manufacturing and Materials Processing Methods
Characterizations, Applications, and Design
Edited by Sarbjeet Kaushal, Sandeep Bansal, Chander Prakash, Bhupinder Singh and Dheeraj Gupta

Advanced Manufacturing Processes
Integration of Sustainable Approaches
Edited by Hitesh Vasudev, Chander Prakash, Mohammad Khalid, and Kavindra Kesari

Industry 5.0
Concepts and Strategies for Digital Transformation
Edited by Mahender Singh Kaswan, Rajeev Rathi and Jose Arturo Garza-Reyes

Advanced Manufacturing Technologies in Biomedical Science
Practical Applications, Case Studies, and Future Trends
Edited by Jashanpreet Singh, Hitesh Vasudev, Chander Prakash, and Manpreet Singh

For more information on this series, please visit: www.routledge.com/Sustainable-Manufacturing-Technologies-Additive-Subtractive-and-Hybrid/book-series/CRCSMTASH

Advanced Manufacturing Technologies in Biomedical Science

Practical Applications, Case Studies, and Future Trends

Edited by Jashanpreet Singh, Hitesh Vasudev,
Chander Prakash, and Manpreet Singh

CRC Press
Taylor & Francis Group
Boca Raton London New York

CRC Press is an imprint of the
Taylor & Francis Group, an **informa** business

Designed cover image: Shutterstock

First edition published 2026
by CRC Press
2385 NW Executive Center Drive, Suite 320, Boca Raton FL 33431

and by CRC Press
4 Park Square, Milton Park, Abingdon, Oxon, OX14 4RN

CRC Press is an imprint of Taylor & Francis Group, LLC

ISBN: 978-1-032-84916-4 (hbk)
ISBN: 978-1-032-84998-0 (pbk)
ISBN: 978-1-003-51606-4 (ebk)

DOI: 10.1201/9781003516064

Typeset in Times
by Apex CoVantage, LLC

This book is dedicated to our families,
friends, teachers, and research supervisors.

Contents

Preface

Advanced Manufacturing Technologies in Biomedical Science: Practical Applications, Case Studies, and Future Trends is a comprehensive book that explores the latest advancements and innovations in the field of biomedical manufacturing. The book covers a wide range of topics, from microfabrication techniques to bioprinting and tissue engineering, providing essential knowledge for researchers, engineers, and professionals in the biomedical industry. The book begins with an introduction to advanced manufacturing technologies in biomedical science, setting the stage for the subsequent chapters. It then delves into the various techniques and technologies used in biomedical manufacturing, such as microfabrication, 3D printing, nanotechnology, and biodegradable materials. Also, the book discusses advanced coating technologies, additive manufacturing in tissue engineering, robotics and automation, smart materials, and bioprinting. It highlights the importance of quality control and regulatory compliance in biomedical manufacturing and explores sustainable manufacturing practices. The book concludes with case studies that demonstrate the practical applications of advanced manufacturing technologies in biomedical science, as well as future trends and challenges in the field. This book serves as a valuable resource for researchers, engineers, and professionals seeking to stay updated on the latest advancements and innovations in biomedical manufacturing.

About the Editors

Dr. Jashanpreet Singh is currently working as Assistant Professor in 'University Center for Research and Development' at Chandigarh University, Mohali, Punjab, India. He obtained his PhD in the field of slurry erosion and thermal spray coatings from Thapar Institute of Engineering and Technology, Patiala, India, in 2019. He has teaching experience of more than five years and industry experience of more than two years. His areas of research include tribology-solid particle erosion, power plant engineering, ash conveying, thermal spray coatings, CFD simulation, composites, and material characterization. He has contributed comprehensively on thermal spray coatings and tribology in reputed journals including *Wear, Tribology International, Ceramics International, Applied Surface Science Advances, Particulate Science and Technology, Engineering Failure Analysis, ASME: Journal of Tribology, ASCE Journal of Pipeline Systems—Engineering and Practice, Coating*s, *Proceedings of IMeche Part J: Journal of Engineering Tribology, Part E: Journal of Process Mechanical Engineering, Surface Review and Letters, Materials Science and Engineering B*, and *Industrial Lubrication and Tribology*, under the flagship of various publishers. He has authored 85+ research publications in which 52 publications are indexed in SCIE/ESCI (Web of Science) and 76 are indexed in Scopus database in various international journals, books, and conferences of repute. He has authored a book with CRC Press and chapters in six different CRC Press books. He is a reviewer for various journals such as *Ceramics International, Surface Coatings and Technology, Tribology in Industry, Surface Topography: Metrology and Properties, Vacuum, IMeche Part E: Journal of Process Mechanical Engineering, Material Research Express, Surface Review and Letters, International Journal of Interactive Design and Manufacturing, Industrial Lubrication and Tribology, and Materials Today: Proceedings.* He serves as a guest editor or section editor on numerous scientific journals. He is listed in World's Top 2% Scientists by Stanford University from 2022 to 2024. He has received "Trusted Reviewer Status" from the Institute of Physics (IOP) in 2020. He has been awarded the "Outstanding Reviewer Award 2021" by the Institute of Physics (IOP) for the journal *Surface Topography: Metrology and Properties.* He is a life member of AICTSD, IAENG, and NITTSD.

Dr. Hitesh Vasudev is working as Professor in the School of Mechanical Engineering, Lovely Professional University, Phagwara, Punjab, India. He received his PhD from Guru Nanak Dev Engineering College, Ludhiana, Punjab, India, in 2018, under the guidance of Prof. (Dr.) Harmeet Singh, GNDEC, Ludhiana, and Dr. Lalit Thakur, NIT, Kurukshetra. His research areas include surface engineering/thermal spraying (HVOF, flame spray, cold and plasma spray, and microwave claddings). He is currently working on the development of nanostructured, multi-modal, and high-entropy alloy coatings for high-temperature oxidation- and corrosion-resistance thermal barrier coatings (TBCs) and microwave processing of materials. Recently, he has been listed in World's Top 2% Scientists published by Stanford University and Elsevier (2023 and 2024). He has contributed extensively on thermal spray coatings in reputable journals, which include *Surface Coatings and Technology*, *Materials Today Communications*, *Engineering Failure Analysis*, *Journal of Cleaner Production*, *Surface Topography: Metrology and Properties*, *Journal of Failure Analysis and Prevention*, *International Journal of Surface Engineering*, and *Interdisciplinary Materials Science*, under the flagship of various publication groups. Moreover, he is a dedicated reviewer of reputed journals such as *Surface Coatings and Technology*, *Journal of Thermal Spray and Technology*, *Ceramics International*, *Journal of Material Engineering Performance*, *Engineering Failure Analysis*, *Surface Topography: Metrology and Properties*, *Material Research Express*, *Engineering Research Express*, and *IGI Global* journals. He has been awarded "Top Cited Paper Awards India 2022" by IOP Publishing, the UK, in Review Category. He has won Research Excellence Award in 2019, 2020, 2021, and 2023 from Lovely Professional University, India. He has 40+ SCI-indexed papers, 100 Scopus-indexed papers, 15 conference papers, 5 books (1 self-authored and 4 edited books), and 25 book chapters. He has been granted a patent titled "High-Temperature Oxidation and Erosion Resistant Alloy-718/Al2O3 Composite Coatings." He has organized one national conference and many international conferences. He has received seed money for a project tilted "Fabrication of Coatings for Bio-Medical Applications," Project Number: LPU/DRD/SEED/SAC/140222/24804, from Lovely Professional University. He has received a grant from Scientific Engineering and Research Board (SERB), New Delhi, Government of India, to conduct a conference in 2023.

Prof. Chander Prakash is Group Pro-Vice Chancellor of Rayat Bahra University, Mohali, Punjab, India. He is an accomplished academic leader with over 18 years of extensive experience in academic administration, research, and global university rankings. A visionary professional, he has driven transformative initiatives in higher education, focusing on elevating institutional reputation and cultivating a thriving research ecosystem. He is a passionate researcher with diversified research interests such as developing materials for biomedical and healthcare applications and additive manufacturing and developing and exploring new cost-effective manufacturing technologies for biomedical industries. He has published over 397 (326 SCI/Scopus) scientific articles in peer-reviewed, reputable, top-notch journals, conferences, and books. Dr. Prakash is a highly cited researcher at the international level, with 8,010 citations, an H-index of 50, and an i-10 index of 173. He is among India's Top 1% of leading mechanical and aerospace engineering scientists, as per Research.com. He holds the 38th rank in India and 1,590th rank in the world. He also consistently appeared in the top 2% of researchers as per Stanford Study in 2021, 2022, 2023, and 2024. As a prolific author, Prof. Prakash has edited or authored 35 books, served as Series Editor for 3 book series, and contributed as Guest Editor for leading journals. He currently serves as the Editor-in-Chief of prestigious international journal *IECE Transactions on Advanced Functional Materials and Processing*. He is also an editorial board member of highly reputed journals. Beyond publications, Prof. Prakash has significantly contributed to Intellectual Property Rights (IPR), with 18 patents filed, 6 granted, and has successfully raised $1.2 million in research grants from bodies like DSTSERB, UKIERI-DST, and the Ministry of Science and Technology, Government of India. His outstanding contributions have earned him the Research

Excellence Award (2019, 2020, 2021). He has actively contributed to institutional accreditation as an NAAC Assessor and Chairperson, ensuring academic quality and excellence.

Dr. Manpreet Singh is Computational Research Scientist at the Henry M. Jackson Foundation for the Advancement of Military Medicine, Inc. (HJF), Bethesda, Maryland, USA, in support of the Department of Defense Biotechnology High Performance Computing Software Applications Institute (DOD-BHSAI), Telemedicine and Advanced Technology Research Center (TATRC), United States Army Medical Research and Development Command (USAMRDC), Fort Detrick, Maryland, USA. Dr. Singh received his PhD in mechanical engineering (thermo-fluids sciences specialization) from the University of Maryland. During his PhD, Dr. Singh worked on a National Science Foundation (NSF-1705538)-funded project titled "Mild Hyperthermia to Enhance Delivery of Therapeutic Nanocarriers in Tumors: Imaging, In Vivo Study, and Simulation." He is one of the few leading interdisciplinary experts in the fields of thermal engineering and mathematics and is well known for developing mathematical models of biological systems and medical devices to identify novel diagnostic and treatment strategies to improve the care available for chronic diseases, such as cancer and type-1 diabetes, and cold-related injuries, such as frostbite and loss of dexterity, hypothermia, and so on. Most importantly, Dr. Singh's work in developing novel medical devices is exemplary, as the multi-orifice insulin delivery device that he developed is currently undergoing human clinical trials in the United States and Europe to obtain Food and Drug Administration 510K approval and CE Mark approval. His multi-hole cannula design being commercialized for insulin delivery demonstrates the impact of Dr. Singh's work. Moreover, his open-source algorithm for magnetic coil design has been consistently adopted by other researchers to inform their own work. In addition, he has actively engaged his peers in the field of thermal engineering by authoring and coauthoring 35 peer-reviewed scientific publications, including 8 peer-reviewed journal articles, 2 peer-reviewed conference proceedings articles, 3 book chapters, and 22 peer-reviewed conference abstracts that have been published in leading international research journals such as *International Journal of Heat and Mass Transfer, International Communications in Heat and Mass Transfer, ASME Journal of Heat Transfer, Computers in Biology and Medicine*, and *International Journal of Thermal Sciences*. More recently, he has received early career recognition with the "AMMCS-2023 Kolmogorov-Wiener Young Researcher Award" at the VIth International Conference on Applied Mathematics, Modeling and Computational Science held at Wilfrid Laurier University, Waterloo, Ontario, Canada, from August 14 to 18, 2023, for improving the prominent mathematical model (Pennes Bioheat Transfer Equation 1948) to predict temperature distribution in cancerous tissues. Dr. Singh has studied the heterogeneous blood perfusion using medical imaging at each pixel location to relax the uniform blood perfusion assumption. Additionally, Dr. Singh is a recipient of three more research awards during his doctoral degree program at the University of Maryland, including the "Dissertation Fellowship Award," "Student Researcher of the Quarter Award," and "Graduate Student of the Month Award," and three times "GSA Professional Development Grantee." Such awards hold higher recognition as these awards were received from an "R1" doctoral university, classified as Research Extensive or Very High Research Activity (VHRA) university under Carnegie Classification of Institutions of Higher Recognition in the United States. Furthermore, Dr. Singh's appointment as an academic editor for *PLOS One*, Guest Associate Editor for *Frontiers in Thermal Engineering*, Co-Guest Editor for *Bioengineering* and moreover, unsolicited invitations to review book proposals as a subject matter expert for Taylor & Francis Group, Judge for Senior Capstone Projects and International Conferences such as 10th American Society of Thermal and Fluids Engineering Conference, Topic Coordinator for Specialized research topics, review invitations for international journals such as *Case Studies in Thermal Engineering*, *Thermal Science and Engineering Progress*, *Heat and Mass Transfer*, *Frontiers in Oncology*, and many more topical advisor positions for journals testify to his high stature in the field of computational heat and mass transfer and mathematics.

Contributors

Esther Titilayo Akinlabi
Faculty of Engineering and Environment
Northumbria University
Newcastle upon Tyne
United Kingdom

Anavadya K. K.
Department of Chemistry
Vellore Institute of Technology
Vellore, Tamil Nadu, India

Shinar Athwal
Thapar Institute of Science and Technology
Patiala, Punjab, India

Dileep Singh Baghel
School of Pharmaceutical Sciences
Lovely Professional University
Phagwara, Punjab, India

Ranjit Bariki
Department of Chemical and Petroleum Engineering University
United Arab Emirates University
Abu Dhabi, UAE

Anand Kumar Chaudhary
Department of Rasa Shastra and Bhaishjya Kalpana (Ayurvedic Pharmaceutics)
Faculty of Ayurveda, Institute of Medical Sciences
Banaras Hindu University
Varanasi, Uttar Pradesh, India

Saumya Das
Noida Institute of Engineering and Technology (Pharmacy Institute)
Greater Noida, Uttar Pradesh, India

Srinithi Shankar Ganesh
Department of Mechanical Engineering
K. S. Rangasamy College of Technology
Namakkal, Tamil Nadu, India

Kashish Garg
University Institute of Biotechnology
Chandigarh University
Mohali, Punjab, India

Sachin Gupta
Department of Robotics and Control
School of Electronics and Electrical Engineering
Lovely Professional University
Phagwara, Punjab, India

Shivali Gupta
Department of Chemistry
School of Chemical and Physical Education
Lovely Professional University
Phagwara, Punjab, India

Abdul Wahab Hashmi
School of Mechanical Engineering
Shandong University of Technology
Zibo, Shandon, China

Minhaz Husain
Department of Mechanical Engineering
National Institute of Technical Teachers Training and Research
Chandigarh, Punjab, India

Vishnu Jayakumar
Department of Food Technology, K. S. Rangasamy
College of Technology
Namakkal, Tamil Nadu, India

N. Jeyaprakash
School of Mechanical and Electrical Engineering
China University of Mining and Technology
Xuzhou City, Jiangsu, China

Aeimy Mary Jose
School of Bioengineering and Biosciences,
Lovely Professional University
Phagwara, Punjab, India

Kardam Joshi
Topical Research and Development
Amneal Pharmaceuticals
Piscataway, New Jersey, United States

Sahil Kainth
Department of Mechanical Engineering
Rayat Bahra Institute of Engineering and Nano Technology
Hoshiarpur, Punjab, India

Gurmeet Kaur
Department of Computer Science and Engineering
Punjabi University
Patiala, Punjab, India

Gursimran Kaur
Mittal School of Business
Lovely Professional University
Phagwara, Punjab, India

Hardeep Kaur
University Institute of Biotechnology
Chandigarh University
Mohali, Punjab, India

Karuna Khajuria
Department of Health and Medical Education
Jammu and Kashmir, India

Anish Kumar
School of Bioengineering and Biosciences
Lovely Professional University
Phagwara, Punjab, India

Bimlesh Kumar
School of Pharmaceutical Sciences
Lovely Professional University
Phagwara, Punjab, India

Manoj Kumar
Department of Mechanical Engineering
Chitkara University Institute of Engineering and Technology
Rajpura, Punjab, India

Sanjeev Kumar
Department of Mechanical Engineering, UIET
Panjab University
Chandigarh, Punjab, India

Anshika Mahajan
Jammu University,
Jammu, Jammu and Kashmir, India

Avijit Mazumder
Noida Institute of Engineering and Technology (Pharmacy Institute)
Greater Noida, Uttar Pradesh, India

Rupa Mazumder
Noida Institute of Engineering and Technology (Pharmacy Institute)
Greater Noida, Uttar Pradesh, India

Amrinder Mehta
Research and Development Cell
School of Mechanical Engineering
Lovely Professional University
Phagwara, Punjab, India

Chandra Mohan
Department of Chemistry
School of Basic and Applied Sciences
K. R. Mangalam University
Gurugram, Haryana, India

Saraswathy Nagendran
Mithibai College of Arts
Chauhan Institute of Science and Amrutben
Jivanlal College of Commerce and Economics
Mumbai, Maharashtra, India

Sunday Ayoola OKE
Department of Mechanical Engineering
University of Lagos, Faculty of Engineering
Akoka-Yaba, Lagos, Nigeria

Narendra Kumar Pandey
School of Pharmaceutical Sciences
Lovely Professional University
Jalandhar, Punjab, India

Dhara Patel
Topical Research and Development
Amneal Pharmaceuticals
Piscataway, New Jersey, United States

Baburam Pokhrel
School of Pharmaceutical Sciences
Lovely Professional University
Jalandhar, Punjab, India

Gaurav Prashar
Department of Mechanical Engineering
Rayat Bahra Institute of Engineering and Nano Technology
Hoshiarpur, Punjab, India

Yokenthira Ramasamy
Department of Food Technology
K. S. Rangasamy College of Technology
Namakkal, Tamil Nadu, India

Ruby Celsia Arul Selvaraj
Department of Food Technology
K. S. Rangasamy College of Technology
Namakkal, Tamil Nadu, India

Jeet Shah
Mithibai College of Arts
Chauhan Institute of Science and Amrutben Jivanlal College of Commerce and Economics
Mumbai, Maharashtra, India

Shruti Sharma
School of Pharmaceutical Sciences
Lovely Professional University
Jalandhar, Punjab, India

Vikas Sharma
University Centre for Research and Development
Chandigarh University
Mohali, Punjab, India

Amrinderpal Singh
Department of Mechanical Engineering, UIET
Panjab University, Chandigarh, Punjab, India

Bhupinder Singh
Department of Chemical and Environmental Engineering
University of Nottingham, University Park
Nottingham, United Kingdom

Gurpreet Singh
Department of Mechanical Engineering
Rayat Bahra Institute of Engineering and Nano Technology
Hoshiarpur, Punjab, India

Gurwinder Singh
Department of Mechanical Engineering
National Institute of Technical Teachers Training and Research
Chandigarh, Punjab, India

Jashanpreet Singh
University Centre for Research and Development
Chandigarh University
Mohali, Punjab, India

Manpreet Singh
Department of Defense Biotechnology High Performance Computing Software Applications Institute, Telemedicine and Advanced Technology Research Center
United States
Army Medical Research and Development Command
Fort Detrick, Maryland
The Henry M. Jackson Foundation for the Advancement of Military Medicine, Inc.,
Bethesda, Maryland, United States

Rajwinder Singh
Department of Materials Science and Engineering
Uppsala University
Uppsala, Sweden

Rupinder Singh
Department of Mechanical Engineering
National Institute of Technical Teachers Training and Research
Chandigarh, Punjab, India

Saksham Singh
University Institute of Biotechnology
Chandigarh University
Mohali, Punjab, India

Sandeep Singh
Department of Policy Research
Panjab University
Chandigarh, Punjab, India

Saurabh Singh
School of Pharmaceutical Sciences
Lovely Professional University
Jalandhar, Punjab, India

Ruchira Srivastava
Department of Mechanical Engineering
Amity University
Greater Noida, Uttar Pradesh, India

Ayushi Thakur
Department of Mechanical Engineering
Amity University
Greater Noida, Uttar Pradesh, India

Rimika Thakur
University Institute of Biotechnology
Chandigarh University
Mohali, Punjab, India

Hitesh Vasudev
Research and Development Cell, School of Mechanical Engineering
Lovely Professional University
Phagwara, Punjab, India

Praveen Kumar Verma
Research and Development Cell, School of Mechanical Engineering
Lovely Professional University
Phagwara, Punjab, India

Sunil Verma
Department of Management Information System
Webster University
Tashkent, Uzbekistan

Vijayalakshmi U.
Department of Chemistry
Vellore Institute of Technology
Vellore, Tamil Nadu, India

Noushi Zaidi
Department of Basic Science, College of Science
King Faisal University
Hofuf, Saudi Arabia

1 Introduction to Advanced Manufacturing Technologies in Biomedical Science

Jashanpreet Singh, Vikas Sharma, and Manpreet Singh

CONTENTS

1.1 INTRODUCTION TO ADVANCED MANUFACTURING TECHNOLOGIES

Integrated manufacturing technology refers to a variety of applications and equipment commonly used to improve manufacturing performance for the production of goods [1]. Based on the theory of smart manufacturing, the concepts

DOI: 10.1201/9781003516064-1

of elements of advanced manufacturing are put forward, which includes automation, big data and analyzing system, artificial intelligence, 3D printing, and so on [2,3]. In this chapter, a number of technologies have been discussed that have evolved over the years and gained acceptance in the business environment thereby leading to enhanced performance, efficient results as well as improved profitability among the companies that have embraced the relevant technologies. Applying modern technologies such as robotics, nanotechnology, laser cutting or machining, networking, and IT integration offers five specific benefits. The advantage lies in improving the efficiency of production operation, cutting costs, raising production and quality, and better meeting the needs of customers [4–8]. A variety of industries adopt advanced manufacturing which is used in automaking, aerospace, drugs and pharmaceuticals, electrical and electronics, and medical instrument manufacturing [1,9,10]. Advanced manufacturing is a progressive and ongoing process with the goal of improving upon an existing technology of manufacturing to help organizations maintain relevance and value. This is done through invention, embodiment, and innovation, leading to Robert's third proposition that generates further opportunities within the business reality context [11]. Some examples are adaptive manufacturing, also known as 3D printing technology, robotics and automation, smart twin technology, laser cutting or welding, and nanotechnology [12,13].

Additive manufacturing (AM), or 3D printing, is a process where an object is gradually constructed from a source material by depositing successive layers of the material on top of one another to form an object, which has the physical characteristics and purpose that cannot be easily produced by conventional manufacturing processes [14–19]. Lesser material is required in AM processes which helps in improving the precision and which makes it fit for utilization not only in the mentioned industries but also in almost any field including technology, aerospace, medical, and so on [20,21]. Automate means minimizing cycle time not considering inherent variability resulting due to fatigue or other factors, when performing a complicated operation. Robots are mostly incorporated in the automobile industry, aerospace, and consumer industries [22,23]. Digital twin technology creates virtual representations of physical objects, processes, and assets for sensing, inspecting, and optimizing. Also, it increases capacity and time and improves function [24]. Laser technology applied to welding and machining ensures easier and safer working and processing and quick production of parts which causes less heat to the material being used [25]. Methods like proximity sensor welding, battery welding, and electronics manufacturing need it [26]. Through nanotechnology, the property of used material is improved, depending on the light-emitting and light-absorbing action and the management of chemical reaction. The key characteristic of nanotechnology is the increase of density, which means that as many as possible of any object in an area or space is produced, thus miniaturizing systems applied in AM. All of these technologies are a sample of the powerful new instruments within AM and the new revolutionary tools and methods for making the production processes more effective and high quality.

1.2 IMPORTANCE OF ADVANCED MANUFACTURING IN BIOMEDICAL SCIENCE

This section assesses the manner by which new manufacturing technologies have influenced biomedical science. This has helped in the development of better medical equipment, custom-made implants, and best treatment plans. Some of the advanced manufacturing processes are shown in Figure 1.1. Thus, it is necessary to consider the conventional manufacturing process and the associated disadvantages and challenges as well as the new manufacturing methods that enable to address them. Traditional techniques of production have been widely used in manufacturing organizations for quite some time now. Such methods usually entail steps such as machining, injection moulding, casting, and so on [27]. Machining is a process in which cutting or application of any force is exercised to produce a material with components and shapes. On the other hand, the injection moulding processes involve the use of moulds to force the material to take certain shapes. These are the tried-and-tested, high-volume production methods that assist manufacturers in developing similar products in a short time and for a relatively low cost. Traditional manufacturing makes use of many tools and moulds, nearly all of which are costly and take a long time to develop. Such subordinate sequencing also constrains flexibility where change of the design is concerned and the ability to provide a customized product to a client, as such manoeuvres are always expensive and time-consuming. While applied to complex technology or rigid machines, such approaches allow for solving a plethora of simple tasks at a very high quality, but they cannot cope with the new demands of the constantly evolving medical business or personalization of therapies.

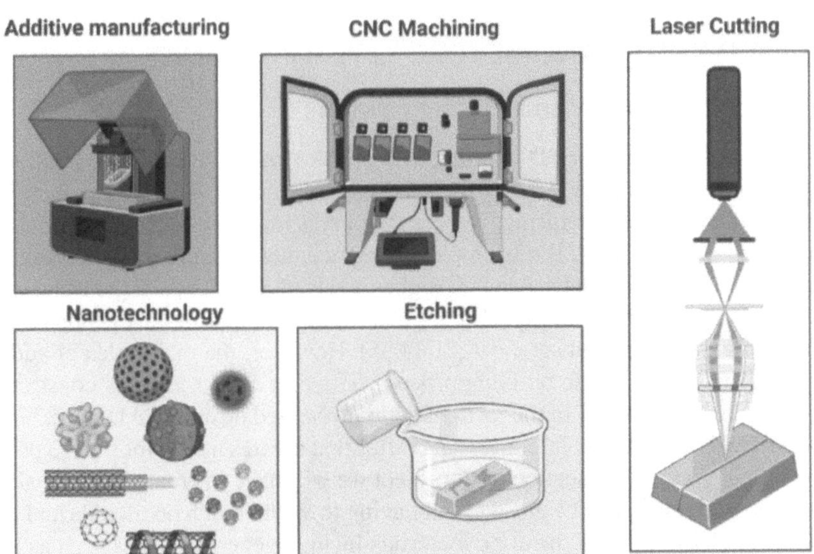

FIGURE 1.1 Various advanced manufacturing processes.

This section also investigates the issues arising from the utilization of conventional manufacturing engineering approaches in biomedical applications. However, like every other method, conventional methods also have their demerits and/or challenges as seen here. The first of the identified gaps is when creating products using the subtraction technique, which often results in the loss of excessive materials. For instance, during material conversion where we specify and cut material for the actual end product, in machining, waste in the form of chips and scrap is normally produced. Also, it results in high cost of production, and it has a number of implications for the environment and its sustainability. Another issue inherent in the use of the AM processes is that once the tooling is defined, the initial designs cannot be altered at all. Traditionally executed manufacturing processes have fixed longer cycle time for mould preparation or tooling modification; hence bringing about design change or low volume production is costly. This rigidity can be particularly deleterious to the string biomedical marketplace, where bespoke implants are continually needed.

In addition, traditional engineering methods are often cheaper when integrated in mass production but are not suitable for medium-product quantity production, which is often the case in healthcare systems. It is quite clear that a majority of mould or tooling costs have massive initial expenditures that are not ideal for low-volume production; therefore, they come with per-piece costs that are very costly for custom medical devices. However, based on the aforementioned operating challenges, conventional manufacturing may not be in a good place to deal with the geometric difficulties related to comparison of forms and shapes that stimulate osseointegration or enhance the use for further generations of dental implants forms that cannot even be manually sculpted.

1.3 ADVANCED MANUFACTURING TECHNOLOGIES

1.3.1 Additive Manufacturing (3D Printing)

Additive manufacturing or 3D printing is a process of constructing objects, using layers from computer models [28–31]. A more conventional method of part making is the "subtractive manufacturing," where the part is made by reducing the material from a solid billet [32,33]. For example, aerospace, automobile, medical, and consumer product industries have adopted higher levels of advanced 3D printing, where both chemistry and engineering come together to offer superior part geometry with a very low level of rejected scrap [10,21,34,35]. However, the major idea of additive manufacturing is layer-wise building process. The first aspect towards construction of this structure is a model in the form of computer-aided design (CAD) [36]. Slicing software divides the model into layers and after that creates a path for the 3D printer. Each of them applies to a section of the object we will have to create, and it is simple to come up with intricate designs without having to spend much on moulds and other formalities. Most of the 3D printing materials include generic plastics such as PLA, ABS, and PET-G; metals such as aluminum and steel; ceramics; and biological matter [37]. Different requirements like strength, flexibility, and thermal conductivity among others will cause the material to be used to be different [38]. Such versatility makes it possible to come up with a number of designs that are scientifically attractive and at the same time useful in one way or the other.

As mentioned earlier, AM comprises a range of manufacturing processes, as shown in **Figure 1.2,** wherein every manufacturing process has its own process and technique. Among the numerous types of 3D printing, fused deposition modelling (FDM) is the oldest but also the simplest of its kind [39]. The working process of the machine involves extruding thermoplastic and melting a filament with the help of a heated nozzle and depositing it in a desired pattern in layers. This makes FDM ideal for developing models or actual, usable parts since the method is affordable and easy to control [40]. The process of stereolithography (SLA) involves the use of a UV laser to trigger the curing of liquid photopolymer resin into layers of solid plastics [41]. It involves the use of a digital model to guide the fusing of the liquid resin when building the laser. It yields high-solution end-products as well as precisely polished curved surfaces, but they require subsequent stages of processing such as washing besides last hardening. Selective laser sintering or SLS is one of the most widely used processes in this category: a high-energy laser melts and fuses material particles in powdered form (nylon or polymer, for instance) layered on top of each other [42]. SLS is ideal for functional prototypes and end-use applications since it can produce non-support material structures and geometrically very complex structures [43]. The material jetting technology dispenses droplets of a liquid photopolymer onto a build platform and then exposes it. Material jetting is a process of manufacturing an object in multiple materials and hues with great precision, but the manufacturing costs are on the higher side compared to other techniques [44,45]. In binder jetting, we use a liquid binder to selectively impregnate the powder material thus bonding the two together. After the part is printed, it is customary to sinter or

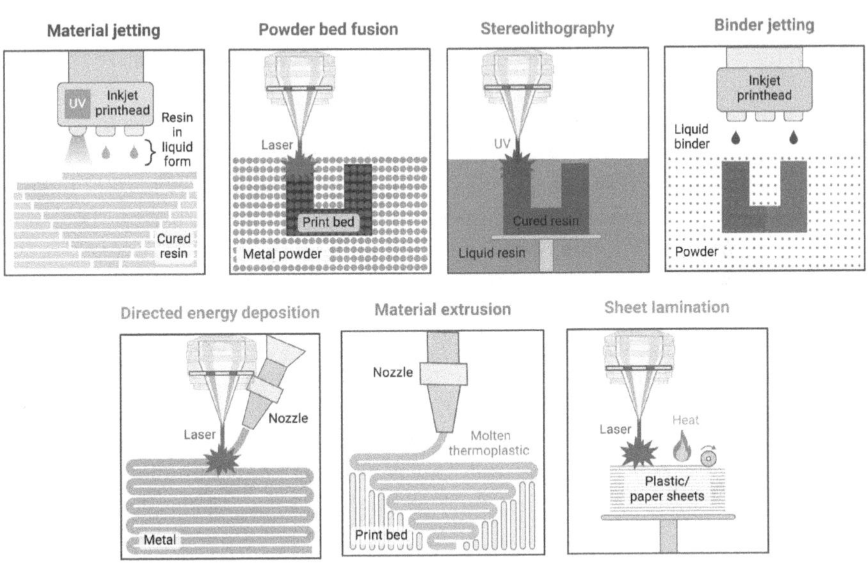

FIGURE 1.2 Various additive manufacturing processes.

infiltrate the part to achieve acceptable mechanical properties. With direct energy deposition (DED), energy sources used include lasers or electron beams, and these are used to melt material during its deposition [46].

1.3.1.1 Applications of Additive Manufacturing

The application of 3D printing technology has to a great extent expanded numerous sectors of biomedical science and healthcare. The concept of the tailored—making medical product from the technology of nanotechnology has significantly impacted the future of surgery, prosthetics, and manufacture of medical equipment. Different applications of AM in the biomedical industry are also described with special reference to patient and healthcare centres' impact. A significant application of 3D printers within the biomedical field is in the production of anatomical models for surgical purposes. MRI- or CT-scanned images can be taken, and doctors can come up with exact model of the patient, especially if the surgery is complex in nature. This way, operations and problems related to it are given more attention in preparation, which enhances its efficiency and surgical accuracy and reduces operation time. Computerized restoration of material enables development of implants and prosthetics that are unique to each client [47]. This is useful in orthopaedic and dental implantation since the implant/prosthetic has to fit into a particular place to its maximum. Hospitals continue to acquire 3D printers that can directly produce highly specialized tools such as orthopaedic implants, cranial plates, and even dental restorations like crowns and bridges [48,49].

The capacity to design and produce such devices effectively and swiftly improves patients' satisfaction and therapeutic outcomes and reduces the risk of receiving adverse effects due to wrong anatomical matching. Its subgroup, bioprinting, is based on the arrangement of live cells which construct tissues or an organ. That is why the provided technology can be used for the production of tissues for transplantation or investigation of drug quality. Organ constructs through bioprinting present tissue architecture in humans which a future research could revolutionize regenerative medicine. Altogether, bioprinting is still in its infancy while at the same time it possesses many opportunities to free the transplantology from the lack of donors, and increase the chances of successful transplant operations. The main approaches to the bioprinting processes can be visualized in the form of a structural diagram which is shown in **Figure 1.3**. In addition, when it comes to the use of 3D printing technology, particularly in the development of medical instruments, enhanced rates of production have been realized, some of which can be attributed to proper modelling of the device designs on the printer.

3D printing enables the fabrication of surgical instruments, medicine, and diagnostic equipment for individual use with specific patients or in special operations. For instance, vaccination involves the 3D-printed microneedles, which are shown to have greater immunogenicity than the traditional techniques [50,51]. Additionally, 3D printing is slightly elastic so that the healthcare providers can easily show revisions or amendments that may come up as the practice of the designs begins. Advancement in the production of medical products is point-of-care manufacturing. When implemented within the facility, the clinician is able to design and develop needed devices or models specifically within the facilities and at the right time due to

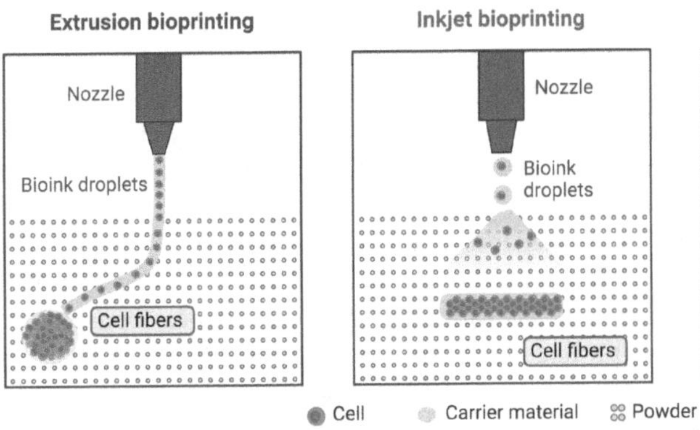

FIGURE 1.3 Different types of bioprinting processes.

patients' status. Besides, the demonstrated capability also balances the length of the waiting time within patient populations with regard to revitalizing a dynamic pace of change contingent on certain clinical realities [52]. When more facilities develop fabrication centres in hospitals, more rapid manufacturing takes place. Nevertheless, as with any innovation, there are issues that relate to integration of additive manufacturing in biomedical science. The two major themes of regulation have always been the safety of the medical products and the effectiveness of the 3D printing process. These problems have been brewing, and the US Food and Drug Administration (FDA) has sought to address them through approval and regulation of these technologies [53]. Nevertheless, the FDA also demands qualified staff's education while operating such improved instruments.

Moreover, materials science developments themselves will define more extensive additive technologies' usage in medicine in the future. Innovative developments in biodegradable material technology are expected to make temporary implantation and controlled delivery for drugs safer and efficient [54,55]. Searching for development of research, it can be stated that additive manufacturing will keep its significant position in the framework of the concept of "personalized medicine" and tailor-made solutions for patients, enhancing efficacy in different branches of medicine. The main advantage of 3D printing in achieving a high degree of customization of products is that this technology allows subjects to create goods that meet customer needs at minimal time. In addition, 3D printing can be effectively used for the formation of a rapid prototype which may be opportune for many manufacturing enterprises. The technology offers design flexibility for creating complex designs of components and products with sophisticated geometry, lighter structure, specially designed structure, fewer numbers of parts, and even deposition of multiple material at once [56,57]. With the 3D printing technology, organizations can continue holding tools for hours rather than days and return it in manufacturing depots and reduce its costs, as well as increase the effectiveness of organizational functioning [58]. 3D printing decreases the possibility of an error or losses at the stage of printing as compared to traditional printing that affects redesigning of prototype or change in the design [59]. 3D printing is turning into an important factor contributing to advanced manufacturing in terms of innovation, cost, and efficiency as well as offering new possibilities of manufacturing products of different types across numerous sectors and industries.

3D manufacturing supply chain in the current generation of manufacturing systems adds a lot of improvements to the existing manufacturing supply chain in many ways to transform the traditional manufacturing systems through 3D manufacturing printing [60]. Just like 3D printing, the idea of concentrating manufacturing at the demand centres promotes cut on transportation and storage costs. This strategy dramatically minimizes the multiple complex supply chain webs, and furthermore, decreases the time and inventory expense. Since 3D printing involves considerable control in the designing process, product design can be customized and personalized to fit each client's individual needs and desires. This capability allows companies to design for the needs of customer within the market, thereby offering more customer satisfaction especially given the market trend on downsizing [61]. They pointed out that additive manufacturing offers a solution to what they consider a classic supply chain management question—how to manage the first and second tiers for the supply of spares. They argued that organizations can use 3D printing to manufacture spare as required without having to establish and stock large inventories of blanks. Furthermore, mid and end life cycle stocks are also kept; this is generally necessary to replace breaks and minimize customer waiting time hence improving satisfaction levels [62]. 3D printing should assist the organization to make the supply chain more reactive so that, in the event some of these sources of disruption occur like natural disasters, political instabilities or, pandemics, then the supply chain has to be able to print those critical parts or products in those regions. Amorphous manufacturing paradigm is less centralized compared to the conventional supply chain system, and risks brought by specific occurrences are fully minimized to retain functionality [63,64]. Nevertheless, small manufacturers based in the United States may face several challenges in the application of 3D printing technology like customers' demand is uncertain. So it is difficult to receive cheap credit, and the use of new technologies requires proper knowledge and training. The following barriers need to be discussed to increase the role of additive manufacturing technology for improving the supply chain operations and performance in the context of small- and medium-sized business organizations. Therefore, 3D printing is suitable to be made one at a time in localized complex manufacturing supply chain that has a good search engine for spare parts and is less prone to breakdown and possesses SM traits.

1.3.2 Computer Numerical Control (CNC) Machining

CNC machining is a critical technology for advanced manufacturing processes that have characterized the fabrication of biomedical devices and implants [65]. The computer controls the tools and equipment in this process, enabling precise cutting, shaping, and material manipulation. The process begins with the creation of a computer-aided design, or CAD, model of the desired component, also known as a CAM or computer-aided manufacturing model [66]. The computer control system then converts this digital model into a form it understands, enabling the CNC machine to perform the desired operations accurately. CNC machining comes in different categories, some of which are milling, turning, and drilling. All these methods use an assortment of cutting tools and procedures for getting the required shapes and surface finishes. For instance, CNC milling uses rotating cutting tools to cut a workpiece, whereas in CNC turning, the workpiece rotates against a stationary cutting tool. Accuracy is important in biomedical applications, for it determines whether a given component will be safe and perform optimally within the human body given the stringent tolerances.

The biomedical industry highly benefits from CNC machining because of the need to produce small components with tight tolerances required in the construction of medical technology equipment or implantation in the human body. **Figure 1.4** illustrates the various applications of CNC machining in biomedical applications. It has a key use in the creation of orthopaedic components like hips and knee replacements. These implants require precise measurements to conform to the patient's anatomy, ensuring significant comfort and structural integrity following surgery. The customization is possible due to information entering the CNC machining process, which is formed by data about the patient retrieved from imaging devices such as MRIs or CT scans. Next to orthopaedic uses, it is applied to create surgical instruments that require the highest level of accuracy in production. CNC technology produces surgical instruments such as scalpels, forceps, and retractors, which are sharp, reliable, and capable of reproducing subsequent modifications in surgery. Design complexity consolidated at the microscale reduces variability and improves the surgical tools' quality. The manufacturing of microfluidic systems is a major application of CNC machining in the biomedical domain [67,68]. These devices are known as microscale manipulators, and they manipulate fluids for diagnostic purposes, proof

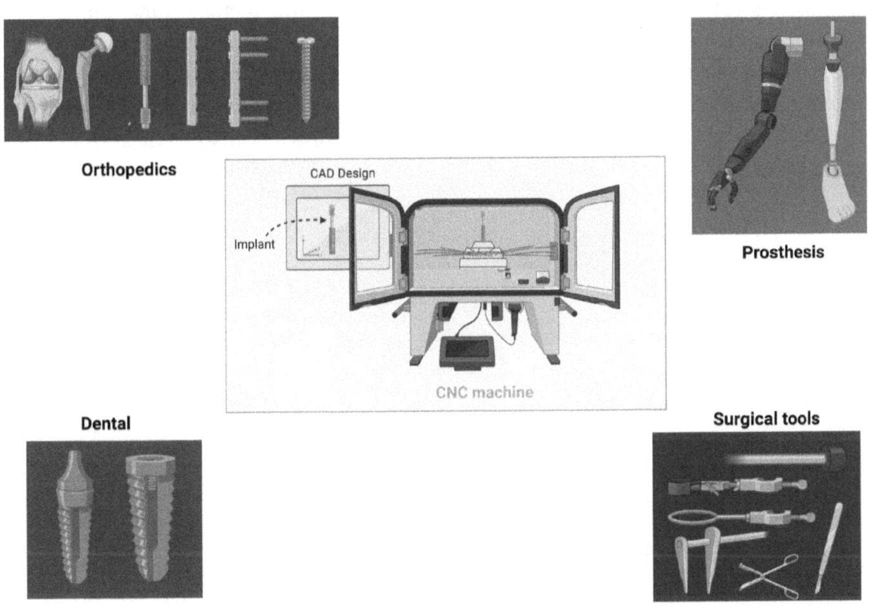

FIGURE 1.4 Applications of CNC in biomedical applications.

of concept, and drug delivery. Machining flexibility that results from the accuracy of CNC equipment is aided in manufacturing tight channels and chambers necessary for functional fluid controls. Furthermore, CNC machining is useful in the manufacturing of bioresorbable implants that corrode in the body after accomplishing their work. It is possible to use biocompatible materials, such as titanium and certain polymers, to create implants that will help provide temporary support without causing further problems associated with permanent implants.

1.3.3 Laser Cutting and Etching

Laser cutting and etching are sophisticated processes that involve applying a focused laser to alter the properties of materials [69,70]. Many sectors, particularly biomedical science, have witnessed a surge in the popularity of these processes, as they play a crucial role in the design of medical equipment and instruments as well as the development of customized medical treatments. This section focuses on the concept and technique of laser cutting and etching, along with the various uses in the biomedical sector.

Laser cutting (LC) is a thermal parting process that employs a high-power laser beam directed at the material to be cut [71]. Therefore, laser heat melts or evaporates the material for easy and accurate cutting. You can adjust the power, speed, and focus of these patterns, and with the laser's ability to cut in any direction, you can create intricate designs and shapes at a faster pace. LC process is applicable to a wide range of materials, such as metals, plastics, woods, and ceramics [72,73]. On the other hand, laser etching involves using a laser light to melt the surface of an object without causing significant material removal, as illustrated in **Figure 1.5**. This process forms an elevated mark or a pattern on the surface. One can apply it for aesthetic purposes or identification, such as numbering serials or logos. While engraving carves a deeper pit to fit the tool, etching alters only the surface layer of the material [74,75]. Laser etching is beneficial in situations where deep, easily readable markings are required, as the laser's burning process results in high-contrast marks [76,77].

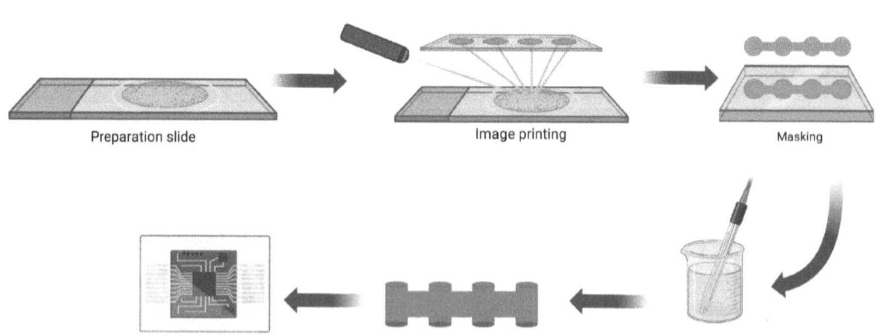

FIGURE 1.5 Schematic diagram of etching process for biosensor applications.

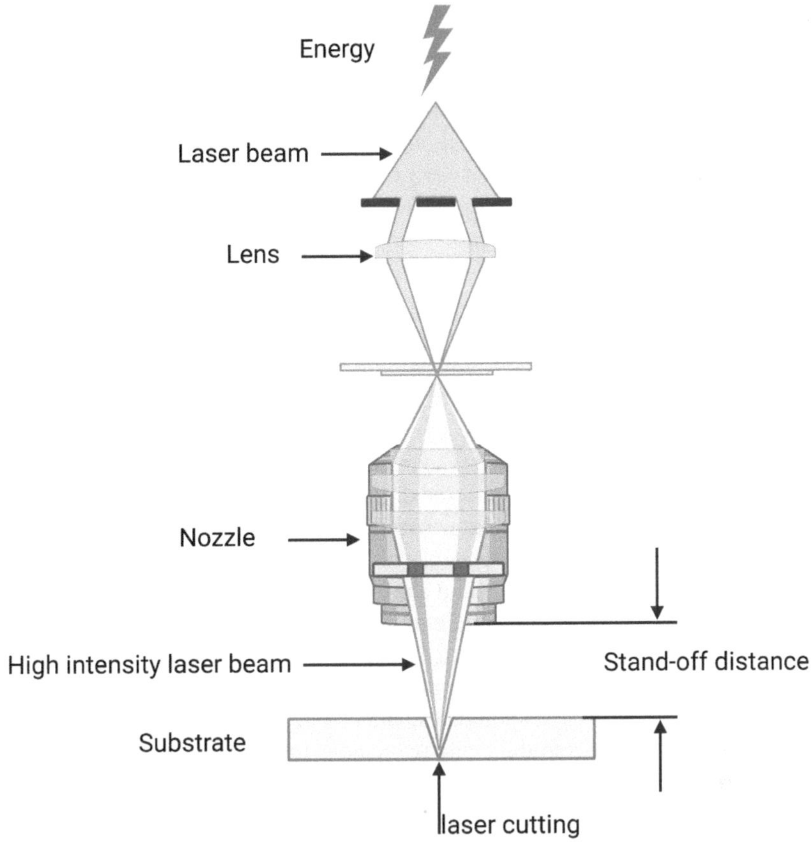

FIGURE 1.6 Schematic diagram of laser cutting technique.

Figure 1.6 illustrates a schematic diagram of the laser cutting technique. Laser cutting and etching are complex techniques that make use of laser beams to change the properties of materials. These subsequent processes have in the recent past gained acceptance in many industries and particularly in biomedical science in designing medical tools and equipment and in the creation of personalized medical treatments.

Processes of Laser Cutting and Etching

The processes for both laser cutting and etching involve several key steps:

- *Design Creation*: The first process is designing a digital model based on CAD or computer-aided design applications. The cutting or etching process uses this design as a positive to produce the negative.
- *Material Preparation*: We select the material for processing based on its compatibility with the laser technique. It can be made using acrylic and metals like stainless steel or polymers.

- *Laser Set-Up*: Adjust the laser cutter or engraver based on the material type and the desired outcome. Fine-tuning power intensity, movement speed, and focus depths are necessary to enhance the performance.
- *Execution*: The machine operates according to the agreed-upon design, in which the laser beam follows the outline of the material to either cut through it or inscribe a desired design on it.
- *Post-processing*: After cutting or etching, you may use subprocesses like rinsing or applying a protective layer [78,79].

Biomedical sciences have greatly benefitted from laser cutting and etching in several ways. The application of laser cutting enables the production of slender surgical instruments with intricate shapes that conventional milling could not accomplish. Precision in the creation of surgical instruments such as scalpels and forceps enhances operations. Some medical devices require specific structures to function correctly [80,81]. Hence, the use of laser cutting enables the fast manufacturing of these small devices, such as stents and catheters, which require specific dimensions to function within the body. The integration of AM technology and laser cutting significantly reduces the manufacturability of implants designed to fit a patient's anatomical structure. This personalization of garments makes them more fitting and comfy while increasing clinical effectiveness. Regenerative medicine can also use laser cutting to design scaffolds that aid cells in tissue regeneration processes. Therefore, we can design these scaffolds to align with the desired tissue. Laser etching finds its application in the proper branding of medical instruments, serial numbers, bar codes, expiration dates, and so on. This provides some traceability into the process and adheres to the many regulations in place while also keeping products sterile. Biologists employ laser etching for writing on surfaces of biomaterials to improve biocompatibility or induce the ability to support cell adhesion. This change can profoundly alter the process of implant/tissue interaction.

1.3.4 Nanotechnology in Manufacturing

Nanotechnology is simply the realization that matter at the atomic and molecular levels behaves differently than when it exists in macroscopic form and typically works at a scale between 1 and 100 nm [82,83]. It is fast becoming an important field of research and development in manufacturing since it brings properties and characteristics that improve material manufacture performance, accuracy, and reliability. Medical applications of nanotechnology are revolutionary in biomedical science, pushing advancements in drug delivery, diagnostics, and devices. This section focuses on detailed knowledge with regard to nanotechnology in manufacturing processes as well as its utilization in the biomedical industry.

1.3.4.1 Principles of Nanotechnology

Bottom-up and top-down are the main concepts of nanotechnology. A bottom-up approach is the creation of many materials from the basic and fundamental components, such as molecular or atomic. Indeed, it encompasses the construction of nanoparticles or nanostructures either chemically or physically. Such methods are CVD, PVD, ALD, and the top-down approach (**Figure 1.7**). Chemical vapour deposition (CVD) is a deposition technique that produces various materials with an

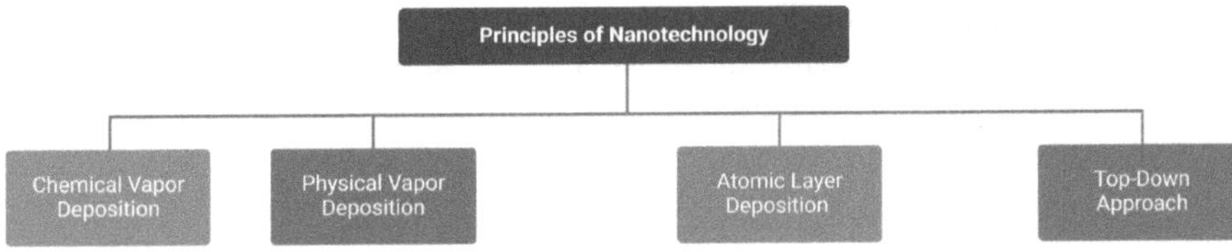

FIGURE 1.7 Flowchart for principles of nanotechnology.

exclusive solid phase from gaseous precursors on a substrate [84]. Physical vapour deposition (PVD) involves evapourizing a solid material in vacuum to form a thin film [85]. The process of atomic layer deposition (ALD) grows thin films one atomic layer at a time, providing ultimate control over thickness and material composition [86]. Using large-volume materials, the top-down approach mills them to nanosize using mechanical, thermal, or chemical methods. Some of these methods include grinding, milling, and laser ablation. However, in one-vendor creation, a much higher amount of nanoparticles can be produced; nevertheless, the size distribution will be much more varied compared to the bottom-up formation.

1.3.4.2 Applications of Nanotechnology in Biomedical Science

It shows how nanotechnology has a comprehensive and significant impact on biomedical science and its ability to present fresh and creative solutions for executing diagnostics, treatments, and caring for patients. The application of nanoparticles can target the specific drug delivery to the cells or tissues of choice. This specific targeting of the treatment, as opposed to general treatment, has fewer side effects and works better. For instance, researchers employ liposomal and dendritic structures to create spatial reservoirs for drug delivery, based on controlled release laws. Nanoscale materials enhance the capability in terms of sensitivity and specificity of diagnostic tests. Imaging strategies use dots of quantum and gold nanoparticles to enhance differentiation in imaging procedures like MRI and CT scans. They allow diagnosing diseases in their initial stages, such as at the molecular level. Nanotechnology increases the efficiency of medical devices by modifying their compatibility with living tissues and their utility. For instance, a thin protective layer at the nanoscale is effective in preventing bacteria from attaching themselves to implants, thus minimizing related infection. Similarly, nanosensors can measure physiological parameters with optimum resolution [87,88]. We incorporate cellulose-based nanomaterials to fabricate scaffolds that mimic the topography of the extracellular matrix (ECM). These scaffolds help in the growth of cells and tissue regeneration to effectively replace damaged tissues or organs [89]. Medical instruments and wound dressings use levelling silver nanoparticles, which exhibit high antimicrobial efficacy, to prevent microbial colonization.

1.4 INTEGRATION OF ADVANCED MANUFACTURING IN BIOMEDICAL RESEARCH

Among all of the AM technologies, especially additive manufacturing, or 3D printing, the application's impact on biomedical research and healthcare services has been dramatic. These changes contribute to the enhancement and optimization of medical device innovation, medical device individualization, tissue engineering, regenerative medicine progression, targeted drug delivery systems and implants, as well as the creation of biomaterials. This section is dedicated to these major topics, showcasing how AM is revolutionizing biomedical science.

1.4.1 Customization of Medical Devices

Smart technologies allow producing individualized medical devices meeting the specific needs of the patient in terms of anatomical and physiological features. Compared to the conventional approaches to manufacturing that involve developing equipment of particular standard sizes and shapes, modern technologies can produce devices that conform to individual patients' requirements. We can categorize customized medical devices into three broad categories: custom devices, patient-matched devices, and adaptable devices. A doctor's prescription specifically tailors custom-made appliances to fit a specific patient. Small lots produce telescoped patient-matched devices that are unique to each patient's anatomy, provided they adhere to the design envelope.

Large-scale manufacturing produces standard commodities for multipurpose devices, but during usage, specific modifications may be necessary to meet the patient's needs. In general, the advantages of personalized medical devices are better accuracy during operations, shorter surgery time, and better results for patients. First, when planning to manufacture implants, it is possible to choose specific shapes to match the outlines of the bone structure, which would enable better prospects for the integration and functionality of the implant. When incorporated into this usage, AM not only streamlines the production process but also reduces the cost associated with standard manufacturing practices, thereby enabling providers to access affordable, customized solutions for healthcare management. **Figure 1.8** illustrates a schematic diagram for various components of tissue engineering.

1.4.2 Tissue Engineering and Regenerative Medicine

New manufacturing technologies have elevated tissue engineering and regenerative medicine to new heights [90–92]. Therefore, 3D printing is considered an efficient approach to creating scaffolds that resemble natural tissues, as it allows for the design and construction of controllers that create sophisticated three-dimensional structures. These scaffolds have the potential to facilitate cell attachment and stimulate tissue formation, crucial for the repair of organs or specific tissues [93,94]. Recent advancements involve the utilization of bioprinting technologies, which deposit living cells and bio-inks to construct functional tissue structures. For instance, researchers are developing 3D-printed mesh to complement stem cells, which can aid in the reconstruction of new bone or cartilage [95–97]. It also has the advantage of accelerating the healing process while simultaneously reducing the need for autologous grafts, which could potentially be extremely painful and dangerous for patients. The use of smart materials in tissue engineering scaffolds enables the tissue to respond actively to its environment and provide engineered tissue a higher utility in applications related to the body [98]. As these technologies advance, there are optimistic chances of creating healthy organs for transplantation which is enough to address the critical scarcity of donor organs.

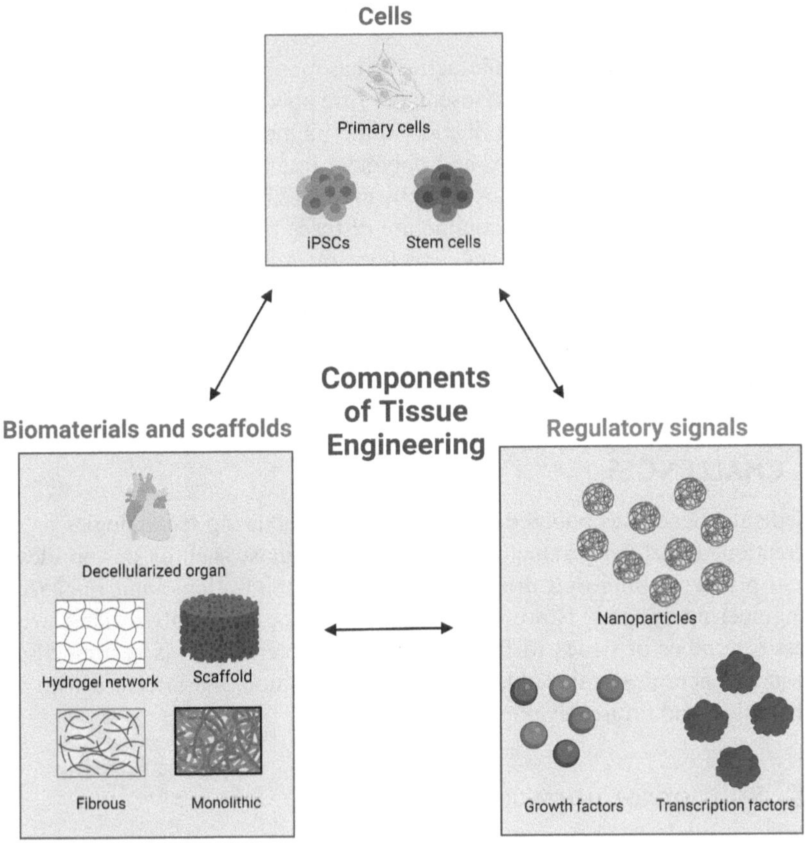

FIGURE 1.8 Schematic diagram for various components of tissue engineering.

1.4.3 Implants and Drug Delivery Systems

Manufacturing has also used new technologies to modify delivery systems, enhancing their efficiency and reducing complications. Nanotechnology plays a crucial role in this situation, as it enables the design of nanoparticles that can transport drugs and distribute them to specific body tissues. For instance, 3D printing makes it possible to design drug-releasing implants that can administer the drug directly at the target site in a gradual and sustained manner. It does more than just improve the healing process; it also increases patient compliance because of the fewer number of times one needs to administer the drug [5]. Also, implants contain active agents that can be encapsulated in ways that allow their controlled release according to the subject's needs [99–105]. Moreover, advanced manufacturing enables the development of complex devices that combine technologies of both drug delivery and medicine implantation. These radical advancements are especially helpful in chronic illnesses, where constant dissolution of the drug through continuous release is critical to the management of the disorder [106,107].

1.4.4 Development and Testing of New Biomaterials

Another area where advanced manufacturing has made contributions is the development of new biomaterials. Instead, researchers are now able to produce material with desired properties for a given application in the biomedical field. For instance, it is possible to align bioactive glasses and polymers in a way that they encourage cell attachment and proliferation and are friendly to tissues in the human body. Innovative methodologies enable the pilot manufacture of these biomaterials and their characterization under different conditions, which means a faster rate of innovation. This capability holds significant value in verifying the regulatory compliance of newly developed materials prior to their patient use. Further, intricate structures achieved through 3D printing also provide researchers with the opportunity to develop novel geometries that improve the behaviour of the material in a living organism.

1.5 CHALLENGES

Biomedical science has adopted progressive manufacturing technologies as a new age creation model for producing biomedical products, such as custom-designed medical products, improved drug delivery system innovations, and improved tissue engineering systems. However, as these technologies rapidly expand, we must address a number of issues to fully utilize their potential. This section discusses key issues concerning stakeholders, including regulation, the interface with digital health, ethics, and future developments.

1.5.1 Regulatory Challenges and Standards

The most crucial issue that advanced manufacturing in biomedical science has to overcome is the strict legislation of the field. The FDA and EMA have strict guidelines that prohibit the marketing of a medical device or product without their approval. This is quite This is evident in the frequent introduction of new technology, leading to numerous questions regarding legal compliance. The process of obtaining approval for new medical devices is both time-consuming and complex. 3D-printed medical equipment could not conform to the conventional regulatory structures that apply to manufacturing. This may result in a delay in the release of advanced products on the consumer market, as manufacturers often face difficulties in demonstrating their products' compliance with safety and effectiveness standards, particularly in the absence of new manufacturing methods.

1.5.2 Integration with Digital Health Technologies

The emergence of socio-technical technologies like telemedicine, wearable devices, and numerous health smart applications has necessitated the development of integrated systems that can seamlessly share the real-time health status of patients. Making that transition will require overcoming the technical obstacles that impede data compatibility. We must accomplish this by facilitating advanced communication between medical devices and digital health platforms, all while safeguarding the identities of patients. The issue lies in the lack of a clear communication protocol in most of these systems, which can lead to their isolation. Furthermore, networked or connected medical devices are more vulnerable to cyber threats than their non-connected counterparts. Implementing cybersecurity measures with health IT systems is a proactive measure to prevent privacy and security breaches that could endanger patients' lives.

1.5.3 Ethical Considerations

This section aims to propose an ethical agenda concerning the future use of advanced manufacturing technologies in biomedical science. This aspect of customized medical devices makes people question the equity in the provision of medical devices. If some individuals cannot afford additional therapies, or cannot access them in geographically deprived regions, or cannot afford them solely due to their economic status, personalized medicine may lead to new forms of inequality. It is therefore critical that population groups attain equal access to these innovations, which is important for health equity. Moreover, bioprinting technologies for creating tissues to be used in engineering offer some concerns in terms of getting tissues and cells out there. It remains unclear who has permission to donate their bodily fluids for bioprinting and whether the created tissues can be branded and sold to the public or used in experimental procedures for animals or possessed by any individual or organization.

1.6 FUTURE SCOPE

The application of technologies in the field of manufacturing systems is changing the direction of biomedical sciences and the clinical course of patients' treatments. Advanced system integration has reshaped customization, impacting personalized medical devices, bioprinted tissues, and advanced drug delivery systems. Laser cutting and etching improve precision in general surgical tools and specifically MD manufacturing, whereas nanotechnology enables contributions to diagnostics, tissue engineering, and biomaterials. However, there are still regulatory, ethical, and technical requirements that must be addressed to fully utilize these technologies, as outlined later. Over time, as research and regulatory environments change, the biomedical sector is set to adopt advanced manufacturing as the main driver of personalized medicine. Not only will the integration of blockchain into the medical industry improve the availability and quality of healthcare for patients, but it will also create a system that will eventually optimize the need for personalized healthcare treatment around the world, making healthcare more efficient.

1.7 CONCLUSION

The application of technologies in the field of manufacturing systems is changing the direction of the biomedical sciences and the clinical course of the treatments of the patients. Advanced systems integration has reshaped customization impacting on personalized medical devices, bioprinted tissues, and advanced systems of drug delivery. Laser cutting and etching improve precision in general surgical tools and specifically

MD manufacturing, whereas nanotechnology enables contributions to diagnostics, tissue engineering, and biomaterials. There are still issues of regulatory, ethical, and technical requirements that should be met to fully leverage such technologies as focused in the following manner. The biomedical sector may integrate advanced manufacturing as a central force behind personalized medicine because research advancements and regulatory changes may take place in the future. The medical industry can achieve enhanced patient health care access with quality improvements as blockchain implementation builds a system which optimizes personalized treatment worldwide for medical efficiency.

REFERENCES

[1] Ashima R, Haleem A, Bahl S, et al. Automation and manufacturing of smart materials in additive manufacturing technologies using Internet of Things towards the adoption of Industry 4.0. *Mater Today Proc*. 2021;45:5081–88.

[2] Sahoo S, Lo C-Y. Smart manufacturing powered by recent technological advancements: A review. *J Manuf Syst*. 2022;64:236–50.

[3] Majeed A, Zhang Y, Ren S, et al. A big data-driven framework for sustainable and smart additive manufacturing. *Robot Comput Integr Manuf.* 2021;67:102026.

[4] Sharma V, Kumar V. Application of Box-Behnken design and response surface methodology for multi-optimization of laser cutting of AA5052/ZrO2 metal– matrix composites. *Proc Inst Mech Eng Part L J Mater Des Appl*. 2018;232:652–68.

[5] Sharma V, Kumar V. Comparison of machining characteristics of metal matrix composites using CO2 laser curve cutting process. *Proc Inst Mech Eng Part E J Process Mech Eng*. 2018;232:349–68.

[6] Sharma V, Kumar V. Investigating the quality characteristics of Al5052/SiC metal matrix composites machined by CO2 laser curve cutting. *Proc Inst Mech Eng Part L J Mater Des Appl*. 2018;232:3–19.

[7] Sharma V, Kumar V, Bist A. Investigations on morphology and material removal rate of various MMCs using CO 2 laser technique. *J Brazilian Soc Mech Sci Eng*. 2020;42:1–14.

[8] Sharma V, Singh JP, Raman R, et al. Machine learning approach for prediction analysis of aluminium alloy on the surface roughness using CO2 laser machining. *Proc Inst Mech Eng Part E J Process Mech Eng*. 2024. https://doi.org/10.1177/09544089241231093.

[9] Fidan I, Huseynov O, Ali MA, et al. Recent inventions in additive manufacturing: Holistic review. *Inventions*. 2023;8:103.

[10] Ford SLN. Additive manufacturing technology: Potential implications for US manufacturing competitiveness. *J Int'l Com Econ*. 2014;6:40.

[11] Thrift N. Re-inventing invention: New tendencies in capitalist commodification. *Econ Soc*. 2006;35:279–306.

[12] Melton T. The benefits of lean manufacturing: What lean thinking has to offer the process industries. *Chem Eng Res Des*. 2005;83:662–73.

[13] Wheelwright SC, Clark KB. *Revolutionizing product development: Quantum leaps in speed, efficiency, and quality*. Simon and Schuster; 1992.

[14] Singh R, Toseef M, Kumar J, et al. Benefits and challenges in additive manufacturing and its applications. In: Kaushal S, Singh I, Singh S, et al., editors. *Sustainable advanced manufacturing and materials processing [Internet]*. 1st ed. Boca Raton: CRC Press; 2022. pp. 137–57. Available from: www.taylorfrancis.com/books/9781003269298/chapters/10.1201/9781003269298-8.

[15] Singh J. Sustainability issues in laser-based additive manufacturing. In: *Handbook of laser-based sustainable surface modification and manufacturing techniques*. CRC Press; 2023. p. 167–89.

[16] Ahmad S, Hashmi AW, Singh J, et al. Innovations in additive manufacturing of shape memory alloys: Alloys, microstructures, treatments, applications. *J Mater Res Technol.* 2024;32:4136–97.

[17] Sharma V, Singh JP, Hussan K, et al. Machine learning approach for predicting the machining characteristics of additive manufactured ABS material. *Proc Inst Mech Eng Part C J Mech Eng Sci.* 2024. https://doi.org/10.1177/09544062241283330.

[18] Chohan JS, Mittal N, Kumar R, et al. Mechanical strength enhancement of 3D printed acrylonitrile butadiene styrene polymer components using neural network optimization algorithm. *Polymers.* 2020;12(10):2250.

[19] Singh JIP, Sharma V, Singh S, et al. Impact of molding temperature, fiber loading and chemical modifications on the physicomechanical, and microstructural morphology properties of woven kenaf fiber/PLA composites for non-structural applications. *J Nat Fibers.* 2024;21:2326586.

[20] Oladele IO, Adelani SO, Agbabiaka OG, et al. Applications and disposal of polymers and polymer composites: A review. *Eur J Adv Eng Technol.* 2022;9:65–89.

[21] Rouf S, Malik A, Singh N, et al. Additive manufacturing technologies: Industrial and medical applications. *Sustain Oper Comput.* 2022;3:258–74.

[22] Pillai R, Sivathanu B, Mariani M, et al. Adoption of AI-empowered industrial robots in auto component manufacturing companies. *Prod Plan Control.* 2022;33:1517–33.

[23] Javaid M, Haleem A, Singh RP, et al. Substantial capabilities of robotics in enhancing industry 4.0 implementation. *Cogn Robot.* 2021;1:58–75.

[24] Javaid M, Haleem A, Suman R. Digital twin applications toward industry 4.0: A review. *Cogn Robot.* 2023;3:71–92.

[25] Moskvitin G V, Polyakov AN, Birger EM. Application of laser welding methods in industrial production. *Weld Int.* 2013;27:572–80.

[26] Saariluoma H, Piiroinen A, Unt A, et al. Overview of optical digital measuring challenges and technologies in laser welded components in EV battery module design and manufacturing. *Batteries.* 2020;6:47.

[27] Rajput RK. *A textbook of manufacturing technology: Manufacturing processes.* Firewall Media; 2007.

[28] Roohpour N, Wasikiewicz JM, Moshaverinia A, et al. Polyurethane membranes modified with isopropyl myristate as a potential candidate for encapsulating electronic implants: A study of biocompatibility and water permeability. *Polymers (Basel).* 2010;2:102–19.

[29] Parry L, Ashcroft IA, Wildman RD. Understanding the effect of laser scan strategy on residual stress in selective laser melting through thermo-mechanical simulation. *Addit Manuf [Internet].* 2016;12:1–15. Available from: https://linkinghub.elsevier.com/retrieve/pii/S2214860416300987.

[30] Gärtner E, Meyenborg I, Toenjes A. Adapting Fe–Mn–Si–Cr shape memory alloy for laser powder bed fusion by adjusting the Mn content. *Prog Addit Manuf.* 2023;1–10.

[31] Chang C, Chen C, Wang J, et al. Metallic and bone tissue advancements: Materials, applications, and case studies. In: *Additive manufacturing materials and technology.* Elsevier; 2024. pp. 413–44.

[32] Priarone PC, Ingarao G. Towards criteria for sustainable process selection: On the modelling of pure subtractive versus additive/subtractive integrated manufacturing approaches. *J Clean Prod.* 2017;144:57–68.

[33] Sathish K, Kumar SS, Magal RT, et al. A comparative study on subtractive manufacturing and additive manufacturing. *Adv Mater Sci Eng.* 2022;2022:6892641.

[34] Goh GD, Agarwala S, Goh GL, et al. Additive manufacturing in unmanned aerial vehicles (UAVs): Challenges and potential. *Aerosp Sci Technol [Internet].* 2017;63:140–51. Available from: http://doi.org/10.1016/j.ast.2016.12.019.

[35] Aboutaleb AM, Bian L, Shamsaei N, et al. Systematic optimization of Laser-based Additive Manufacturing for multiple mechanical properties. In: *2016 IEEE International Conference on Automation Science and Engineering [Internet]*. IEEE; 2016. pp. 780–5. Available from: http://ieeexplore.ieee.org/document/7743481/.

[36] Gao W, Zhang Y, Ramanujan D, et al. The status, challenges, and future of additive manufacturing in engineering. *Comput Des*. 2015;69:65–89.

[37] Pelin G, Sonmez M, Pelin C-E. The use of additive manufacturing techniques in the development of polymeric molds: A review. *Polymers (Basel)*. 2024;16:1055.

[38] Lin Y, Jia Y, Alva G, et al. Review on thermal conductivity enhancement, thermal properties and applications of phase change materials in thermal energy storage. *Renew Sust Energy Rev*. 2018;82:2730–42.

[39] Ayodele BE. *Modeling of FDM 3D printing for improved performance*. Texas A&M University-Kingsville; 2015.

[40] Baran EH, Erbil HY. Surface modification of 3D printed PLA objects by fused deposition modeling: A review. *Colloids and Interfaces*. 2019;3:43.

[41] Zakeri S, Vippola M, Levänen E. A comprehensive review of the photopolymerization of ceramic resins used in stereolithography. *Addit Manuf*. 2020;35:101177.

[42] Lupone F, Padovano E, Casamento F, et al. Process phenomena and material properties in selective laser sintering of polymers: A review. *Materials (Basel)*. 2021;15:183.

[43] Xu J, Gao M, Zhan J, et al. Towards support-free design for 3D printing of thin-walled composite based on stratified manufacturability reinforcement. *CIRP J Manuf Sci Technol*. 2022;38:457–72.

[44] Gibson I, Rosen D, Stucker B, et al. Material jetting. *Addit Manuf Technol*. 2021; 203–35.

[45] Gülcan O, Günaydın K, Tamer A. The state of the art of material jetting—A critical review. *Polymers (Basel)*. 2021;13:2829.

[46] Svetlizky D, Zheng B, Vyatskikh A, et al. Laser-based directed energy deposition (DED-LB) of advanced materials. *Mater Sci Eng A*. 2022;840:142967.

[47] Dobrzański LA, Dobrzański LB. Dentistry 4.0 concept in the design and manufacturing of prosthetic dental restorations. *Processes*. 2020;8:525.

[48] Lin L, Fang Y, Liao Y, et al. 3D printing and digital processing techniques in dentistry: A review of literature. *Adv Eng Mater*. 2019;21:1801013.

[49] Pillai S, Upadhyay A, Khayambashi P, et al. Dental 3D-printing: Transferring art from the laboratories to the clinics. *Polymers (Basel)*. 2021;13:157.

[50] Parhi R. Recent advances in 3D printed microneedles and their skin delivery application in the treatment of various diseases. *J Drug Deliv Sci Technol*. 2023;84:104395.

[51] Al-Nimry SS, Daghmash RM. Three dimensional printing and its applications focusing on microneedles for drug delivery. *Pharmaceutics*. 2023;15:1597.

[52] McNulty T, Ferlie E. *Reengineering health care: The complexities of organizational transformation*. OUP Oxford; 2002.

[53] Hackett JL, Gutman SI. Introduction to the Food and Drug Administration (FDA) regulatory process. *J Proteome Res*. 2005;4:1110–13.

[54] Tofail SAM, Koumoulos EP, Bandyopadhyay A, et al. Additive manufacturing: Scientific and technological challenges, market uptake and opportunities. *Mater Today [Internet]*. 2018;21:22–37. Available from: https://linkinghub.elsevier.com/retrieve/pii/S1369702117301773.

[55] Li N, Huang S, Zhang G, et al. Progress in additive manufacturing on new materials: A review. *J Mater Sci Technol*. 2019;35:242–69.

[56] Yang L, Hsu K, Baughman B, et al. *Additive manufacturing of metals: The technology, materials, design and production*. Springer Cham; 2017.

[57] Vaezi M, Chianrabutra S, Mellor B, et al. Multiple material additive manufacturing–Part 1: A review: This review paper covers a decade of research on multiple material additive manufacturing technologies which can produce complex geometry parts with different materials. *Virtual Phys Prototyp*. 2013;8:19–50.

[58] Ben-Ner A, Siemsen E. Decentralization and localization of production: The organizational and economic consequences of additive manufacturing (3D printing). *Calif Manage Rev*. 2017;59:5–23.

[59] Attaran M. The rise of 3-D printing: The advantages of additive manufacturing over traditional manufacturing. *Bus Horiz*. 2017;60:677–88.

[60] Alogla AA, Baumers M, Tuck C, et al. The impact of additive manufacturing on the flexibility of a manufacturing supply chain. *Appl Sci*. 2021;11:3707.

[61] Habel J, Klarmann M. Customer reactions to downsizing: When and how is satisfaction affected? *J Acad Mark Sci*. 2015;43:768–89.

[62] Amini MM, Retzlaff-Roberts D, Bienstock CC. Designing a reverse logistics operation for short cycle time repair services. *Int J Prod Econ*. 2005;96:367–80.

[63] Kassab A, Al Nabhani D, Mohanty P, et al. Advancing plastic recycling: Challenges and opportunities in the integration of 3d printing and distributed recycling for a circular economy. *Polymers (Basel)*. 2023;15:3881.

[64] Rantanen J, Khinast J. The future of pharmaceutical manufacturing sciences. *J Pharm Sci*. 2015;104:3612–38.

[65] Pathak C, Kumari S. CNC machines in production and manufacturing of medical devices. *Artif Intell Biomed Mod Healthc Informatics*. 2025;393–401.

[66] Sarcar MMM, Rao KM, Narayan KL. *Computer aided design and manufacturing*. PHI Learning Pvt. Ltd.; 2008.

[67] Jiang Z, Chen D, Sun K, et al. A systematic review of micro-texture formation based on milling: From mechanism, existing techniques, characterization to typical applications. *Int J Adv Manuf Technol*. 2024;134:2151–77.

[68] Luttge R. *Nano-and microfabrication for industrial and biomedical applications*. William Andrew; 2016.

[69] Shanjin L V, Yang W. An investigation of pulsed laser cutting of titanium alloy sheet. *Opt Lasers Eng*. 2006;44:1067–77.

[70] Demir AG, Previtali B, Biffi CA. Fibre laser cutting and chemical etching of AZ31 for manufacturing biodegradable stents. *Adv Mater Sci Eng*. 2013;2013:692635.

[71] Steen WM, Kamalu JN. Laser cutting. In: *Materials processing: Theory and practice*. Elsevier; 1983. pp. 15–111.

[72] Grigoriev SN, Fedorov SV, Hamdy K. Materials, properties, manufacturing methods and cutting performance of innovative ceramic cutting tools– A review. *Manuf Rev*. 2019;6:19.

[73] Khatak P. Laser cutting technique: A literature review. *Mater Today Proc*. 2022;56:2484–89.

[74] Li M, Li L, Fan Y, et al. From top to down—Recent advances in etching of 2D materials. *Adv Mater Interfaces*. 2022;9:2201334.

[75] Donovan TE, Eidson RS. Instruments and equipment for tooth preparation. *Sturdevant's Art Sci Oper Dent Sturdevant's Art Sci Oper Dent*. 2012;164.

[76] Lazov L, Deneva H, Narica P. Laser marking methods. In: *Environment. Technology. Resources. Proceedings of the International Scientific and Practical Conference*. 2015. pp. 108–15.

[77] McKee TJ. Laser marking. In: *Handbook of laser technology and applications*. CRC Press; 2021. pp. 35–45.

[78] Singh J. Applications of laser technology for processing and post-treatments of powders and coatings. *Handb Laser-Based Sustain Surf Modif Manuf Tech*. 2023;135–66.

[79] Sunitha K, Vasudev H. A short note on the various thermal spray coating processes and effect of post-treatment on Ni-based coatings. *Mater Today Proc [Internet]*. 2022;50:1452–7. Available from: https://linkinghub.elsevier.com/retrieve/pii/S2214785321058132.

[80] Lee HC, Pacheco NE, Fichera L, et al. When the end effector is a laser: A review of robotics in laser surgery. *Adv Intell Syst*. 2022;4:2200130.

[81] Steen WM, Mazumder J, Steen WM, et al. Biomedical laser processes and equipment. *Laser Mater Process*. 2010;441–84.

[82] Binns C. *Introduction to nanoscience and nanotechnology*. John Wiley & Sons; 2021.

[83] Whitesides GM. Nanoscience, nanotechnology, and chemistry. *Small*. 2005;1:172–79.

[84] Vargas Garcia JR, Goto T. Thermal barrier coatings produced by chemical vapor deposition. *Sci Technol Adv Mater*. 2003;4:397–402.

[85] Krella AK. Degradation of protective PVD coatings. In: *Handbook of material failure analysis with case studies from the chemicals, concrete, and power industries*. Elsevier; 2016. pp. 411–40.

[86] Leskelä M, Ritala M. Atomic layer deposition (ALD): From precursors to thin film structures. *Thin Solid Films*. 2002;409:138–46.

[87] Harun-Ur-Rashid M, Jahan I, Foyez T, et al. Bio-inspired nanomaterials for micro/nanodevices: A new era in biomedical applications. *Micromachines*. 2023;14:1786.

[88] Kromer C. *Nanoscale tools for biosensing and treatment of bacterial biofilms and eukaryotic cells*. 2024. Available from: http://dx.doi.org/10.17169/refubium-44048

[89] Bružauskaitė I, Bironaitė D, Bagdonas E, et al. Scaffolds and cells for tissue regeneration: Different scaffold pore sizes—different cell effects. *Cytotechnology*. 2016;68:355–69.

[90] Shafiee A, Atala A. Tissue engineering: Toward a new era of medicine. *Annu Rev Med*. 2017;68:29–40.

[91] Fisher MB, Mauck RL. Tissue engineering and regenerative medicine: Recent innovations and the transition to translation. *Tissue Eng Part B Rev*. 2013;19:1–13.

[92] Bajaj P, Schweller RM, Khademhosseini A, et al. 3D biofabrication strategies for tissue engineering and regenerative medicine. *Annu Rev Biomed Eng*. 2014;16:247–76.

[93] Yarlagadda PKDV. Chandrasekharan M, Shyan JYM. Recent advances and current developments in tissue scaffolding. *Biomed Mater Eng*. 2005;15:159–77.

[94] Kim TG, Shin H, Lim DW. Biomimetic scaffolds for tissue engineering. *Adv Funct Mater*. 2012;22:2446–68.

[95] Deptuła M, Zawrzykraj M, Sawicka J, et al. Application of 3D-printed hydrogels in wound healing and regenerative medicine. *Biomed Pharmacother*. 2023;167:115416.

[96] Wang Z, Wang Y, Yan J, et al. Pharmaceutical electrospinning and 3D printing scaffold design for bone regeneration. *Adv Drug Deliv Rev*. 2021;174:504–34.

[97] Ivanovski S, Breik O, Carluccio D, et al. 3D printing for bone regeneration: Challenges and opportunities for achieving predictability. *Periodontol 2000*. 2023;93:358–84.

[98] Khan F, Tanaka M. Designing smart biomaterials for tissue engineering. *Int J Mol Sci*. 2017;19:17.

[99] Singh J, Singh S, Verma A. Artificial intelligence in use of ZrO2 material in biomedical science. *J Electrochem Sci Eng [Internet]*. 2022;13:83–97. Available from: https://pub.iapchem.org/ojs/index.php/JESE/article/view/1498.

[100] Singh J, Hashmi AW, Behra A, et al. Review of Mg alloys for bio-implants protected by the deposition of chemical conversion coatings. In: *AIP Conference Proceedings*. AIP Publishing; 2024.

[101] Singh J, Singh S, Gill R. Applications of biopolymer coatings in biomedical engineering. *J Electrochem Sci Eng*. 2022;13:63–81.

[102] Singh CJ, Ram B, Singh J, et al. Experimental investigation on characterization of friction stir processed AZ31-based composite. *Sci Rep*. 2024;14:15453.
[103] Singh J, Hashmi AW, Ahmad S, et al. Critical review on biodegradable and biocompatibility magnesium alloys: Progress and prospects in bio-implant applications. *Inorg Chem Commun*. 2024;169:113111.
[104] Hashmi AW, Singh J, Ahmad S. Future perspective of self-healing nano-coatings for corrosion protection. *Discov Disruption, Futur Implic Nanomater*. 2024;597–624.
[105] Singh J, Hashmi AW, Kumar A, et al. Review on protection of Mg alloys bioimplants by deposition of micro-arc oxidation coatings. In: *AIP Conference Proceedings*. AIP Publishing; 2024.
[106] Rai VK, Mishra N, Agrawal AK, et al. Novel drug delivery system: An immense hope for diabetics. *Drug Deliv*. 2016;23:2371–90.
[107] Mandal AS, Biswas N, Karim KM, et al. Drug delivery system based on chronobiology—A review. *J Control Release*. 2010;147:314–25.

2 Recent Progress in Manufacturing Techniques Utilized in Biomedical Science

Significance, Advances, and Applications

Praveen Kumar Verma, Hitesh Vasudev, and Bhupinder Singh

CONTENTS

2.1 INTRODUCTION

The rise of advanced manufacturing technologies (AMT) in biomedical science could be considered a new milestone in contemporary medicine. AMTs are redefining how medical devices, implants, and prosthetics are designed, developed, and deployed. These are times when precision, customization, and efficiency are crucial; thus, these solutions are transformative for catering to the diverse and complex needs of patients. From giving life to implants that have saved many lives to producing engineered prosthetics that represent patients to the world, these technologies are revolutionizing healthcare delivery and improving the quality of life for millions. Biomedical science inherently demands high precision, biocompatibility,

DOI: 10.1201/9781003516064-2

and adaptability, as applied cases must interact with living organisms often under dynamic physiological conditions. Traditionally, conventional manufacturing techniques have been suited to the industry, but they are not adequate when it comes to dealing with complex geometries, diversity in material properties, and custom requirements. Advanced manufacturing technologies fill these gaps by offering a level of control unrivaled in terms of material properties, intricacies in design, or scalability in production. This has led to the creation of impossible devices and systems [1–3].

Additive manufacturing allows for the generation of structures that are highly complex and resemble native tissues or optimizes device performance by building components directly from digital models layer by layer. Such has proven to be the game changer in applications such as tissue engineering where scaffolds with tailored porosity and geometry are essential for cell growth and tissue regeneration. Similarly, AM has enabled the production of custom orthopedic and dental implants, enhancing patient outcomes by ensuring a perfect fit and reducing the risk of postoperative complications [4]. **Figure 2.1** shows the medical model parts and implants.

Subtractive manufacturing technologies, which include CNC machining, continue to hold a large share of the biomedical industry. The quality produced by subtractive manufacturing is unbeatable in terms of precision and surface characteristics that can be attained with such techniques, making them suitable for a medical instrument or diagnostic equipment. The workability of such techniques over many different materials, including metals and ceramics, means that subtractive manufacturing holds a continued position in advanced biomedical manufacture [6].

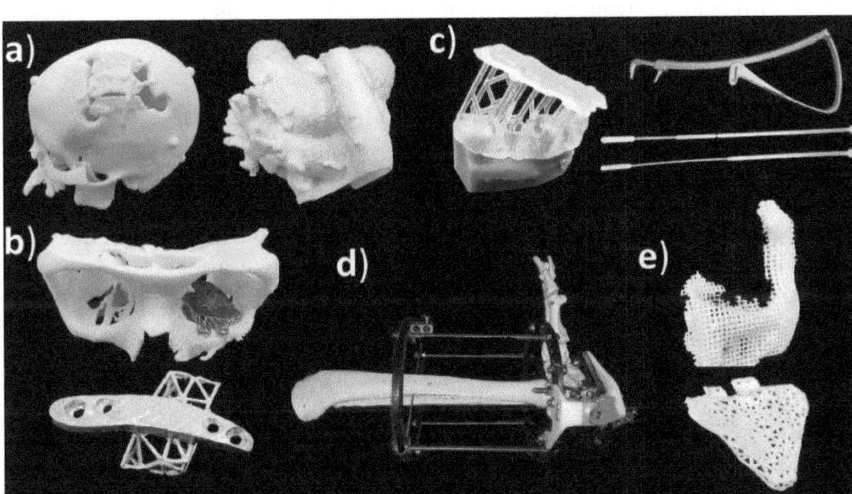

FIGURE 2.1 (**a**) Medical models; (**b**) implants; (**c**) tools, instruments, and parts for medical devices; (**d**) medical aids, supportive guides, splints, and prostheses; (**e**) biomanufacturing [5] (CC By 4.0 Attribution).

Materials used for advanced manufacturing in biomedical applications are also revolutionary. From biocompatible metals, such as titanium and cobalt-chromium alloys, to biodegradable polymers and bioactive ceramics such as hydroxyapatite, the materials' selection has increased dramatically. Such materials can manufacture the outputted devices not only structurally sound but also capable of being integrated or even mimicked with biological tissues. For example, bioresorbable polymers are now more frequently used for functions such as temporary scaffolds and drug delivery systems, where the material essentially degrades once it serves its purpose [7].

Advanced manufacturing technologies also enable personalized medical solutions, an area becoming more and more critical in advanced healthcare. Personalization is far more important in areas such as prosthetics, where anatomy and functional requirements vary from patient to patient. With AMTs, prosthetics can now be developed to custom-fit the patient, ensuring comfort and functionality, hence improving the quality of life for the user. Furthermore, the speed and efficiency of the technologies have reduced the timelines for production significantly, hence bettering the ability to get these devices to the patients within the fastest time possible. The impact of advanced manufacturing, while touching the lives of patients, extends to the general care ecosystem. Streamlining production processes and cutting down material wastage not only reduce costs, thereby increasing the accessibility of high-quality medical devices, but also allow for rapid prototyping and iterative design due to the flexibility of the techniques used in advanced manufacturing [8].

Advanced manufacturing technologies in biomedical science have immense potential, but they face many challenges from material limitations and problems related to a high cost of implementation to regulatory hurdles. These issues will require continued collaboration between researchers' industry stakeholders and regulatory bodies. Emerging trends—including bio fabrication, nanomanufacturing, and artificial intelligence integration—will further enhance the capabilities and applications of AMTs in healthcare as the technology continues to evolve [9].

2.2 SIGNIFICANCE OF ADVANCED MANUFACTURING IN BIOMEDICAL SCIENCE

In the biomedical domain, precision, reliability, and adaptability are paramount because solutions need to be different for every patient due to their unique physiological demands. However, through traditional manufacturing processes, often though historically successful, present difficulties in effectively addressing the needs of biomedical applications, since challenges come from the constraints of material handling, getting the accuracy required, and scaling the production process. AMTs have emerged as a revolutionary solution, breaking these barriers to be able to produce innovative, efficient, and patient-specific medical devices and implants [10].

One of the most significant contributions made by AMTs is that it allows for customized solutions. Advanced manufacturing, especially additive manufacturing (AM), permits the creation of implants and prosthetics according to the precise anatomy that characterizes each patient. By using highly detailed imaging data such as CT or MRI scans, AMTs create digital models upon which they can fabricate devices of near-absolute accuracy. That kind of precision enhances fit, functionality, and comfort for implants and prosthetics that will reduce complications and improve outcomes for patients. The benefit in such capability is significant, especially in very complex cases, as with reconstructive surgery, where every patient's needs are unique [11].

Another critical advantage of AMTs is their ability to fabricate complex geometries that mimic natural tissues or enhance the functionality of medical devices. Traditional methods often struggle with intricate designs, especially those involving porous structures or internal cavities required for tissue engineering scaffolds or drug delivery systems. AMTs excel in this regard, as they enable layer-by-layer construction of intricate designs, ensuring optimal performance and biological integration. For example, scaffolds fabricated with these techniques can have controlled porosity and microarchitecture that allow cell attachment, proliferation, and regeneration of tissue [12]. **Figure 2.2** shows the applications in advanced biomedical hydrogels.

Material flexibility is another building block of AMTs allowing for the incorporation of a wide array of biocompatible materials in biomedical applications. Techniques that have been developed can handle materials as diverse as titanium alloys, magnesium alloys, ceramics, and polymers, each with unique property sets applicable to unique applications. For example, titanium and its alloys are the most widely applied biomaterial for orthopedic and dental implants. This is because these alloys offer great strength with excellent corrosion resistance and biocompatibility. Polymers are ideal in applications such as drug delivery systems and biodegradable sutures, where flexibility and control over degradation are important requirements. Hybrid methods allow for layers of materials to be combined, and this capability further extends the scale of applications where devices meet structural and functional demands [14].

Moreover, high-end manufacturing technologies have drastically reduced time-to-market for new medical devices. Fast prototyping ability makes it easy to generate

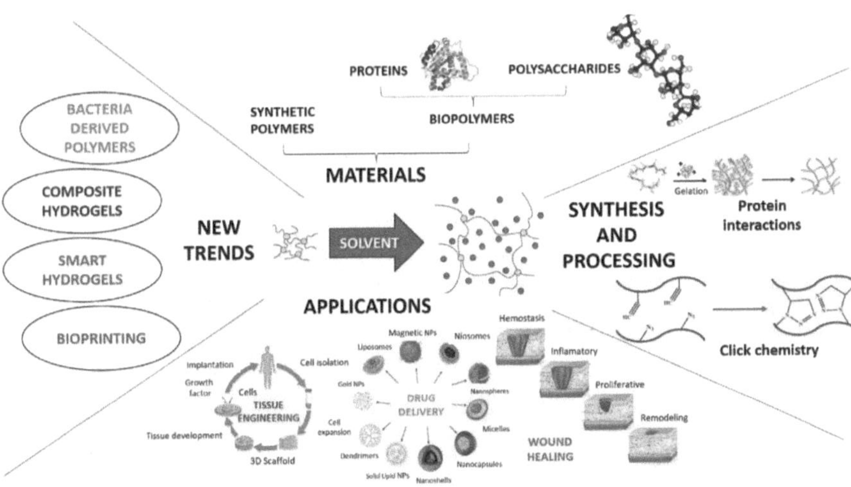

FIGURE 2.2 Trends, materials, synthesis, and applications in advanced biomedical hydrogel [13]. (CC By 4.0 Attribution)

several iterations of the same device for testing, therefore, hastening the development cycle. Thus, for instance, this pace enhances innovation speed while making sure that treatments and life-saving devices reach patients faster than ever. Indeed, the production aspect is promoted by scalability so these technologies can benefit either massive production or any small-batch, highly customized production [15].

Advanced manufacturing technologies break the limitation cycle of conventional manufacturing by allowing for unparalleled precision, adaptability, and efficiency in biomedical applications. Customization, complex geometries, material versatility, and reduced production timelines are some of the factors driving paradigmatic shifts in patient care, thanks to these technologies. This is because manufacturing capabilities that can be aligned with the demands of modern medicine are indeed setting a framework for a new era of innovation in the biomedical field [16].

2.3 ADVANCED MANUFACTURING TECHNOLOGIES

2.3.1 Additive Manufacturing (AM)

Additive manufacturing (AM), also commonly referred to as 3D printing, is a transforming technology in the field of biomedical science offering unprecedented capabilities to produce highly intricate and customizable medical devices. Unlike traditional manufacturing methods, AM builds up structures layer on layer following digital designs that enable the precise fabrication of complex geometries or shapes, often impossible or cost-prohibitive with conventional methods. This innovative approach has a wide spectrum of applications in biomedical science, ranging from implants and prosthetics to tissue engineering scaffolds, each with significant contributions to improving patient outcomes and advancing healthcare solutions [17,18]. **Figure 2.3** shows the process flow for tools, instruments, and parts for medical devices.

AM applications in biomedicine have had the most impactful application in producing implants. Orthopedic and dental implants manufactured using AM are designed to closely match the anatomy, thus providing a superior fit and functionality. Moreover, AM enables the integration of advanced features, such as porous structures that promote osseointegration—the natural process by which bone

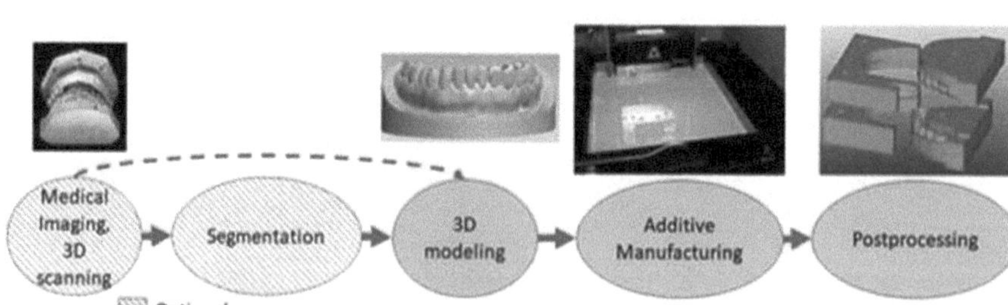

FIGURE 2.3 Typical process flow for tools, instruments, and parts for medical devices [5]. (CC By 4.0 Attribution)

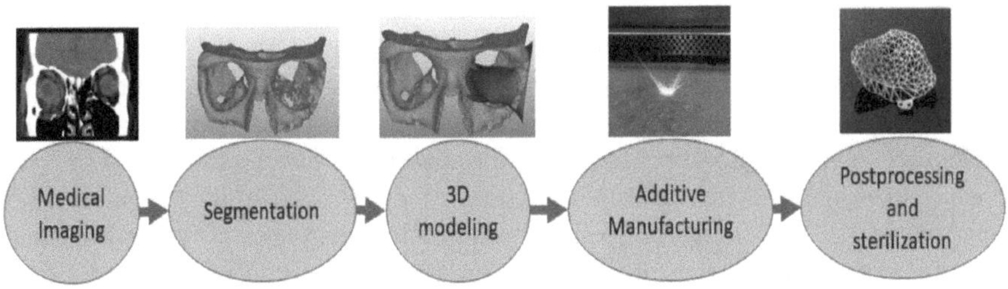

FIGURE 2.4 Typical process flow for implants [5]. (CC By 4.0 Attribution)

integrates with an implant. This enhanced osseointegration not only improves the stability of the implant but also reduces recovery time and the risk of complications. For example, customized titanium implants with specific surface topographies can provide superior cell adhesion and bone tissue development, providing advantages over traditionally produced counterparts [19,20]. **Figure 2.4** shows the process flow for implants.

Additive manufacturing has also revolutionized the prosthetics of different types. Traditional prosthetics are too lengthy to produce and are very costly as well. They fail to provide adequate customization under the requirements for unique patients. With AM, prosthetics will now be done in very few hours with more accuracy. Digital scanning technologies make it possible to design lightweight and ergonomic prosthetics to the precise dimension of the patient's anatomy. This customization mainly makes them more comfortable and practical while improving the quality of life of the consumer. For example, prosthetic limbs that are produced using AM can be lightweight but strong to reduce the physical burden on the user while staying durable and effective [21].

Another revolutionary application of AM in the biomedical field is in the fabrication of tissue engineering scaffolds. Tissue engineering aims at restoring damaged tissues or organs, and scaffolds find a critical role in this because they provide a temporary structure for cell anchorage, proliferation, and tissue growth. Precision, controlled porosity, intricate microarchitecture, and biomimetic properties closely resembling those of natural tissues require AM. The scaffolds can be formulated using a range of biocompatible materials. These include biodegradable polymers and bioactive ceramics, based upon the specific application. For instance, hydroxyapatite-based scaffolds are quite often used for bone regeneration, while polymeric scaffolds are chosen for soft tissue applications. The ability to engineer such precise structures has advanced the field of regenerative medicine to the extent that solutions for what was once considered untreatable conditions can now be developed [22].

2.3.2 Subtractive Manufacturing

Subtractive manufacturing is an important process in modern manufacturing where material is removed from an original workpiece to produce desired shapes and components. Unlike AM, which accumulates a product layer by layer, subtractive manufacturing removes material from a solid block to obtain the desired shape and product. Some common techniques include milling, turning, and drilling, each tailored for applications and material properties. Milling requires rotary cutters to remove material from a workpiece with various shapes and features such as slots, holes, and contours. It is very versatile and can produce complex geometries within tight tolerances, which makes it suitable for precision parts. Turning is carried out when the workpiece is rotated about its axis while a cutting tool removes some material to create cylindrical shapes, like shafts and pistons. This method is specifically good for producing symmetrical components with high surface quality. Drilling, as the term applied to it, is a process used to obtain precise holes in a workpiece, which may or may not subsequently have machining done upon them, using processes like reaming or tapping, for specific dimensions and finishes [23].

This way, subtractive manufacturing is very helpful in working with tough materials such as titanium and stainless steel that often must be used in industries with stringent strength and durability requirements. Titanium, with its outstanding strength-to-weight ratio and strong corrosion resistance, is commonly used in high-strength applications involving aerospace, while stainless steel holds an excellent record in the production of surgical instruments and components in high-performance applications due to its premium mechanical properties and resistance to oxidation and staining. The subtractive manufacturing process is used in the manufacturing of precision surgical instruments. These instruments must have the finest and most precise standards of accuracy and finish so that they can perform reliably in any surgical practice. The elimination of complex shapes and fine details with high accuracy are helpful in making subtractive manufacturing ideal for this application. Diagnostic devices also benefit from subtractive manufacturing processes, as they will quite often contain high-performance components, including housings, connectors, or mechanical parts [24].

Subtractive manufacturing continues to be the backbone of modern manufacturing, as it provides the necessary precision and material compatibility for a range of applications that demand high performance. Its capacity to generate complex designs from tough materials makes it relevant in sectors where quality and precision are of paramount importance [25].

2.3.3 Hybrid Manufacturing

Hybrid manufacturing takes additive and subtractive processes in one single process which now is a step ahead in the new inventions made related to manufacturing. Hybrid manufacturing can produce parts having excellent precision, surface finish of excellent quality, and complex geometries that have been otherwise achievable only with a multitude of manufacturing processes. AM, or 3D printing, excels at making complex shapes and internal structures by adding material layer by layer. It affords a lot of design freedom because one can have intricate features that would be impossible to make in the first place with subtractive processes alone. However, AM sometimes fails when surface finish and tight tolerances need to be developed for certain applications [26].

The other category is subtraction manufacturing, which includes milling, turning, and drilling material removal processes known for their accuracy and high-quality surface finishes of the parts. This effectively improves the surface quality and dimensional accuracies of parts produced through AM. Hybrid manufacturing offers a comprehensive approach by combining both methods to reap both benefits. The most valuable application of hybrid manufacturing has been the creation of multifunctional implants. Medical implants often require complex geometries to replace or support the anatomical structures that they target. Additive manufacturing is particularly useful to produce such complex shapes with customized features, while subtractive manufacturing can be utilized to fine-tune the surface finish to ensure the precise fit and functionality of the implant. This ensures implants that are tailored to patient needs but also meet the stringent quality and performance requirements that exist in the medical field [27].

Hybrid manufacturing can also be used for repairing damaged biomedical components. Any biomedical device or implant will wear out or damage over time, and the replacement of the damaged components is costly in terms of time and resources. Hybrid manufacturing offers the solution of allowing parts that have reached their end to be repaired and refurbished, thus building back up the worn parts by additive methods and subtractive methods to return the part to its original dimension and surface quality. This would not only ensure an extended life for biomedical components, but it would also diminish the total cost and usage of resources involved in maintaining and replacing these components [28].

2.4 ADVANCED MATERIALS IN BIOMEDICAL MANUFACTURING

Advanced manufacturing technologies have hugely expanded the limits of materials used in biomedical applications so that highly specialized solutions for delicate needs are achieved to fulfill stringent demands placed upon the medical community. Metallic biomaterials, such as titanium and magnesium alloys, are considered implants because they possess higher strength and durability plus greater biocompatibility. Titanium alloys have a high strength-to-weight ratio, corrosion resistance, and excellent osseointegration; thus, they are appropriate for orthopedic, dental, and cardiovascular implants. Biodegradable magnesium alloys can be applied for temporary implants that degrade gradually within the organism, eliminating the requirement for secondary surgery. Biodegradable polymers, such as PLA, PGA, and their copolymers, PLGA, are widely used in drug delivery systems and tissue engineering. Such polymers are designed to degrade and release therapeutic agents in a controlled fashion. This is crucial for sustained drug delivery and temporary scaffolds for tissue regeneration. In both bone repair and coating applications, hydroxyapatite, zirconia, and other ceramic materials are unavoidable. Hydroxyapatite, being similar in composition to the mineral part of the bone, has extensive applications in bone grafts, coatings on implants, and tissue engineering scaffolds because of its high biocompatibility. Dental implants and prosthetics, especially those made of zirconia, with high strength, toughness, and wear resistance, yield excellent biocompatibility and aesthetic properties. Composite materials consisting of polymers combined with fibers or particles of ceramics, metals, or other polymers provide enhanced mechanical

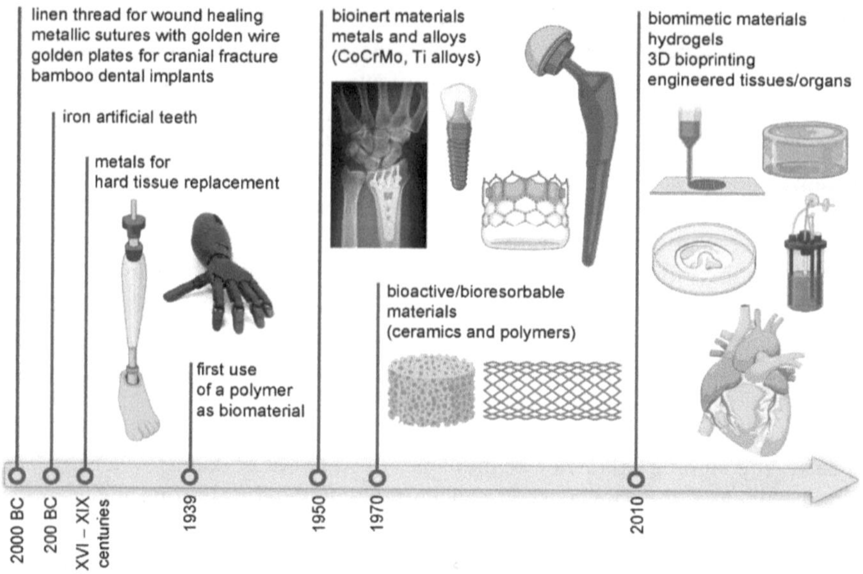

FIGURE 2.5 The history of biomaterials: from replacement to regeneration [31]. (CC By 4.0 Attribution)

properties such as increased strength, stiffness, and toughness while maintaining the required biocompatibility. For instance, the composites of hydroxyapatite and biodegradable polymers create scaffolds for bones with improved mechanical integrity and bioactivity, thus facilitating the growth and healing of bones. Generally, the wide variety of materials used in AMTs ensures an innovative biomedical solution that always leads to better patient outcomes and advances medical science. Each class of materials offers properties tailored to specific applications, achieving just the optimal balance of strength, biocompatibility, and functionality required for various medical devices and treatments [29, 30]. **Figure 2.5** shows the historical timeline of advances in biomaterials for medical applications.

2.5 EMERGING TRENDS IN BIOMEDICAL MANUFACTURING

Biomedical manufacturing is changing and developing, in an enormous manner, following various emerging trends. These are vast trends that are therefore reshaping the development and production of medical devices, implants, and treatments. They range from fabrication to nanomanufacturing and AI integration, with a significantly increased focus on sustainability. Each has unique advancements and challenges along this path and holds the potential for significantly better healthcare outcomes and patient experience [32].

Biofabrication integrates living cells in AMTs to fabricate functional tissues and organs. It connects 3D printing with biological materials to place cells, biomaterials, and growth factors into a specific composition resembling the architecture of natural tissues. Biofabrication holds great promise for applications in regenerative medicine, offering solutions toward organ transplantation scarcity through the production of custom-made biocompatible organs tailored for an individual patient. It has also been shown to be useful in tissue engineering, where damaged tissues can be repaired or replaced, offering new hopes in the treatment of burn injuries, heart disease, and osteoarthritis, among others. The possibility of creating tissues and organs that closely replicate natural physiology ushers new avenues for personalized medicine, with promises of more efficient and targeted therapies [33].

Nanomanufacturing is another important trend in biomedical manufacturing that could mainly be represented by the production of nanoscale devices and materials intended for drug delivery and diagnostics. At the nanoscale, materials exhibit unique properties useful for medical applications. For example, nanoparticles can be designed to specifically release drugs at the site of the targeted cells, thus reducing side effects and increasing treatment efficacy. This precision targeting is particularly useful in chemotherapy, where nanocarriers enable chemotherapy drugs to directly target cancer cells while preserving healthy tissue. Furthermore, nanomanufacturing opens new avenues for designing superior diagnostic equipment, such as nanosensors that can detect disease-related biomarkers at the earliest stages. These nanoscale devices can provide rapid, accurate, and minimally invasive diagnostic options, significantly improving disease management and patient outcomes [34].

The integration of artificial intelligence (AI) into biomedical manufacturing is revolutionizing the design and optimization of medical devices and implants. AI-driven algorithms can analyze vast amounts of data to identify optimal design parameters, predict performance, and personalize devices to individual patient anatomies. This increased level of personalization will ensure a more accurate fit, improved functionality, and increased patient comfort. For example, AI could be used to create uniquely tailored orthopedic implants to match the exact bone structure of a patient for reduced risks of problems and faster recovery time. Moreover, optimization through AI will optimize the manufacturing process with faster production time and cost-cutting measures while preserving the quality. The second is predictive capability; AI ensures the development of new materials and structures that can more closely emulate natural tissues, hence strengthening the effectiveness of implants and prosthetics [35].

A very important consideration in biomedical manufacturing is sustainability. It is primarily to reduce environmental impact and to improve the overall ecological footprint of medical products. The lead in this regard is in the development of eco-friendly manufacturing processes and biodegradable materials. Key sustainability manufacturing practices include the use of renewable energy sources, reducing waste through efficient production techniques, and recycling materials wherever possible. Biodegradable materials, such as certain polymers and composites, are increasingly used in medical devices and implants. Materials used here degrade safely within the body or environment, which means less waste over the long term or even an end to surgical removal of some implants. The development of sustainable practices in biomedical manufacturing, therefore, not only addresses environmental concerns but also enhances the biocompatibility and safety of medical products [36]. **Figure 2.6** shows the diagram linking the UN Sustainable Development Goals with selected detailed aspects of good health and well-being of people, including the organization of medical care and the design and production of medical devices necessary in these activities.

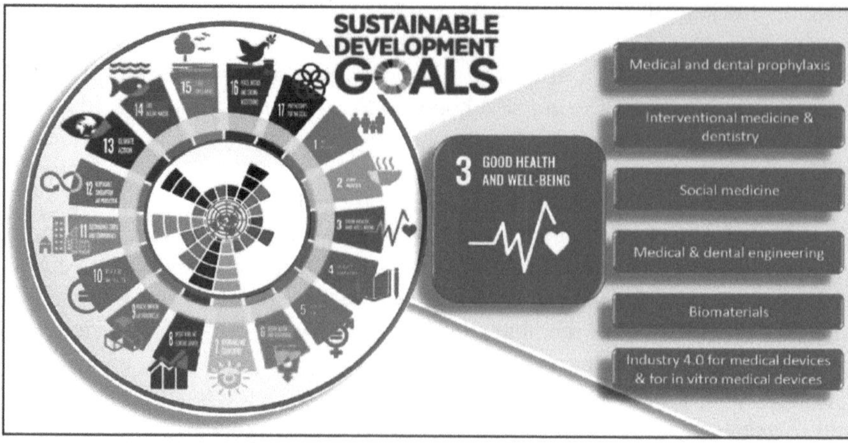

FIGURE 2.6 Diagram linking the UN Sustainable Development Goals to key aspects of health, medical care organization, and medical device design and production [37]. (CC By 4.0 Attribution)

2.6 CHALLENGES AND FUTURE DIRECTIONS

Advanced manufacturing technologies that offer such a wide set of advantages to biomedical science have been faced with numerous significant challenges that have not allowed the widespread adoption and full utilization of these technologies. These are mainly regulatory hurdles, high costs, and material issues, each of which has unique obstacles that must be addressed for the effective implementation of these technologies in clinical settings. Overcoming these challenges will require increased research–industry–clinical collaboration, standardization of manufacturing and quality control processes, and continued investments in the development of material science and digital design tools [38].

The regulatory obstacles are one of the biggest challenges in adopting advanced manufacturing in the biomedical sector. Stringent requirements for safety, efficacy, and quality as outlined by regulatory agencies such as the U.S. Food and Drug Administration (FDA) and the European Medicines Agency (EMA) can slow down the approval process for new technologies and products. Navigating these regulatory landscapes requires a deep understanding of compliance requirements and the ability to demonstrate consistent product quality and performance. Enhanced collaboration between researchers, clinicians, and industry stakeholders is essential to streamline this process. Collaborative efforts by these groups ensure that new manufacturing methods and materials possess regulatory compliance from the outset, thereby saving these time- and cost-consuming aspects of introducing new biomedical products in the market. High costs are another major challenge hindering the adoption of AMTs in the biomedical sector. The initial investment in new equipment such as 3D printers and nanomanufacturing tools is exceptionally high for many organizations. Moreover, the costs of the development and validation of new materials and processes can contribute to the total expense. Standardization of manufacturing and quality control processes is very important for consistency in production and waste reduction. While processes are standardized, manufacturers can obtain economies of scale, thus decreasing the overall cost of production and making highly advanced biomedical products more attainable [39].

Material limitations are another significant challenge in advanced biomedical manufacturing. New biomaterials that are biocompatible yet appropriate for advanced manufacturing processes must be developed. Today, most of the materials that have been developed are found to either not possess the required properties for the desired applications or not yet cleared for medical applications. Material science needs to continue building on this progress to overcome the material limitations. Advancing the understanding of how materials interact with biological systems can lead to researchers creating more effective and versatile biomedical products by developing new compounds with enhanced properties. Going digital with design tools makes it easier to rapidly prototype and test new materials and devices, rapidly improving development time [40–43].

Also, the laser technology finds wide usage throughout multiple applications such as machining operations and additive manufacturing techniques together with post-processing procedures and coating skills. Researchers have examined metal matrix composite (MMC) laser machining through CO_2 laser approaches to study material removal rate together with surface morphology and roughness qualities [44–48]. Research on AM technology has advanced substantially in the field of laser-based AM sustainability issues and shape memory alloys for AM applications [49–51]. Technological breakthroughs in machine learning allow manufacturers to optimize machining features of AM systems alongside the improvement of mechanical properties in 3D-printed products [52–54]. Post-processing applications that use laser technologies serve as fundamental procedures for enhancing powder-based materials alongside coatings [55, 56]. The mechanical and wear resistance characteristics of cladding [57, 58] and coatings [59–64] are investigated in recent studies. Thermal spray coatings are found also feasible in case of protecting exterior components of larger machines in erosion and corrosion environment [65–71]. Researchers have dedicated attention to biocoatings together with bioimplants [72–74].

Another important issue is the incorporation of digital design tools, including CAD software and AI, within the development process. Such tools allow for faithful modeling and simulation of new devices so that designs can be optimized before prototypes are produced. This not only reduces the time and expense related to product design but also makes sure that the final products meet the specifications and standards required for performance. Continued investment in these technologies will drive innovation and efficiency in the biomedical manufacturing sector.

2.7 CONCLUSION

Advanced manufacturing technologies fundamentally change the landscape of biomedical science, as they usher a new degree of breakthroughs in patient care and medical innovation. By unleashing precision, customization, and versatility about materials, these technologies are perfectly responding to some of the most formidable challenges facing healthcare. Techniques like 3D printing, nanomanufacturing, and biofabrication make it possible to create extremely personalized medical devices, implants, and even functional tissues and organs, tailored to the needs of individual patients. This level of customizing treatment not only ensures better patient outcomes but also amplifies the efficacy and functionality of medical interventions. Besides, with advanced manufacturing offering materials ranging from biocompatible polymers and metals to advanced composites, the possibility is there to tailor the creation of new treatments and devices to both effect and safety in an unprecedented way [42].

Advanced manufacturing will also interact powerfully with emerging fields such as bioinformatics and AI. Bioinformatics brings along considerable amounts of data that can be useful in preparing and developing medical devices so they are adequately geared to treat or mitigate numerous diseases. AI, on the other hand, provides powerful tools for design optimization, predictive modeling, and automation of processes, thereby creating very fast and efficient production of complex biomedical products. In line with this, AI can simplify the processes involved in production to reduce costs and enhance quality control such that the final products achieve high standards of safety and performance. All these synergies open the door to next-generation solutions in biomedical science which may revolutionize everything from diagnostic tools and therapeutic devices to regenerative medicine and personalized treatments. AMTs continue to evolve, coupled with research and interaction among disciplines and professionals, and hold out the promise to unlock unprecedented capabilities in healthcare. As these technologies mature and become more integrated into clinical practice, they have the potential to significantly improve patient outcomes, reduce the costs of healthcare, and drive forward frontiers of medical science. In conclusion, AMTs are not just enhancing current biomedical capabilities but are also laying the groundwork for a future where medical solutions are more precise, personalized, and effective than ever before [43].

REFERENCES

1. Ventola CL. Medical applications for 3D printing: Current and projected uses. *P T.* 2014;39(10):704–11.
2. Rengier F, Mehndiratta A, von Tengg-Kobligk H, Zechmann CM, Unterhinninghofen R, Kauczor HU, Giesel FL. 3D printing based on imaging data: Review of medical applications. *International Journal of Computer Assisted Radiology and Surgery.* 2010;5(4):335–41.
3. Javaid M, Haleem A. Additive manufacturing applications in medical cases: A literature-based review. *Alexandria Journal of Medicine.* 2018;54(4):411–22.
4. Bose S, Vahabzadeh S, Bandyopadhyay A. Bone tissue engineering using 3D printing. *Materials Today.* 2013;16(12):496–504.
5. Salmi M. Additive manufacturing processes in medical applications. *Materials.* 2021;14(1):191.
6. Levy GN, Schindel R, Kruth JP. Rapid manufacturing and rapid tooling with layer manufacturing (LM) technologies, state of the art and future perspectives. *CIRP Annals.* 2003;52(2):589–609.
7. Wang W, Yeung KW. Bone grafts and biomaterials substitutes for bone defect repair: A review. *Bioactive Materials.* 2017;2(4):224–47.
8. Ventola CL. Medical applications for 3D printing: Current and projected uses. *P T.* 2014;39(10):704–11.

9. Chen M, Le DQ, Hein S, Wang X, Xie Y, Hui J, Geris L. Recent advances in 3D biofabrication techniques for bone tissue engineering. *Biofabrication.* 2019;11(4):043001.
10. Javaid M, Haleem A. Additive manufacturing applications in medical cases: A literature based review. *Alexandria Journal of Medicine.* 2018;54(4):411–22.
11. Rengier F, Mehndiratta A, von Tengg-Kobligk H, Zechmann CM, Unterhinninghofen R, Kauczor HU, Giesel FL. 3D printing based on imaging data: Review of medical applications. *International Journal of Computer Assisted Radiology and Surgery.* 2010;5(4):335–41.
12. Bose S, Vahabzadeh S, Bandyopadhyay A. Bone tissue engineering using 3D printing. *Materials Today.* 2013;16(12):496–504.
13. Sánchez-Cid P, Jiménez-Rosado M, Romero A, Pérez-Puyana V. Novel trends in hydrogel development for biomedical applications: A review. *Polymers.* 2022;14(15):3023.
14. Verma PK, Singh S, Kapoor M, Singh S. A review on the surface topography and corrosion behavior of Mg-alloy coatings for biomedical implants. *Results in Surfaces and Interfaces.* 2024;15:100227.
15. Gibson I, Rosen DW, Stucker B. *Additive Manufacturing Technologies: 3D Printing, Rapid Prototyping, and Direct Digital Manufacturing.* Springer; 2014.
16. Melchels FP, Domingos MA, Klein TJ, Malda J, Bartolo PJ, Hutmacher DW. Additive manufacturing of tissues and organs. *Progress in Polymer Science.* 2012;37(8):1079–104.
17. Chia HN, Wu BM. Recent advances in 3D printing of biomaterials. *Journal of Biological Engineering.* 2015;9(1):4.
18. Gross BC, Erkal JL, Lockwood SY, Chen C, Spence DM. Evaluation of 3D printing and its potential impact on biotechnology and the chemical sciences. *Analytical Chemistry.* 2014;86(7):3240–53.
19. Parthasarathy J, Starly B, Raman S, Christensen A. A design for the additive manufacture of functionally graded porous structures with tailored mechanical properties for biomedical applications. *Journal of Manufacturing Processes.* 2010;12(1):8–19.
20. Verma PK, Vasudev H, Singh G, Singh S. A review on the microstructural and biomedical properties of implants manufactured using additive manufacturing. *Journal of The Institution of Engineers (India): Series D.* 2024:1–5.
21. Wang X, Xu S, Zhou S, Xu W, Leary M, Choong P, Qian M, Brandt M, Xie YM. Topological design and additive manufacturing of porous metals for bone scaffolds and orthopaedic implants: A review. *Biomaterials.* 2016;83:127–41.
22. Van der Stok J, Wang H, Amin Yavari S, Siebelt M, Sandker M, Waarsing JH, Verhaar JA, Jahr H, Zadpoor AA, Weinans H. Enhanced bone regeneration through temporary presence of a 3D printed polymeric scaffold in a mechanically loaded segmental defect. *European Cells and Materials.* 2013;26(1):133–45.
23. Moroni L, Boland T, Burdick JA, De Maria C, Derby B, Forgacs G, Groll J, Li Q, Malda J, Mironov VA, Nakamura M. Biofabrication: A guide to technology and terminology. *Trends in Biotechnology.* 2018;36(4):384–402.
24. Bertol LS, Júnior WV, da Silva FP, Aumund-Kopp C. Medical design: Direct metal laser sintering of Ti–6Al–4V. *Materials & Design.* 2010;31(8):3982–8.
25. Gibson I, Rosen DW, Stucker B. *Additive Manufacturing Technologies: 3D Printing, Rapid Prototyping, and Direct Digital Manufacturing.* Springer; 2014.
26. Nguyen DT, Lewandowski JJ, Seifi M. Mechanical properties of 316L stainless steel manufactured by laser powder bed fusion: Effects of process parameters and heat treatment. *Materials Science and Engineering: A.* 2020;769:138455.
27. Xu F, Wee B, Mao H, Liu J. Overview of hybrid additive-subtractive manufacturing processes for high-quality metal parts. *Engineering.* 2021;7(5):653–63.
28. Zhang Y, Li S, Cao J, Zhang D, Qin E, Wang S. Design and fabrication of a hybrid structure for mandibular defect repair based on 3D printing technology. *Scientific Reports.* 2018;8(1):1–9.

29. Flynn JM, Shokrani A, Newman ST, Dhokia V. Hybrid additive and subtractive machine tools–research and industrial developments. *International Journal of Machine Tools and Manufacture*. 2016;101:79–101.
30. Balla VK, Bodhak S, Bose S, Bandyopadhyay A. Porous tantalum structures for bone implants: Fabrication, mechanical and in vitro biological properties. *Acta Biomaterialia*. 2010;6(8):3349–59.
31. Todros S, Todesco M, Bagno A. Biomaterials and their biomedical applications: From replacement to regeneration. *Processes*. 2021;9(11):1949.
32. Yuan B, Zhou S, Dong J, Shen Y, Yang J, Zhou Y, Xie Y, Zhou J, Zhang Z, Liu C. Novel multifunctional scaffold with core–shell fibers for bone regeneration application. *Materials Science and Engineering: C*. 2019;94:1–11.
33. Murphy SV, Atala A. 3D bioprinting of tissues and organs. *Nature Biotechnology*. 2014;32(8):773–85.
34. Riehemann K, Schneider SW, Luger TA, Godin B, Ferrari M, Fuchs H. Nanomedicine—challenge and perspectives. *Angewandte Chemie International Edition*. 2009;48(5):872–97.
35. Choi JW, Kim J. AI-based design of personalized biomedical devices. *Journal of Computational Design and Engineering*. 2019;6(4):489–96.
36. Anastas PT, Zimmerman JB. Design through the 12 principles of green engineering. *Environmental Science & Technology*. 2003;37(5):94A–101A.
37. Dobrzański LA, Dobrzańska-Danikiewicz AD, Dobrzański LB. Effect of biomedical materials in the implementation of a long and healthy life policy. *Processes*. 2021;9(5):865.
38. Ventola CL. Medical applications for 3D printing: Current and projected uses. *Pharmacy and Therapeutics*. 2014;39(10):704–11.
39. Ventola CL. The pharmaceutical industry and 3D printing: Promises and hurdles. *Pharmacy and Therapeutics*. 2014;39(12):830–5.
40. Bose S, Roy M, Bandyopadhyay A. Recent advances in bone tissue engineering scaffolds. *Trends in Biotechnology*. 2012;30(10):546–54.
41. Waran V, Narayanan V, Karuppiah R, Owen SL, Aziz T. *Advanced Medical Prototyping and 3D Modeling in Neurosurgery*. Springer; 2017.
42. Murphy SV, Atala A. 3D bioprinting of tissues and organs. *Nature Biotechnology*. 2014;32(8):773–85.
43. Pandey PM, Reddy NV, Dhande SG. Real time adaptive slicing for fused deposition modeling. *International Journal of Machine Tools and Manufacture*. 2003;43(1):61–71.
44. Sharma V, Kumar V. Application of Box-Behnken design and response surface methodology for multi-optimization of laser cutting of AA5052/ZrO2 metal–matrix composites. *Proceedings of the Institution of Mechanical Engineers, Part L: Journal of Materials: Design and Applications*. 2018;232(8):652–68.
45. Sharma V, Kumar V. Comparison of machining characteristics of metal matrix composites using CO2 laser curve cutting process. *Proceedings of the Institution of Mechanical Engineers, Part E: Journal of Process Mechanical Engineering*. 2018;232(3):349–68.
46. Sharma V, Kumar V. Investigating the quality characteristics of Al5052/SiC metal matrix composites machined by CO2 laser curve cutting. *Proceedings of the Institution of Mechanical Engineers, Part L: Journal of Materials: Design and Applications*. 2018;232(1):3–19.
47. Sharma V, Kumar V, Bist A. Investigations on morphology and material removal rate of various MMCs using CO2 laser technique. *Journal of the Brazilian Society of Mechanical Sciences and Engineering*. 2020;42:1–14.
48. Sharma V, Singh JP, Raman R, Bathla G, Saini A. Machine learning approach for prediction analysis of aluminium alloy on the surface roughness using CO2 laser machining. *Proceedings of the Institution of Mechanical Engineers, Part E: Journal of Process Mechanical Engineering*. 2024;09544089241231093.

49. Singh R, Toseef M, Kumar J, Singh J. Benefits and challenges in additive manufacturing and its applications. In: Kaushal S, Singh I, Singh S, Gupta A, editors. *Sustainable Advanced Manufacturing and Materials Processing.* 1st ed. Boca Raton: CRC Press; 2022. pp. 137–57. https://doi.org/10.1201/9781003269298-8.
50. Singh J. Sustainability issues in laser-based additive manufacturing. In: *Handbook of Laser-Based Sustainable Surface Modification and Manufacturing Techniques.* CRC Press; 2023. pp. 167–89.
51. Ahmad, S., et al. Innovations in additive manufacturing of shape memory alloys: Alloys, microstructures, treatments, applications. *Journal of Materials Research and Technology.* 2024;32:4136–97.
52. Sharma V, Singh JP, Hussan K, Kumar R. Machine learning approach for predicting the machining characteristics of additive manufactured ABS material. *Proceedings of the Institution of Mechanical Engineers, Part C: Journal of Mechanical Engineering Science.* 2024;09544062241283330.
53. Chohan JS, et al. Mechanical strength enhancement of 3D printed acrylonitrile butadiene styrene polymer components using neural network optimization algorithm. *Polymers.* 2020;12(10). https://doi.org/10.3390/polym12102250.
54. Singh J, et al. Impact of molding temperature, fiber loading and chemical modifications on the physicomechanical, and microstructural morphology properties of woven kenaf fiber/PLA composites for non-structural applications. *Journal of Natural Fibers.* 2024;21(1):2326586.
55. Singh J. Applications of laser technology for processing and post-treatments of powders and coatings. In: *Handbook of Laser-Based Sustainable Surface Modification and Manufacturing Techniques.* CRC Press; 2023. pp. 135–66.
56. Sunitha K, Vasudev H. A short note on the various thermal spray coating processes and effect of post-treatment on Ni-based coatings. *Materials Today: Proceedings.* 2022;50:1452–7. https://doi.org/10.1016/j.matpr.2021.09.017.
57. Sharanabasava H, et al. Microstructure, mechanical and wear properties of SiC and Mo reinforced NiCr microwave cladding. *Advanced Materials and Processing Technologies.*2024;10:3620–33.
58. Singh J, Gill HS. Evolution of nickel-based superalloy claddings for against high-temperature oxidation and wear. In: *Thermal Claddings for Engineering Applications.* CRC Press; 2024. pp. 160–81.
59. Singh J, Kumar S, Kumar R, Mohapatra SK. Machine learning regression tools for erosion prediction of WC-10Co4Cr thermal spray coating. *Results Surfaces Interfaces.* 2023;13:100156. https://doi.org/10.1016/j.rsurfi.2023.100156.
60. Yedida VVS, Vasudev H. A review on the development of thermal barrier coatings by using thermal spray techniques. *Materials Today: Proceedings.* 2022;50:1458–64.
61. Singh J, Singh S. Support vector machine learning on slurry erosion characteristics analysis of Ni- and Co-alloy coatings. *Surface Review and Letters.* 2023. https://doi.org/10.1142/S0218625X23400061.
62. Prashar G, Vasudev H. A review on the influence of process parameters and heat treatment on the corrosion performance of Ni-based thermal spray coatings. *Surface Review and Letters.* 2022;29(1):2230001.
63. Singh J, Vasudev H, Szala M, Gill HS. Neural computing for erosion assessment in Al-20TiO2 HVOF thermal spray coating. *International Journal on Interactive Design and Manufacturing.* 2024;18:2321–32.
64. Singh J, Vasudev H, Kumar R, Ubaidullah M. Study on wear analysis of Ni-20Al2O3 HVOF micron layers using artificial neural network technique. *International Journal on Interactive Design and Manufacturing.* 2023;18:5925–38. https://doi.org/10.1007/s12008-023-01433-2.

65. Prashar G, Vasudev H. Surface topology analysis of plasma sprayed Inconel625-Al2O3 composite coating. *Materials Today: Proceedings*. 2022;50:607–11. https://doi.org/10.1016/j.matpr.2021.03.090.
66. Thakur L, Vasudev H, Singh J, Prashar G. *Artificial Intelligence and Machine Learning in the Thermal Spray Industry: Practices, Implementation, and Challenges*. CRC Press; 2023.
67. Dutta V, Thakur L, Singh B, Vasudev H. A study of erosion–corrosion behaviour of friction stir-processed chromium-reinforced NiAl bronze composite. *Materials (Basel)*. 2022;15(15):5401. https://doi.org/10.3390/ma15155401.
68. Singh J, Singh S, Vasudev H, Chohan JS, Kumar S. Neural computing and Taguchi's method-based study on erosion of advanced Mo2C–WC10Co4Cr coating for the centrifugal pump. *Advances in Materials and Processing Technologies*. 2024;10(3):2569–81.
69. Singh J, Singh S, Vasudev H, Katiyar JK. Artificial neural network model for wear characteristic analysis of WC-10Co4Cr and Stellite 6 thermal spray coatings. *Tribology International*. 2024;199:109924.
70. Majji BGR, Vasudev H, Bansal A. A review on the oxidation and wear behavior of the thermally sprayed high-entropy alloys. *Materials Today: Proceedings*. 2022;50:1447–51.
71. Singh J, Singh S, Verma A. Artificial intelligence in use of ZrO2 material in biomedical science. *Journal of Electrochemical Science and Engineering*. 2022;13(1):83–97. https://doi.org/10.5599/jese.1498.
72. Singh J, Hashmi AW, Behra A, Kumar A, Dogra N, Kumar P. Review of Mg alloys for bio-implants protected by the deposition of chemical conversion coatings. In *AIP Conference Proceedings*. AIP Publishing; 2024.
73. Singh J, Singh S, Gill R. Applications of biopolymer coatings in biomedical engineering. *Journal of Electrochemical Science and Engineering*. 2022;13(1):63–81. https://doi.org/10.5599/jese.1460.
74. Singh CJ, Ram B, Singh J, Prakash C, Paramasivam P, Kumar R. Experimental investigation on characterization of friction stir processed AZ31-based composite. *Scientific Reports*. 2024;14(1):15453.

3 Significance of Additive Manufacturing in Biological Applications

Amrinder Mehta and Hitesh Vasudev

CONTENTS

3.1 INTRODUCTION

Additive manufacturing (AM) is a revolutionary technology that has revolutionized many industries one of which is biology. In this process, objects are created by adding layers to an object constructed from digital design plans. AM has expanded the potential of generating new forms in tissue engineering and the modeling of organs like tissue scaffolds. It makes it possible to fashion detailed medical replacements, including implants, prosthetics, as well as living tissue [1]. This effectiveness helps the researcher develop complex geometries that resemble natural biological systems and improve tissue engineering and regenerative medicine. In its current form, AM is yet to realize its full potential in the healthcare industry, but it holds even greater possibilities, as it holds the key to the future of medicine, that is, targeted treatments and fast-forwarded drug development [2]. The chapter illustrates the fabrication of PCL porous scaffolds and waxy structures by electric field-driven jet deposition for fused deposition 3D printing with micron-scale

DOI: 10.1201/9781003516064-3

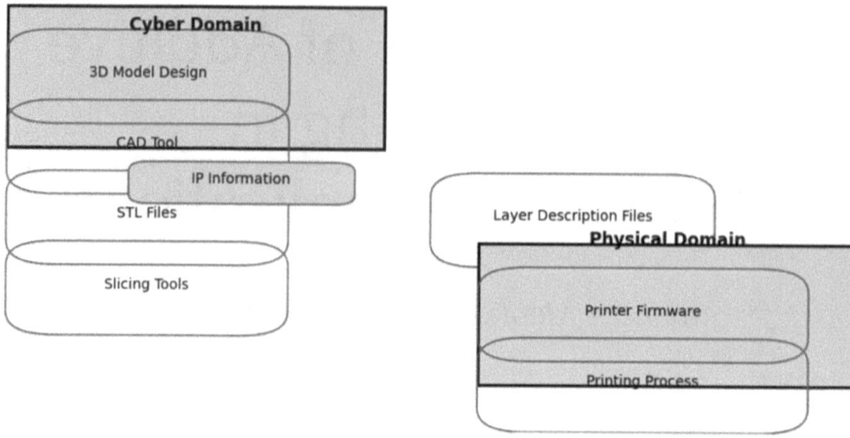

FIGURE 3.1 Phases in AM process. (No permission required: Created by authors)

resolution. This technique is a distinct innovation in using 3D printable technology especially for biomedical uses [3].

Figure 3.1 captures the mutual behavior of the cyber domain and physical domain during the 3D printing process. In the cyber domain, the first step is to create a 3D model using CAD software and then move to generate STL files and slice the models. This phase contains information relating to intellectual property (IP) [4]. The physical domain comprises layer description files, firmware of the printer, and physical printing. The red ovals illustrate the crucial milestone that are data and process transition points, which demonstrate the flow of digital designs into physical objects by technologies such as 3D printing [5].

At the same time, materials processing based on laminated object manufacturing using laser has been developed, especially laser powder bed fusion (LPBF). Over the years, research has concentrated on the application of mesh layouts, increasing materials characteristics, and application of process techniques. They include the enhancement of the BCCZ lattice and the diamond lattice structures, as well as the mechanical properties of AlSi10Mg alloy [6]. The changing techniques of electric field and laser used in the process of 3D printing as represented by these two categories of printers are enough to show how fast the technology is improving. These approaches reveal a lot of potential for enhancing many sectors such as biomedical engineering, aerospace, and others due to their ability to build multifaceted structures schemed with proper characteristics and efficiency [7]. In this chapter, the role of additive manufacturing in biological applications is examined, with the focus on its essential role in changing the image of medical science, tissue engineering, and personalized approach in healthcare.

3.2 ADDITIVE MANUFACTURING TECHNIQUES

3.2.1 Vat Photopolymerization

Digital light processing (DLP) is a sophisticated 3D printing process that belongs to the vat photopolymerization type, essential in medicine. In its essence, DLP employs a digital micromirror device to reflect the light projected on a photosensitive resin [8].

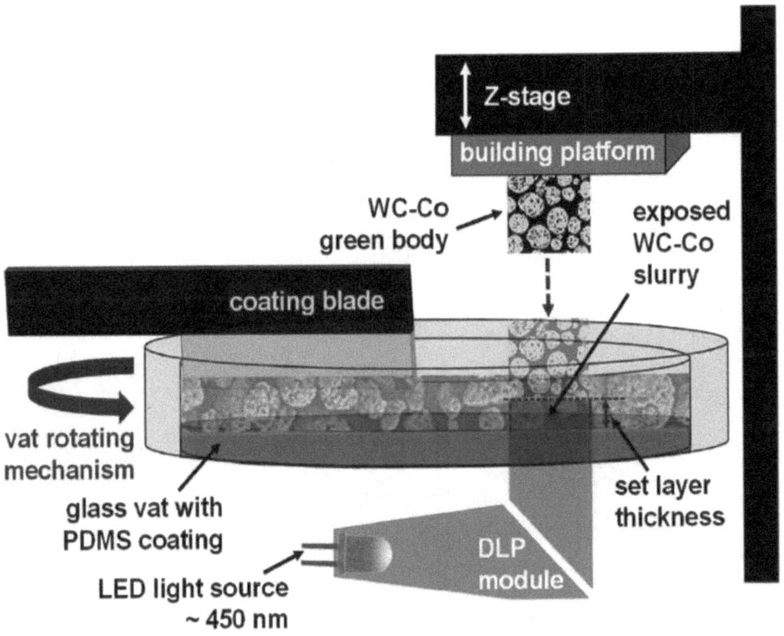

FIGURE 3.2 Schematic representation of vat photopolymerization. [10] (Under CC 4.0 Attribution)

This process facilitates control of the degree of cure of the resin successively for each layer providing highly accurate print. Thus, the principal benefits of DLP are complex structures with geometrically smooth surfaces and relatively short time for its completion. These attributes make DLP particularly suitable for generation of individual medical parts, dental implants, and anatomical models for planning of operations [9].

Figure 3.2 shows an example of an additive manufacturing for DLP based on the fabrication of the WC-Co parts. A glass container with a rotating system allows slurry of WC-Co particles to be spread into thin layers using a coating blade. In the DLP module, 450 nm light is used to solidify each layer of the slurry and produce a green body. As each layer is built, only the building platform needs to move in the vertical plane or the Z-stage. Again, the PDMS coating of the development vat helps to separate the layers easily from one another, and the rotating blade helps in spreading the slurry for a complete and accurate layer formation [10].

3.2.2 Laser-based Techniques

Organic synthesis techniques, in particular the selective laser melting (SLM) also known as laser powder bed fusion (LPBF), have shown potential in manufacturing biodegradable magnesium alloys for orthopedic implants. These techniques provide several advantages for biomedical applications: the creation of intricate architecture and free-form structures for sufficient osteoconductive properties needed porous structures to improve bone-to-implant bonding [11]. LPBF provides the versatility of controlling the implant geometry to produce patient-specific implant with efficient mechanical characteristics and degradation kinetics.

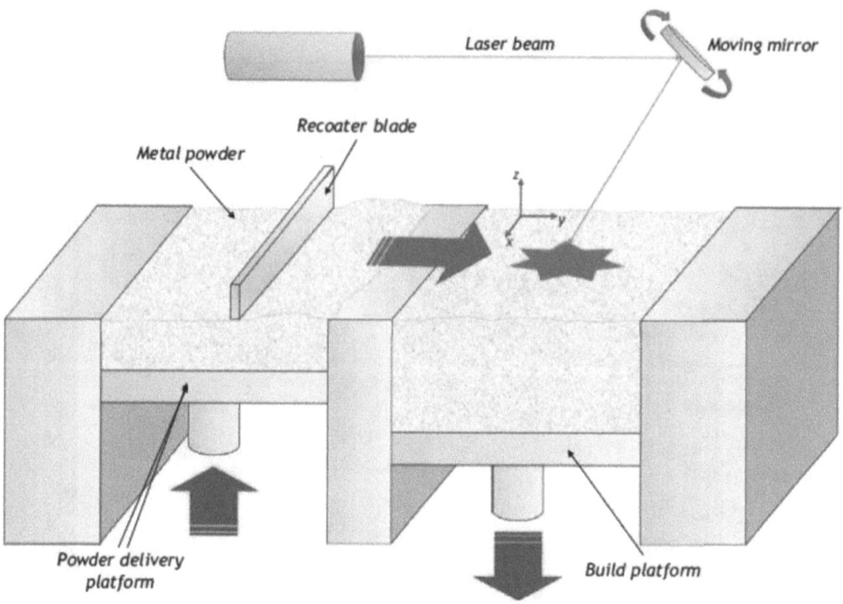

FIGURE 3.3 The laser powder bed fusion (LPBF) process [12]. (Under CC 4.0 Attribution)

Figure 3.3 explains SLM known as a type of additive manufacturing technology. The recoater blade is utilized in spreading metal powder over the build platform. Laser beam is guided by a moving mirror to selectively fuse the powder layer based on the required design. The powder delivery platform moves up to current more material, while the build platform lowers down after every layer has been sintered. This layer-by-layer process goes on until the structure of the complete object is created. The active laser can be moved only in X and/or Y axes while the build platform moves only in the z axis for layering [12].

Stress shielding and the requirement of the successive surgical interventions are another two problems solved by means of these techniques using magnesium alloys with the properties close to the bone [13]. Nevertheless, there are some issues that retard the fast degradation of magnesium and the need to enhance the corrosion rate to make magnesium successfully used in long-term implant applications.

3.2.3 Extrusion-based Methods

Two of the most promising classes of AM methods are direct ink write (DIW) and fused filament fabrication (FFF) for the fabrication of polyurethanes and other biomaterials. These techniques include the process of material deposition through a nozzle to develop a three-dimensional structure one layer at a time [14]. DIW uses an ink that can be in liquid or paste-like consistency, while FFF melts the filament inside a heated nozzle and extrudes them. Each has pros and outs in terms of creating intricate shapes and tailored structures within the biomedical sector including implantation materials or medication delivery systems [15]. So flexible are these techniques that fine-tuning to an array of material characteristics and system layout is possible, and as such these techniques form a handy resource if not a necessity in the biomaterials field.

3.3 APPLICATIONS IN BIOLOGICAL RESEARCH AND MEDICINE

3.3.1 Tissue Engineering and Regenerative Medicine

AM has revolutionized tissue engineering (TE) and regenerative medicine (Re-M) by allowing the construction of architecturally complex, bioinspired scaffolds that replicate native tissues. This technology offers flexibility and control in terms of scaffolding design and structure, porosity, and material selection for cell attachment, differentiation, and tissue regeneration. Since 3D printing technology processes and prescribes the form of the tissue and implant required, it can create biomimetic scaffolds and thereby have immense application in personalized medicine [16]. Additional techniques have also been developed which makes it possible to directly pattern cells and bioactive molecules into scaffold, hence forming more intricate and active tissue construct. These advancements have dramatically enhanced the opportunity to develop tissues for transplanting, pharmaceutical screening, and representation of diseases and states, creating fresh horizons in regenerative medicine and opportunities for treatment to patients with tissue pathology or organ dysfunction [17].

3.3.2 Bioinspired Structural Designs

When put together with deep learning techniques, additive manufacturing has transformed how bioinspired structural designs are made. These synergisms enable the engineers to imitate the various intricate nature's formations to outstanding level of accuracy. It is perhaps worthy of note that this has often involved the creation of a graph-oriented deep learning framework to understand the complex design paradigms of the spider web architectures [18].

Figure 3.4 shows different categories of implants that can be developed in the structural design of bioinspired materials. A 3D printing machine is at the core of the design, highlighting modern manufacturing processes that are used to create these implants [19]. The four types of implants illustrated include the orthopedic implants used in bones and joints, knee implants for knee joint arthroplasty, shoulder implants for shoulder joint arthroplasty, and dental implants for dental prosthesis. It focuses on suggesting that the bioinspired structures that imitate some biological forms can improve performance and interaction of those medical devices within the human body [20].

Through this method, an attempt is made to understand the efficiency and robustness of the spider web and to reproduce it. Artificial intelligence can involve making observations of nature and translating the observation results into new and improved physical configurations; thus, by exploring the designs in the natural world and how these can be translated to create novel structures with superior properties as strength, flexibility, and lightness [21]. In addition to broadening the knowledge of natural systems, this strategy also offers the opportunity for the development of new engineering solutions in various areas that include construction up to aerospace engineering.

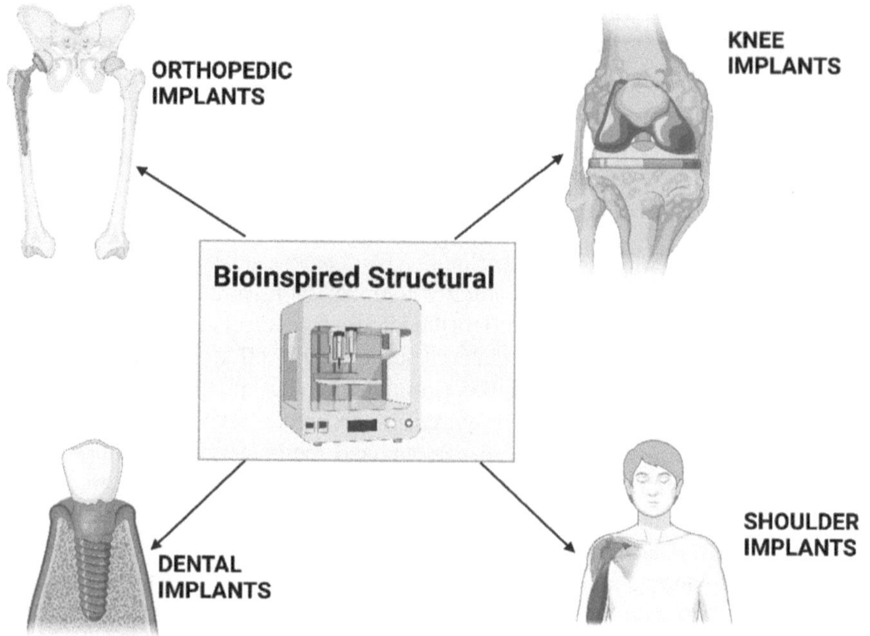

FIGURE 3.4 AM bioinspired structural designs. (Created by authors)

3.3.3 Engineered Living Materials

Additive manufacturing when coupled with synthetic biology has produced engineered living materials (ELMs) that are the new generation of biohybrid structures which explore the conceptual interconnectivity between 3D printing and living systems. Smart materials are composites that include living cells or biological parts with other artificial structures; adaptive systems, life-like materials, and functional structures [22]. As we shall see later, ELMs that have been developed may be able to synthesize desired substances, detect toxic substances, or reproduce and increase their ability as time passes.

Two 3D printed objects are displayed in the **Figure 3.5**. The object on the left can be estimated as a certain form of nodal formation which resembles a torus knot or trefoil knot of a certain type, created with the further addition of a peculiar porous or textured material. The object on the right is an empty sphere with six rings each of which containing a circular opening; thus, suggesting it could be a lattice or organic-like structure. Both objects consist of fine geometries that are usually achieved by rapidly prototyping techniques and additive manufacturing that creates geometries difficult to produce through other manufacturing methods [23].

It extends new opportunities in the fields like green construction, biomedical application, and in environmental management among others with the help of engineered biological systems as well as modern techniques of manufacturing [24]. ELMs are a major advance in designing materials that are alive and smart in nature but border on just that side of alive.

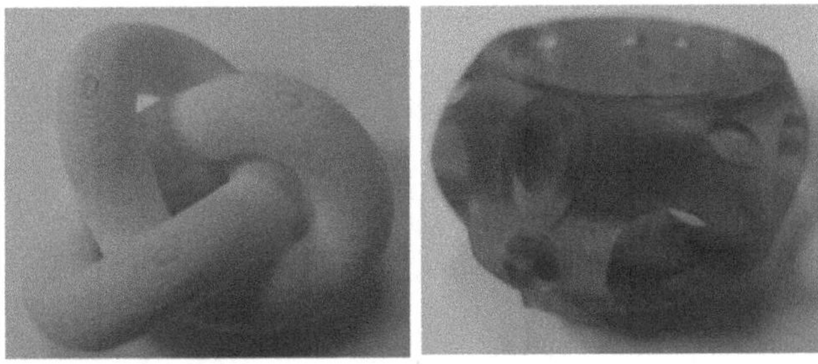

FIGURE 3.5 Artistic models fabricated using AM technology [23]. (Reproduction permission by Taylor and Francis under CC 4.0 Attribution)

3.3.4 Soft Robotics in Medicine

AM has had a major positive impact on soft robotics in medicine by providing very accurate and functional custom-made manufacturing. This approach enables production of compliant structures that can function on, interface, and interact with human tissues and organs: Material extrusion, vat photopolymerization and material jetting technologies have been used to manufacture soft robotic actuators, grippers, and prosthetics with integrated sensors [25]. Such devices might be designed to conform to the shape of the human anatomy, which should help to reduce tissue damage during surgery or during the process of rehabilitation. Further, 3DP enables fast prototyping and part customization of soft robots for medical applications including minimally invasive surgical instruments, wearable orthopedic appliances, and artificial muscles for organs [26].

3.4 CHALLENGES

Despite the huge opportunity that lies in the use of additive manufacturing in biological applications, the technology is faced with several core challenges. The final important challenge, it is currently a major problem for mass production scale to meet the requirements for application in a wide range of clinical contexts because existing processes require significant time and are expensive for large-scale utilization [27]. **Figure 3.6** is a fishbone (Ishikawa) diagram which shows the difficulty in a process. It categorizes issues into six areas: People (no process [control]map), Methods (no basic concept of design), Machines (poor parts quality), Materials (no material characterization norms), Measurements (no constant monitoring system), and Environment (using less energy than optimum) [28].

While 3D printing biomedical tools have the potential of reducing costs and producing highly specialized equipment, the protocols for approval of tissues for use in medical and for devices which use printed biological parts are slow and prolonged, presenting great challenges to the use of 3D printing in clinical care [29]. The overall enhancement of the printed materials characteristics, especially biocompatibility and long-term stability, is of the greatest importance for the purpose of using the printed materials in the biological environment [30]. Table 3.1 gives an insight of the

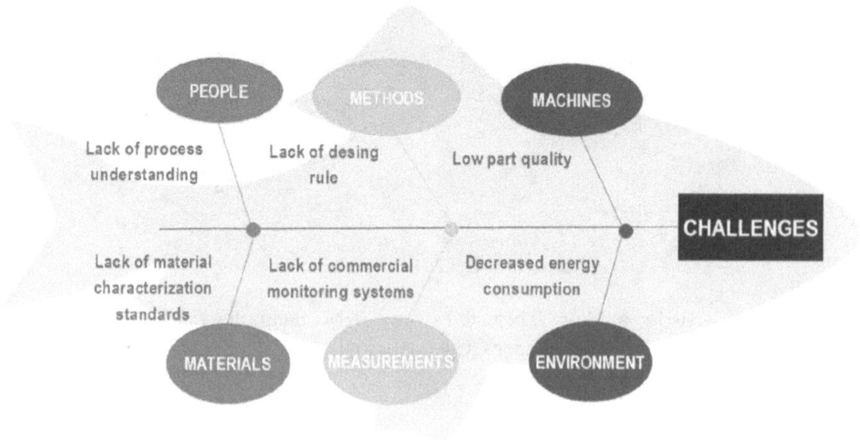

FIGURE 3.6 Challenges in AM [28]. (Reproduction permission by Springer Nature)

TABLE 3.1
Table Summarizing the Challenges of Additive Manufacturing in Orthopedics

Method	Challenges	Description	Ref.
General AM	Lack of data	Insufficient long-term clinical data on the performance and outcomes of 3D-printed orthopedic implants	[32]
General AM	Regulatory hurdles	Absence of established government regulations for 3D-printed medical devices	[33]
General AM	Cost considerations	High initial investment and production costs, especially for small production runs	[34]
General AM	Quality control	Ensuring consistent product quality and meeting medical standards	[35]
General AM	Limited material range	Restricted selection of biocompatible materials suitable for orthopedic applications	[36]
SLM/EBM	Post-processing requirements	Need for additional treatments to improve surface finish and mechanical properties	[37]
SLM/EBM	Biomechanical considerations	Ensuring proper mechanical strength and fatigue resistance of printed implants	[38]
General AM	Design complexity	Requirement for expert CAD modelers to design patient-specific implants	[39]
General AM	Production volume	Limited capacity for large-scale manufacturing compared to traditional methods	[40]
General AM	Maintenance	Specialized equipment maintenance and calibration requirements	[41]
General AM	Sterilization compatibility	Ensuring 3D-printed implants can withstand standard sterilization processes	[42]
General AM	Material characterization	Need for comprehensive understanding of printed materials' properties in vivo	[43]

major issues regarding the application of AM in orthopedics. The limitations cover the following areas of endeavor: legal and permissions, technology, finance, and therapeutic. Overcoming such challenges becomes paramount to the advancement and development of the AM technologies in orthopedic applications [31].

There remains a growing need to enhance the complexity of the biomaterials to be used to repair human tissues and organs and the bio-inks to be used for tissue printing. Improving accuracy and clarity focusing on challenging biological samples is critical for manufacturing highly detailed tissue and organ models [44]. Therefore, further research, interdisciplinary cooperation, and regulatory changes must be carried out to get to the optimal level of translating this innovative technology in biology and medicine.

3.5 FUTURE PERSPECTIVES

Expected advancements in additive manufacturing of biological structures will therefore aim at overcoming existing constraints and achieving raised functionality. Integration of the next-generation biomimetic designs will therefore seek to enhance structures that somewhat mimic natural biological systems [45]. Combining more than one material and the incorporation of more than one cell kind will make it possible to produce sophisticated tissues and organs in a single print. This means that better approaches to in vivo tracking and localization of soft robots will help improve medical procedures and interventions.

Laser technology integration in manufacturing is found helpful in improvement with AM and coating techniques. Studies that investigate laser machining techniques for composites have been focusing on methods to enhance material removal rates along with cutting quality [46–50]. The AM field has experienced research momentum because of sustainability requirements and shape memory alloy innovations [51–53]. Machine learning applications have started to forecast manufacturing traits and strengthen the mechanical features of three-dimensional printed materials according to studies [54–56]. Laser-based post-processing treatments are helpful in enhancing material performance and surface characteristics [57, 58]. The research examines cladding technologies with microwave and nickel-based superalloy claddings to understand their microstructural and mechanical properties [59, 60]. Studies into thermal spray coatings have gained extensive attention because researchers analyze erosion resistance and apply neural computing systems for wear analysis and optimize processes with AI technologies [61–72].

AM shows great promise in biomedical applications because researchers use it to create bioimplants and surface coatings with improved mechanical properties and enhanced compatibility to human tissue. Research on zirconia-based biomedical materials has accelerated because of their excellent durability and low wear properties thanks to AI optimization efforts [73]. Researchers have extensively investigated protective coatings for magnesium-based bioimplants through conversion coatings and micro-arc oxidation for enhancing their endurance along with resistance to corrosion [74]. Bioimplant surface modifications have become more efficient because of the combined use of biopolymer coatings within AM technology [75]. Researchers have developed next-generation medical implants which offer better self-healing properties and biofunctionality [76–77].

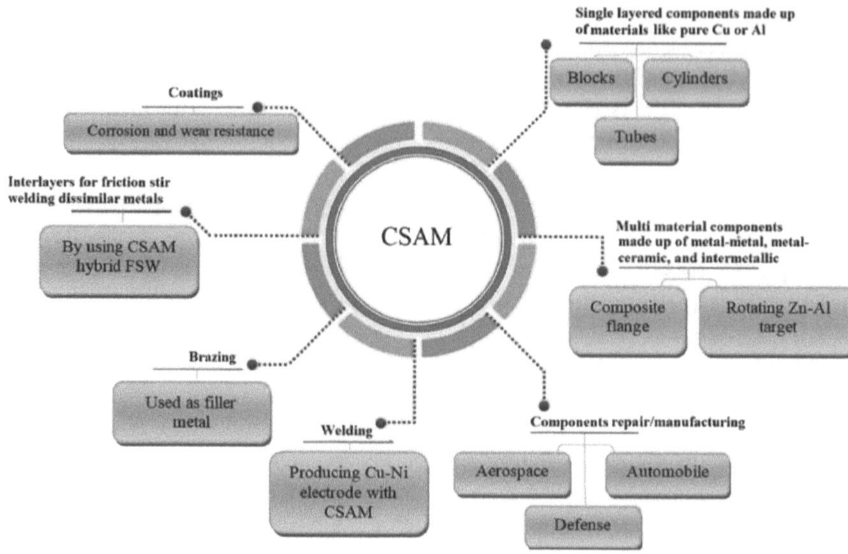

FIGURE 3.7 The major areas of CSAM [78]. (Reproduction permission by Elsevier)

Figure 3.7 shows all the possible uses of cold spray additive manufacturing (CSAM). It also describes CSAM in producing single-layered components, blocks, cylinders, tubes, from copper or aluminum and multi-material; composite flanges, rotating Zn-Al targets. CSAM is also utilized in applications where coatings, corrosion, and wear improvement are needed, in friction stir welding of dissimilar metals and as filler metals in brazing. Also, it assists in making Cu-Ni electrodes and is used in aerospace, defense, automobile industries for parts refurbishment and fabrication [78].

Investigation of further stimuli-responsive structures will advance the development of other biological systems that can adapt to the environment. Tomorrow's engineering knowledge will enhance tissue engineering and development, future medical usage, and state-of-art technology in the production of medical devices [78]. Over time, such technologies can cause revolutionary changes in the field of regenerative medicine, drugs development, and personalized medicine, which will help to enhance the quality of patients' life.

3.6 CONCLUSION

AM is applied in a wide variety of fields ranging from biology, through aerospace and automobile to the fashion industry, because it empowers the production of structure designs with complicated aerodynamic shapes that mimic natural biosystems. This technology has opened up the possibility to create new forms in the fields of tissue engineering, organ mimicry, and biomedical replacements—including implants and prosthetics, as well as living tissue. AM techniques such as vat photopolymerization, laser-based methods, and extrusion-based methods have been used in the fabrication of scaffold, implants, and biomaterials with desired characteristics. AM has also been used in tissue engineering and regenerative medicine to develop bioinspired scaffolds or representative tissue for personalized medicine. It combines with several deep learning methods to enhance the development of biomimetic structural designs of complex natural patterns. Furthermore, AM in tandem with synthetic biology has fabricated engineered living materials (ELMs), which investigate the relationship between additive manufacturing and living organisms. Nevertheless, AM has the following challenges: Need to work on biomaterials, improving the accuracy and tailored adjustments to regulatory barriers. The challenges of present-day AM are predicted to be addressed to adapt enhanced biomimetic designs and fabricate complex tissues and organs in a single print run, which is expected to redefine the fields of regenerative medicine, drug manufacturing, and genomics.

REFERENCES

1. Allaire G, Bogosel B. Optimizing supports for additive manufacturing. *Structural Multidisciplinary Optimization*. 2018;58:2493–515.
2. Altıparmak SC, Yardley VA, Shi Z, Lin J. Challenges in additive manufacturing of high-strength aluminium alloys and current developments in hybrid additive manufacturing. *International Journal of Lightweight Materials Manufacture*. 2021;4:246–61.
3. Ansari P, Salamci MU. On the selective laser melting based additive manufacturing of AlSi10Mg: The process parameter investigation through multiphysics simulation and experimental validation. *Journal of Alloys Compounds*. 2022;890:161873.
4. Buchanan C, Gardner L. Metal 3D printing in construction: A review of methods, research, applications, opportunities and challenges. *Engineering Structures*. 2019;180:332–48.
5. Chen H, Guo L, Zhu W, Li C. Recent advances in multi-material 3D printing of functional ceramic devices. *Polymers*. 2022;14:4635.
6. Dilip J, Miyanaji H, Lassell A, Starr TL, Stucker B. A novel method to fabricate TiAl intermetallic alloy 3D parts using additive manufacturing. *Defence Technology*. 2017;13:72–6.
7. Goh GD, Sing SL, Yeong WY. A review on machine learning in 3D printing: Applications, potential, and challenges. *Artificial Intelligence Review*. 2021;54:63–94.
8. Goyanes A, Fina F, Martorana A, Sedough D, Gaisford S, Basit AW. Development of modified release 3D printed tablets (printlets) with pharmaceutical excipients using additive manufacturing. *International Journal of Pharmaceutics*. 2017;527:21–30.
9. Guttridge C, Shannon A, O'Sullivan A, O'Sullivan KJ, O'Sullivan LW. Biocompatible 3D printing resins for medical applications: A review of marketed intended use, biocompatibility certification, and post-processing guidance. *Annals of 3D Printed Medicine*. 2022;5:100044.
10. Rieger T, Schubert T, Schurr J, Kopp A, Schwenkel M, Sellmer D, Wolff A, Meese-Marktscheffel J, Bernthaler T, Schneider G. Vat photopolymerization of cemented carbide specimen. *Materials*. 2021;14:7631.
11. Han Y, Yang Z, Ding T, Xiao J. Environmental and economic assessment on 3D printed buildings with recycled concrete. *Journal of Cleaner Production*. 2021;278:123884.
12. Cobbinah PV, Nzeukou RA, Onawale OT, Matizamhuka WR. Laser powder bed fusion of potential superalloys: A review. *Metals*. 2020;11:58.
13. Khosravani MR, Reinicke T. On the environmental impacts of 3D printing technology. *Applied Materials Today*. 2020;20:100689.
14. Layani M, Wang X, Magdassi S. Novel materials for 3D printing by photopolymerization. *Advanced Materials*. 2018;30:1706344.

15. Liu S, Lu B, Li H, Pan Z, Jiang J, Qian S. A comparative study on environmental performance of 3D printing and conventional casting of concrete products with industrial wastes. *Chemosphere*. 2022;298:134310.
16. Saade MRM, Yahia A, Amor B. How has LCA been applied to 3D printing? A systematic literature review and recommendations for future studies. *Journal of Cleaner Production*. 2020;244:118803.
17. Sochol R, Sweet E, Glick C, Venkatesh S, Avetisyan A, Ekman K, Raulinaitis A, Tsai A, Wienkers A, Korner K. 3D printed microfluidic circuitry via multijet-based additive manufacturing. *Lab on a Chip*. 2016;16:668–78.
18. Tam K-MM, Mueller CT. Additive manufacturing along principal stress lines. *3D Printing Additive Manufacturing*. 2017;4:63–81.
19. Tinoco MP, de Mendonça ÉM, Fernandez LIC, Caldas LR, Reales OAM, Toledo Filho RD. Life cycle assessment (LCA) and environmental sustainability of cementitious materials for 3D concrete printing: A systematic literature review. *Journal of Building Engineering*. 2022;52:104456.
20. Xing W, Ouyang D, Li N, Liu L. Insight into micro-cracking in 3D-printed Fe-based BMGs by selective laser melting. *Intermetallics*. 2018;103:101–6.
21. Zhang X, Chu D, Zhao X, Gao C, Lu L, He Y, Bai W. Machine learning-driven 3D printing: A review. *Applied Materials Today*. 2024;39:102306.
22. Barragan De Los Rios GA, Ferreira R, Mariani FE, da Silva EJ, Coelho RT. Study of the surface roughness of a remanufactured bimetallic AISI 1045 and 316L SS part obtained by hybrid manufacturing (DED/HSM). *The International Journal of Advanced Manufacturing Technology*. 2023;124:3185–99.
23. Petrovic V, Vicente Haro Gonzalez J, Jordá Ferrando O, Delgado Gordillo J, Ramón Blasco Puchades J, Portolés Griñan L. Additive layered manufacturing: Sectors of industrial application shown through case studies. *International Journal of Production Research*. 2011;49:1061–79.
24. Baumers M, Dickens P, Tuck C, Hague R. The cost of additive manufacturing: Machine productivity, economies of scale and technology-push. *Technological Forecasting Social Change*. 2016;102:193–201.
25. Bayat M, Dong W, Thorborg J, To AC, Hattel JH. A review of multi-scale and multi-physics simulations of metal additive manufacturing processes with focus on modeling strategies. *Additive Manufacturing*. 2021;47:102278.
26. Benoist V, Arnaud L, Baili M. A new method of design for additive manufacturing including machining constraints. *The International Journal of Advanced Manufacturing Technology*. 2020;111:25–36.
27. Bourell D, Kruth JP, Leu M, Levy G, Rosen D, Beese AM, Clare A. Materials for additive manufacturing. *CIRP Annals*. 2017;66:659–81.
28. Singh G, Mehta A, Vasudev HJPiAM. Sustainability of additive manufacturing: A comprehensive review. *Progress in Additive Manufacturing*. 2024:1–24.
29. Bremen S, Meiners W, Diatlov A. Selective laser melting: A manufacturing technology for the future? *Laser Technik Journal*. 2012;9:33–8.
30. Chen C, Xie Y, Yin S, Li W, Luo X, Xie X, Zhao R, Deng C, Wang J, Liao H. Ductile and high strength Cu fabricated by solid-state cold spray additive manufacturing. *Journal of Materials Science Technology*. 2023;134:234–43.
31. Cheng B, Chou K. Melt pool evolution study in selective laser melting. In *26th Annual International Solid Freeform Fabrication Symposium – An Additive Manufacturing Conference*. Austin, TX; 2015.
32. Levesque JN, Shah A, Ekhtiari S, Yan JR, Thornley P, Williams DS. Three-dimensional printing in orthopaedic surgery: A scoping review. *EFORT Open Reviews*. 2020;5:430–41.

33. Pathak K, Saikia R, Das A, Das D, Islam MA, Pramanik P, Parasar A, Borthakur PP, Sarmah P, Saikia M. 3D printing in biomedicine: Advancing personalized care through additive manufacturing. *Exploration of Medicine.* 2023;4:1135–67.
34. Srivastava AK, Kumar A, Kumar P, Gautam P, Dogra N. Research progress in metal additive manufacturing: Challenges and opportunities. *International Journal on Interactive Design Manufacturing.* 2023:1–17.
35. Wazeer A, Das A, Sinha A, Inaba K, Ziyi S, Karmakar A. Additive manufacturing in biomedical field: A critical review on fabrication method, materials used, applications, challenges, and future prospects. *Progress in Additive Manufacturing.* 2023;8:857–89.
36. Sing SL, An J, Yeong WY, Wiria FE. Laser and electron-beam powder-bed additive manufacturing of metallic implants: A review on processes, materials and designs. *Journal of Orthopaedic Research.* 2016;34:369–85.
37. Mohanty S, Gokuldoss Prashanth K. Metallic coatings through additive manufacturing: A review. *Materials.* 2023;16:2325.
38. Monzón M, Ortega Z, Martínez A, Ortega F. Standardization in additive manufacturing: Activities carried out by international organizations and projects. *The International Journal of Advanced Manufacturing Technology.* 2015;76:1111–21.
39. Murmura F, Bravi L. Additive manufacturing in the wood-furniture sector: Sustainability of the technology, benefits and limitations of adoption. *Journal of Manufacturing Technology Management.* 2018;29:350–71.
40. Nguyen HD, Pramanik A, Basak A, Dong Y, Prakash C, Debnath S, Shankar S, Jawahir I, Dixit S, Buddhi DJJoMR. Technology. A critical review on additive manufacturing of Ti-6Al-4V alloy: Microstructure and mechanical properties. *Journal of Materials Research Technology.* 2022;18:4641–61.
41. Ullah F, Othman MBH, Javed F, Ahmad Z, Akil HM. Classification, processing and application of hydrogels: A review. *Materials Science Engineering: C.* 2015;57:414–33.
42. Virgin L. Enhancing the teaching of linear structural analysis using additive manufacturing. *Engineering Structures.* 2017;150:135–42.
43. White BC, Garland A, Alberdi R, Boyce BL. Interpenetrating lattices with enhanced mechanical functionality. *Additive Manufacturing.* 2021;38:101741.
44. Wu H, Liu S, Zhang Y, Liao H, Raoelison R-N, Deng S. New process implementation to enhance cold spray-based additive manufacturing. *Journal of Thermal Spray Technology.* 2021;30:1284–93.
45. Xu X, Luo D, Guo C, Rong Q. A custom-made temporomandibular joint prosthesis for fabrication by selective laser melting: Finite element analysis. *Medical Engineering Physics.* 2017;46:1–11.
46. Sharma V, Kumar V. Application of Box-Behnken design and response surface methodology for multi-optimization of laser cutting of AA5052/ZrO2 metal–matrix composites. *Proceedings of the Institution of Mechanical Engineers, Part L: Journal of Materials: Design and Applications.* 2018;232(8):652–68.
47. Sharma V, Kumar V. Comparison of machining characteristics of metal matrix composites using CO2 laser curve cutting process. *Proceedings of the Institution of Mechanical Engineers, Part E: Journal of Process Mechanical Engineering.* 2018;232(3):349–68.
48. Sharma V, Kumar V. Investigating the quality characteristics of Al5052/SiC metal matrix composites machined by CO2 laser curve cutting. *Proceedings of the Institution of Mechanical Engineers, Part L: Journal of Materials: Design and Applications.* 2018;232(1):3–19.
49. Sharma V, Kumar V, Bist A. Investigations on morphology and material removal rate of various MMCs using CO2 laser technique. *Journal of the Brazilian Society of Mechanical Sciences and Engineering.* 2020;42:1–14.

50. Sharma V, Singh JP, Raman R, Bathla G, Saini A. Machine learning approach for prediction analysis of aluminium alloy on the surface roughness using CO2 laser machining. *Proceedings of the Institution of Mechanical Engineers, Part E: Journal of Process Mechanical Engineering*. 2024;09544089241231093.
51. Singh R, Toseef M, Kumar J, Singh J. Benefits and challenges in additive manufacturing and its applications. In: Kaushal S, Singh I, Singh S, Gupta A, editors. *Sustainable Advanced Manufacturing and Materials Processing*. 1st ed. Boca Raton: CRC Press; 2022. pp. 137–57. https://doi.org/10.1201/9781003269298-8.
52. Singh J. Sustainability issues in laser-based additive manufacturing. In: *Handbook of Laser-Based Sustainable Surface Modification and Manufacturing Techniques*. CRC Press; 2023. pp. 167–89.
53. Ahmad S, et al. Innovations in additive manufacturing of shape memory alloys: Alloys, microstructures, treatments, applications. *Journal of Materials Research and Technology*. 2024;32:4136–97.
54. Sharma V, Singh JP, Hussan K, Kumar R. Machine learning approach for predicting the machining characteristics of additive manufactured ABS material. *Proceedings of the Institution of Mechanical Engineers, Part C: Journal of Mechanical Engineering Science*. 2024;09544062241283330.
55. Chohan JS, et al. Mechanical strength enhancement of 3D printed acrylonitrile butadiene styrene polymer components using neural network optimization algorithm. *Polymers*. 2020;12(10). https://doi.org/10.3390/polym12102250.
56. Singh J, et al. Impact of molding temperature, fiber loading and chemical modifications on the physicomechanical, and microstructural morphology properties of woven kenaf Fiber/PLA composites for non-structural applications. *Journal of Natural Fibers*. 2024;21(1):2326586.
57. Singh J. Applications of laser technology for processing and post-treatments of powders and coatings. In: *Handbook of Laser-Based Sustainable Surface Modification and Manufacturing Techniques*. CRC Press; 2023. pp. 135–66.
58. Sunitha K, Vasudev H. A short note on the various thermal spray coating processes and effect of post-treatment on Ni-based coatings. *Materials Today: Proceedings*. 2022;50:1452–7. https://doi.org/10.1016/j.matpr.2021.09.017.
59. Sharanabasava H, et al. Microstructure, mechanical and wear properties of SiC and Mo reinforced NiCr microwave cladding. *Advanced Materials and Processing Technologies*. 2024;10:3620–33.
60. Singh J, Gill HS. Evolution of nickel-based superalloy claddings for against high-temperature oxidation and wear. In: *Thermal Claddings for Engineering Applications*. CRC Press; 2024. pp. 160–81.
61. Singh J, Kumar S, Kumar R, Mohapatra SK. Machine learning regression tools for erosion prediction of WC-10Co4Cr thermal spray coating. *Results Surfaces Interfaces*. 2023;13:100156. https://doi.org/10.1016/j.rsurfi.2023.100156.
62. Yedida VVS, Vasudev H. A review on the development of thermal barrier coatings by using thermal spray techniques. *Materials Today: Proceedings*. 2022;50:1458–64.
63. Singh J, Singh S. Support vector machine learning on slurry erosion characteristics analysis of Ni- and Co-alloy coatings. *Surface Review and Letters*. 2023. https://doi.org/10.1142/S0218625X23400061.
64. Prashar G, Vasudev H. A review on the influence of process parameters and heat treatment on the corrosion performance of Ni-based thermal spray coatings. *Surface Review and Letters*. 2022;29(1):2230001.
65. Singh J, Vasudev H, Szala M, Gill HS. Neural computing for erosion assessment in Al-20TiO2 HVOF thermal spray coating. *International Journal on Interactive Design and Manufacturing*. 2024;18:2321–32.

66. Singh J, Vasudev H, Kumar R, Ubaidullah M. Study on wear analysis of Ni-20Al2O3 HVOF micron layers using artificial neural network technique. *The International Journal on Interactive Design and Manufacturing.* 2023;18:5925–38. https://doi.org/10.1007/s12008-023-01433-2.
67. Prashar G, Vasudev H. Surface topology analysis of plasma sprayed Inconel625-Al2O3 composite coating. *Materials Today: Proceedings.* 2022;50:607–11. https://doi.org/10.1016/j.matpr.2021.03.090.
68. Thakur L, Vasudev H, Singh J, Prashar G. *Artificial Intelligence and Machine Learning in the Thermal Spray Industry: Practices, Implementation, and Challenges.* CRC Press; 2023.
69. Dutta V, Thakur L, Singh B, Vasudev H. A study of erosion–corrosion behaviour of friction stir-processed chromium-reinforced NiAl bronze composite. *Materials (Basel).* 2022;15(15):5401. https://doi.org/10.3390/ma15155401.
70. Singh J, Singh S, Vasudev H, Chohan JS, Kumar S. Neural computing and Taguchi's method-based study on erosion of advanced Mo2C–WC10Co4Cr coating for the centrifugal pump. *Advances in Materials and Processing Technologies.* 2024;10(3):2569–81.
71. Singh J, Singh S, Vasudev H, Katiyar JK. Artificial neural network model for wear characteristic analysis of WC-10Co4Cr and Stellite 6 thermal spray coatings. *Tribology International.* 2024;199:109924.
72. Majji BGR, Vasudev H, Bansal A. A review on the oxidation and wear behavior of the thermally sprayed high-entropy alloys. *Materials Today: Proceedings.* 2022;50:1447–51.
73. Singh J, Singh S, Verma A. Artificial intelligence in use of ZrO2 material in biomedical science. *Journal of Electrochemical Science and Engineering.* 2022;13(1):83–97. https://doi.org/10.5599/jese.1498.
74. Singh J, Hashmi AW, Behra A, Kumar A, Dogra N, Kumar P. Review of Mg alloys for bio-implants protected by the deposition of chemical conversion coatings. In *AIP Conference Proceedings.* AIP Publishing; 2024.
75. Singh J, Singh S, Gill R. Applications of biopolymer coatings in biomedical engineering. *Journal of Electrochemical Science and Engineering.* 2022;13(1):63–81. https://doi.org/10.5599/jese.1460.
76. Singh CJ, Ram B, Singh J, Prakash C, Paramasivam P, Kumar R. Experimental investigation on characterization of friction stir processed AZ31-based composite. *Scientific Reports.* 2024;14(1):15453.
77. Prashar G, Vasudev H. A comprehensive review on sustainable cold spray additive manufacturing: State of the art, challenges and future challenges. *Journal of Cleaner Production.* 2021;310:127606.
78. Assadi H, Kreye H, Gärtner F, Klassen T. Cold spraying–A materials perspective. *Acta Materialia.* 2016;116:382–407.

4 Advanced Additive Manufacturing Techniques for Sustainable Remanufacturing

Praveen Kumar Verma, Hitesh Vasudev, and N. Jeyaprakash

CONTENTS

4.1 INTRODUCTION

Sustainable remanufacturing is rapidly becoming a keystone for circular economy models; so it offers an ideal route for minimizing waste, preserving resources, and lengthening the life of products while being efficient. Traditional manufacturing usually involves extraction and thereby produces enormous waste; rather, remanufacturing focuses on refurbishing end-of-life products into like-new or even upgraded

 DOI: 10.1201/9781003516064-4

states. This approach reduces the environmental impact and supports the economics of sustainability by reducing procurement costs and disposal costs of materials. In this light, remanufacturing has emerged as a strategic approach toward increasing global demand for resource efficiency and environmental stewardship [1].

Additive manufacturing (AM), which is simply known as 3D printing, has dramatically altered the field of remanufacturing. Flexibility, precision, and customized items are what distinguish AM from subtractive processes; it constructs its parts layer by layer, unlike any other process, making near-net-shape production very efficient in material use for repairing and refurbishing complex components. In this case, AM becomes ideal for applications such as in aerospace, automotive, and healthcare, where the high-value parts require much more attention to detail. One of the key features associated with AM in remanufacturing is its flexibility in accommodating a wide range of materials, such as metals, polymers, and composites. This enables various components with different mechanical, thermal, and chemical properties to be restored. Moreover, technologies such as directed energy deposition (DED) and powder bed fusion (PBF) in AM enable manufacturers to accurately control material deposition. That way, they can repair the worn or damaged area of a component without impairing the integrity of the original component. Such technologies are of particular importance to those industries where the performance and reliability of components are a matter of critical concern: repairing turbine blades in the aerospace industry or repairing parts of an engine in the automotive industry. Beyond its technical capabilities, AM aligns closely with the principles of sustainability. Reducing material wastage, allowing for the use of recycled or bio-based materials, and minimizing the need for extensive tooling all contribute to lower environmental footprints. For instance, remanufacturing components using AM techniques can significantly reduce greenhouse gas emissions compared to manufacturing new parts from raw materials. Further, the localized nature of AM manufacturing allows on-demand manufacturing by having low transportation costs and correlated emissions [2]. Additive manufacturing workflow is shown in **Figure 4.1**.

This chapter explores AM's transformative role in the sustainable remanufacturing process by exploring technological, economic, and ecological aspects. Following

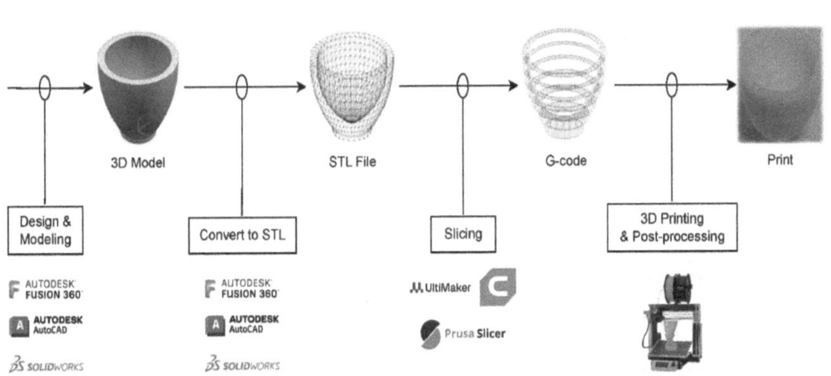

FIGURE 4.1 The overall workflow of the additive manufacturing process [3]. (CC By 4.0 Attribution)

an overview of the basics of AM technology in remanufacturing processes and their technical capabilities, limitations, and ranges of application across the different manufacturing industries, this chapter discusses various material considerations important for conducting sustainable remanufacturing work, including innovation in recyclable and biodegradable feedstocks. LCA, or life cycle analysis, measures the environmental impact of remanufactured components against newly manufactured ones and thus provides a further ecological evaluation of the benefits of AM in remanufacturing. The results of such analysis reveal significant energy consumption and resource usage reductions that are critical for the achievement of global sustainability goals [4, 5].

However, there are also several challenges in integrating AM into remanufacturing. Some of these challenges include high energy consumption in some AM processes, material compatibility with existing components, and the economic feasibility of large-scale implementation. In addition, regulatory and quality assurance standards are significant barriers to the wide-scale adoption of AM in remanufacturing, especially in safety-critical industries. Emerging trends in AM, like applying digital twins, AI-enabled process optimization, and hybrid manufacturing systems, will continue to be discussed for how the efficiency and sustainability of the process can be improved in terms of remanufacturing. These innovations are the future, and they will help push this technology forward to better circumvent current limitations and find potential new applications in sustainable remanufacturing [6–8].

4.2 ADDITIVE MANUFACTURING IN REMANUFACTURING

With its ability to restore components with exactness, less material wasting, and design flexibility, AM has become an up-and-coming remanufacturing technology. Because different AM techniques can support various needs of remanufacturing in different industries by providing different advantages according to the type of component to be repaired, the extent of repair, and the material used, they can be applied accordingly. This section explores the most popular AM techniques utilized in remanufacturing, including powder bed fusion (PBF), directed energy deposition (DED), material extrusion (ME), and binder jetting [9].

4.2.1 Powder Bed Fusion (PBF)

PBF is a class of AM processes where thermal energy, such as that provided by a laser or electron beam, is selectively melted and fused layer by layer onto material powders. This makes it particularly suitable for repairing parts of intricate designs and complex geometries, including turbine blades, medical implants, and microelectronics of very high resolution and precision. In remanufacturing, PBF has superiority in restoring fine details in parts that require very high tolerances. For instance, an aerospace company using a turbine blade may experience localized wear or damage under their operational temperatures and stresses. PBF can selectively repair those areas and restore the intact integrity and performance of the original part. Similarly, in the biomedical industry, PBF is used to restore or tailor implants and prostheses so as to achieve individual patient-based solutions [10].

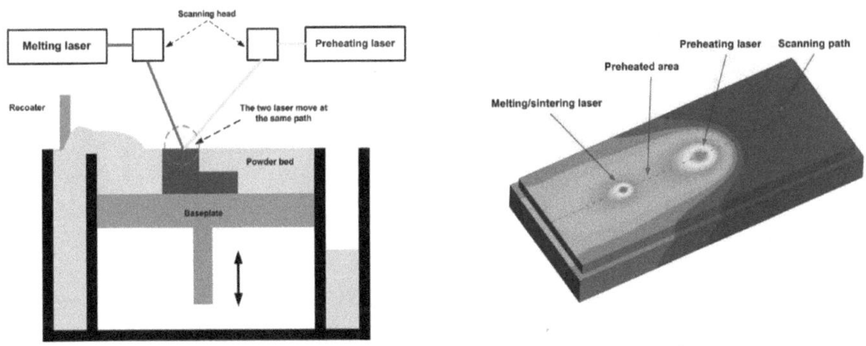

(a) (b)

FIGURE 4.2 The preheating system developed in this study; (**a**) schematic diagram for the system, (**b**) simulation of the two lasers moving at the same scanning path. [11] (CC By 4.0 Attribution)

A key advantage of PBF in remanufacturing is its material efficiency. The process permits recycling of unused powders and minimizes the wastage of materials. This attribute is particularly useful in working with high-cost materials such as titanium alloys and cobalt-chrome alloys. **Figure 4.2** shows the setup diagram of PBF.

Additionally, PBF's ability to process a wide range of materials, including metals, ceramics, and polymers, makes it versatile for many applications. Despite its advantages, PBF has challenges in remanufacturing. The process is energy-intensive and requires stringent control of environmental conditions, such as inert atmospheres, to prevent oxidation and contamination. Moreover, the layer-by-layer approach can result in residual stresses, which may compromise the mechanical properties of the repaired component if not properly managed. Advances in post-processing techniques, such as heat treatment and surface finishing, are critical to addressing these issues [12, 13].

4.2.2 Directed Energy Deposition (DED)

DED is an open-ended AM technique that utilizes a focused energy source like a laser, electron beam, or plasma arc to deposit material onto a substrate. The technique best applies large-scale repair processes, which are mainly observed in industries related to aerospace, heavy machinery, and energy as their parts are often large in size and extremely eroded in nature due to the nature of their operations. The direct advantages of DED include the ability to repair or rebuild worn or damaged parts directly onto an existing substrate. For example, in the aerospace industry, DED is applied to refurbish critical components, such as engine casings and landing gear, which are exposed to high mechanical stresses. It enables manufacturers to restore these components to their initial specifications, thereby maximizing their operational life and reducing the demand for replacement parts. DED is specifically beneficial when dealing with expensive materials because it minimizes material loss by depositing material only at the point of need. It can be used with multiple

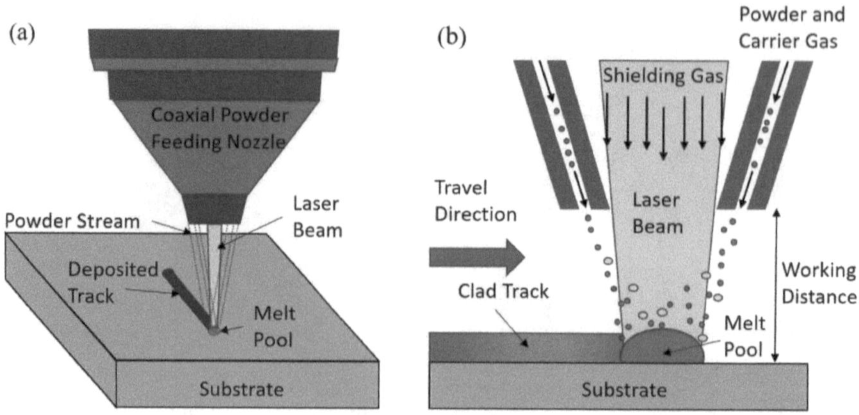

FIGURE 4.3 Principle of directed energy deposition with powder as the feedstock material: (**a**) overview, and (**b**) detail. [15] (CC By 4.0 Attribution)

materials, such as metals, ceramics, and composites, making it versatile for different applications. Moreover, DED enables in situ repair of components, which means that entire disassembly is not required and, therefore, reduces time and cost [14]. **Figure 4.3** shows the principle of directed energy deposition with powder as the feedstock material.

However, DED also poses certain limitations. The process demands strict control over the heat input to avoid warping or residual stresses in the repaired part. Additionally, parts manufactured by DED are characterized by a rough surface finish that requires post-processing such as machining or polishing. Improvements in hybrid manufacturing systems that integrate DED with subtractive techniques can overcome these limitations by offering smoother and more accurate repairs. This has helped ensure that sustainable DED benefits by utilizing reused costly parts while preventing a great percentage of its detrimental effects on the environment when fresh components are made. Advances in DED hardware, monitoring, and materials that this industry employs are set to propel remanufacturing forward on this road toward sustainable use in industries [16, 17].

4.2.3 Material Extrusion (ME)

Material extrusion (ME) is the most common and lowest-cost AM technique associated with fused deposition modeling (FDM). In this technique, a thermoplastic material is extruded through a heated nozzle and deposited on top of another layer to form a three-dimensional component. Although often perceived as the most elementary compared to other AM methods, the versatility and low cost of ME make it particularly useful for some remanufacturing applications [18].

In remanufacturing, ME is mainly used to produce replacement parts for repair, plastic component repair, or jigs and fixtures needed for other repair processes. For instance, in automotive, ME can be employed to repair or replace dashboards, panels, or housings. The method is also used in the consumer electronics industry to rehabilitate casings and other plastic parts. The affordability and ease of ME systems have made them available to SMEs and even single users. Moreover, ME accommodates a broad spectrum of materials, including biodegradable polymers like polylactic acid (PLA) and thermoplastics with carbon or glass fibers, which provide additional mechanical strength. These can be applied in ways that allow the remanufacturing solutions tailored to specific requirements and cost-effectively. Still, ME has limitations. Mainly, it is limited to only thermoplastic materials which means repair to metal or ceramic components could be impossible with this process. The resolution achievable with the layer of ME is also not high enough for PBF or DED technique, and it might jeopardize the dimensional accuracy of repaired parts. However, ME has an important place in sustainable remanufacturing because it reutilizes materials that already exist while minimizing waste. Innovations include multi-material extrusion, nozzle designs, and advanced slicing algorithms for ME systems that further increase the capability of such ME systems and make them more readily applicable to a wider range of remanufacturing processes [19–21].

4.2.4 Binder Jetting

Binder jetting is an AM process in which a liquid binding agent is used to selectively join powder particles layer by layer to form a solid structure. Unlike processes that rely on heat or lasers, binder jetting operates at ambient temperatures, thus offering unique benefits for a remanufacturing application. It is one of the most suited, especially for producing replacement parts and restoring components in terms of industries such as those in the automotive, aerospace, and consumer goods spaces. Binder jetting has very good applications in remanufacturing, where parts contain intricate geometries that traditional methods would be expensive and difficult to produce. With this technique, complicated lattice structures or internal channels can be very efficiently reproduced as they would be found in heat exchangers and fluid control systems. Binder jetting also enables the creation of lightweight parts through optimized designs, which will enhance energy efficiency in applications like aerospace [22, 23].

A significant advantage of binder jetting is its ability to process vast material spectra, including metals, ceramics, and even sand. This is important for remanufacturing since the material of the replacement parts often requires the same composition as the original components. Binder jetting also allows for multiple-material printing, where combining different properties within a part can be achieved, allowing strength to be combined with thermal conductivity. Binder jetting is thus aligned with sustainability goals by minimizing material wastage. In the process, only binder and powder used in making the final part are consumed, and unused powder is often recyclable. Moreover, since it does not require high temperatures, it consumes less energy than any other AM technique such as PBF or DED. Another ecological benefit is that it is compatible with sustainable materials, such as bio-based binders and recycled powders. This would open opportunities for industries looking to integrate remanufacturing with green manufacturing practices. Moreover, near-net-shape parts production reduces the need for post-processing, which saves even more energy and resources [24, 25].

4.3 MATERIALS IN ADDITIVE REMANUFACTURING

Materials are at the heart of additive remanufacturing success, and it is their functionality, sustainability, and economic viability that determine the success of the process. Choosing the right material ensures compatibility with the original component and has a bearing on the environmental impact of remanufacturing [26].

4.3.1 Metal Powders (Titanium, Nickel Alloys)

The additive remanufacturing process includes PBF and DED. The process mainly relies on the precision of metal powders for critical component restoration through high precision and mechanical integrity. Of these, titanium and nickel alloys are the most outstanding ones [27].

These include titanium powders that have a high strength, are light in weight, and are known for excellent corrosion resistance. Thus, the use of such powders is quite popular in aerospace and biomedical remanufacturing applications. It is an excellent choice for repairing turbine blades and biomedical implants. It's used to extend the life cycle of medical devices, such as hip and knee replacements, due to its biocompatibility. Nickel alloys, however, have an excellent performance in high-temperature applications because of their high thermal stability and oxidation resistance. They are primarily applied to the rejuvenation of parts in the energy and aerospace industries, which includes casings of engines and heat exchangers. These benefits notwithstanding, there still are issues such as the expensive nature of high-purity powders and contamination in processing. Innovations in powder recycling as well as innovative atomization methods have reduced the burden of the issues that previously plagued this product, hence making the product more viable and more economical for remanufacturing [28, 29].

4.3.2 Biodegradable Polymers (PLA, PHA)

The most recent biodegradable polymers to be used in additive remanufacturing are polylactic acid (PLA) and polyhydroxyalkanoates (PHA) due to their eco-friendly properties. These materials are best suited for repairing or replacing parts in industries where lightweight, low-cost, and sustainable solutions are the norm, such as consumer goods and packaging. Among the most used biodegradable polymers, PLA is sourced from renewable resources such as corn starch. Such processing and compatibility with material extrusion (ME) techniques make it very suitable for producing low-stress replacement parts, such as housings, fixtures, and prototypes. Additionally, PLA's composability aligns with sustainability goals, reducing the environmental impact of discarded materials. PHA exhibits superior mechanical properties than PLA, with increased toughness and flexibility, thus suitable for harsher applications. It is also produced from bacterial fermentation, which aligns with the goal of waste-to-resource by converting organic waste into feedstock [30]. **Figure 4.4** shows the biodegradable polymers and their applications.

Although biodegradable polymers are environmentally advantageous, they suffer from lower durability and thermal resistance than other polymers, making them

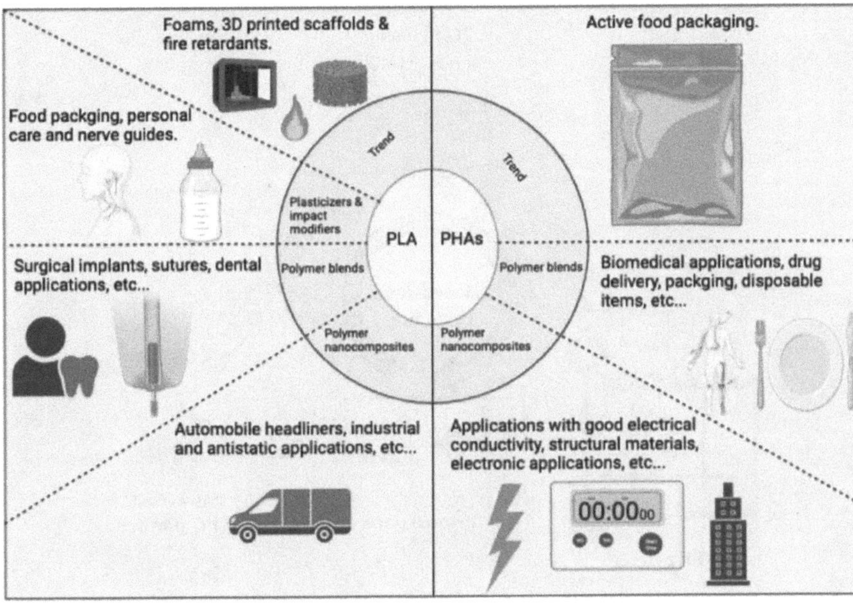

FIGURE 4.4 Biodegradable polymers and their applications [31]. (CC By 4.0 Attribution)

unsuitable for high-performance applications. Increasingly, research into polymer blends and reinforcements is expanding their applicability to open remanufacturing to their use [32].

4.3.3 Composite Materials Tailored for Enhanced Mechanical Properties

The most common use of additive remanufacturing in modern times is composite materials that involve two or more distinct phases, which can provide enhanced mechanical, thermal, and chemical properties. Composite materials are specifically designed for performance requirements and thus are used to repair high-stress components across industries. Fiber-reinforced composites, which include carbon fiber or glass fiber in a polymer matrix, are widely used to repair lightweight yet strong components in the automotive and aerospace sectors. Such composites offer superior strength-to-weight ratios, thus allowing for the restoration of structural parts without adding much mass.

Metal matrix composites (MMCs) are another new class of materials that is gaining ground. For instance, an aluminum composite with silicon carbide as the reinforcing element is used for the remanufacturing of engine parts, which improves wear resistance and thermal stability. The major problem with composites is the complexity of processing, which may cause defects like delamination because of the difference in thermal and mechanical properties between phases. Innovations in AM techniques, such as multi-material printing and optimized deposition strategies, are overcoming these problems and enabling the production of defect-free composite repairs [33].

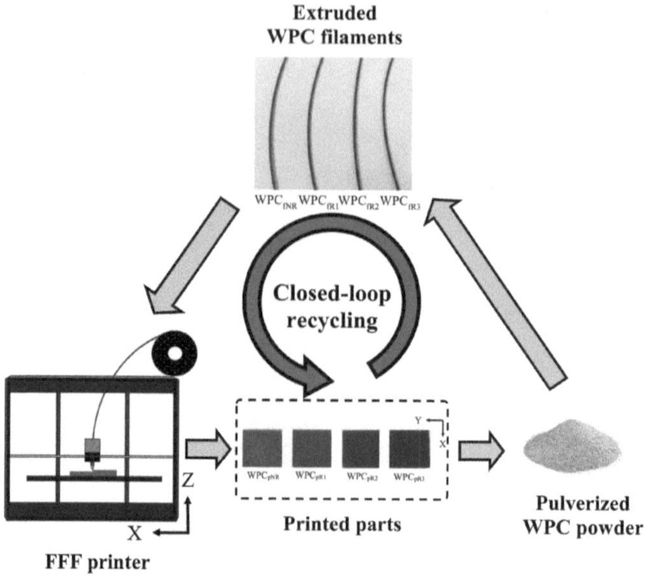

FIGURE 4.5 Closed-loop recycling [35]. (CC By 4.0 Attribution)

4.3.4 Material Recovery and Reuse

Material recovery and reuse are important to reduce the carbon footprint of additive remanufacturing. Advances in material processing have allowed the recycling of powders, supports, and excess materials to make remanufacturing more sustainable and cost-effective. In metal-based AM processes, unused powders can be sieved, cleaned, and reused in subsequent builds. Improvements in powder recycling techniques, including plasma spheroidization, restore the morphology and flowability of used powders, allowing them to be reused without compromising quality [34]. **Figure 4.5** shows the closed-loop recycling system.

Polymers used in ME processes can also be recycled through grinding and re-extrusion. Closed-loop systems are emerging, where waste material from one build is reprocessed into feedstock for another, minimizing waste generation. The development of such green binders and recyclable support materials further enhances sustainability because these innovations not only cost less in terms of the material but also reduce the energy consumed while using raw materials when extracted and processed [36].

4.4 ENVIRONMENTAL IMPACT OF AM IN REMANUFACTURING

AM offers great potential for improving the sustainability of remanufacturing through reduced material waste, enabling the reuse of high-value components, and minimizing environmental impacts. However, its implementation does come with environmental trade-offs, especially regarding energy consumption and overall resource efficiency. This section explores the environmental impact of AM in remanufacturing by focusing on energy efficiency, waste reduction, and LCA [37].

4.4.1 Energy Efficiency

Though the AM process is material-efficient, it is energy-consuming. Energy-intensive techniques, such as PBF and DED, in which lasers or electron beams are used, involve extremely high temperatures in the process of melting and fusing materials. Unless proper control over energy consumption is maintained, this can undermine the potential environmental advantages associated with minimizing the amount of waste material involved. In the context of remanufacturing, energy efficiency is especially relevant for large-scale repairs or restoration of high-value components. For example, while DED saves resources through targeted repairs, extended periods of operation of high-energy equipment can increase the carbon footprint of the process. Binder jetting, though operated at ambient temperatures, also requires sintering or infiltration post-processing, thus adding to energy consumption [38].

Improving energy efficiency in AM is achieved through process parameters optimization, such as the power of the laser or scan speed, and implementation of hybrid manufacturing systems using a combination of AM and energy-efficient subtractive technologies. Another approach is the development of low-energy AM systems, such as ultrasonic or cold spray technologies, to address these challenges. Despite these advancements, achieving an equilibrium between material efficiency and consumption of energy is still widely researched. Another promising potential pathway toward the reduction in environmental impact through further integration into renewable energy systems is from powering AM systems with either solar or wind energy sources [39].

4.4.2 Waste Reduction

One of the most important environmental benefits of AM in remanufacturing is zero waste. AM techniques can inherently enable near-net shape manufacturing, where material gets deposited only where it's needed, thereby reducing waste generation. This is important when working with high-cost materials like titanium or nickel alloys typically used in aerospace and biomedical remanufacturing. For instance, in traditional subtractive manufacturing, up to 70% of the original material can be lost as waste during machining. In contrast, AM processes such as PBF or ME can achieve material utilization rates exceeding 90%, significantly reducing scrap. Unused powders from metal-based AM processes can often be sieved and reused, further enhancing material efficiency [40, 41].

In addition to material savings, AM allows for the repair of parts that would otherwise be scrapped. For example, worn turbine blades or damaged engine casings can be restored to their original specifications using AM techniques, thereby extending their lifespan and reducing the demand for new raw materials. AM reduces material waste to a significant degree but is not waste-free. Waste generation from support structures created during printing and other post-processing activities such as cleaning and finishing also contribute to this. Topology optimization and support-free printing techniques in AM design help reduce auxiliary material usage to a considerable extent [42].

4.4.3 Life Cycle Analysis (LCA)

Life cycle analysis or LCA constitutes an important tool for understanding AM's environmental impact in the remanufacturing process. LCA counts energy intake, material yield, and emission at the most comprehensive phase of the item's whole life cycle—raw material extractions until post-processing into end-of-product processing. Studies have demonstrated that AM can reduce the environmental impact of remanufacturing in certain contexts. For example, the capability to repair or restore high-value components instead of manufacturing new ones reduces the demand for raw materials and related mining activities. Moreover, the localized nature of AM processes can lower transportation emissions by enabling on-site or regional remanufacturing [43].

However, LCA also reveals the environmental trade-offs associated with AM, such as the energy-intensive nature of certain processes. For instance, though PBF provides high precision and material efficiency, its energy consumption during the build phase and post-processing can increase its overall carbon footprint. LCA tools continue evolving to include factors related to the recycling of powders, renewable energy, and improving material recovery. Such a feature can dramatically change the environmental impact of AM processes. For instance, closed-loop material systems and practices such as green manufacturing alleviate the energy and emission prices of AM [44].

4.5 CHALLENGES AND LIMITATIONS

Additive manufacturing has revolutionized remanufacturing, offering unprecedented possibilities for extending the life cycle of products and minimizing waste. However, a series of technical, economic, and regulatory challenges have hindered its widespread adoption, and these need to be overcome to fully realize its potential. One significant technical barrier is managing residual stresses and ensuring material compatibility in repaired components. Residual stresses, usually introduced in AM processes involving fast cooling and solidification of the deposited material, can negatively affect the mechanical integrity of repaired parts. Such stresses cause warping, cracking, and fatigue failure over time and are significant in high-performance applications, such as in aerospace and biomedical implants. Material compatibility between the substrate and the AM-deposited material is also critical, but this is challenging. These could include mismatches at interfaces due to differences in the thermal expansion coefficients, chemical composition, or microstructural properties, leading to weak interfaces or phase mismatches in remanufactured components. Such problems are increasingly being addressed with advanced techniques, such as preheating, in-situ monitoring, and post-processing treatments, but add complexity and cost to the process [45, 46].

Economic viability is one of the main barriers to the adoption of AM for remanufacturing purposes. The initial investment of AM equipment, for instance, laser-based systems or high-precision deposition setups, is quite high. It can also be very expensive when specialized materials, powder preparation, and maintenance are added into the equation, which deters small and medium enterprises. Although AM provides significant savings in the long term, it reduces waste and provides local production, the higher the upfront costs, the lesser the likelihood of companies integrating the process into their operations. AM scalability is still low compared to other conventional manufacturing methods, which limits the economic viability of AM in terms of mass production. Further key enablers include reducing the costs of equipment, improving the efficiency of the process, and formulating cost-effective materials that are needed to make AM accessible and economically viable. Moreover, regulatory and quality standards also pose a critical challenge. Unlike traditional manufacturing, where well-established standards guide material properties and performance metrics, AM lacks universal guidelines for the certification of remanufactured parts. This gap creates uncertainty for industries operating in highly regulated sectors such as aerospace, healthcare, and defense, where safety and reliability are paramount. For example, remanufactured parts should be subjected to extremely rigorous standards of dimensional accuracy, mechanical strength, and fatigue resistance, while a lack of standardized testing and certification protocols complicates the approval and market acceptance. Variability inherent in the AM processes, influenced by factors such as machine settings, material properties, and environmental conditions, further complicates quality assurance. This challenge will necessitate cooperation among industry stakeholders, standardization bodies, and regulatory agencies in developing comprehensive guidelines and certification frameworks tailored to AM in remanufacturing [47, 48].

However, despite these limitations, the prospects of technological improvement and policy action are expected to continue in opening doors toward overcoming the hurdles. Innovation into new techniques of AM by cold spray and hybrid manufacturing reduces the residual stresses and improves material compatibility, overcoming the technical limitations of AM. Efforts at affordable systems and recycled materials of AM have been improving on the economic feasibility. On the regulatory side, organizations such as ASTM International and ISO are striving for the development of standards for AM processes and materials that would facilitate more widespread implementation [49].

4.6 FUTURE PROSPECTS

Prospects for sustainable manufacturing technologies in additive manufacturing are encouraging and promising. This is all because of a combination of policy intervention, technological advancements, and global impact. The governments in the various countries are becoming more conscious of the need to promote friendly, environment-friendly manufacturing processes. It is policy interventions that take on this role by offering grants, tax incentives, and more regulatory support. These policies spur companies to invest in greener technologies, thus pushing the process of shifting to greener manufacturing practices even more rapidly. These policies encourage environmental sustainability but also raise industry competitiveness due to lower costs and higher efficiency [50].

Besides policy support, another great opportunity for the implementation of AI and ML into AM is in optimizing the manufacturing process. AI and ML can analyze vast amounts of data to identify patterns and trends that human operators might overlook. This data-driven approach enables manufacturers to fine-tune their processes for better resource utilization and less material waste and energy consumption. For example, algorithms of AI can predict maintenance needs of equipment to avoid downtime and extend the service life of machinery. In its turn, ML models will optimize all production parameters to have products of quality standards with absolutely minimum usage of raw material inputs, thus improving sustainability and saving operational costs on AM techniques. The adoption of sustainable technologies in AM could help ameliorate urgent environmental crises, especially in developing areas. One of the major problems these regions face is the management of electronic waste or e-waste. E-waste contains hazardous materials that could harm the environment and human health if not managed appropriately. However, it also contains valuable materials that can be recovered and reused. Sustainable AM technologies provide innovative solutions for recycling and repurposing electronic components, transforming e-waste into valuable resources. The potential advanced recycling techniques extract precious metals from discarded electronics, lessen the need to mine the earth, and conserve our resources [51, 52].

In addition, sustainable AM can contribute to economic growth in developing regions by creating new business opportunities and jobs. It can be used by local entrepreneurs to establish recycling facilities and manufacturing plants that are based on recycled materials and thus promote economic growth together with environmental sustainability. It can also make supply chains more resilient by allowing for the on-demand production of parts and components, reducing dependence on imports, and mitigating global supply chain disruptions. Apart from this, sustainable AM can prove a potential benefit for not just developing regions but even developed countries. Reduction in material waste and lowering energy consumption will certainly aid the industries in becoming environmentally friendly and achieving all levels of corporate sustainability. Plus, with the ability to provide high-quality customized products at high speed on demand, the market opening is bound to increase in many directions and customer satisfaction increases as well. However, the full potential of sustainable AM can be achieved only through the concerted efforts of all the stakeholders. Governments must continue implementing and expanding policy incentives that encourage the adoption of sustainable technologies. Industry leaders must invest in research and development to advance AM capabilities and integrate AI and ML into their processes. Educational institutions have a critical role in training the next generation of engineers and technicians to apply the principles of sustainable manufacturing and advanced technologies [53–56].

When combined with AM and coating processes, laser technology has shown to be an asset in manufacturing. Research on laser machining methods for composites has been centered on ways to improve cutting quality and material removal rates [54–58]. Due to advancements in shape memory alloys and sustainability standards, the AM area has seen a surge in research activity [59–61]. Research indicates that machine learning technologies have begun to improve the mechanical properties of 3D printed materials and predict manufacturing attributes [62–64]. One way to improve the material's performance and surface properties is to use a laser for post-processing treatments [65, 66]. The microstructural and mechanical features of nickel-based superalloy claddings and cladding methods are investigated in this study [67–72]. Because of the growing interest in erosion resistance, wear analysis using neural computing systems, and process optimization using artificial intelligence technologies, thermal spray coatings have been the subject of several studies [73–80].

Because it allows scientists to make surface coatings and bioimplants with better mechanical qualities and increased compatibility to human tissue, AM has a lot of potential in the biomedical field [81–83]. Due to their low wear qualities and exceptional durability, zirconia-based biomedical materials have been the subject of expedited research as a result of AI optimization efforts [84]. To increase the durability and corrosion resistance of magnesium-based bioimplants, researchers have looked at protective coatings such as conversion coatings and micro-arc oxidation [85]. The use of biopolymer coatings with AM technology allows for more efficient surface alterations to bioimplants [86–87]. New medical implants with enhanced biofunctionality and self-healing capabilities have been created by researchers [87].

4.7 CONCLUSION

The advanced additive manufacturing technique has come to represent an important solution for sustainable remanufacturing. Innovative approaches toward dealing with issues concerning resource scarcity, environmental degradation, and increasing demand for greater production efficiency are realized through such technologies. The contribution that AM techniques make to the circular economy is the embedding of sustainable practices in the remanufacturing sector. Such an economy involves materials and products that are continually being reused, refurbished, and recycled to minimize waste as well as conserve natural resources. Among the major advantages of advanced AM techniques lies the significant reduction of material waste. Traditional manufacturing usually involves subtractive methods, cutting away excess material in which substantial waste occurs. In contrast, AM constructs the product layer by layer using just the amount of material that is necessary. This will ensure accuracy in waste generation, and it further enhances the efficiency of materials usage by allowing the possibility of the use of recycled and sustainable materials. AM also facilitates the customization and repair of existing components so that they can be made to last longer and diminish the intake of new raw materials. Energy efficiency is another important benefit of advanced AM techniques in sustainable remanufacturing. AM processes consume relatively less energy compared to traditional manufacturing techniques, which involve several stages of production and transportation of parts. By enabling localized production, AM reduces the carbon footprint associated with the global supply chain. This would further enable complex geometries and lightweight structures achievable by AM to reduce the energy use by significant margins in the later use phase of the products, especially in industries related to aerospace and automotive, where such reductions in weight are often crucial. Additional advancement of AM techniques through their combination with digital technologies like AI and the Internet of Things contributes to higher sustainability in the remanufacturing process. For instance, such technologies may provide real-time monitoring for predictive maintenance, optimizing production parameters to use as many as resources possible and get the highest possible quality in product and durability.

REFERENCES

1. Nasr N, Thurston M. Remanufacturing: A key enabler to sustainable product systems. *Proc CIRP.* 2015;29:15–20.
2. Ngo TD, Kashani A, Imbalzano G, Nguyen KTQ, Hui D. Additive manufacturing (3D printing): A review of materials, methods, applications, and challenges. *Compos Part B Eng.* 2018;143:172–96.
3. Zhou L, Miller J, Vezza J, Mayster M, Raffay M, Justice Q, Al Tamimi Z, Hansotte G, Sunkara LD, Bernat J. Additive manufacturing: A comprehensive review. *Sensors.* 2024;24(9):2668.
4. Bhaskar S, Arunachalam R, Walunj AR, Kandasubramanian B. Sustainable additive manufacturing—New perspectives and applications. *J Clean Prod.* 2020;256:120704.
5. Khajavi SH, Partanen J, Holmström J. Additive manufacturing in the spare parts supply chain: Hub configuration and technology maturity. *Rapid Prototyp J.* 2014;20(5):336–43.
6. Kellens K, Baumers M, Gutowski T, Flanagan W, Lifset R, Duflou JR. Environmental dimensions of additive manufacturing: Mapping application domains and their environmental implications. *J Ind Ecol.* 2017;21(S1):S49–S68.
7. Ford S, Despeisse M. Additive manufacturing and sustainability: An exploratory study of the advantages and challenges. *J Clean Prod.* 2016;137:1573–87.
8. Gao W, Zhang Y, Ramanujan D, Ramani K, Chen Y, Williams CB, et al. The status, challenges, and future of additive manufacturing in engineering. *CAD Comput Aided Des.* 2015;69:65–89.
9. Tang Y, Mak KH, Zhao Y, Guo Y, Li J. Current status and future trends in additive manufacturing for remanufacturing. *Manuf Lett.* 2020;25:93–7.
10. Frazier WE. Metal additive manufacturing: A review. *J Mater Eng Perform.* 2014;23(6):1917–28.
11. Kaya D, Abdelmoula M, Küçüktürk G, Grossin D, Stamboulis A. A novel approach for powder bed fusion of ceramics using two laser systems. *Materials.* 2023;16(6):2507.
12. Murr LE, Gaytan SM, Ramirez DA, Shindo PW, Martinez E, Medina F, et al. Metal fabrication by additive manufacturing using laser and electron beam melting technologies. *J Mater Sci Technol.* 2012;28(1):1–14.
13. Kruth JP, Leu MC, Nakagawa T. Progress in additive manufacturing and rapid prototyping. *CIRP Ann.* 1998;47(2):525–40.
14. Gu D, Meiners W, Wissenbach K, Poprawe R. Laser additive manufacturing of metallic components: Materials, processes and mechanisms. *Int Mater Rev.* 2012;57(3):133–64.
15. Scherm F, Daoud H, Glatzel U. Influence of printing strategies on the microstructure and mechanical properties of additively manufactured alloy 625 using directed energy deposition (DED-LB-p). *Metals.* 2024;14(9):1041.
16. DebRoy T, Wei HL, Zuback JS, Mukherjee T, Elmer JW, Milewski JO, et al. Additive manufacturing of metallic components—Process, structure and properties. *Prog Mater Sci.* 2018;92:112–224.
17. Herderick E. Additive manufacturing of metals: A review. *Mater Sci Technol.* 2011;27(7):606–14.
18. Manogharan G, Wysk R, Harrysson O, Aman R. AIMS–a metal additive-hybrid manufacturing system: System architecture and attributes. *Procedia Manuf.* 2015;1:273–86.
19. Gibson I, Rosen DW, Stucker B. *Additive Manufacturing Technologies.* 3rd ed. New York: Springer; 2021.
20. Leicht A, Duflou JR, Dewulf W. Low-energy hybrid repair techniques for high-value metal components: A state-of-the-art. *CIRP J Manuf Sci Technol.* 2018;22:33–46.
21. Turner BN, Strong R, Gold SA. A review of melt extrusion additive manufacturing processes: I. Process design and modeling. *Rapid Prototyp J.* 2014;20(3):192–204.

22. Wang Y, Yu W, Ma J, Liu Z, Zhang S. An investigation of multi-material 3D printing of PLA and carbon fiber-reinforced PLA using FDM. *J Mater Process Technol.* 2017;250:23–31.
23. Jiang J, Xu X, Stringer J. Optimization of multimaterial structures for additive manufacturing: A review. *Addit Manuf.* 2021;37:101607.
24. Peng T, Kellens K, Tang R, Chen C, Chen G. Sustainability of additive manufacturing: An overview on its energy demand and environmental impact. *Addit Manuf.* 2018;21:694–704.
25. Gibson I, Rosen DW, Stucker B. *Additive Manufacturing Technologies.* 3rd ed. New York: Springer; 2021.
26. Yap CY, Wang Y, Sing SL, et al. Review of selective laser melting: Materials and applications. *Appl Phys Rev.* 2015;2(4):041101.
27. Wang X, Jiang M, Zhou Z, Gou J, Hui D. 3D printing of polymer matrix composites: A review and prospective. *Compos Part B Eng.* 2017;110:442–58.
28. Kruth JP, Leu MC, Nakagawa T. Progress in additive manufacturing and rapid prototyping. *CIRP Ann.* 1998;47(2):525–40.
29. Tao Y, Zhang D, Liu Z, et al. Additive manufacturing-based hybrid techniques for high-value metal component remanufacturing. *J Manuf Proc.* 2019;38:125–37.
30. DebRoy T, Wei HL, Zuback JS, Mukherjee T, Elmer JW, Milewski JO, et al. Additive manufacturing of metallic components—Process, structure and properties. *Prog Mater Sci.* 2018;92:112–224.
31. Naser AZ, Deiab I, Defersha F, Yang S. Expanding poly (lactic acid)(PLA) and polyhydroxyalkanoates (PHAs) applications: A review on modifications and effects. *Polymers.* 2021;13(23):4271.
32. Herderick E. Additive manufacturing of metals: A review. *Mater Sci Technol.* 2011;27(7):606–14.
33. Gu D, Meiners W, Wissenbach K, Poprawe R. Laser additive manufacturing of metallic components: Materials, processes and mechanisms. *Int Mater Rev.* 2012;57(3):133–64.
34. Korpela A, Zimmermann T, Deegan G. Biodegradable polymers for industrial applications. In: Kalia S, Averous L, editors. *Biodegradable and Biobased Polymers for Environmental and Biomedical Applications.* New York: John Wiley & Sons; 2011. pp. 231–49.
35. Chien YC, Wu JH, Shu CH, Lo JT, Yang TC. Closed-loop recycling of 3D-printed wood–PLA composite parts: Effects on mechanical and structural properties via fused filament fabrication. *Polymers.* 2024;16(21):3002.
36. Tan E, Rahman M. A review on the use of biodegradable polymers in food packaging. *J Polym Environ.* 2017;25(1):23–31.
37. Chua CK, Leong KF. *3D Printing and Additive Manufacturing: Principles and Applications.* 5th ed. Singapore: World Scientific; 2017.
38. Fiedler T, Belnoue JP, Richardson MOW, Stommel M, Fernández Villegas I. Polymer composite additive manufacturing: A materials perspective. *Compos Part A Appl Sci Manuf.* 2021;149:106529.
39. Goh GD, Agarwala S, Goh GL, Dikshit V, Sing SL, Yeong WY. Additive manufacturing in biomedical device design and development. In: Wimpenny DI, Pandey PM, Kumar LJP, editors. *Advances in 3D Printing & Additive Manufacturing Technologies.* Singapore: Springer; 2017. pp. 281–303.
40. Leicht A, Duflou JR, Dewulf W. Low-energy hybrid repair techniques for high-value metal components: A state-of-the-art. *CIRP J Manuf Sci Technol.* 2018;22:33–46.
41. Ngo TD, Kashani A, Imbalzano G, Nguyen KTQ, Hui D. Additive manufacturing (3D printing): A review of materials, methods, applications, and challenges. *Compos Part B Eng.* 2018;143:172–96.

42. Morrow WR, Qi H, Kim I, Mazumder J, Skerlos SJ. Environmental aspects of laser-based and conventional tool and die manufacturing. *J Clean Prod.* 2007;15(10):932–43.
43. Kellens K, Mertens R, Paraskevas D, Dewulf W, Duflou JR. Environmental impact of additive manufacturing processes: Does AM contribute to a more sustainable way of part manufacturing? *Proc CIRP.* 2017;61:582–7.
44. Ford S, Despeisse M. Additive manufacturing and sustainability: An exploratory study of the advantages and challenges. *J Clean Prod.* 2016;137:1573–87.
45. Li X, Wang H, Chen X, Liu Y, Li J, Tang H, et al. Near-net shape manufacturing of high-performance Ti-6Al-4V alloy using selective laser melting: A review. *J Mater Process Technol.* 2018;255:35–49. https://doi.org/10.1016/j.jmatprotec.2017.12.029.
46. DebRoy T, Wei HL, Zuback JS, Mukherjee T, Elmer JW, Milewski JO, et al. Additive manufacturing of metallic components—Process, structure and properties. *Prog Mater Sci.* 2018;92:112–224. https://doi.org/10.1016/j.pmatsci.2017.10.001.
47. Zhang Y, Jiang Z, Ling H, Zhou Y, Wang J, Zhang P. Material efficiency and recycling rate of metal-based additive manufacturing: A review. *J Manuf Process.* 2021;63:99–117. https://doi.org/10.1016/j.jmapro.2021.01.020.
48. Peng T, Kellens K, Tang R, Chen C, Chen G. Sustainability of additive manufacturing: An overview on its energy demand and environmental impact. *Addit Manuf.* 2018;21:694–704. https://doi.org/10.1016/j.addma.2018.04.022.
49. Yang S, Yang Y, Fu J, Bai J, Li X. Reusability of waste Ti-6Al-4V powders in additive manufacturing. *J Mater Sci Technol.* 2020;41:72–83. https://doi.org/10.1016/j.jmst.2019.11.030.
50. Kellens K, Baumers M, Gutowski T, Flanagan W, Lifset R, Duflou JR. Environmental dimensions of additive manufacturing: Mapping application domains and their environmental implications. *J Ind Ecol.* 2017;21(S1):S49–S68. https://doi.org/10.1111/jiec.12629.
51. Khajavi SH, Partanen J, Holmström J. Additive manufacturing in the spare parts supply chain: Hub configuration and technology maturity. *Rapid Prototyp J.* 2014;20(3):216–27. https://doi.org/10.1108/RPJ-07-2012-0067.
52. Vayre B, Vignat F, Villeneuve F. Metallic additive manufacturing: State-of-the-art review and prospects. *Mech Ind.* 2012;13(2):89–96. https://doi.org/10.1051/meca/2012003.
53. Gibson I, Rosen DW, Stucker B. *Additive Manufacturing Technologies: Rapid Prototyping to Direct Digital Manufacturing.* 2nd ed. New York: Springer; 2015.
54. Frazier WE. Metal additive manufacturing: A review. *J Mater Eng Perform.* 2014;23(6):1917–28. https://doi.org/10.1007/s11665-014-0958-z.
55. Kumar R, Singh R, Ahuja IPS. Investigations of mechanical, thermal and morphological properties of FDM fabricated parts for elevated temperature applications. *J Manuf Process.* 2019;42:120–36. https://doi.org/10.1016/j.jmapro.2019.05.034.
56. Lockett H, Smith C, Wang T, Cooper DR. Topological optimization and freeform fabrication: A review. *Struct Multidisc Optim.* 2014;50(4):597–616. https://doi.org/10.1007/s00158-014-1067-5.
57. Sharma V, Kumar V. Application of Box-Behnken design and response surface methodology for multi-optimization of laser cutting of AA5052/ZrO2 metal–matrix composites. *Proc Inst Mech Eng Part L J Mater Des Appl.* 2018;232(8):652–68.
58. Sharma V, Kumar V. Comparison of machining characteristics of metal matrix composites using CO2 laser curve cutting process. *Proc Inst Mech Eng Part E J Process Mech Eng.* 2018;232(3):349–68.
59. Sharma V, Kumar V. Investigating the quality characteristics of Al5052/SiC metal matrix composites machined by CO2 laser curve cutting. *Proc Inst Mech Eng Part L J Mater Des Appl.* 2018;232(1):3–19.

60. Sharma V, Kumar V, Bist A. Investigations on morphology and material removal rate of various MMCs using CO2 laser technique. *J Braz Soc Mech Sci Eng*. 2020;42:1–14.
61. Sharma V, Singh JP, Raman R, Bathla G, Saini A. Machine learning approach for prediction analysis of aluminium alloy on the surface roughness using CO2 laser machining. *Proc Inst Mech Eng Part E J Process Mech Eng*. 2024;09544089241231093.
62. Singh R, Toseef M, Kumar J, Singh J. Benefits and challenges in additive manufacturing and its applications. In: Kaushal S, Singh I, Singh S, Gupta A, editors. *Sustainable Advanced Manufacturing and Materials Processing*. 1st ed. Boca Raton: CRC Press; 2022. pp. 137–57. https://doi.org/10.1201/9781003269298-8.
63. Singh J. Sustainability issues in laser-based additive manufacturing. In: *Handbook of Laser-Based Sustainable Surface Modification and Manufacturing Techniques*. CRC Press; 2023. pp. 167–89.
64. Ahmad S, et al. Innovations in additive manufacturing of shape memory alloys: Alloys, microstructures, treatments, applications. *J Mater Res Technol*. 2024;32:4136–97.
65. Sharma V, Singh JP, Hussan K, Kumar R. Machine learning approach for predicting the machining characteristics of additive manufactured ABS material. *Proc Inst Mech Eng Part C J Mech Eng Sci*. 2024;09544062241283330.
66. Chohan JS, et al. Mechanical strength enhancement of 3D printed acrylonitrile butadiene styrene polymer components using neural network optimization algorithm. *Polymers*. 2020;12(10). https://doi.org/10.3390/polym12102250.
67. Singh J, et al. Impact of molding temperature, fiber loading and chemical modifications on the physicomechanical, and microstructural morphology properties of woven kenaf Fiber/PLA composites for non-structural applications. *J Nat Fibers*. 2024;21(1):2326586.
68. Singh J. Applications of laser technology for processing and post-treatments of powders and coatings. In: *Handbook of Laser-Based Sustainable Surface Modification and Manufacturing Techniques*. CRC Press; 2023. pp. 135–66.
69. Sunitha K, Vasudev H. A short note on the various thermal spray coating processes and effect of post-treatment on Ni-based coatings. *Mater Today Proc*. 2022;50:1452–7. https://doi.org/10.1016/j.matpr.2021.09.017.
70. Sharanabasava H, et al. Microstructure, mechanical and wear properties of SiC and Mo reinforced NiCr microwave cladding. *Adv Mater Process Technol*. 2024;10:3620–33.
71. Singh J, Gill HS. Evolution of nickel-based superalloy claddings for against high-temperature oxidation and wear. In: *Thermal Claddings for Engineering Applications*. CRC Press; 2024. pp. 160–81.
72. Singh J, Kumar S, Kumar R, Mohapatra SK. Machine learning regression tools for erosion prediction of WC-10Co4Cr thermal spray coating. Results Surfa Interfaces. 2023;13:100156. https://doi.org/10.1016/j.rsurfi.2023.100156.
73. Yedida VVS, Vasudev H. A review on the development of thermal barrier coatings by using thermal spray techniques. *Mater Today Proc*. 2022;50:1458–64.
74. Singh J, Singh S. Support vector machine learning on slurry erosion characteristics analysis of Ni- and Co-alloy coatings. *Surf Rev Lett*. 2023. https://doi.org/10.1142/S0218625X23400061.
75. Prashar G, Vasudev H. A review on the influence of process parameters and heat treatment on the corrosion performance of Ni-based thermal spray coatings. *Surf Rev Lett*. 2022;29(1):2230001.
76. Singh J, Vasudev H, Szala M, Gill HS. Neural computing for erosion assessment in Al-20TiO2 HVOF thermal spray coating. *Int J Interact Des Manuf*. 2024;18:2321–32.
77. Singh J, Vasudev H, Kumar R, Ubaidullah M. Study on wear analysis of Ni-20Al2O3 HVOF micron layers using artificial neural network technique. *Int J Interact Des Manuf*. 2023;18:5925–38. https://doi.org/10.1007/s12008-023-01433-2.

78. Prashar G, Vasudev H. Surface topology analysis of plasma sprayed Inconel625-Al2O3 composite coating. *Mater Today Proc.* 2022;50:607–11. https://doi.org/10.1016/j.matpr.2021.03.090.
79. Thakur L, Vasudev H, Singh J, Prashar G. *Artificial Intelligence and Machine Learning in the Thermal Spray Industry: Practices, Implementation, and Challenges.* CRC Press; 2023.
80. Dutta V, Thakur L, Singh B, Vasudev H. A study of erosion–corrosion behaviour of friction stir-processed chromium-reinforced NiAl bronze composite. *Materials (Basel).* 2022;15(15):5401. https://doi.org/10.3390/ma15155401.
81. Singh J, Singh S, Vasudev H, Chohan JS, Kumar S. Neural computing and Taguchi's method-based study on erosion of advanced Mo2C–WC10Co4Cr coating for the centrifugal pump. *Adv Mater Process Technol.* 2024;10(3):2569–81.
82. Singh J, Singh S, Vasudev H, Katiyar JK. Artificial neural network model for wear characteristic analysis of WC-10Co4Cr and Stellite 6 thermal spray coatings. *Tribol Int.* 2024;199:109924.
83. Majji BGR, Vasudev H, Bansal A. A review on the oxidation and wear behavior of the thermally sprayed high-entropy alloys. *Mater Today Proc.* 2022;50:1447–51.
84. Singh J, Singh S, Verma A. Artificial intelligence in use of ZrO2 material in biomedical science. *J Electrochem Sci Eng.* 2022;13(1):83–97. https://doi.org/10.5599/jese.1498.
85. Singh J, Hashmi AW, Behra A, Kumar A, Dogra N, Kumar P. Review of Mg alloys for bio-implants protected by the deposition of chemical conversion coatings. In *AIP Conference Proceedings.* AIP Publishing; 2024.
86. Singh J, Singh S, Gill R. Applications of biopolymer coatings in biomedical engineering. *J Electrochem Sci Eng.* 2022;13(1):63–81. https://doi.org/10.5599/jese.1460.
87. Singh CJ, Ram B, Singh J, Prakash C, Paramasivam P, Kumar R. Experimental investigation on characterization of friction stir processed AZ31-based composite. *Sci Rep.* 2024;14(1):15453.

5 Advanced Coating Technology in Biomedical Science

Challenges and Perspectives for Smart Material

Amrinder Mehta and Hitesh Vasudev

CONTENTS

5.1 INTRODUCTION

The limited coatings technology advancement has been steadily growing rapidly over the last few decades in the biomedical science sector that is involved in the manufacturing of medical equipment, implants, and drug delivery systems. One of the nanocarriers used as the novel methodology in the delivery of RNA and antisense oligonucleotides is cell membrane-coated nanoparticles (CMCNPs), which have biomimetic characters to avoid immune surveillance and mimic cellular [1].

Figure 5.1 outlines a sequential three-step method for the synthesis of MEM-protected nanoparticles. Step 1 deals with isolation of the cell membrane: hypotonic

DOI: 10.1201/9781003516064-5

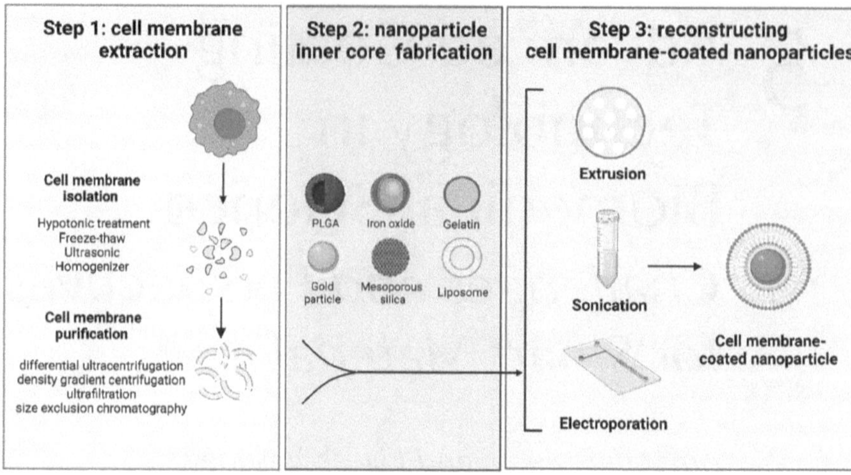

FIGURE 5.1 A schematic diagram of preparing monotypic cell membrane-coated nanoparticles. Step 1 includes two processes of harvesting cell membrane fragments; step 2 requires cautious selection and fabrication of the inner core according to the purpose; step 3 is the final step to coat the cell membrane onto a template [2]. (Reproduction permissions by Springer Nature)

treatment, freeze–thaw cycles, ultrasonic processing, and different purification methods such as ultracentrifugation. Step 2 shows various forms of nanoparticle core which can be prepared, such as PLGA, iron oxides, gelatin, gold particle, mesoporous silica, and liposome. As it is illustrated on the flowchart of the third step, it depicts the final reconstruction phase wherein the purified cell membrane is reassembled with the nanoparticle core through various techniques, namely extrusion, sonication, or electroporation to afford the final cell membrane-coated nanoparticle structure [2].

AMP coatings have been reported to provide a solution for implant-related infection and biofilm development. Micro-arc oxidation (MAO) has conferred placement of active metal ions at titanium implants for the betterment of bactericidal, anti-inflammatory and osteogenic features [3]. Moreover, microneedle (MN) technology has enhanced the techniques of drug delivery system, which includes poor absorption and skin permeation restrictions. Combined, these coating technologies assist in getting increased biocompatibility function, precise delivery, and even enhanced therapy in numerous biomedical applications [4]. This chapter attempts to discuss the recent development in a field of coating technology in biomedical science by highlighting the issues encountered and potentials of smart material.

5.2 CURRENT STATE OF ADVANCED COATING TECHNOLOGY

5.2.1 Biocompatible Coatings

Biocompatible coatings have now reached the point where they cannot be overlooked for use in medical implant and device applications as they function as an intermediate layer between materials and tissue. These coatings are developed so that the body does not react negatively by inflammation or reject the coating and its interaction with the surrounding tissues [5]. Superiority in coatings include the use of active proteins and peptides, growth factors, and antimicrobial properties to stimulate tissue regeneration, minimize infection, and ultimately increase implant stability [6]. **Figure 5.2** has highlighted biomimetic coatings used in dental implants based on two profiles. To the left on the picture, they include such coatings as hydroxyapatite, nanoceramics, growth factors, and extracellular matrix to increase osseointegration. On the right side, the image shows strategies to combat peri-implant inflammation through different coating types: Examples are drug coatings, peptide coatings, polysaccharide coatings, and metal coatings with ions such as Ag^{+}, $Cu^{2+,}$ and Zn^{2+}. These anti-inflammatory coatings help to either eradicate or remove bacteria from the surface of the implant. The central image illustrates a dental implant and the aspect related to the threads of the implant and the bone tissues [7].

Some coatings imitate native extracellular matrix (ECM) and promote cell interaction, as well as tissue remodeling. Some apply nanotechnology in the development of antimicrobial surfaces while others apply nanotechnology in developing antimicrobial coatings. Alterations in the surface make biocompatible coatings a pivotal boost to the function, length, and safety of implants that in turn culminates in better patient experiences and minimal complications in different surgical procedures [8]. Recent advancements include hydrophilic and antimicrobial coatings.

Hydrophilic coatings introduced a good change in the medics and medical instruments, especially the catheters and the guidewires. In these coatings, their primary function includes the ability to interrogate and selectively adhere to water molecules to present a slippery interface when in contact with body fluids. The information

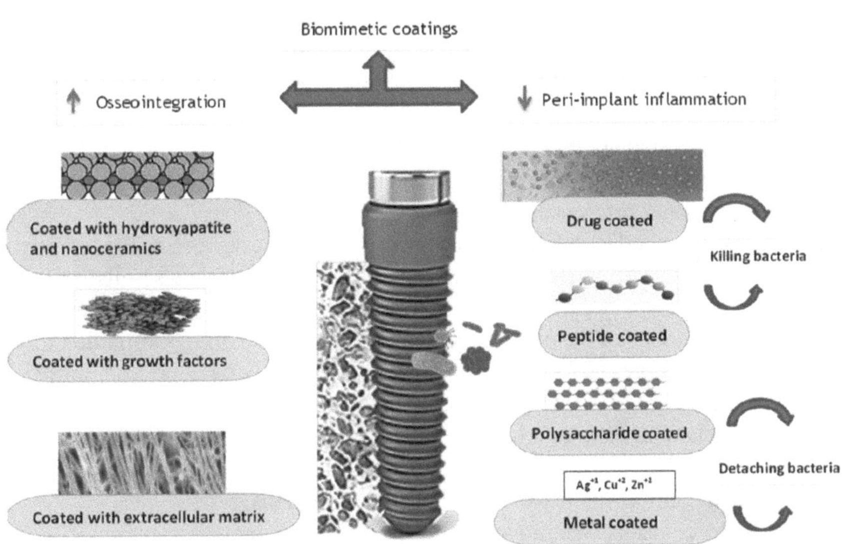

FIGURE 5.2 Overview of biocompatible coatings [7]. (Creative Commons Attribution 4.0)

TABLE 5.1
Information about Hydrophilic Coatings

S. No.	Surface Properties	Materials Used	Contact/ Tilt Angles (Degrees)	Comments
1.	Enhanced lubricity for medical devices	Hydrophilic polymers (e.g., polyethylene glycol)	70	The coatings improve biocompatibility, reduce friction during device insertion, and help prevent infections commonly associated with urinary catheters [9].
2.	Reduction in bacterial adhesion	Polyethylene glycol (PEG), zwitterionic polymers, hyaluronic acid (HA), sodium alginate		Improvements in device maneuverability, reduced infections, and biocompatibility due to the hydrophilic coating help in associating medical device surfaces with lower bacterial colonization rates [10].
3.	Transparent coatings	Polymethyl methacrylate (PMMA), silica nanoparticles	1.7	These improve biocompatibility, reduce unwanted cell adhesion, and used in medical devices for anti-biofouling applications [11].
4.	Biocompatibility through advanced material use	Polymers such as PEG, polyvinyl alcohol (PVA), and others known for their hydrophilicity	35	These coatings are essential for reducing thrombosis, improving biocompatibility, and enhancing the water wettability of surfaces, crucial in biomedical applications [12].
5.	Improved reduction of thrombus formation	Heparin sodium, phosphorylcholine, polyvinylpyrrolidone (PVP)	153.6	These coatings significantly reduce thrombogenicity and are suitable for medical devices, enhancing hemocompatibility while preventing thrombus formation effectively [13].

about hydrophilic coatings which is given in **Table 5.1** has been created based on the results of the search. Information on the surface properties, materials, contact/tilt angles, comments, and references is given in **Table 5.1**.

This property alone reduces the force of contact between the device and the tissues surrounding it making it easier to insert. The elimination of friction decreases discomfort to the patients during the procedure, reduces tissue damages, and increases the ease-of-use and precision of the tools for the medical personnel [13]. Further, the hydrophilic finishes enable avoidance of thrombus formation and the adhesion of bacteria, hence minimizing other complications. Some of the more developed hydrophilic coatings also contain the self-disinfecting element or drug-releasing characteristic to expand the utilization abilities of the coatings [14]. These coatings have gained the importance to enhance safety, effectiveness, and comfort to the patient in many interventional procedures.

Antimicrobial coatings which can incorporate silver nanoparticles or antibiotics have been developed as a strong approach to combating infections linked to devices. Silver nanoparticles are some of the most effective because they are effective in

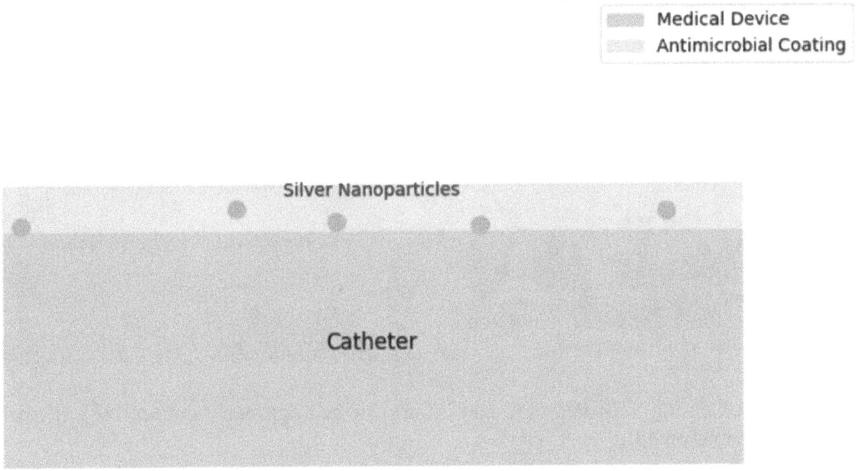

FIGURE 5.3 Antimicrobial coating on medical devices with silver nanoparticles. (Created by authors)

killing bacteria, fungi, and viruses. **Figure 5.3** is simple and clearly explains the antimicrobial coatings in medical devices especially using silver nanoparticles [15].

Such nanoparticles gradually release silver ions that affect the bacterial structure and functions: there is inhibition of adhesion and biofilm formation. Coatings can be applied to numerous medical devices such as catheters, implants, or drug delivery systems as well as to wound dressings. The authors established that silver nanoparticles have a higher potential compared to common antibiotics since they are less likely to lead to bacterial resistance [16]. More modern kinds of such coatings also contain not only silver nanoparticles but polymers or other antimicrobial substances as well to intensify their effectiveness. Such coatings substantially decrease the rates of HAIs, which enhances the quality of patients' recovery and decreases the expenses on the device-related infections' treatment.

Cell-adhesive coatings are important in facilitating the attachment of cells to the surface of the implant and proliferation of neighboring tissues. These coatings, extracellular matrix proteins, peptides, or growth factors, which represent the biological cell substrate, are commonly incorporated into the material surface [17]. As diagrammed in **Figure 5.4**, Prevelex is a polymer coating technology, whose structure and application are outlined here. In part (a) the chemical formula of Prevelex with its phosphate groups and functional groups (R1, R2, R3) are shown, and this part also demonstrates how Prevelex spreads over multiple layers of the material and makes it water loving and electrostatic neutral. In part (b), the figure illustrates how the coated surface resists proteins and cell adhesion through electrostatic repulsion with the charged surface striped pattern. In part (c), conformal coating is applied on microstructures with a particular pitch of 200 μm which prove how the coating adapts to various geometries on the surface as well as the nano-repellent nature of the material [18].

The coatings with RGD (arginine–glycine–aspartic acid) peptides have demonstrated better adhesion and proliferation of cells on the surface of implants than have previously

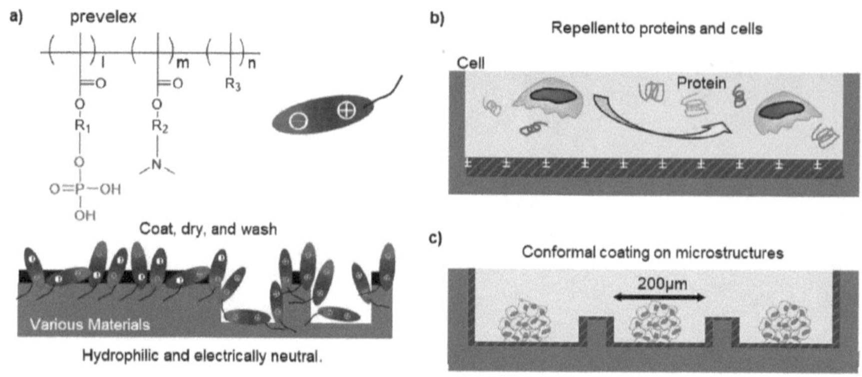

FIGURE 5.4 Coating with Prevelex and its use for cell aggregate culture [18]. (Creative Commons Attribution 4.0)

been seen. Higher generation coatings have been developed to incorporate nanostructured features that provide a surface profile suitable for cell adhesion. Positive features on the surface of the implant may increase the rate of tissue growth, improve mechanical properties of the impacted tissues, and decrease the likelihood of rejection. This technology has successfully been applied in orthopedic implants, dental implants, and tissue engineering scaffolds greatly improving the longevity and efficiency of the implants [19].

5.2.2 Drug-Eluting Coatings

Drug-eluting coatings have revolutionized controlled drug delivery and provided a complex method for delivering therapeutic agents for an enhanced length of time. Such coatings are designed to encapsulate and release drugs over time, making treatment much more effective as it reduces side effects. The methods of manipulation of these coatings allow sustaining the ensured drug concentrations in the target site, whereby frequent administrations of the drug are thus avoided [20]. This has widely been used in implantable technology in areas such as stent technology, implantations, and in wound dressings. The coatings may be designed to sustain single or multiple drug release over time depending on the physiologic condition prevailing at the site of placement of the coatings. This characteristic of drug delivery enhances patients' concordance, besides enabling selective treatment and decreasing possible systemic effects and their consequences that contribute to the overall enhancement of the therapeutic results and, in general, the patients' quality of life [21].

Biodegradable polymers have heralded polymer-based coatings in drug delivery systems through controlling the release kinetics of drugs. Figure 5.5 explains the main processes of drug delivery through the system based on polymers. The different transport phenomena are depicted in the diagram, where a lumen has particles and a polymer matrix. On the left side, two primary processes are highlighted: diffusion and advection. The polymer section in the middle demonstrates five crucial mechanisms: diffusion, swelling, dissolution, degradation (erosion), and osmosis. On the right side, three processes are shown occurring in the tissue: Convection in the porous medium, diffusion, and receptor binding are the possible mechanisms

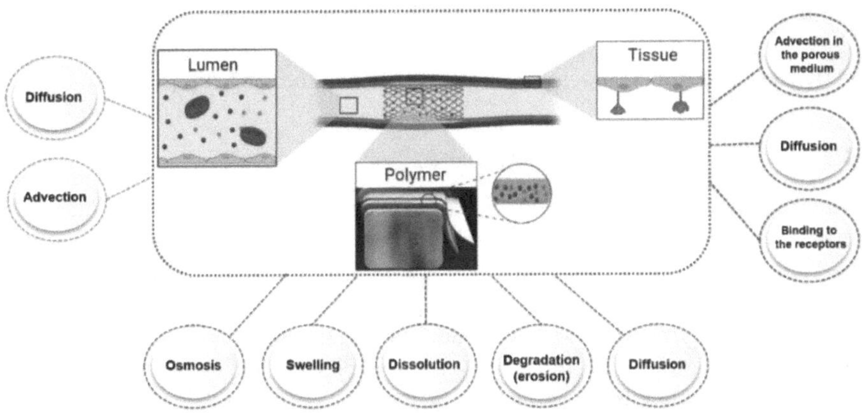

FIGURE 5.5 Polymer-based coatings [22]. (Creative Commons Attribution 4.0)

of drug transport in tissues. This can be regarded as a complete perspective on the process by which drugs go from delivery systems to biological tissues [22].

These coatings encase the therapeutic agents in a polymer matrix although the polymer gradually dissolves in the body to release the drug at a controlled rate. Some of the familiar biodegradable polymers include poly (lactic-co-glycolic acid) (PLGA), polycaprolactone (PCL), and poly (lactic acid) (PLA). As for the containers, the release rate regulated by polymer composition, molecular weight, or crystallinity. Advanced systems include stimuli-sensitive polymers that are capable of sensitive response to certain physiological signals for drug-controlled release [23]. Polymer-based coatings can be applied to a plurality of medical equipment including stents, implants, and nanoparticles. This technology makes therapy more effective by keeping the level of drugs constantly high, has a lower toxicity, and increases patient compliance. Such polymers are also biodegradable, meaning that there are no requirements for their removal and beneficial for long-term use [24].

5.3 CHALLENGES IN ADVANCED COATING TECHNOLOGY

There are a number of obstacles to overcome, notwithstanding the enormous development that has been made in advanced coating technology.

5.3.1 Durability and Long-Term Stability

Maintenance of the coating's hardness and stability for long term in biological environment is one of the most significant problems in biomedical applications. These coatings have to resist the conditions present inside the human body as well as enzymes, pH changes, and mechanical loadings and remain functional for long time durations. New and improved materials and methods for tougher coatings are being researched, and attempts are made to improve the polymer cross-link density, the use of nanoparticles and the layering of materials [25]. The ultimate target is to design coatings that cannot degrade, become weakened to a certain level, or fail on delivering their functions of drug elution, bacteria and fungi killing, or integrating with the tissues. Stability remains a critical parameter for implantable devices and drug-eluting systems, as well as other biomedical applications, as it influences the effectiveness and safety of delivered interventions in the long run [26].

5.3.2 Scalability and Manufacturing

It is also a major challenge to produce cost-efficient and reproducible manufacturing routes for enhanced coatings for biomedical engineering. Due to the multilayering, nanoscale fabrication or bioactivity, the fabrication processes of such coatings are challenging and cannot be easily translated from the laboratory to mass production level [27, 28]. Thus, challenges that include standardization, replicability, and stability of the products with vulnerable biological components during production become crucial. However, high initial and operating costs as a result of the special equipment and material make it difficult to popularize [29]. Some of the challenges have been met by employing deposition from solution methods and using new techniques such as automated deposition systems, roll-to-roll processing, and 3D printing methods. It is also necessary to define those areas where it is possible to adhere to high quality standards but also be as effective as possible; naturally, it is also possible to work closely when the organization is creating protocols and procedures that meet strict external demands [30]. These are the manufacturing drawbacks that need to be addressed to bring improved advanced coatings to a variety of medical uses while making them affordable. Facing strict legal standards concerning safety and effectiveness may be costly as well as take a great deal of time.

5.3.3 Biocompatibility and Immune Response

Biomedical applications, particularly those involving patients with multiple conditions, creating solutions that can reduce problematic reactions to coating remains a major challenge. Self-made by humans immune system can detect foreign substances such as coatings of medical devices that can cause inflammation, rejection, or failure of the devices [31]. To address biocompatibility issues, strategies include the use biomimetic ways, whereby synthetic materials can be engineered to resemble tissues, incorporation of anti-inflammatory compounds, and creation of coatings that can mobilize immune responses. The fluorinated polymers appear to have potential for decreasing stent thrombosis, since they have more affinity for albumin than for platelets [32]. Moreover, it has been ascertained that certain quorum-quenching molecules can be effective in preventing biofilm formation on medical instruments. Nevertheless, development of universally biocompatible coatings for effective and safe functioning throughout various patient populations with different genotypes and diseases still pose technical challenges and requires further research and development [33]. Using polymeric coatings as multifunctional and multitasking is challenging, as the wanted properties and functions may require different material characteristics.

5.4 PERSPECTIVES FOR SMART MATERIALS

The main direction for further development of modern coating technology in biomedical science is to create intelligent and adaptive coatings. These coatings will be able to change their property or deliver certain therapeutic agents in response to certain biological signals. This development means better and individualized medical devices and therapies which improve patient experiences in all conceivable uses.

5.4.1 Self-Healing Coatings

Manufactured coatings gaining self-healing capabilities are the innovative achievement in the medical device and implant industry that could help to boost the maximal lifespan and performance rates of used devices. These advanced coatings are designed to help them incorporate techniques including microcapsules or vascular networks that contain healing compounds. In case of any harm in the coating, then these systems self-part fill the healing agents so as to start the healing process [34]. The course, this self-repairing feature, is capable of preventing or at least mitigating problems like micro-crack, scratches, or wear that would otherwise impede the device's efficiency or cause total failure. Thus, the integrity of the coating layer of the device is preserved by these systems, as well as the biocompatibility, drug elution, or protection they provide [35].

This is a technical illustration that demonstrates how autonomously healing materials can be applied in the situation of robotic prosthetics. **Figure 5.6** is divided into three sections: a modulus scale ranging from metals 1011 Pa to soft hydrogels 103

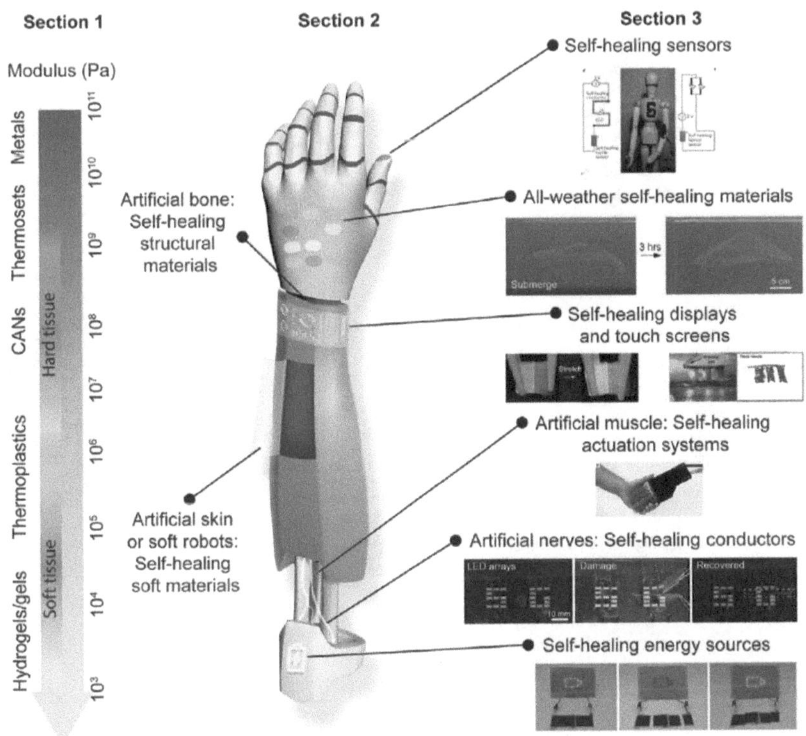

FIGURE 5.6 Self-healing materials and components for smart robotics [36]. (Reproduction permissions by Wiley)

Pa, an ideal central robotic arm design, and several self-healing applications. The robotic arm has several self-repair elements of flesh, bones, skin, muscles, and nerves incorporated into its design. The third and final part illustrates applications which include self-healing sensors, all-weather materials, touch, and energy applications. Such a complex design would represent one of the most sophisticated biomimetic technologies that could repair and maintain themselves; therefore, the prosthetic technology [36]. Self-healing coatings not only enhance the durability of medical implants but also reduce the need for invasive replacement procedures, potentially improving patient outcomes and reducing healthcare costs.

5.4.2 Nanostructured Coatings

In the field of biomedical science, nanostructured coatings are considered a new and innovative development as they provide greater properties and utilities at the nanoscale layer. **Figure 5.7** is helpful to visualize how these six factors relate and are equally significant for controlling properties and performance of nanostructured coatings [37, 38]. Each parameter in the coating process serves unique functions that determine the properties of the applied coating. That is, nodes are hexagonal

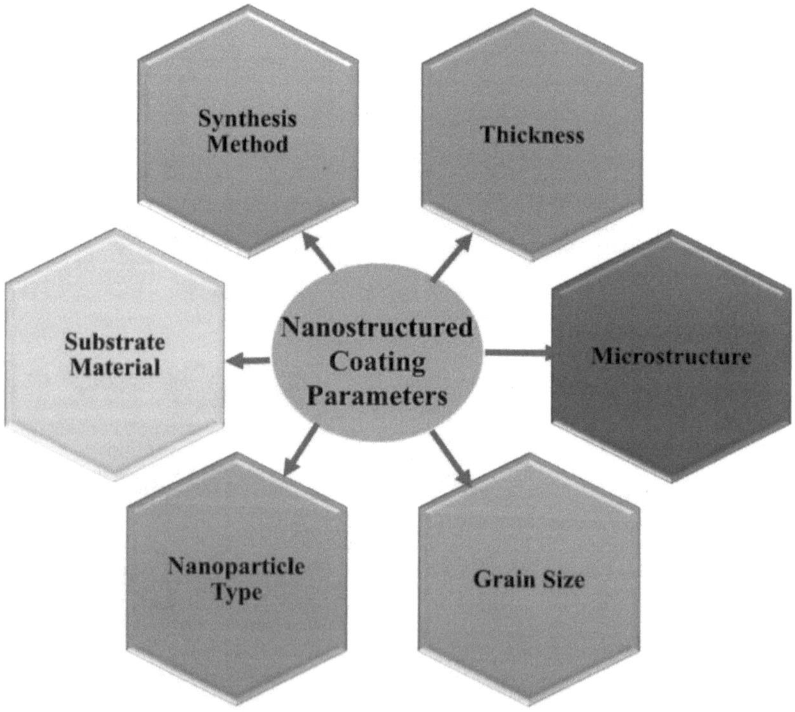

FIGURE 5.7 Various parameters influencing nanostructured coating formation [38]. (Creative Commons Attribution 4.0)

and placed around the central concept in a radial manner, and thus, it is easy to find the organization of these crucial coating parameters. Such systematic arrangement proves itself beneficial when one studies the complex process involved in developing and optimizing nanostructured coatings [39].

These coatings can be made with the exact topographical characteristics of the tissue to which they are being implanted and thus have low rejection rates by the body. It has been postulated that through the control of surface features and chemical composition at the nanometer-length scale, more desirable coatings for tissue engineering applications could be developed with improved cell attachment, proliferation, and differentiation. For instance, the applications of nanostructured surface in titanium dental implants have produced enhanced osseointegration [40]. Also, it can be possible that such coatings will add the nanoparticle functionality for developing intentional drug delivery or antibacterial functionality. This level of surface organization provides medical engineers and researchers a high degree of control over the biological response of the human body to transplanted or inserted devices and a better chance for faster-healing and longer-lasting implants.

5.4.3 Bioinspired Coatings

The field of biomedical science has an interesting twenty-first-century solution to address the problems of bioinspired coatings. These coatings are designed to imitate the function of biological surfaces to provide additional functional improvements. The phenomenon is the mobility that has been encouraged in the field of manufacture of coatings that mimic the shark skin, which is known to be antimicrobial. One of these coatings contains microscopic surface patterns that were copied from the ridges of a shark skin, and the surface closely resists bacterial attachment and biofilm development. It has the potential to eliminate hospital-acquired infection on such devices and implants [41]. Bioinspired coatings mimic designs seen in nature and can offer far greater antibacterial activity, optimized drag, and increased endurance—all of which could dramatically alter the way medical devices are coated and, in turn, benefit patients' lives.

5.4.4 Smart Drug Delivery Systems

Coating technology is moving toward the future of adaptive drug delivery systems, where these drug delivery systems can recognize one or more biochemical or physiologic signals. **Figure 5.8** represents the drug-loaded smart hydrogels and their uses in medicinal field. The diagram illustrates how these hydrogels can be made to respond to such stimuli as temperature, pH, electricity magnetic field, light, glucose, and enzymes. When stimulated, the hydrogel matrix dispenses with its drug content, indicated by the red spheres moving away from a complex lattice. The types of use are illustrated to the right and next to it with reference to wound dressing, use on bone implants, osteoporosis, cancer, and contact lenses among others. The smart hydrogel system also exemplifies the effectiveness of a new model of delivering drugs in many treatments in the field of medicine [42].

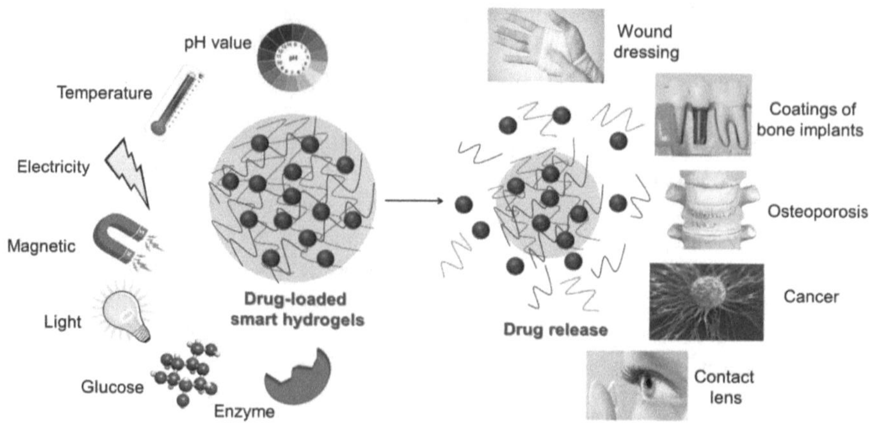

FIGURE 5.8 Hydrogels with intelligence for use in advanced drug delivery systems [42]. (Creative Commons Attribution 4.0)

Such coatings can be designed to release therapeutic agents when exposed to specific changes in pH or temperature, or when specific enzymes are active, or indeed when they are exposed to light. The pH-sensitive polymers can release drugs in response to acidic tumor microenvironments, while thermo-sensitive coatings can release drugs upon exposure to localized heat. Advanced systems include those in which molecular recognition is embedded at the structural level. The polymers used to deliver the drug are designed to selectively identify a given biomarker [43]. This is useful for the precise delivery of medicine, using smart coatings in a way that can reform individually tailored treatment by targeting drugs at disease-stricken tissues only when they are required, and where they are needed, thus harnessing the full potential therapeutic effects while avoiding the negative impact of systemic drug delivery on healthy tissues. This approach could enhance the efficacy of nearly every known affliction, from malignant tumors to chronic illnesses by personalizing medications administration to a particular patient's need or conditions.

5.5 FUTURE SCOPE

Smart materials have revolutionized the biomedical sector using different cutting-edge technologies such as thermal spray coating and additive manufacturing. The laser machining of composites has been investigated to develop complete surface control and precise material removal capabilities that aid biomedical high-performance coating fabrication [44–48]. The additive manufacturing technology for shape memory alloys has led to the development of smart biomedical products, which offer better functionality and customization possibilities [49–51]. The use of machine learning techniques continues to grow in number because they help forecast machining characteristics along with optimizing the mechanical properties of 3D-printed materials, which ensures components can satisfy the demanding standards of biomedical applications [52–54]. Post-processing treatments that incorporate laser-based techniques enhance biomedical implants by creating better bioimplant bonds as well as increasing wear durability [55, 56]. The life of biomedical implants can be increased by deposition of thermal spray coatings [57–70].

Medical implants exhibit enhanced performance outcomes due to the adoption of zirconia-based materials with added special biopolymer coatings and new surface treatment methods [71–74]. Modern coating solutions enable the manufacture of implants with enhanced qualities and higher dependability. Scientists develop reactive coatings that detect body changes and external environment conditions through automatic response mechanisms. Real-time health tracking sensors integrated into these medical coatings would permit doctors to find early implant abnormalities leading to better patient safety. Scientists need to address various challenges about coating longevity while the materials show body safety and mass production scalability to implement these coatings in real-world applications.

5.6 CONCLUSION

Some recent developments of advanced coating technology in biomedical science include cell membrane-coated nanoparticles for drug delivery and antimicrobial peptides coatings for implant. Hydrophilic, antimicrobial, and cell-adhesive coatings have enhanced function, durability, and safety of medical implants and devices. Polymer-based coatings as well as stimuli-responsive coatings for sustained drug delivery have emerged as state-of-the-art technology. But there are several issues left to address, more specifically durability, long-term stability, capacity extension, manufacturability, biocompatibility, and immune response. The next generation of coating technology therefore holds potential in smart and adaptive coatings, self-healing coatings, nanostructured coatings, bio-mimicking coatings, and smart drug delivery and target coatings which are responsive to living tissue signals.

REFERENCES

1. Abbady HE, Klinkenberg ET, de Moel L, Nicolai N, van der Stelt M, Verhulst AC, Maal TJ, Brouwers L. 3D-printed prostheses in developing countries: A systematic review. *Prosthetics Orthotics International*. 2022;46:19–30.
2. Liu H, Su Y-Y, Jiang X-C, Gao J-Q. Cell membrane-coated nanoparticles: A novel multifunctional biomimetic drug delivery system. *Drug Delivery Translational Research*. 2023;13:716–37.
3. Liu L, Wang S, Zhang B, Jiang G, Liu H, Yang J, Wang J, Liu W. Present status and prospects of nanostructured thermal barrier coatings and their performance improvement strategies: A review. *Journal of Manufacturing Processes*. 2023;97:12–34.
4. Mehta A, Singh G. Consequences of hydroxyapatite doping using plasma spray to implant biomaterials. *Journal of Electrochemical Science Engineering Failure Analysis*. 2023;13:5–23.
5. Mehta A, Vasudev H, Jeyaprakash N. Role of sustainable manufacturing approach: Microwave processing of materials. *International Journal on Interactive Design Manufacturing*. 2023:1–17.
6. Mehta A, Vasudev H, Singh S. Sustainable manufacturing approach with novel thermal barrier coatings in lowering CO2 emissions: Performance analysis with probable solutions. *International Journal on Interactive Design Manufacturing*. 2023:1–13.

7. Abdulghafor MA, Mahmood MK, Tassery H, Tardivo D, Falguiere A, Lan R. Biomimetic coatings in implant dentistry: A quick update. *Journal of Functional Biomaterials*. 2023;15:15.
8. Abdullah JY, Abdullah AM, Hadi H, Husein A, Rajion ZA. Comparison of STL skull models produced using open-source software versus commercial software. *Rapid Prototyping Journal*. 2019;25:1585–91.
9. Faustino CM, Lemos SM, Monge N, Ribeiro IA. A scope at antifouling strategies to prevent catheter-associated infections. *Advances in Colloid Interface Science*. 2020;284:102230.
10. Abdelgawad M, Park P, Wheeler AR. Optimization of device geometry in single-plate digital microfluidics. *Journal of Applied Physics*. 2009;105.
11. Ali T, Najam-ul-Haq M, Mohyuddin A, Musharraf SG, Hussain D. Next-generation functional nanotextiles—Prospects and challenges. *Sustainable Materials Technologies*. 2023:e00640.
12. Allahdini A, Jafari R, Momen G. Transparent non-fluorinated superhydrophobic coating with enhanced anti-icing performance. *Progress in Organic Coatings*. 2022;165:106758.
13. Asadollahi S, Profili J, Farzaneh M, Stafford L. Development of organosilicon-based superhydrophobic coatings through atmospheric pressure plasma polymerization of HMDSO in nitrogen plasma. *Materials*. 2019;12:219.
14. Attarzadeh R, Dolatabadi A. Icephobic performance of superhydrophobic coatings: A numerical analysis. *International Journal of Heat Mass Transfer*. 2019;136:1327–37.
15. Knetsch ML, Koole LH. New strategies in the development of antimicrobial coatings: The example of increasing usage of silver and silver nanoparticles. *Polymers*. 2011;3:340–66.
16. Su Q, Chang S, Zhao Y, Zheng H, Dang C. A review of loop heat pipes for aircraft anti-icing applications. *Applied Thermal Engineering*. 2018;130:528–40.
17. Missirlis D, Spatz JP. Combined effects of PEG hydrogel elasticity and cell-adhesive coating on fibroblast adhesion and persistent migration. *Biomacromolecules*. 2014;15: 195–205.
18. Suzuki K, Hiroi Y, Abe-Fukasawa N, Nishino T, Shouji T, Katayama J, Kageyama T, Fukuda J. Cell-repellent polyampholyte for conformal coating on microstructures. *Scientific Reports*. 2022;12:10815.
19. Kovacs B, Patko D, Szekacs I, Orgovan N, Kurunczi S, Sulyok A, Khanh NQ, Toth B, Vonderviszt F, Horvath R. Flagellin based biomimetic coatings: From cell-repellent surfaces to highly adhesive coatings. *Acta Biomaterialia*. 2016;42:66–76.
20. Rykowska I, Nowak I, Nowak R. Drug-eluting stents and balloons—materials, structure designs, and coating techniques: A review. *Molecules*. 2020;25:4624.
21. Wang Y, Zhang W, Zhang J, Sun W, Zhang R, Gu H. Fabrication of a novel polymer-free nanostructured drug-eluting coating for cardiovascular stents. *ACS Applied Materials Interfaces*. 2013;5:10337–45.
22. Abbasnezhad N, Zirak N, Champmartin S, Shirinbayan M, Bakir F. An overview of in vitro drug release methods for drug-eluting stents. *Polymers*. 2022;14:2751.
23. McKittrick C, Cardona M, Black R, McCormick C. Development of a bioactive polymeric drug eluting coronary stent coating using electrospraying. *Annals of Biomedical Engineering*. 2020;48:271–81.
24. Hu T, Lin S, Du R, Fu M, Rao Q, Yin T, Huang Y, Wang G. Design, preparation and performance of a novel drug-eluting stent with multiple layer coatings. *Biomaterials Science*. 2017;5:1845–57.
25. Mehmood A, Scibioh MA, Prabhuram J, An M-G, Ha HY. A review on durability issues and restoration techniques in long-term operations of direct methanol fuel cells. *Journal of Power Sources*. 2015;297:224–41.

26. Boinovich L, Emelyanenko AM, Pashinin AS. Analysis of long-term durability of superhydrophobic properties under continuous contact with water. *ACS Applied Materials Interfaces*. 2010;2:1754–8.
27. Nasiri S, Khosravani MR. Machine learning in predicting mechanical behavior of additively manufactured parts. *Journal of Materials Research Technology*. 2021;14:1137–53.
28. Sharma Y, Mehta A, Vasudev H, Jeyaprakash N, Prashar G, Prakash C. Analysis of friction stir welds using numerical modelling approach: A comprehensive review. *International Journal on Interactive Design Manufacturing*. 2023:1–14.
29. Prashar G, Vasudev H, Mehta A. Application of Bimodal structured thermal sprayed coatings in power plant components. *Advanced Ceramic Coatings for Energy Applications*. 2024:273–87.
30. Saxena A, Mehta A, Vasudev H, Prashar G, Jasim NY. A short review on machine learning for the purpose of optimizing and predicting the properties of polymeric nanocomposites. *Materials Today: Proceedings*. 2023. https://doi.org/10.1016/j.matpr.2023.07.347
31. Yedida VS, Mehta A, Vasudev H, Singh S. Role of numerical modeling in predicting the oxidation behavior of thermal barrier coatings. *International Journal on Interactive Design Manufacturing*. 2024;18:5653–62.
32. Al-Turjman F, Zahmatkesh H. A comprehensive review on the use of AI in UAV communications: Enabling technologies, applications, and challenges. *Unmanned Aerial Vehicles in Smart Cities*. 2020:1–26.
33. Alves T, Das R, Morris T. Embedding encryption and machine learning intrusion prevention systems on programmable logic controllers. *IEEE Embedded Systems Letters*. 2018;10:99–102.
34. Allaire G, Bogosel B. Optimizing supports for additive manufacturing. *Structural Multidisciplinary Optimization*. 2018;58:2493–515.
35. Altıparmak SC YV, Shi Z, Lin J. Challenges in additive manufacturing of high-strength aluminium alloys and current developments in hybrid additive manufacturing. *International Journal of Lightweight Materials Manufacture*. 2021;4:246–61.
36. Tan YJ, Susanto GJ, Anwar Ali HP, Tee BC. Progress and roadmap for intelligent self-healing materials in autonomous robotics. *Advanced Materials*. 2021;33:2002800.
37. Ataie A, Mostaghimi J, Pershin L, Xu P. Fabrication of nanostructured cobalt ferrite coatings using suspension plasma spraying (SPS) technique. *Surface Coatings Technology*. 2017;328:451–61.
38. Farooq SA, Raina A, Mohan S, Arvind Singh R, Jayalakshmi S, Irfan Ul Haq M. Nanostructured coatings: Review on processing techniques, corrosion behaviour and tribological performance. *Nanomaterials*. 2022;12:1323.
39. Bakhsheshi-Rad H, Najafinezhad A, Hadisi Z, Iqbal N, Daroonparvar M, Sharif S, Ismail AF, Akbari M, RamaKrishna S, Berto F. Characterization and biological properties of nanostructured clinoenstatite scaffolds for bone tissue engineering applications. *Materials Chemistry Physics*. 2021;259:123969.
40. Sezavar A, Sajjadi SA, Babakhani A, Peng RL, Yuan K. Oxidation behavior of a nanostructured compositionally graded layer (CGL) thermal barrier coating (TBC) deposited on IN-738LC. *Surface Coatings Technology*. 2019;374:374–82.
41. Zhang L, Tang Z, Fang J, Jiang X, Jiang Y-P, Sun Q-J, Fan J-M, Tang X-G, Zhong G. Synaptic and resistive switching behaviors in NiO/Cu2O heterojunction memristor for bioinspired neuromorphic computing. *Applied Surface Science*. 2022;606:154718.
42. Bordbar-Khiabani A, Gasik MJIJoMS. Smart hydrogels for advanced drug delivery systems. *International Journal of Molecular Sciences*. 2022;23:3665.
43. Karimi M, Bahrami S, Ravari SB, Zangabad PS, Mirshekari H, Bozorgomid M, Shahreza S, Sori M, Hamblin MR. Albumin nanostructures as advanced drug delivery systems. *Expert Opinion on Drug Delivery*. 2016;13:1609–23.

44. Sharma V, Kumar V. Application of Box-Behnken design and response surface methodology for multi-optimization of laser cutting of AA5052/ZrO2 metal–matrix composites. *Proceedings of the Institution of Mechanical Engineers, Part L: Journal of Materials: Design and Applications*. 2018;232(8):652–68.
45. Sharma V, Kumar V. Comparison of machining characteristics of metal matrix composites using CO2 laser curve cutting process. *Proceedings of the Institution of Mechanical Engineers, Part E: Journal of Process Mechanical Engineering*. 2018;232(3):349–68.
46. Sharma V, Kumar V. Investigating the quality characteristics of Al5052/SiC metal matrix composites machined by CO2 laser curve cutting. *Proceedings of the Institution of Mechanical Engineers, Part L: Journal of Materials: Design and Applications*. 2018;232(1):3–19.
47. Sharma V, Kumar V, Bist A. Investigations on morphology and material removal rate of various MMCs using CO2 laser technique. *Journal of the Brazilian Society of Mechanical Sciences and Engineering*. 2020;42:1–14.
48. Sharma V, Singh JP, Raman R, Bathla G, Saini A. Machine learning approach for prediction analysis of aluminium alloy on the surface roughness using CO2 laser machining. *Proceedings of the Institution of Mechanical Engineers, Part E: Journal of Process Mechanical Engineering*. 2024;09544089241231093.
49. Singh R, Toseef M, Kumar J, Singh J. Benefits and challenges in additive manufacturing and its applications. In: Kaushal S, Singh I, Singh S, Gupta A, editors. *Sustainable Advanced Manufacturing and Materials Processing*. 1st ed. Boca Raton: CRC Press; 2022. pp. 137–57. https://doi.org/10.1201/9781003269298-8.
50. Singh J. Sustainability issues in laser-based additive manufacturing. In: *Handbook of Laser-Based Sustainable Surface Modification and Manufacturing Techniques*. CRC Press; 2023. pp. 167–89.
51. Ahmad S, et al. Innovations in additive manufacturing of shape memory alloys: Alloys, microstructures, treatments, applications. *Journal of Materials Research and Technology*. 2024;32:4136–97.
52. Sharma V, Singh JP, Hussan K, Kumar R. Machine learning approach for predicting the machining characteristics of additive manufactured ABS material. *Proceedings of the Institution of Mechanical Engineers, Part C: Journal of Mechanical Engineering Science*. 2024;09544062241283330.
53. Chohan JS, et al. Mechanical strength enhancement of 3D printed acrylonitrile butadiene styrene polymer components using neural network optimization algorithm. *Polymers*. 2020;12(10). https://doi.org/10.3390/polym12102250.
54. Singh J, et al. Impact of molding temperature, fiber loading and chemical modifications on the physicomechanical, and microstructural morphology properties of woven kenaf Fiber/PLA composites for non-structural applications. *Journal of Natural Fibers*. 2024;21(1):2326586.
55. Singh J. Applications of laser technology for processing and post-treatments of powders and coatings. In: *Handbook of Laser-Based Sustainable Surface Modification and Manufacturing Techniques*. CRC Press; 2023. pp. 135–66.
56. Sunitha K, Vasudev H. A short note on the various thermal spray coating processes and effect of post-treatment on Ni-based coatings. *Materials Today: Proceedings*. 2022;50:1452–7. https://doi.org/10.1016/j.matpr.2021.09.017.
57. Sharanabasava H, et al. Microstructure, mechanical and wear properties of SiC and Mo reinforced NiCr microwave cladding. *Advanced Materials and Processing Technologies*. 2024;10:3620–33.
58. Singh J, Gill HS. Evolution of nickel-based superalloy claddings for against high-temperature oxidation and wear. In: *Thermal Claddings for Engineering Applications*. CRC Press; 2024. pp. 160–81.

59. Singh J, Kumar S, Kumar R, Mohapatra SK. Machine learning regression tools for erosion prediction of WC-10Co4Cr thermal spray coating. *Results Surfaces Interfaces.* 2023;13:100156. https://doi.org/10.1016/j.rsurfi.2023.100156.
60. Yedida VVS, Vasudev H. A review on the development of thermal barrier coatings by using thermal spray techniques. *Materials Today: Proceedings.* 2022;50:1458–64.
61. Singh J, Singh S. Support vector machine learning on slurry erosion characteristics analysis of Ni- and Co-alloy coatings. *Surface Review and Letters.* 2023. https://doi.org/10.1142/S0218625X23400061.
62. Prashar G, Vasudev H. A review on the influence of process parameters and heat treatment on the corrosion performance of Ni-based thermal spray coatings. *Surface Review and Letters.* 2022;29(1):2230001.
63. Singh J, Vasudev H, Szala M, Gill HS. Neural computing for erosion assessment in Al-20TiO2 HVOF thermal spray coating. *International Journal on Interactive Design and Manufacturing.* 2024;18:2321–32.
64. Singh J, Vasudev H, Kumar R, Ubaidullah M. Study on wear analysis of Ni-20Al2O3 HVOF micron layers using artificial neural network technique. *The International Journal on Interactive Design and Manufacturing.* 2023;18:5925–38. https://doi.org/10.1007/s12008-023-01433-2.
65. Prashar G, Vasudev H. Surface topology analysis of plasma sprayed Inconel625-Al2O3 composite coating. *Materials Today: Proceedings.* 2022;50:607–11. https://doi.org/10.1016/j.matpr.2021.03.090.
66. Thakur L, Vasudev H, Singh J, Prashar G. *Artificial Intelligence and Machine Learning in the Thermal Spray Industry: Practices, Implementation, and Challenges.* CRC Press; 2023.
67. Dutta V, Thakur L, Singh B, Vasudev H. A study of erosion–corrosion behaviour of friction stir-processed chromium-reinforced NiAl bronze composite. *Materials (Basel).* 2022;15(15):5401. https://doi.org/10.3390/ma15155401.
68. Singh J, Singh S, Vasudev H, Chohan JS, Kumar S. Neural computing and Taguchi's method-based study on erosion of advanced Mo2C–WC10Co4Cr coating for the centrifugal pump. *Advances in Materials and Processing Technologies.* 2024;10(3):2569–81.
69. Singh J, Singh S, Vasudev H, Katiyar JK. Artificial neural network model for wear characteristic analysis of WC-10Co4Cr and Stellite 6 thermal spray coatings. *Tribology International.* 2024;199:109924.
70. Majji BGR, Vasudev H, Bansal A. A review on the oxidation and wear behavior of the thermally sprayed high-entropy alloys. *Materials Today: Proceedings.* 2022;50:1447–51.
71. Singh J, Singh S, Verma A. Artificial intelligence in use of ZrO2 material in biomedical science. *Journal of Electrochemical Science and Engineering.* 2022;13(1):83–97. https://doi.org/10.5599/jese.1498.
72. Singh J, Hashmi AW, Behra A, Kumar A, Dogra N, Kumar P. Review of Mg alloys for bio-implants protected by the deposition of chemical conversion coatings. In *AIP Conference Proceedings.* AIP Publishing; 2024.
73. Singh J, Singh S, Gill R. Applications of biopolymer coatings in biomedical engineering. *Journal of Electrochemical Science and Engineering.* 2022;13(1):63–81. https://doi.org/10.5599/jese.1460.
74. Singh CJ, Ram B, Singh J, Prakash C, Paramasivam P, Kumar R. Experimental investigation on characterization of friction stir processed AZ31-based composite. *Scientific Reports.* 2024;14(1):15453.

6 Development of Biodegradable Materials and Advanced Coating Technologies for Biomedical Devices

Hardeep Kaur, Kashish Garg, Shinar Athwal, Rimika Thakur, Saksham Singh, Sandeep Singh, Ranjit Bariki, and Chandra Mohan

CONTENTS

6.1 INTRODUCTION

Technological breakthroughs have highly impacted human existence, leading to the modification of numerous procedures and modern healing methods that have significantly enhanced the standard of living [1,2]. Nevertheless, the innovation

 DOI: 10.1201/9781003516064-6

of biomaterials has revolutionized healthcare by providing a greener alternative solution for numerous illnesses and diseases [3–6]. For instance, in the United States alone, numerous implantable medical devices have been equipped to perform various revisionary surgeries for millions of people [7]. Additionally, these biodegradable materials fabricated by various manufacturing processes like 3D printing (**Figure 6.1**) have been exercised in various bioimplants and biomedical devices that have become a significant part of modern medicine [8–10], performing various therapeutic, diagnostic, and regenerative functions, which have led to the development of various clinical procedures, like percutaneous coronary intervention, total bone replacement, vital-sign monitoring, treating cardiovascular diseases, tissue repair, fracture fixation, dental screws, hip replacement, controlled drug delivery, cardiac stunts, joint arthrodesis, and electronic pacing [7,10–17]. Further, the efficiency of these biomedical devices is highly impacted by their surface coatings and bulk attributes of the materials that are utilized in the formation of the biomedical devices resulting in the modernization of these biomedical devices, which had touched the threshold of choosing the specific materials based upon their properties [14,17–20]

Owing to the osteoconductivity, toughness, non-infectivity, biocompatibility, mechanical and thermal properties, high strength, ease of processing, and low immunogenicity, material based upon polymers, composites, chitosan, ceramics, and metal alloys such as platinum alloy (pacemaker), titanium-hydroxyapatite (dental restorations),

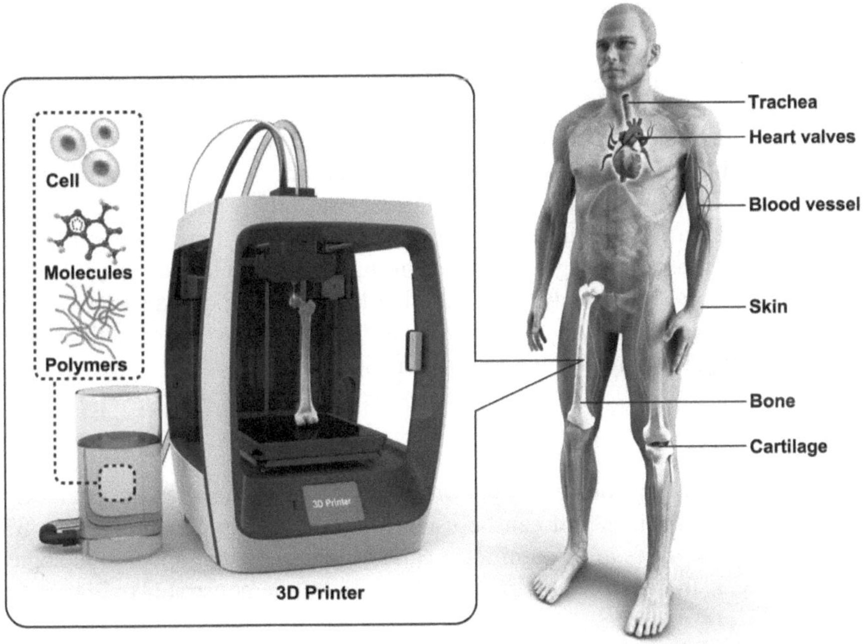

FIGURE 6.1 Representation of a 3D printing machine used for grafting various human organs [36]. (Permissions under Creative Commons Attribution 4.0 International License)

magnesium alloys (orthopedics), and so on have been employed for the formation of the biomedical devices [3,10,18,21–27]. Nonetheless, these materials encountered major setbacks, like poor interface bonding, corrosion, low stimulation toward foreign bodies and inflammation, lower mechanical strength, liberation of H_2 gas, ferromagnetic behavior, poor contrast, high density, poor vascularization, transparency, swelling, accumulation of by-products, and degradation [1,23,24,28]. However, innovation of the cutting-edge coating technologies, such as anodizing, dip-coating, Langmuir-Blodgett deposition, sputtering, electrochemical plating, spray coating, chemical grafting, surface-tethered polymers, self-assembled monolayers, electrophoretic deposition method, spin coating, and chemical vapor deposition have been equipped to seize the impacting limitations [3,24,29,30]. Indeed, these coatings are made up of smart self-healing materials (heparin, fibrin, titanium, layered double hydroxide, fluoride-based, graphene oxide, hyaluronic acid, endothelial cells, magnesium, phosphate, and ceramics), which not only create the physical barrier along with the increase in wear and tear resistance but also act as the antifouling agent [31–33]. Moreover, these coatings are flexible and can be exploited for biomimetic surfaces and controlled release of hydrophobic and hydrophilic drugs [34], which can be further used for the enhancement of biomedical devices [35]. This chapter discusses various techniques and materials that can contribute toward the development of advanced biomedical devices.

6.2 BIODEGRADABLE MATERIALS

By the action of microorganisms, these biodegradable substances are intended to convert itself into numerous environmental-friendly substances such as the biomass residues, water, and carbon dioxide. For waste reduction and environmental impact mitigation, these materials are essential. Biodegradable substances can be categorized as polymers, natural biodegradable materials, and biodegradable composites that are exploited in numerous methods which are illustrated in **Figure 6.2.**

Biodegradable polymers are a significant class of materials that undergo biological decomposition in their natural environment. Naturally occurring biodegradable materials that form from renewable resources are becoming more and more important because of their advantages for the environment and their uses in a variety of industries and biomedicine. Advanced materials known as biodegradable composites combine biodegradable polymers with reinforcing materials to improve the materials' functionality, biocompatibility, and mechanical qualities.

6.2.1 Polymers

Polymers are important biodegradable materials because they can be engineered to have specific attributes and can be used in a vast variety of applications [37]. Biodegradable polymers are a significant class of materials that undergo biological decomposition in their natural environment [19] which is demonstrated in **Figure 6.3.**

6.2.1.1 Polylactic Acid (PLA)

Polylactic acid (PLA) is defined as the aliphatic thermoplastic that is generated from renewable resources like sugarcane or corn starch. PLA is perfect for

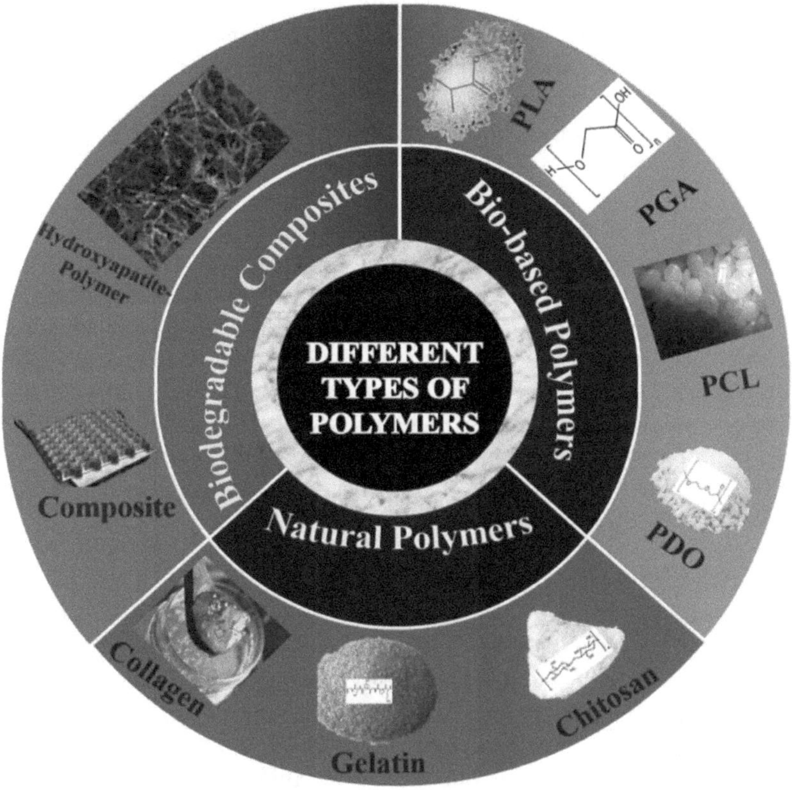

FIGURE 6.2 Different types of polymers.

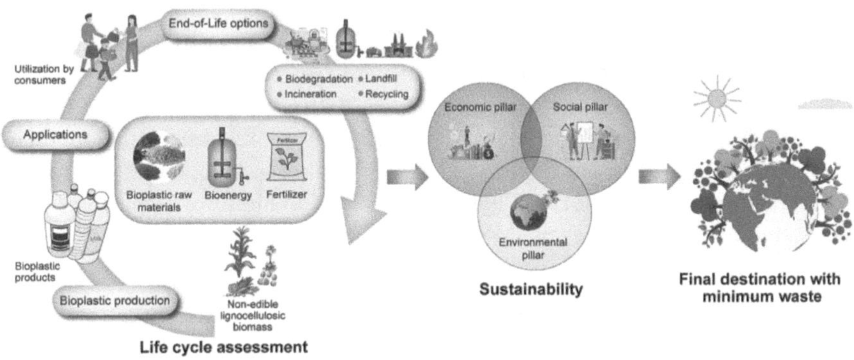

FIGURE 6.3 Systematic representation of the life cycle of biodegradable plastic [38]. (Permissions under Creative Commons Attribution 4.0 International License)

packaging, disposable tableware, medical implants, and 3D printing because of its advantageous properties (transparency and good mechanical strength) highlighted in recent studies [39–42]. However, the biodegradation of these PLA generates the natural lactic acid under optimized conditions [43]. Furthermore, the PLA composites and blends are employed to increase its applicability and working performance [44].

6.2.1.2 Polyglycolic Acid (PGA)

Another type of biodegradable thermoplastic polymer, polyglycolic acid (PGA) is mostly employed in the medical field like medical sutures, tissue engineering, and drug delivery systems owing to its high tensile strength, biocompatible nature, high crystallinity, and quick rate of degradation [19]. Generally, glycolic acid is obtained by hydrolyzing PGA, which is further converted to carbon dioxide and water, making it a suitable candidate for temporary implants [43]. Despite having such properties, this bioplastic faces setback due to its poor degradation rates and low mechanical qualities, leading to find the various ways to overcome these limitations and expand the applicability of these plastics [45].

6.2.1.3 Polycaprolactone (PCL)

Polycaprolactone (PCL) is a biodegradable polyester that is flexible and possesses lower melting point along with high elongation and easy processability that makes it compatible to use with other materials. However, owing to its high degradation stability, this material usually find its way in various long-term applications such as biodegradable composites, medical devices, and drug delivery systems [46]. During its hydrolysis under physiological conditions, PCL gets transformed into caproic acid due to the internal breakdown of the ester linkages. Recent research has uncovered PCL's potential in the field of sustained drug release and tissue engineering scaffolds [7,43].

6.2.1.4 Polydioxanone (PDO)

Another biodegradable polymer polydioxanone, with its crystalline structure, flexibility, and good tensile strength, is used in various medical applications. The degradation rate of PDO is lower when compared to that of PGA and faster than that of PCL [47]. This polymer when employed with various materials gives the biocompatibility and the good knot security. These PDO polymers can be used in various scaffolds in tissue engineering and surgical procedures due to the generation p-dioxanone by the action of hydrolyses, which further get metabolized into water and carbon dioxide. This research is needed to develop more sophisticated medical devices, and to improve mechanical properties [43].

6.2.2 Natural Biodegradable Materials

Polymeric materials obtained from natural, renewable source that can be easily decomposed in the environment are becoming increasingly popular because of the advantages associated with their usage in different sectors of economy such as biomedical science. In these polymers, collagen, gelatin, and chitosan are of prime consideration due to their versatile characteristics.

6.2.2.1 Collagen and Gelatin

Some of the practical polymers include gelatin, which is a polymer of the collagen protein that has undergone hydrolytic degradation, for medical use due to its excellent amino acid composition. It is accessible in forms of tablets, granules, or powder and can be ingested by dissolving in water [48]. Recent findings focus on its value in serving as a substrate for three-dimensional cell culture and in composites intended for tissue engineering constructs. High in proteins and low in calories, this food substance has no fats or cholesterol; thus, gelatin is a protective colloid. It binds well with oil and water phases preventing casein and soy protein clotting in stomach acid enhancing digestion [49]. It happens mainly due to the gelling and texturizing properties of gelatin that it finds significant application in the food industry. It is used to improve the texture of dessert, as a stabilizer in shrink-packaged meats, and as an ingredient in fruits salads and ice cream production among others. It also finds uses in producing edible films and coatings [50]. Significant other uses extend to the cosmetic and health industries and skincare on behalf of film-forming alongside nutritional attributes. In medicine, gelatin plays a role in hydrogels, pharmaceutical preparations, cell transplantation, and vehicles [51]. An example is collagen, a structural protein that possesses high tensile strength, biocompatibility, and biodegradability, found in high concentrations in animals' extracellular matrix (ECM) [48]. It is a unique matrix that finds useful application in areas such as tissue engineering and several pharmacy and medical uses. Collagen-based scaffolds demonstrate high potential for use in vascular tissue engineering, bone regeneration, and skin tissue engineering [52]. These scaffolds are perfect for producing biomimetic tissue because they offer an environment that promotes cell differentiation, adhesion, and proliferation. Collagen nanofibers are made that imitate the ECM found in nature and improve cell interactions and tissue integration (**Figure 6.4**), for instance, by electro-spinning methods [53].

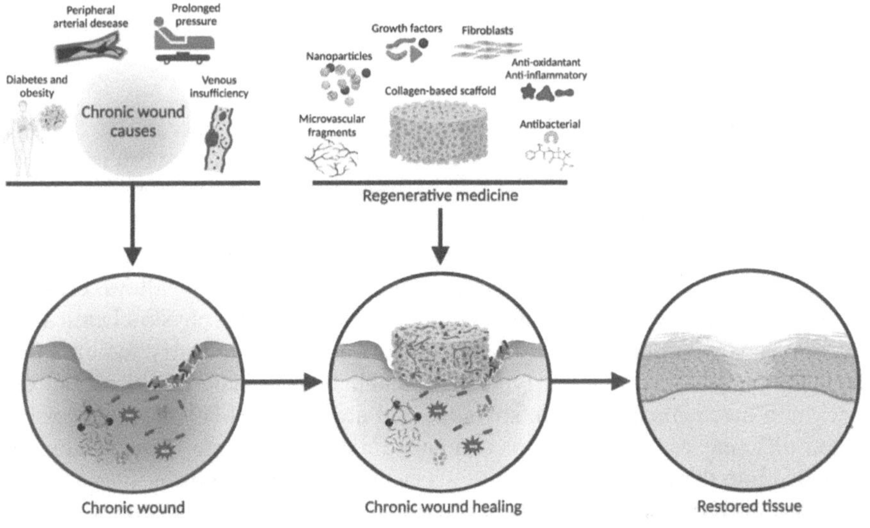

FIGURE 6.4 Collagen-based scaffold used in chronic wound healing [54]. (Permissions under Creative Commons Attribution 4.0 International License)

6.2.2.2 Chitosan

Chitosan, derived from chitin, is a copolymer that consists of glucosamine and its substitute (N-acetyl glucosamine). It is becoming a popular raw material for various products such as food, industry, medical appliances, pharmaceutical, agriculture, and so on [55]. This is because of the presence of the amino group and hydroxyl functional moieties, which give chitosan multiple properties such as a poly-electrolysis, antimicrobial activity, antioxidant activity, gel-foaming, biocompatibility, metal chelation, and eased processability [56].

The biopolymer chitin is the parent compound of chitosan, which is found in a wide variety of organisms, such as in the exoskeletons of crustaceans, insects, and mollusks; algae; and fungal cell walls [57]. Industrial applications primarily use chitosan sourced from crustaceans such as crabs, prawns, and shrimp shells [58]. These exoskeletons are abundant waste products from the food manufacturing plants. The United States Food and Drug Administration (USFDA) has already approved commercial products that produce the homeostatic agents that are exploited for the healing and management of wounds and is most well-known applications of chitosan [59]. Moreover, the antimicrobial property against numerous infectious organisms like bacteria, filamentous fungi, and yeast is observed by the action of chitosan and its derivatives. Bacteria cannot grow even after discarding the polymer from the media, suggesting that chitosan possesses growth-inhibitory activities. This becomes essential due to the fact that the resistance populations may emerge if the cells adapt to chitosan.

6.2.3 Biodegradable Composites

Advanced materials known as biodegradable composites combine biodegradable polymers with reinforcing materials to improve the materials' functionality, biocompatibility, and mechanical qualities. Recent studies focus on optimizing these composites for various applications, especially in the environment and biomedical domains.

6.2.3.1 Composite Materials

Composite materials are composed of two or more constituent materials with distinct physio-chemical properties. They combine to form a material with unique characteristics that differ from that of individual components [60]. According to Chawla (2012), the future of technological advancements hinges upon composite substances. These materials offer numerous benefits over metals, alloys, ceramics, and polymers, as they can be engineered to possess specific physio-chemical and thermo-mechanism properties. For example, the aerospace industry requires lightweight materials with properties typically found in heavier materials like wear resistance, high mechanical strength, stiffness, and abrasion [61]. Various authors have created different classifications for composite materials. These classifications can be divided into three main categories: particle-reinforced composites that use inclusions with uniform axes, fiber-reinforced composites that use fiber-like inclusions, and structural composites that combine composites with homogenous materials. The major differentiation between the first two categories is the shape of dispersed phase particles. Particle-type composites typically have spherical particles, while fiber-type composites have irregular geometries but higher length-to-diameter ratios, similar to natural fibers [62,63].

6.2.3.2 Hydroxyapatite-Polymer Composites

Hydroxyapatite (HA)-polymer composites stand out particularly in the field of biodegradable materials owing to their superior osteoconductivity and biocompatibility [64]. Mixing biodegradable polymers with hydroxyapatite (HA0, a significant constituent of natural bone), results in a composite material that facilitates bone regrowth and blends seamlessly with native bone tissue [65]. There is an extensive use of these composite materials in dental implants, orthopedic devices, and bone tissue engineering [66–69]. When the polymer matrix gradually breaks down and makes way for new bone tissue to grow in its place, the HA acts as scaffold to increase the attachment and proliferation of bone cells [70]. Progress in recent times has been directed toward strengthening bonding between HA particles and the polymer matrix at the interface to augment mechanical characteristics and guarantee the stability and efficacy of the composite in biomedical settings.

6.3 ADVANCED COATING TECHNOLOGIES

6.3.1 Bioactive Coatings

Medical implants integrate and function better when coated with bioactive materials that have a positive interaction with biological tissues (**Figure 6.5**). The enhancement of implants' biocompatibility and effectiveness in diverse medical applications is contingent upon their critical roles [71].

The controlled release and encapsulation of pharmaceuticals is achieved by polymeric coating, which employs biodegradable polymers like PGA and PLA. To improve treatment efficacy and minimize systemic side effects, drug-eluting coatings are made to deliver therapeutic agents at controlled rates right at the site of implantation. To improve the way medical implants interact with biological tissues, surface enhancement techniques are used to change the surface properties of the implants. With dynamic control over their properties and functions, smart coatings are engineered to react to the environmental stimuli. The innovation of intelligent biomedical devices that can adjust to shifting bodily conditions has advanced significantly with the help of these coatings.

6.3.1.1 Hydroxyapatite Coatings

Hydroxyapatite (HA) is made up of calcium phosphate, which is exploited as the bioactive coatings for coating dental and orthopedic implants and closely resembles the mineral component of the bone. The implant-bounded tissues of bone can accelerate the tissue growth and can bind with these implants due to the enhanced osteoconductivity of the HA coatings. Usually applied using methods like plasma spraying (**Figure 6.6**), these coatings produce a surface that enhances the implant's stability and integration with the bone. Studies have shown the significance of the enhancement in the growth of the bone and decrease in the healing times as compared to that of non-coated implants [71].

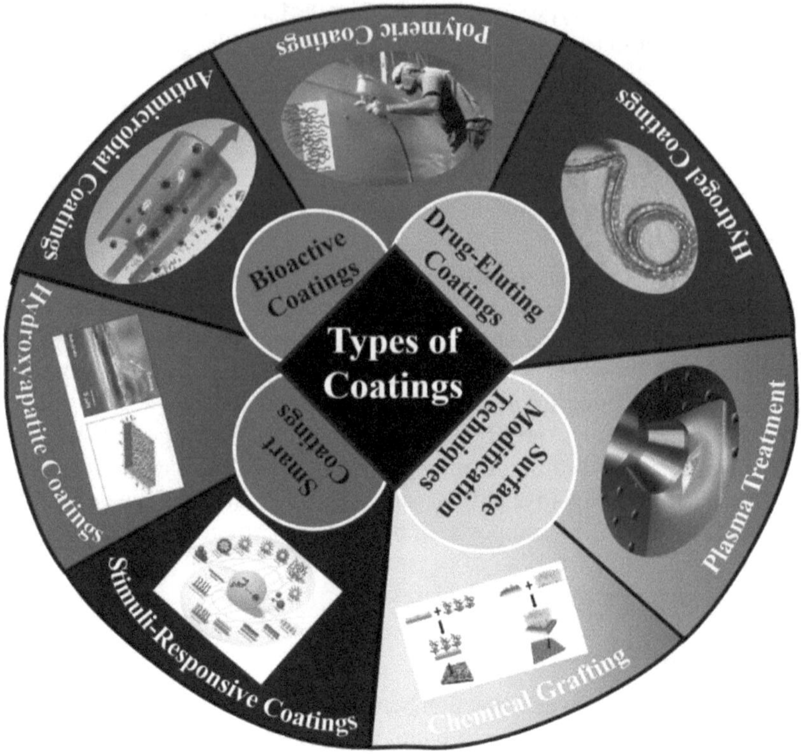

FIGURE 6.5 Types of coatings.

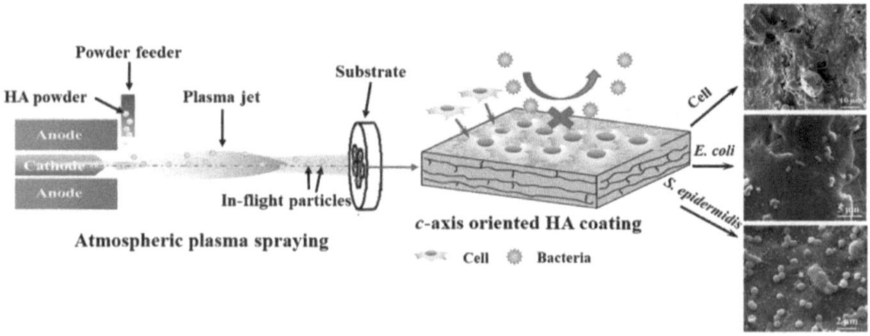

FIGURE 6.6 Illustration of the plasma spraying technique that is employed for carving HA coatings [72]. (Permissions under Creative Commons Attribution 4.0 International License)

6.3.1.2 Antimicrobial Coatings

The invasions of microorganisms in the body lead to various types of infections. Hence, the antimicrobial coatings become crucial. These antimicrobial coatings release the antimicrobial agents such as antimicrobial peptides, silver nanoparticles, and antibiotics, which are responsible for the prevention of bacterial growth upon the implant's surface (**Figure 6.6**). These particles break down the cell wall of bacteria which stops the formation of biofilms [73,74]. Studies based upon recent research have shown that the antimicrobial coatings, having the longer duration of antimicrobial efficacy can reduce the infection rates and increase the shelf-life of the implants, henceforth making it suitable for the applications in various places like the hospitals and surgical rooms, having higher probability of bacterial contamination [75].

6.3.2 Drug-Eluting Coatings

These coatings face various systemic setbacks; so to overcome the same and increase the treatment efficacy, drug-eluting coatings are fabricated that are functionalized to deliver the therapeutic agents at the site of implantation under controlled rates [76,77].

6.3.2.1 Polymeric Coatings

A polymeric coating comprising polylactic acid (PLA) and polyglycolic acids (PGA) is used to achieve the encapsulation and controlled release of pharmaceuticals. This type of coatings find applications in drug-eluting stents, in which they release the anti-proliferative medications, which help in the prevention of restenosis. These coatings improve the patients' outcome by lowering the repeat interventions, reducing the risk of drug-related complications, and ensuring prolonged therapeutic effect [78].

6.3.2.2 Hydrogel Coatings

It has become possible to deliver these pharmaceuticals at controlled rates due to the hydrophilic polymers-based hydrogel coatings that can swell up and hold water in large quantities. Drugs can be released from these coatings, depending upon the elevation in temperature, pH, or other environmental entities by engineering them to respond to particular stimuli. Applications needing sustained and localized drug delivery benefit greatly from hydrogels (**Figure 6.7**). Their biocompatibility and capacity to create a gel-like matrix when in contact with biological fluids make them appropriate for their application in numerous contexts, such as the treatment of cancer and wound healing. Hydrogel's tunable qualities enable the change in drug release profiles to suit the modification of drug release profiles to suit the particular requirements of various medical conditions [76].

6.3.3 Surface Modification Techniques

To improve the way medical implants interact with biological tissues, surface modification techniques are used to change the surface properties of implants [80,81].

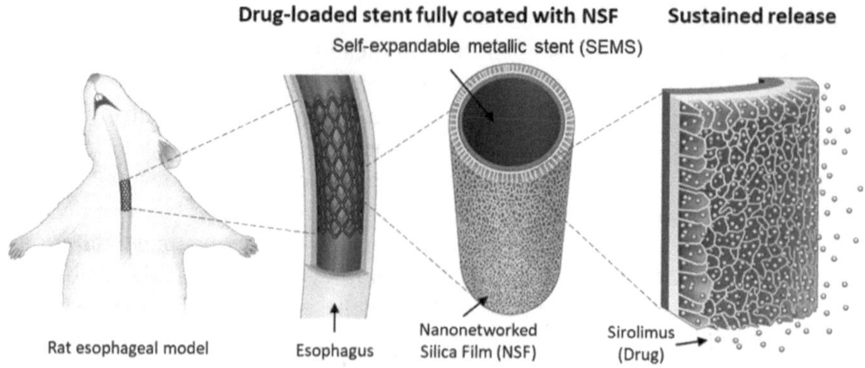

FIGURE 6.7 Representation of drug-releasing hydrogel slant [79]. (Permissions under Creative Commons Attribution 4.0 International License)

6.3.3.1 Plasma Treatment

To modify the physio-chemical characteristics of the implant surface without affecting bulk material, plasma treatment entails subjecting it to a plasma field. This method can introduce functional groups that encourage cell adhesion and proliferation, increase surface roughness, and improve surface wettability. The effectiveness of plasma treatment for improving the bioactivity and osseointegration of titanium implants has been determined, hence being more appropriate for long-term clinical use. Such a process establishes functional groups and enhances the surface roughness that contributes significantly to the early cell adhesion and then cell proliferation, and finally ends up with the implant's integration with the neighboring tissues. In addition, the plasma treatment accustoms the surface to be more hydrophilic thus helping to develop a stable bone implant bond [80].

6.3.3.2 Chemical Grafting

Chemical grafting is a technique in which some active molecules are immobilized on the surface of an implant by using a chemical bond. Thus, by ultimately altering surface chemistry, desired cellular responses can be invoked. For example, coating osteogenic peptides (**Figure 6.8**) can improve bone integration and formation on implant surfaces. Such an approach enables one to fix different biomolecules covalently and thus elaborate multiple functional surfaces appropriate for solving various medical issues. Through this approach the required antibiotic, growth factor, or other bioactive molecule can be incorporated onto the implant surface, enhancing the therapeutic effect and reducing healing time [81,82].

6.3.4 Smart Coatings

Smart coatings are functional and possess dynamic characteristics that may be influenced by the external conditions. Such coatings have become critical in enhancing the advancement of smart biomedical devices that are capable of

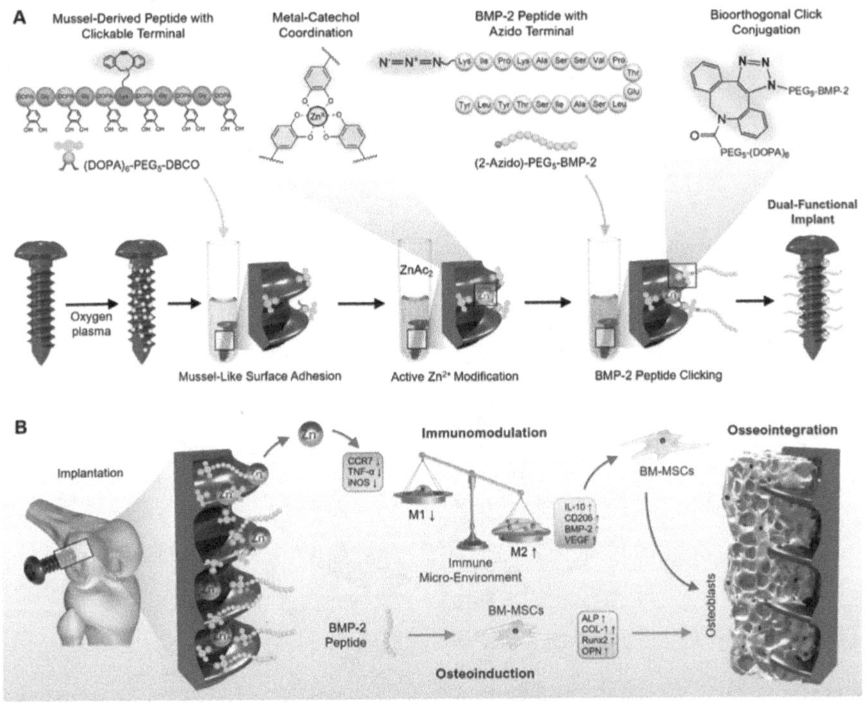

FIGURE 6.8 Illustration of osteogenic peptide grafting [83]. (Permissions under Creative Commons Attribution 4.0 International License)

altering their behaviour in response to the prevailing environment [29,76,84–86]. Stimuli-responsive coatings can transform their chemical or a physical characteristic in response to evoking stimuli such as light, temperature, pH, or even magnetic fields. These coatings are of special importance in controlled release technologies, especially in drug targeting where coatings can be designed to release some therapeutic agents in response to some particular physiological stimulus. This means designing coatings that respond to specific stimuli and lets biomedical engineers create instrumentation that is specific to a patient's requirements. Ranking high in both effectiveness and safety, these coatings help release medications when required, reduce the amount of exposure to the drug, and minimize side reactions [76,84].

6.4 APPLICATIONS OF HYDROXYAPATITE IN BIOMEDICAL ENGINEERING

Different uses of hydroxyapatite (HA) in biomedical engineering are in drug delivery and controlled release, in orthopedic and dental implant applications, and in tissue engineering (as shown in **Figure 6.9**). The biomedical applications of HA are summarized in **Table 6.1**.

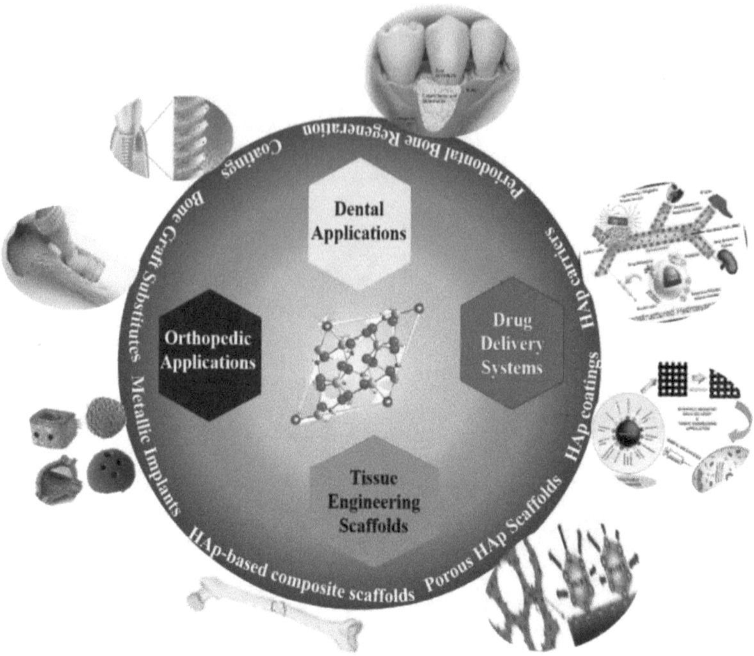

FIGURE 6.9 Various applications of hydroxyapatite in biomedical engineering like drug delivery, drug release, orthopedic usage, dental implants, and tissue engineering.

TABLE 6.1
A Summary of the Biomedical Application of Hydroxyapatite

HA type	Substrate	Synthesis Method	Properties	Application	Ref.
Substituted HA with silicon, magnesium, and zinc ions	Stainless steel substrate 316L	Microwave irradiation	The least bacterial adhesion for magnesium-HA coating was at 30 minutes and 2 h while for silicon-HA coating was at 6 h.	Coating material	[89]
Magnesium-substituted HA	Multi-walled carbon nanotubes and stainless steel	Pyrolysis technique	The composite has spherical-shaped crystals of apatite which are interconnected like a microstructure.	Bone tissue engineering	[98]
Simple HA	Silver	Thermal spraying	Implant coated with silver-containing HA to increase the fusion capacity of bone and prevent infection after surgery.	Bone and spinal implants	[87]
Simple HA	Magnesium alloy	Electrophoretic deposition	In vitro experiments showed that HA coating enhanced Mg alloy corrosion resistance by 25 fold. Moreover, better growth of bone cells was also seen.	Bone graft	[88]

TABLE 6.1 (Continued)
A Summary of the Biomedical Application of Hydroxyapatite

HA type	Substrate	Synthesis Method	Properties	Application	Ref.
Simple HA	Graphene nanosheets	Pulsed layer deposition	Graphene sheets increase the cell activity of human fibroblasts.	Titanium implant coating	[90]
HA	Zirconium	Sol-gel method	HA had adhesion strength greater than 40 MPa, which is suited as a dental implant.	Dental implant	[91]
Fluorine-substituted HA	Ti6Al4V	Sol-gel method	Increased proportions of FHA-enhanced properties like adhesion strength, surface roughness, and hydrophilicity.	Dental implant	[92]
HA/CS	Hyaluronic-reinforced collagenase	Co-precipitation method	The composite exhibited a mechanical strength of approximately 6.69 MPa and had excellent biocompatibility.	Periodontal bone regeneration	[93]
ZA/BMP-2/HA	Calcium sulphate	Thermal treatment	CN/BMP-2/ZA exhibited the highest mineralization compared to other groups.	Bone regeneration	[94]
Carbonated HA	Honeycomb	Co-precipitation method	The porous structure of the scaffold showed increased pore size, porosity, and porogen concentration.	Tissue engineering	[96]
HA-scaffolds	Organic solvents	Stereo-lithography	The compression test confirmed the effectiveness of elastic modulus as the value of the scaffold for the scaffold was about 2.4 GPa to 5.9 GPa, which resembles a cancellous bone well.	Bone-tissue engineering	[97]
Chitosan/l-arginine reinforced HA	Gelatin/acetic acid, genipin	Alkaline treatment and additive manufacturing	The scaffold exhibited a cell-friendly nature and allowed cell adherence along with the long-term maintenance of cell viability.	Tissue engineering	[99]
Mesoporous-HA	HA nanoparticles	Opposite ion core/shell method	Drug-loading efficacy of about 93.7%.	Drug nano vehicle	[100]
Mesoporous HA	$CaCO_3$	Solvent method	HA particles with a size of 20 nm and a specific surface area of 85 m^2/g.	Targeted delivery of drug and regeneration of bone	[101]
Folic acid-HA	Doxorubicin	Hydrothermal and co-precipitation methods	Inhibited the growth of targeted cells.	Drug delivery in cancer treatment	[102]
HA	Chitosan	Ultrasound-assisted precipitation method	Reduced bacteriostatic efficiency.	Drug delivery	[99]

6.4.1 Orthopedic Applications

6.4.1.1 Bone Graft Substitutes

Developing implants with osteoconductive and antimicrobial properties is important to prevent post-operation infection at the surgical sites. So to meet this need, Morimoto et al. in the year 2022 fabricated an implant coated with silver-containing HA to increase the fusion capacity of bone. The implant has gained commercial importance as it is both biocompatible and non-toxic under in vivo and in vitro conditions. So it has been used for spinal inter-body cages and hip prostheses antimicrobial implants and has demonstrated good clinical applicability without adverse effects [87]. Similarly, Kumar et al. [88] performed the HA coating on magnesium alloy (Mg-3Zn) using electrophoretic deposition method. The annealing temperature of HA (the coating) and surface porosity of Mg alloy established the mechanical integrity of the composite. The coating on the alloy was uniform with minimal cracks. In vitro experiments have shown that the HA coating enhanced the Mg alloy corrosion resistance by 25 folds. Moreover, better growth of bone cells was also depicted. HA is a prominent graft substitute as it can regenerate bone cells under an antimicrobial environment and is biocompatible with fewer negative impacts.

6.4.1.2 Coatings for Metallic Implants

Substituted hydroxyapatite can be used as a coating agent, as ion substitution into an apatitic lattice increases antimicrobial activity. Khan et al. in the year 2020 prepared substituted hydroxyapatite with silicon, magnesium, and zinc ions through microwave irradiation method. The substituted HA was coated with 316L-grade stainless steel to avoid high-temperature exposure. Along with this polyvinyl chloride was added as a binding agent. The least bacterial adhesion for magnesium-HA coating was at 30 minutes and 2 h, while for silicon-HA coating was at 6 h. It was observed that electrophoretic deposition exhibited even coating over the stainless steel grade substrate [89]. To overcome the challenge of carbonated HA scaffold, Fathi et al. in the year 2023 integrated an extra layer of graphene nanosheets to develop titanium implants. Graphene sheets have the ability to proliferate, adhere, and spread human fibroblasts. Also, graphene is used to protect the corrosion of titanium implants against the systemic body fluid. The ratio of the bonds between C–C was more than between C–O within the graphene which detected the presence of corrosive ions. The wettability and roughness of titanium were significantly improved by the deposition of a monotonous graphene layer [90]. Therefore, HA is a potential coating material when reinforced with other metals like titanium or stainless steel.

6.4.2 Dental Application

6.4.2.1 Dental Implant Coatings

Some properties of HA like biocompatibility can be compromised due to high-temperature processing. To overcome this, Kim et al. [91] reported the coating of zirconium surface with HA, which was derived by the sol-gel method and then subjected to different temperatures. At 800°C, the only crystalline phase was of zirconium and HA, and the surface depicted a nano-porous structure. Since HA has an adhesion strength greater than 40

MPa, it is best suited for application as a dental implant. The coating of HA over zirconium demonstrated better proliferation and cell attachment than just zirconium alone [91]. Ansari et al. in 2020 worked on improving the in vitro bioactivity and corrosive behaviour of substituted HA. Deposition of polycaprolactone/fluoride substituted-hydroxyapatite (PCL/FHA) on alkali-treated Ti6Al4V increased the overall efficiency of the bio-composite. The results indicated that sol-gel process can generate the crack resistant and compact coating with an even dispersion of fluorine-substituted HA (FHA) in the ceramic phase. Increased proportions of FHA enhanced properties like adhesion strength, surface roughness, and hydrophilicity. PCL/20%wt. FHA coating showed zero cytotoxic effect and enhanced the proliferation of MG63 cells [92]. As a result, HA's inherent strength and biocompatible behaviour increase its use as a dental implant.

6.4.2.2 Periodontal Bone Regeneration

Periodontitis is a medical condition in which alveolar bone is progressively damaged and destroyed. Hydroxyapatite, when combined with other materials, can treat periodontitis and help in bone regeneration. Subramaniam et al. in the year 2016 reported a composite comprising HA, hyaluronic-reinforced collagenase, and calcium sulphate hemihydrate (HA/HA-Col/CS) as the starting material for bone for regenerating periodontal bone. This composite exhibited a mechanical strength of approximately 6.69 MPa and had excellent biocompatibility. H&E staining and micro-CT assays confirmed that collagenase release considerably accelerated the process of bone remodeling. Collagen insured the applicability of composite for the bone regeneration process [93]. Teotia et al. presented another way of bone regeneration by using calcium sulfate and nano-hydroxyapatite (CN) as a bone substitute (**Figure 6.10**). The CN was further substituted with a low concentration of zoledronic acid (ZA) and protein-2 (BMP-2) which acted as bone morphogenetic. After

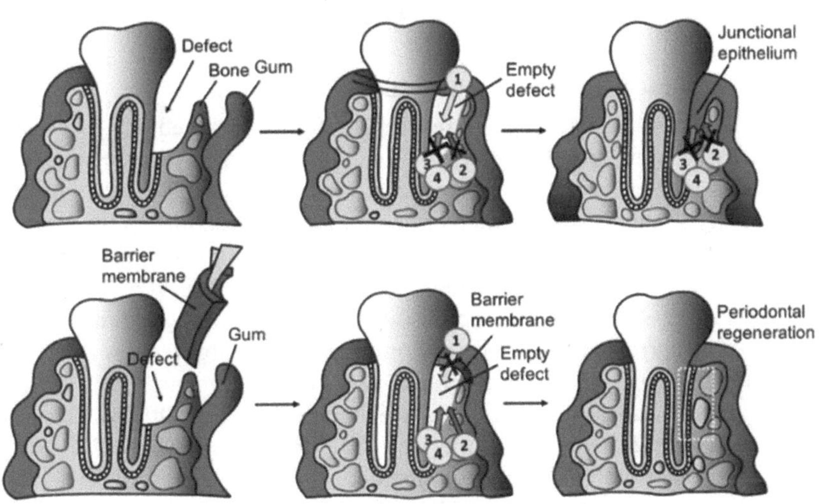

FIGURE 6.10 Representation of periodontal bone regeneration by using nanomaterials [95]. (Permissions under Creative Commons Attribution 4.0 International License)

12 weeks of ex vivo investigation, CN/BMP-2/ZA exhibited the highest mineralization compared to other groups (CN, CN + ZN, and control). Results of micro-CT aligned with the spectroscopic and histological analysis, where the defect was previously present, indicated the qualitative confirmation of new bone [94]. Therefore, HA is excellent for caring the bioactive compounds and when reinforced with other materials improves the overall process of bone regeneration.

6.4.3 Tissue Engineering Scaffolds

6.4.3.1 Porous HAp scaffolds

Porous bio scaffolds have been used for ages to develop biocompatible composites that have potential for biomedical applications. For instance, Sari et al. in the year 2021 synthesized carbonated hydroxyapatite (CHA) bio-ceramic from mussel shells via co-precipitation method where honeycomb was used as a porogen agent. The calcium and phosphorous composition of the developed composite was relatively similar to the natural bone density ratio of the elements. The porous structure of the scaffold showed increased pore size, porosity, and porogen concentration. Honeycomb reduced the crystallite size, which consequently improved bone growth as low crystallinity developed dislocations making cell proliferation easier [96]. Similarly, Wang et al. in the year 2020 created a porous HA structure with a porosity gradient via novel technology. The authors made a ceramic solution through stereo lithography with a better dimension precision of about 60 μm and a minimal pore having a diameter of 500 μm. The effectiveness of elastic modulus was confirmed by the compression test, as the value of the modulus for the scaffold was about 2.4 GPa to 5.9 GPa which resembles a cancellous bone well. The HA bio-ceramic unit showed biocompatibility with bone marrow mesenchymal stem cells and better cell proliferation [97]. So HA composites can be employed in bone tissue engineering without any adverse impact.

6.4.3.2 HAp-Based Composite Scaffolds

Studies have shown that incorporating magnesium-substituted HA with multi-walled carbon nanotubes and its coating over stainless steel implants can be helpful in bone tissue engineering. The composite has spherical-shaped crystals of apatite which are interconnected like a microstructure. Also, magnesium provides a large surface area and decreases the crystallinity of the composite. The nano-composite exhibited enhanced antimicrobial action against G-ve E. coli with 16 mm as the zone of inhibition. Not only this, but also the presence of magnesium revealed a reduced rate of corrosion resistance and improved corrosion resistance. From an electrochemical aspect, the composite was perfect as it demonstrated a reduction in current density and an increase in polarization resistance [98]. By using additive manufacturing, Zaferis et al. in the year 2021 synthesized hybrid HA hydrogels and prepared a scaffold by 3D printing method. The mechanical properties of the hydrogel were enhanced by using genipin as a cross-linking agent, and the rheology was enhanced by utilizing gelatin/acetic acid suspension. Nano-indentation and micro-computed tomography revealed that the modulus values and porosity of the scaffold were relatively similar to the cancellous bone. The scaffold exhibited a cell-friendly nature and allowed cell adherence along with the long-term maintenance of cell viability [99]. Therefore, HA-based scaffolds can be applied to increase the cell population to promote bone tissue engineering.

6.5 FUTURE PROSPECTS

Biodegradable materials and coating technologies for biomedical devices are topics that are developing quickly and have a lot of room to grow in the future. By increasing biocompatibility, future biodegradable materials can lower the likelihood of negative immune responses. The creation of innovative polymers and composites that closely resemble the characteristics of real tissue can help achieve this. Upcoming materials may enable fine-grained control over rates of degradation, customized for particular medical uses. Applications such as tissue engineering and temporary implants can benefit greatly from this. Green chemistry and sustainable manufacturing techniques can improve the environmental friendliness of biodegradable material production. These substances can give cells a temporary framework while they progressively break down to create new tissue. Biomedical device infections can be avoided with coatings that emit antimicrobial compounds. Subsequent coatings will be more durable, suited to certain infections, and more effective. Coatings that react to temperature inflection or pH can release medication on demand or perform other medicinal functions. More flexible and adaptable treatment choices may result from this. These coatings have the potential to upgrade cell differentiation, adhesion, and proliferation. To encourage better tissue integration with implants, they might be utilized. Coatings that incorporate nanotechnology can have better mechanical qualities, higher drug loading capacity, and more accurate therapeutic release control. Therefore, biodegradable materials and coating materials have a bright prospect which can be used to enhance sustainable development in the material industry.

6.6 CONCLUSION

Herein, we have discussed the various techniques and materials that contribute toward the enlargement of advanced biomedical devices. By the action of microorganisms, biodegradable materials are intended to release water, carbon dioxide, and biomass. For waste reduction and environmental impact mitigation, these materials are essential. Biodegradable materials can be differentiated into polymers, natural biodegradable materials, and biodegradable composites. Biodegradable polymers are a significant class of materials that undergo biological decomposition in their natural environment. Advanced materials known as biodegradable composites combine biodegradable polymers with reinforcing materials to improve the materials' functionality, biocompatibility, and mechanical qualities. Naturally occurring biodegradable materials that form from renewable resources are becoming more and more significant because of their advantages for the environment and their uses in a variety of industries and biomedicine. Medical implants integrate and function better when coated with bioactive materials that have a positive interaction with biological tissues. To improve treatment efficacy and minimize systemic side effects, drug-eluting coatings are made to deliver therapeutic agents at controlled rates right at the site of implantation. To improve the way medical implants interact with biological tissues, surface improving techniques are used to change the surface properties of the implants. Hydroxyapatite has various applications in biomedical engineering, as it can be applied in drug delivery, drug release, orthopedic usage, dental implants, and tissue engineering. So a significant improvement has been seen over the years in the biodegradable material and coating technologies in the development of biomedical devices.

REFERENCES

[1] Oriňaková, R., Gorejová, R., Orságová Králová, Z., Oriňak, A. Surface Modifications of Biodegradable Metallic Foams for Medical Applications. Coatings 2020, 10, 819. https://doi.org/10.3390/coatings10090819

[2] Alam F, Ahmed A, Jalal AH, et al. Recent Progress and Challenges of Implantable Biodegradable Biosensors; *Micromachines*. 2024; 15(4):475.

[3] Kaur H, Bhosale A, Shrivastav S. Biosensors: Classification, Fundamental Characterization and New Trends: A Review. *Int J Heal Sci Res*. 2018;8:315.

[4] Hussain T, Mysore M, Patil AY, et al. Apatite Insights: From Synthesis to Biomedical Applications. *Eur Polym J*. 2024;209:112842.

[5] Hu C, Wang L, Liu S, et al. Recent Development of Implantable Chemical Sensors Utilizing Flexible and Biodegradable Materials for Biomedical Applications; *ACS Nano*. 2024;18(5):3969–95.

[6] Ricerca UODDI. *Tailored Polymers for Advanced Biomedical Devices: Electroactive Bioadhesive Coatings for Drug Delivery and Electrospun Scaffolds for Improved Biointegration and Functionality*; 2024; 1–170. https://hdl.handle.net/20.500.14242/85141

[7] Li C, Guo C, Fitzpatrick V, et al. Design of Biodegradable, Implantable Devices Towards Clinical Translation. *Nat Rev Mater*. 2020;5:61–81.

[8] Kong D, Zhang K, Tian J, et al. Biocompatible and Biodegradable Light-Emitting Materials and Devices. *Adv. Mater. Technol*. 2022;2(7):2100006.

[9] Ramzan M, Sabir M, Singh S, et al. Three-Dimensional Hydrogel Bioprinting Technology as a Scaffold of Novel Drug Delivery and Biomedical Devices: A Comprehensive Review; *BIO Web Conf*. 2024;86(27):01013.

[10] Abbasov IB. Biodegradable Polymer Materials in Medicine. *J Compos Biodegrad Polym*. 2021;9:1–6.

[11] Liu CC. Electrochemical Sensors. *Med Devices Syst*. 2006;7:48–1–48–6.

[12] Kaur H, Athwal S, Garg K. Futuristic Approaches in Biofertilizer Industry: Challenges, Opportunities, and Future Directions. In: Kaur S, Dwibedi V, Sahu PK, editors. *Metabolomics, Proteomics Gene Ed Approaches Biofertilizer Ind Vol II*. Singapore: Springer Nature Singapore; 2024. pp. 15–33.

[13] Vipasha S, Hardeep K, Tarun K, et al. Traditional Indian Herb Cathranthus Roseus Used as Cancer Treatment: A Review. *Int J Pharmacogn Phytochem Res*. 2016;8:1926–8.

[14] Amirtharaj Mosas KK, Chandrasekar AR, Dasan A, et al. Recent Advancements in Materials and Coatings for Biomedical Implants. *Gels*. 2022;8(5):323.

[15] Beshchasna N, Saqib M, Kraskiewicz H, et al. Recent Advances in Manufacturing Innovative Stents. *Pharmaceutics*. 2020;12:349.

[16] Wang Y, Li G, Yang L, et al. Development of Innovative Biomaterials and Devices for the Treatment of Cardiovascular Diseases. *Adv Mater*. 2022;34:1–31.

[17] Kaur H, Raveendran AV, Athwal S, et al. Assessment of Diabetes Biomarker Monitoring Via Novel Biosensor Activity. *Results Chem*. 2023;5:100777.

[18] Nagabushanam M, Devade K, Aravind Reddy G, et al. Advance Biomedical Engineering—A Fundamental Review of Composite Materials and Its Applications. *Mater Today Proc.* 2023. https://doi.org/10.1016/j.matpr.2023.08.216
[19] Hosseini ES, Dervin S, Ganguly P, et al. Biodegradable Materials for Sustainable Health Monitoring Devices. *ACS Appl Bio Mater.* 2021;4:163–94.
[20] Kaur H, Athwal S. Paper-Based Microfluidic Devices for Pesticide Detection. In: *Advances in MEMS and Microfluidic Systems.* IGI-Global; 2023. pp. 126–52. https://doi.org/10.4018/978-1-6684-6952-1.ch007
[21] Aziz T, et al. Manufactures of Bio-Degradable and Bio-Based Polymers for Bio-Materials in the Pharmaceutical Field. *J Appl Polym Sci.* 2022;139(29):1–14.
[22] Jasmine S, Krishnamoorthy R. Biodegradable Materials for Bone Defect Repair. *Biodegrad Mater Appl.* 2022;457–70.
[23] Blanco-llamero C, Khouri NG, Bahú JO, et al. Polylactic Acid (PLA): Properties, Synthesis, and Biomedical Applications—A Review of the Literature Polylactic Acid (PLA): Properties, Synthesis, and Biomedical Applications—A Review of the Literature. *J Mol Struct.* 2024;1309:138243.
[24] Tatullo M, Piattelli A, Ruggiero R, et al. Functionalized Magnesium Alloys Obtained by Superplastic Forming Process Retain Osteoinductive and Antibacterial Properties: An In-vitro Study. *Dent Mater.* 2024;40:557–62.
[25] Teo AJT, Mishra A, Park I, et al. Polymeric Biomaterials for Medical Implants and Devices. *ACS Biomater Sci Eng.* 2016;2:454–72.
[26] Kuperkar K, Atanase LI, Bahadur A, et al. Degradable Polymeric Bio (Nano) Materials and Their Biomedical Applications: A Comprehensive Overview and Recent Updates. *Polymers (Basel).* 2024:1–45.
[27] Sharma S, Kaur H, Thakur M, et al. *Engineering 2D Nanomaterials for Biomedical Applications. 2D Nanomater.* John Wiley & Sons, Ltd; 2024. pp. 333–60.
[28] Seitz JM, Durisin M, Goldman J, et al. Recent Advances in Biodegradable Metals for Medical Sutures: A Critical Review. *Adv Healthc Mater.* 2015;4:1915–36.
[29] Singh J, Singh S, Gill R. Applications of Biopolymer Coatings in Biomedical Engineering. *J Electrochem Sci Eng.* 2022;13:63–81.
[30] Visan AI, Popescu-pelin G, Socol G. Degradation Behavior of Polymers Used as Coating Materials for Drug Delivery—A Basic Review. *Polymers (Basel).* 2021;13(8):1272.
[31] Pérez, MB, et al. Creating Anti-Biofouling Surfaces by Degradable Main-Chain Polyphosphoester Polymer Brushes. *Adv Funct Mater.* 2024;34(32):2316201.
[32] Nanocontainer M, Vijayalakshmi S, Jeong Y, et al. Emerging Trends in Smart Self-Healing Coatings: A Focus on Corrosion Protection. *Coatings.* 2024;14(3):324.
[33] Burdus AC, Niculescu A. Coatings for Cardiovascular Stents—An Up-to-Date Review. *Int J Mol Sci.* 2024;25(2):1–28.
[34] Rydz J, Musioł M, Zawidlak-Węgrzyńska B. Polymer-Drug Anti-Thrombogenic and Hemocompatible Coatings as Surface Modifications. *Pharmaceutics.* 2024;16(3):432.
[35] Talebian S, Mendes B, Conniot J, et al. Biopolymeric Coatings for Local Release of Therapeutics from Biomedical Implants. *Adv Sci.* 2023;10:1–25.
[36] Chung JJ, Im H, Kim SH, et al. Toward Biomimetic Scaffolds for Tissue Engineering: 3D Printing Techniques in Regenerative Medicine. *Front Bioeng Biotechnol.* 2020;8:1–12.
[37] Samir A, Ashour FH, Hakim AAA, et al. Recent Advances in Biodegradable Polymers for Sustainable Applications. *NPJ Mater Degrad.* 2022;6.
[38] Ali SS, Abdelkarim EA, Elsamahy T, et al. Bioplastic Production in Terms of Life Cycle Assessment: A State-of-the-Art Review. *Environ Sci Ecotechnol.* 2023;15:100254.
[39] Jiang T, Duan Q, Zhu J, et al. Starch-Based Biodegradable Materials: Challenges and Opportunities. *Adv Ind Eng Polym Res.* 2020;3:8–18.

[40] Singh R, Toseef M, Kumar J, et al. Benefits and Challenges in Additive Manufacturing and Its Applications. In: Kaushal S, Singh I, Singh S, et al., editors. *Sustainable Advanced Manufacturing and Materials Processing* [Internet]. 1st ed. Boca Raton: CRC Press; 2022. pp. 137–57. Available from: www.taylorfrancis.com/books/9781003269298/chapters/10.1201/9781003269298-8.

[41] Singh J. *Sustainability Issues in Laser-Based Additive Manufacturing. Handb Laser-Based Sustain Surf Modif Manuf Tech.* CRC Press; 2023. pp. 167–89.

[42] Ahmad S, Hashmi AW, Singh J, et al. Innovations in Additive Manufacturing of Shape Memory Alloys: Alloys, Microstructures, Treatments, Applications. *J Mater Res Technol.* 2024;32:4136–97.

[43] Magazzini L, Grilli S, Fenni SE, et al. The Blending of Poly(Glycolic Acid) with Polycaprolactone and Poly(l-lactide): Promising Combinations. *Polymers (Basel).* 2021;13.

[44] Jem KJ, Tan B. The Development and Challenges of Poly (Lactic Acid) and Poly (Glycolic Acid). *Adv Ind Eng Polym Res.* 2020;3:60–70.

[45] Schaschke C, Audic JL. Editorial: Biodegradable Materials. *Int J Mol Sci.* 2014;15:21468–75.

[46] Chandran M, Tamilkolundu S, Murugesan C. Conversion of Plastic Waste to Fuel. In: *Plastic Waste and Recycling*. Academic Press; 2020. pp. 385–99.

[47] Panchal SS, Vasava DV. Biodegradable Polymeric Materials: Synthetic Approach. *ACS Omega.* 2020;5:4370–9.

[48] Alipal J, Mohd Pu'ad NAS, Lee TC, et al. A Review of Gelatin: Properties, Sources, Process, Applications, and Commercialisation. *Mater Today Proc.* 2019;42:240–50.

[49] Cao S, Wang Y, Xing L, et al. Structure and Physical Properties of Gelatin from Bovine Bone Collagen Influenced by Acid Pretreatment and Pepsin. *Food Bioprod Process.* 2020;121:213–23.

[50] Perez-Puyana V, Wieringa P, Yuste Y, et al. Fabrication of Hybrid Scaffolds Obtained from Combinations of PCL with Gelatin or Collagen Via Electrospinning for Skeletal Muscle Tissue Engineering. *J Biomed Mater Res—Part A.* 2021;109:1600–12.

[51] Leite ML, Soares DG, Anovazzi G, et al. Fibronectin-Loaded Collagen/Gelatin Hydrogel Is a Potent Signaling Biomaterial for Dental Pulp Regeneration. *J Endod.* 2021;47:1110–17.

[52] Geanaliu-Nicolae RE, Andronescu E. Blended Natural Support Materials—Collagen Based Hydrogels Used in Biomedicine. *Materials (Basel).* 2020;13:1–31.

[53] Naomi R, Bahari H, Ridzuan PM, et al. Natural-Based Biomaterial for Skin Wound Healing (Gelatin vs. Collagen): Expert Review. *Polymers (Basel).* 2021;13:1–20.

[54] La Monica F, Campora S, Ghersi G. Collagen-Based Scaffolds for Chronic Skin Wound Treatment. *Gels.* 2024;10.

[55] Afaf Sarhan, Characterization of Chitosan and Polyethylene glycol Blend Film, *Egypt. J. Chem. 2019;* 62(2):405–12.

[56] Wang W, Meng Q, Li Q, et al. Molecular Sciences Chitosan Derivatives and Their Application in Biomedicine. *Int J Mol Sci.* 2020;21:487.

[57] Kou S (Gabriel), Peters L, Mucalo M. Chitosan: A Review of Molecular Structure, Bioactivities and Interactions with the Human Body and Micro-Organisms. *Carbohydr Polym.* 2022;282:119132.

[58] Kou S (Gabriel), Peters LM, Mucalo MR. Chitosan: A Review of Sources and Preparation Methods. *Int. J. Biol. Macromol.* 2021;169: 85–94.

[59] Pellis A, Guebitz GM, Nyanhongo GS. Chitosan: Sources, Processing and Modification Techniques. *Gels.* 2022;8:5–25.

[60] Krauklis AE, Karl CW, Gagani AI, et al. Composite Material Recycling Technology—State-of-the-Art and Sustainable Development for the 2020s. *J Compos Sci.* 2021;5.

[61] Egbo MK. A Fundamental Review on Composite Materials and Some of Their Applications in Biomedical Engineering. *J King Saud Univ—Eng Sci.* 2021;33:557–68.
[62] Omran AAB, Mohammed AABA, Sapuan SM, et al. Micro-and Nanocellulose in Polymer Composite Materials: A Review. *Polymers (Basel).* 2021;13:1–30.
[63] More CV, Alsayed Z, Badawi MS, et al. Polymeric Composite Materials for Radiation Shielding: A Review. *Environ. Chem. Lett.* 2021;19(3):2057–90.
[64] Tang S, Shen Y, Jiang L, et al. Surface Modification of Nano-Hydroxyapatite/Polymer Composite for Bone Tissue Repair Applications: A Review. *Polymers (Basel).* 2024;16:1–20.
[65] Tabrizian P, Sun H, Jargalsaikhan U, et al. Biomimetic Nacre-like Hydroxyapatite/Polymer Composites for Bone Implants. *J Funct Biomater.* 2023;14:1–17.
[66] Singh CJ, Ram B, Singh J, et al. Experimental Investigation on Characterization of Friction Stir Processed AZ31-Based Composite. *Sci Rep.* 2024;14:15453.
[67] Singh J, Hashmi AW, Ahmad S, et al. Critical Review on Biodegradable and Biocompatibility Magnesium Alloys: Progress and Prospects in Bio-Implant Applications. *Inorg Chem Commun.* 2024;169:113111.
[68] Hashmi AW, Singh J, Ahmad S. Future Perspective of Self-Healing Nano-Coatings for Corrosion Protection. *Discov Disruption, Futur Implic Nanomater.* 2024;597–624.
[69] Singh J, Hashmi AW, Kumar A, et al. Review on protection of Mg alloys bioimplants by deposition of micro-arc oxidation coatings. In *AIP Conference Proceedings.* AIP Publishing; 2024.
[70] Monte JP, Fontes A, Santos BS, et al. Recent Advances in Hydroxyapatite/Polymer/Silver Nanoparticles Scaffolds with Antimicrobial Activity for Bone Regeneration. *Mater Lett.* 2023;338:134027.
[71] Jaafar A, Hecker C, Árki P, et al. Sol-Gel Derived Hydroxyapatite Coatings for Titanium Implants: A Review. *Bioengineering.* 2020;7(4):127.
[72] Liu X, He D, Zhou Z, et al. In Vitro Bioactivity and Antibacterial Performances of Atmospheric Plasma Sprayed C-Axis Preferential Oriented Hydroxyapatite Coatings. *Surf Coatings Technol.* 2021;417:127209.
[73] Paper R, Spectroscopy M, Probes O, et al. Effect of Synthesis Methods and Conditions on Properties and Application of Carbon Dots for the Detection of Potential Water Contaminants: A Review. *Crit Rev Anal Chem.* 2021:1–24.
[74] Kaur H, Athwal S. Application of Nanomaterials for the Removal of Heavy Metal from Wastewater. *Adv Appl Nanotechnol to Ind Wastewater.* 2023;01003:339–51.
[75] Rezi I, Me E, Scholar G. Antimicrobial Coatings for Medical Applications—A Comprehensive Review on Active Nanoparticles Antimicrobial Coatings for Medical Applications—A Comprehensive Review on Active Nanoparticles Characterization. *Coatings.* 2023;13:1830.
[76] Chatterjee S, Hui PC. Stimuli-Responsive Hydrogels—Smart Materials for Biomedical Applications, Edited by Lăcrămioara Popa, Mihaela Violeta Ghica and Cristina-Elena Dinu-Pîrvu, IntechOpen Limited, London, United Kingdom.
[77] Iqbal J, Gunn J, Serruys PW. Coronary Stents: Historical Development, Current Status and Future Directions. *British Med. Bullet.* 2018;193–211.
[78] Ramakrishna S and Adepu S. Controlled Drug Delivery Systems: Current Status and Molecules. *Molecules.* 2021;26:5905.
[79] Jeon E, Kang JM, Bae G, et al. Flexible 3D Nanonetworked Silica Film as a Polymer-Free Drug-Eluting Stent Platform to Effectively Suppress Tissue Hyperplasia in Rat Esophagus (Adv. Healthcare Mater. 14/2022). *Adv Healthc Mater.* 2022;11.
[80] Yan S, Komasa S, Agariguchi A, et al. Osseointegration Properties of Titanium Implants Treated by Nonthermal Atmospheric-Pressure Nitrogen Plasma. *Int J Mol Sci.* 2022;23.

[81] Marcum Zachary A, Sevick MA HS. 基因的改变 NIH Public Access. *JAMA*. 2013;309:2105–6.
[82] Hu X, Wang T, Li F, et al. Surface Modifications of Biomaterials in Different Applied Fields. *RSC Adv*. 2023;13:20495–511.
[83] Wang T, Bai J, Lu M, et al. Engineering Immunomodulatory and Osteoinductive Implant Surfaces Via Mussel Adhesion-Mediated Ion Coordination and Molecular Clicking. *Nat Commun*. 2022;13:1–17.
[84] Deng Z, Yu R, Guo B. Materials Chemistry Frontiers Stimuli-Responsive Conductive Hydrogels: Design, Properties, and Applications. *Mater. Chem. Front*. 2021;2092–123.
[85] Singh J, Singh S, Verma A. Artificial Intelligence in Use of ZrO2 Material in Biomedical Science. *J Electrochem Sci Eng* [Internet]. 2022;13:83–97. Available from: https://pub.iapchem.org/ojs/index.php/JESE/article/view/1498.
[86] Singh J, Hashmi AW, Behra A, et al. Review of Mg Alloys for Bio-Implants Protected by the Deposition of Chemical Conversion Coatings. *AIP Conference Proceedings*. AIP Publishing; 2024.
[87] Morimoto T, Hirata H, Eto S, et al. Development of Silver-Containing Hydroxyapatite-Coated Antimicrobial Implants for Orthopaedic and Spinal Surgery. *Medicina (B Aires)*. 2022;58.
[88] Kumar RM, Kuntal KK, Singh S, et al. Electrophoretic Deposition of Hydroxyapatite Coating on Mg–3Zn Alloy for Orthopaedic Application. *Surf Coatings Technol*. 2016;287:82–92.
[89] Khan AS, Awais M. Low-Cost Deposition of Antibacterial Ion-Substituted Hydroxyapatite Coatings onto 316L Stainless Steel for Biomedical and Dental Applications. *Coatings*. 2020;10.
[90] Fathi AM, Ahmed MK, Afifi M, et al. Taking Hydroxyapatite-Coated Titanium Implants Two Steps Forward: Surface Modification Using Graphene Mesolayers and a Hydroxyapatite-Reinforced Polymeric Scaffold. *ACS Biomater Sci Eng*. 2021;7:360–72.
[91] Kim J, Kang I-G, Cheon K-H, et al. Stable Sol–Gel Hydroxyapatite Coating on Zirconia Dental Implant for Improved Osseointegration. *J Mater Sci Mater Med*. 2021;32:81.
[92] Ansari Z, Kalantar M, Kharaziha M, et al. Polycaprolactone/Fluoride Substituted-Hydroxyapatite (PCL/FHA) Nanocomposite Coatings Prepared by In-situ Sol-gel Process for Dental Implant Applications. *Prog Org Coat*. 2020;147:105873.
[93] Subramaniam S, Fang Y-H, Sivasubramanian S, et al. Hydroxyapatite-Calcium Sulfate-Hyaluronic Acid Composite Encapsulated with Collagenase as Bone Substitute for Alveolar Bone Regeneration. *Biomaterials*. 2016;74:99–108.
[94] Teotia AK, Raina DB, Singh C, et al. Nano-Hydroxyapatite Bone Substitute Functionalized with Bone Active Molecules for Enhanced Cranial Bone Regeneration. *ACS Appl Mater Interfaces*. 2017;9:6816–28.
[95] Soo-Ling B, Abdul Hamid Z. Asymmetric Resorbable-Based Dental Barrier Membrane for Periodontal Guided Tissue Regeneration and Guided Bone Regeneration: A Review. *J Biomed Mater Res Part B Appl Biomater*. 2022;110.
[96] Sari M, Hening P, Chotimah, et al. Porous Structure of Bioceramics Carbonated Hydroxyapatite-Based Honeycomb Scaffold for Bone Tissue Engineering. *Mater Today Commun*. 2021;26:102135.
[97] Wang Z, Huang C, Wang J, et al. Design and Characterization of Hydroxyapatite Scaffolds Fabricated by Stereolithography for Bone Tissue Engineering Application. *Proc CIRP*. 2020;89:170–5.
[98] Sivaraj D, Vijayalakshmi K. Substantial Effect of Magnesium Incorporation on Hydroxyapatite/Carbon Nanotubes Coatings on Metallic Implant Surfaces for Better Anticorrosive Protection and Antibacterial Ability. *J Anal Appl Pyrolysis*. 2018;135:15–21.

[99] Zafeiris K, Brasinika D, Karatza A, et al. Additive Manufacturing of Hydroxyapatite–Chitosan–Genipin Composite Scaffolds for Bone Tissue Engineering Applications. *Mater Sci Eng C*. 2021;119:111639.

[100] Yang Y-H, Liu C-H, Liang Y-H, et al. Hollow Mesoporous Hydroxyapatite Nanoparticles (hmHANPs) with Enhanced Drug Loading and pH-Responsive Release Properties for Intracellular Drug Delivery. *J Mater Chem B*. 2013;1:2447–50.

[101] Safi S, Karimzadeh F, Labbaf S. Mesoporous and Hollow Hydroxyapatite Nanostructured Particles as a Drug Delivery Vehicle for the Local Release of Ibuprofen. *Mater Sci Eng C*. 2018;92:712–19.

[102] Sun W, Fan J, Wang S, et al. Biodegradable Drug-Loaded Hydroxyapatite Nanotherapeutic Agent for Targeted Drug Release in Tumors. *ACS Appl Mater Interfaces*. 2018;10:7832–40.

7 Smart Materials for Biomedical Implant Coatings

A Review of Material Design, Mechanisms, and Clinical Implications

Praveen Kumar Verma and Hitesh Vasudev

CONTENTS

7.1 INTRODUCTION

Biomedical implants have revolutionized healthcare by offering solutions for restoration of bodily functions and improving the quality of life for millions of

DOI: 10.1201/9781003516064-7

patients. Such interventions range from orthopedic implants, including hip and knee replacements, cardiovascular devices such as stents and pacemakers, and are generally critical in managing chronic health conditions and recovery after trauma. These devices are going to be in contact with the human tissue, and hence there are stringent requirements of biocompatibility, mechanical strength, and longevity. Sounding tremendous advancement in implant technology, however, long-term success is still largely due to complications related to infection, rejection of implants, corrosion, and mechanical wear. Hence, the development of coatings that would solve those problems is an intense area of research; it may extend the functional life of the implant and provide for better integration with biological tissues. The application of coatings on implants has been primarily motivated by the need to improve biocompatibility, the ability of a material to perform with an appropriate host response in a specific situation. This kind of reaction can cause a cascade of biological effects, which typically include inflammation, tissue healing, and sometimes detrimental reactions such as fibrous encapsulation or foreign body responses. A coating can be useful in reducing these kinds of reactions by changing the surface properties of the implant to favor cellular attachment, growth, and healing. Coatings also prevent bacterial colonization, which is quite an essential point to be considered in fighting implant-associated infections, which constitute one of the leading causes of failure of implants. Coatings also provide protection as wear and corrosion decrease, causing the failures mechanically or by releasing ions that could prove harmful in the body. Longevity is yet another aspect, and it must be taken quite seriously because most implants are designed to last decades without the requirement of change [1]. Applications of biomedical metal materials are illustrated in **Figure 7.1**.

New biomedical implant coatings may present opportunities for improving the performance of such systems. Smart materials can be broadly defined as those that respond to some external stimulus, such as temperature, pH, electrical signals, or magnetic fields, with some change in their physical or chemical properties. In this way, they can be designed to actively perform in a biological milieu rather than simply furnishing an inactive interface. Smart coatings can be designed to adapt to dynamic physiological environments, thus offering several targeted potential benefits, including drug delivery, real-time monitoring of implant conditions, and on-demand therapeutic interventions [3]. **Figure 7.2** depicts the evolution of biomaterials from regeneration to replacement.

Similar in concept is the research related to shape memory alloys, which would change shape or form with a change in temperature, used in orthopedic implants for improved fixation and stability. For the cardiovascular application, shape memory material will make a device like stent adapt to changes in the diameter of blood vessels, hence reducing complications of restenosis. The driving force behind the interest in smart materials for biomedical coatings is improvement of patient outcomes and reduction of complications associated with traditional implant materials. Despite promising features, clinical translation challenges exist [5]. The coating effects and clinical implications are shown in **Table 7.1**.

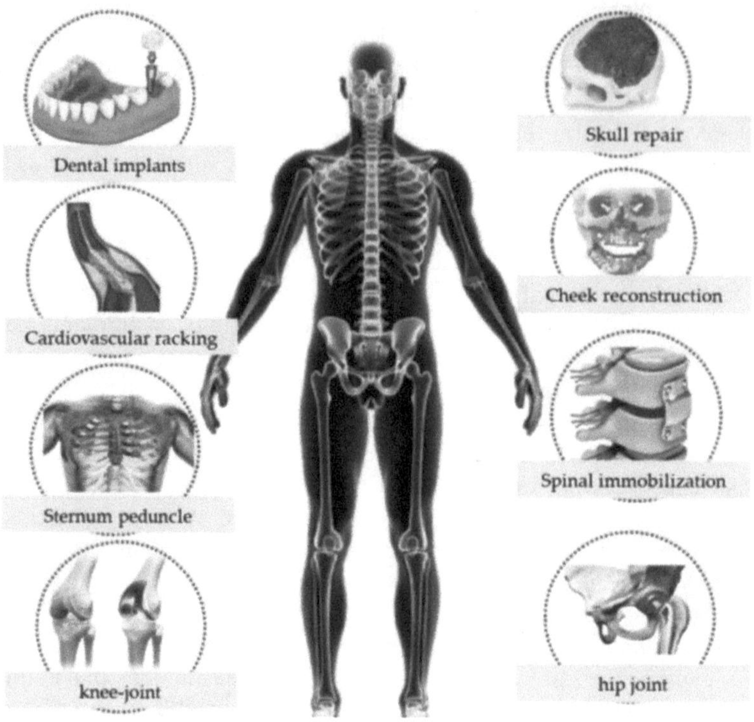

FIGURE 7.1 Biomedical metal materials applications [2]. (Under CC 4.0 Attribution)

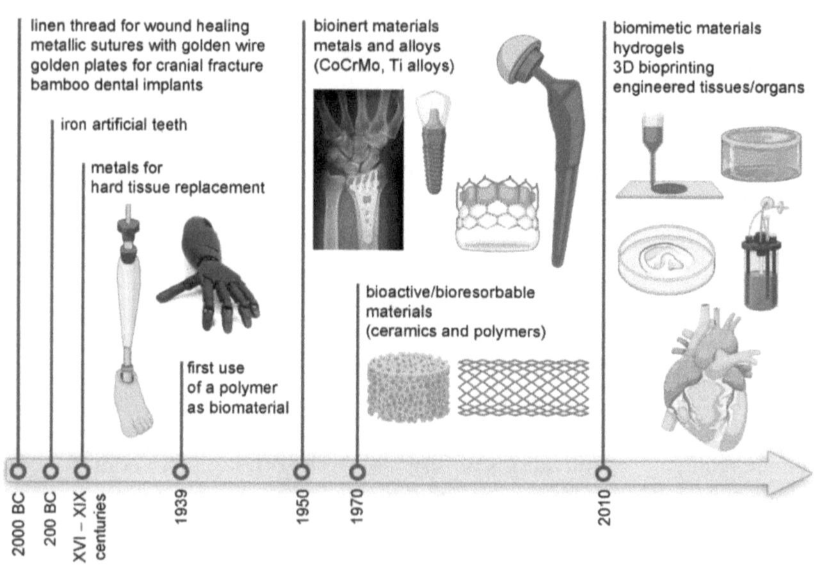

FIGURE 7.2 The evolution of biomaterials from regeneration to replacement [4] (Under CC 4.0 Attribution)

TABLE 7.1
Coating Effects and Clinical Implications

Coating Effect	Outcome	Material Used	Clinical Data
Enhanced Biocompatibility	Promotes better cell adhesion and tissue integration	Hydroxyapatite (HA), smart ceramics	HA coatings improved bone fixation by 40% in orthopedic implants, reducing implant loosening and enhancing osseointegration.
Antibacterial Properties	Reduces infections by releasing antimicrobial agents	Silver nanoparticle coatings	Nanoparticle coatings on hip implants lowered postoperative infection rates by 70% compared to non-coated implants.
Wear and Corrosion Resistance	Reduces wear and degradation in harsh environments	TiN, Mg-based coatings	TiN coatings increased wear resistance by 50% in joint implants under cyclic loading tests.
Enhanced Osteogenesis	Promotes bone growth and faster healing	Piezoelectric materials	Piezoelectric HA coatings increased bone growth in femoral implants by 25% compared to non-coated implants.

7.2 TYPES OF SMART MATERIALS FOR BIOMEDICAL IMPLANT COATINGS

7.2.1 Shape Memory Alloys (SMAs)

Shape memory alloys are a type of smart materials that have gained much attention in biomedical applications of implants based on their property of deformation as well as original shape recoverability upon exposure to some external stimulus, most commonly temperature. The nickel-titanium alloy is the most-studied and applied SMA within the biomedical sector, and it is known by the generic name Nitinol (NiTi). In addition, this alloy possesses not only the remarkable SME but also superelasticity. The latter property postures SMAs as unique candidates to significantly enhance the stability and functionality of implants [6]. **Figure 7.3** illustrates the implant's preparation methods as well as the mechanical and biological characteristics of titanium and its alloy.

The shape memory effect is such a phenomenon in which an SMA can be deformed at relatively low temperatures, and on heating, it recovers its original shape. Such behavior is based on the reversible phase transformation between two crystalline structures: The martensite, stable at low temperature, and austenite, stable at high temperature. In the martensitic phase, SMAs can easily be deformed through the reorientation of twinned martensitic variants, allowing the material to take on any shape. However, as soon as the SMA is heated above its transformation temperature,

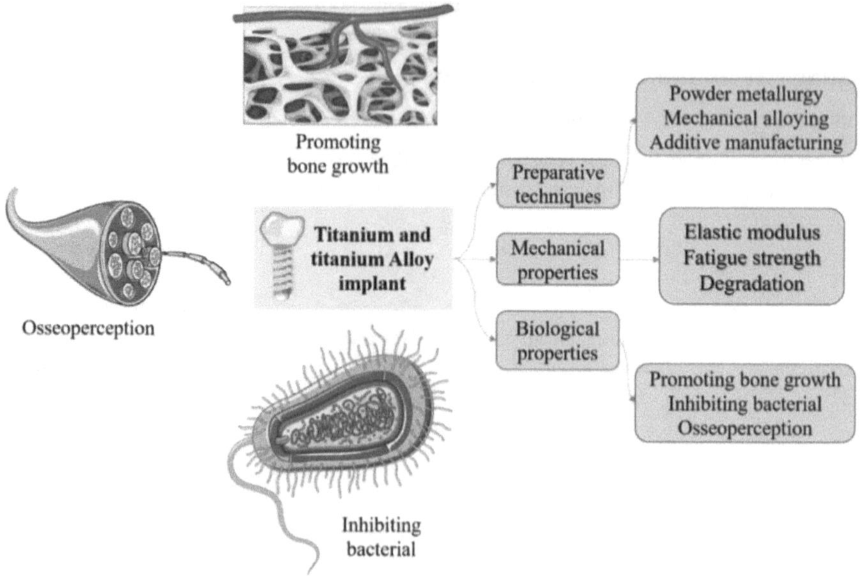

FIGURE 7.3 Preparative techniques and mechanical and biological properties of titanium and its alloy implant [7]. (Under CC 4.0 Attribution)

the alloy returns to an austenitic phase and recovers its original, pre-deformed shape. Transformation is fully reversible; thus, SMAs can be made to "remember" their original shape as well as return to it when heated, and this has several benefits in applications where these implants must accommodate the biological environment as well as retain mechanical integrity. One of the most important properties of SMAs is superelasticity, where they can resist large deformation strains with no permanent deformation. Superelasticity is a characteristic property for stress-induced reversible transformation from an austenitic phase to martensitic phase in mechanically stressed SMA. After the removal of the applied stress, the material goes back to its original form, thereby showing it to be highly flexible and resilient. This property is very useful when the implant must withstand dynamic mechanical stresses. In that case, examples include the cardiovascular system and any other joint movement [8].

Advantages of SMAs in enhancing stability of implants are that they adapt to a physiological environment of a body without losing their structural integrity. An example among orthopedic applications includes the use of SMAs in bone implants or fracture fixation devices. At surgery time, an SMA can be cooled to its martensitic phase, and it will then undergo deformation with the ability of being inserted into the body. Once inside, as the alloy is exposed to body temperature it transforms back to its austenitic phase with force exerted on surrounding tissues or bones, improving fixation and ensuring that healing will occur. It is this shape memory ability that allows it to settle more smoothly into the implant site, decreases micromotion, and favors osseointegration, the biological process by which bone tissue is incorporated with the implant. Applications in cardiovascular areas have already adopted SMAs like NiTi for stents that are small, mesh-like structures used to place inside the blood vessel to keep it open [9].

The SMAs are capable of exhibiting superelastic properties that allow the stent to be compressed sufficiently for insertion in a minimally invasive manner into the narrow or occluded arteries. Upon deployment inside the body, the SMA-based stent expands and recovers its original shape and provides support to the vessel wall, thus restoring blood flow. This superelasticity of SMAs would then be said to enable stents to contend with variations in the diameter of blood vessels due to pulsatile blood flow, which minimizes the possibilities for restenosis and consequently improves long-term follow-up. In addition to this, SMAs have been applied to spinal implants and other load-bearing devices where the ability to recover and withstand large mechanical loads may enhance the performance of an implant over time. For instance, NiTi-based spinal implants could be easily designed to meet the physiological curvature of the spine with the accommodation of micro-movements without any significant stress concentration and wear on the implant. Nevertheless, though these advantages are propounded, SMAs, when used in biomedical applications, pose some challenges as well [10].

Nickel is the primary element used in Nitinol, which has been shown to provoke allergic reactions and cytotoxicity in some individuals. Thus, the most critical parameter followed for safe use in implants is biocompatibility. Surface treatments, coatings, or alloying strategies are generally accepted to reduce the release of nickel ions from SMAs in efforts to enhance their biocompatibility. Moreover, although mechanical properties are promising, long-term stability of materials in biological environments, including corrosion and fatigue resistance, remain research areas [11].

7.2.2 Hydrogels

Highly porous, hydrated polymer networks swell upon environmental stimulation such as pH or temperature and have gained much interest in biomedical applications. They consist of hydrophilic polymer chains and absorb large amounts of water without losing structural integrity. They are promising materials in the biomedical field, particularly for the applications of drug delivery systems, tissue engineering scaffolds, or coatings for biomedical implants.

Hydrogels show a swelling behavior corresponding to the balance between hydrophilic nature and cross-linking structure of polymer chains holding them together. Penetration of water molecules into the polymer matrix leads to an aqueous environment that is reported to cause swelling in the hydrogel. An extent of swelling is perceived by factors which could be linked to the cross-linking degree, the chemical composition of the polymer, and the specific external stimulus [12].

Hydrogels have also gained sensitivity to pH and can be fabricated for biomedical implants that can respond to some local fluctuation in body conditions, including inflammation or infection. Ionizable groups in the polymer network of a pH-sensitive hydrogel, which are carboxyl or amino groups, take protons and donate them depending on the pH environment. If hydrogels contain groups of acids, they release protons in low pH environments and hence give electrostatic repulsion between chains of polymers, resulting in swelling. In basic environments, protonation causes the gel to shrink. Temperature-sensitive gels, such as PNIPAAm-based hydrogels, undergo a phase transition at certain temperatures. Below their critical temperature, hydrogels are swollen and absorb water; above the critical threshold, hydrophobic interactions prevail with the gel expelling water and shrinking. This reversibly swelling response to temperature conditions has been applied to control drug delivery or therapeutic interventions from an implant [13].

7.2.3 Bioactive Glass and Ceramics

Bioactive glass and ceramics have appeared to be critical for coating biomedical implants because of their remarkable capability to initiate bone tissue regeneration based on mechanisms of osteoinduction and bioactivity. These materials are well appreciated in orthopedic and dental applications due to their interaction with biological tissues which effectively enhances the integration of implants with the surrounding bone and encourages healing [14].

7.2.3.1 Osteoinduction

This property is demonstrated by a material where progenitor cells lining the bone surface begin to differentiate into osteoblasts, the cells responsible for the production of bone matrix. Bioactive glass and ceramics, hydroxyapatite (HAp), and bioactive glass (such as Bioglass®) fall into this category based on their composition, which promotes osteogenic activity. The principle is based on the release of biologically active ions from the material, among others being calcium (Ca^{2+}) and phosphate (PO_4^{3-}) and silicon (Si^{4+}), into the surrounding environment. These ions activate pathways that lead to recruitment, proliferation, and differentiation of osteoprogenitor cells thus creating a local biochemical environment favorable to bone formation. Therefore, these biomaterials expedite the healing process at the bone–implant interface by promoting new bone growth [15].

7.2.3.2 Bioactivity

Bioactivity means that it is possible to form a direct chemical bond between the material and living bone tissue. Once this glass or ceramic is implanted in the body, it reacts on its surface with the body fluids where, because of the ion exchange process, the formation of the hydroxycarbonate apatite (HCA) layer is observed that is comparable with the mineral phase of natural bone. This HCA layer provides an optimal surface for osteoblast attachment and proliferation, thus helping to achieve osseointegration in which the implant integrates with the bone. Bioactivity in these materials ensures that they not only act as passive scaffolds but also take an active role in the process of bone regeneration [16].

7.2.4 Magneto-Responsive Materials

Magneto-responsive materials, particularly those containing magnetic nanoparticles, have received great interest in biomedical applications since they respond sensitively to external magnetic fields. Often integrated as a coating of biomedical implants or as drug delivery systems, the materials provided a diverse platform to be able to achieve controlled, non-invasive therapeutic responses. The main principle of such "smart" functionality stems from magnetic properties of nanoparticles, often in the form of iron oxide, which respond to external magnetic fields, thus enabling the tight regulation of biological processes, such as drug release, thermotherapy, or localized stimulation of tissues [17]. **Figure 7.4** presents the various biomedical applications of MNPs.

Magnetic nanoparticles are defined as superparamagnetic; this means magnetization is available only in the presence of an external magnetic field. This ensures the loss of residual magnetism once the field is removed and less chance of agglomeration or interference in surrounding tissues. Once an external magnetic field is applied, it aligns the nanoparticles, which further generates movement or heat based on the strength and type of the applied magnetic stimulus. Targeted drug delivery is a promising use of magneto-responsive materials where therapeutic agents can be released by remote actuation of a magnetic field from the embedded nanoparticles within a hydrogel or polymer matrix coating an implant. The movement of the nanoparticles due to the magnetic field, depending on their interaction with the matrix, will either break bonds within the matrix or cause structural changes that will facilitate the release of encapsulated drugs at the target site. This delivery method results in a localized and controlled administration of the drug and, thus, lowers the need for systemic treatment and reduces side effects [19].

7.2.5 pH-Responsive Polymers

The pH-sensitive polymers are smart materials whose physical and chemical properties have shown a dramatic change with the alteration of pH values in the surrounding environment. These polymers have been explored more for their biomedical applications, particularly for drug delivery systems and coatings on implants, as they can change the behavior of therapeutic agents by adjusting to various pH conditions.

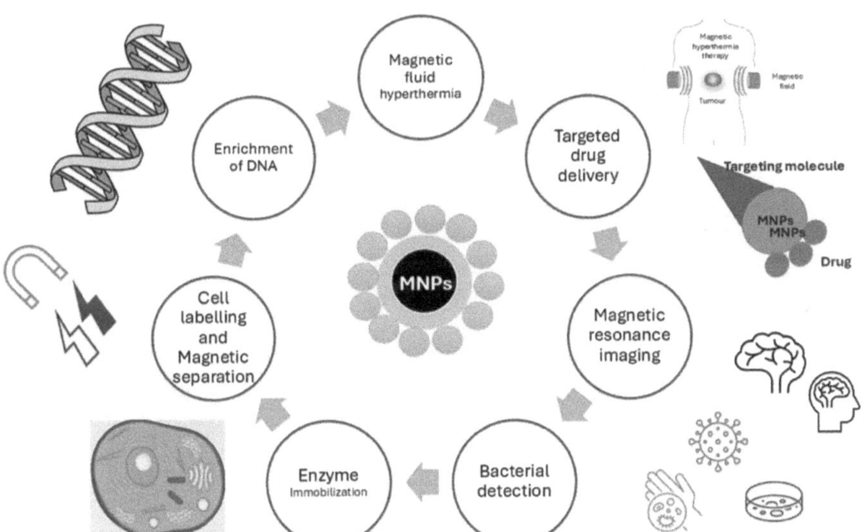

FIGURE 7.4 Various biomedical applications of MNPs [18]. (Under CC 4.0 Attribution)

This adaptive characteristic does make pH-responsive polymers useful for targeted treatments, especially in fields where local pH changes occur, such as inflamed or infected tissues, cancerous regions, or the gastrointestinal tract [20].

The backbone of the responsiveness in these polymers is the presence of ionizable functional groups. These include carboxyl, amino, or sulfonic groups, depending on whether they can donate or accept protons according to the pH environment around them. Charge, solubility, swelling behavior, and structural conformation of the polymer will accordingly change. For instance, under conditions of low pH concentration (acidic conditions), the polymer can become protonated, thus increasing its solubility or swelling capability. On the other hand, under high pH concentrations (basic conditions), it undergoes deprotonation, resulting in collapsing or a reduced swelling of the polymer. The reversible response enables the material to dynamically respond to pH changes in controlled drug delivery or responsive biomedical coatings [21].

In the area of biomedical implants, pH-sensitive polymers may be used as coatings for site-specific release of drugs or bioactive agents once a certain pH threshold is reached. For example, in infected or inflammatory regions by pathogens, whose pH values are generally lower than in normal tissue, the polymer can swell and ensure faster release of antibacterial or anti-inflammatory drugs. The concept of release targeted to areas of drug action reduces drug exposure to the rest of the body while enhancing effectiveness of localized treatment. Similarly, using pH-responsive polymers, it is possible to attain controlled release of chemotherapeutic agents because of the slightly more acidic pH in cancerous tissues. It will ensure that the drugs are targeted at the tumor site and, thus, greatly increase the efficiency of treatment with fewer side effects [22]. **Figure 7.5** shows the types of stimulus-responsive polymers.

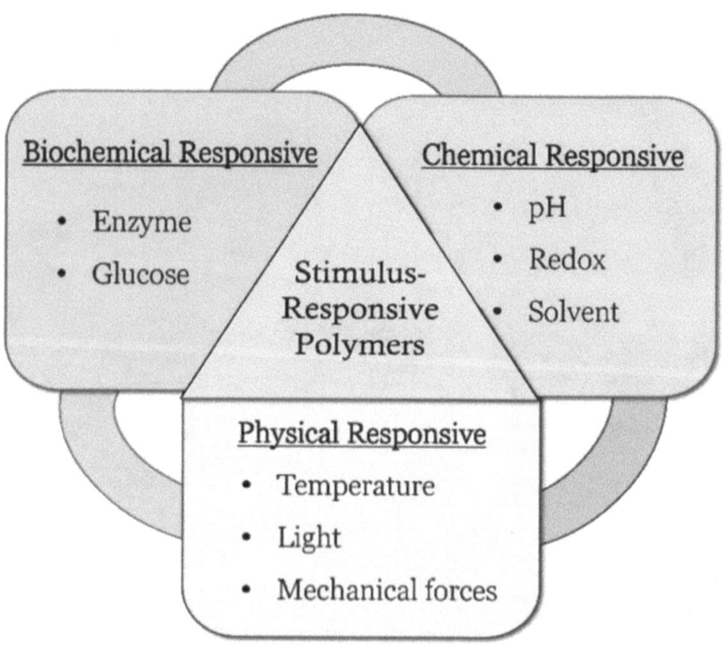

FIGURE 7.5 Types of stimulus-responsive polymers [23]. (Under CC 4.0 Attribution)

Beyond drug delivery applications, these pH-sensitive polymers also may provide protection for implants via adaptive barriers, reducing, for example, biofilm formation, corrosion, or degradation. Their adaptability, biocompatibility, and versatility make these molecules of utmost importance in the development of next-generation biomedical implant coatings [24].

7.3 FUNCTIONAL BENEFITS OF SMART COATINGS

7.3.1 Bioactivity and Osseointegration

Bioactivity and osseointegration are the most critical aspects of the successful development of biomedical implants. These capabilities do not only allow the implant to be stable and well-integrated in the body but, importantly, actively contribute to the healing and regeneration of tissues surrounding it. Bioactivity is thus defined as a material's ability to evoke a biological response that promotes interaction with the living tissue. Osseointegration is the process by which the implant becomes directly bonded to the bone tissue without the formation of any fibrous tissue around it and hence results in long-term stability and functionality [25].

Bioactivity is a property most often associated with materials, such as bioactive glasses, hydroxyapatite (HAp), and some ceramics. These materials can chemically bond into host tissues, particularly bone, by forming a biologically active layer. When bioactive materials are implanted, they initially react to body fluids, which induce a series of surface reactions. The most released ions from these materials include calcium (Ca^{2+}), phosphate (PO_4^{3-}), and silicon (Si^{4+}) in the surrounding environment. Although these ions are involved in signaling pathways that drive osteoblast activity and bone regeneration, these ions can participate in the formation of a HCA layer closely mimicking the mineral composition of natural bone [26].

Cell attachment, proliferation, and differentiation require a substrate that is therefore critical in bioactivity: the formation of the HCA layer. Osteoblasts—the bone forming cells—are bonded to the HCA layer, and this bonding enhances appositional bone around the implant. In addition, materials with bioactive properties, such as hydroxyapatite or bioactive glass, may induce osteoinduction, wherein mesenchymal stem cells are stimulated to differentiate into bone-forming osteoblasts, thus enhancing the regeneration of bone tissue [27].

A synthetic thermoplastic polymer polyetheretherketone (PEEK) is becoming a highly sought component for clinical applications in orthopedic and spinal uses but suffers certain limitations in practical use. PEEK has properties that are desirable, such as being biocompatible, having chemical stability, having low radiolucency, and possessing an elastic modulus close to that of normal human bone. However, it is biologically inert, which precludes good integration with adjacent bone tissues when implanted. The plot of existing approaches to increase PEEK's bioactivity is shown in **Figure 7.6**.

Recent focus has been given on the enhancement of the bioactivity of PEEK to achieve better bone–implant integration. Two approaches have been taken to overcome this inert character of PEEK. The first approach is surface modification by merely treating the PEEK surface or in conjunction with the application of surface coating of activated PEEK. Another strategy is the preparation of bioactive PEEK composites by the impregnation of bioactive materials into the PEEK substrate. Researchers predict wide orthopedic applications for the modified bioactive PEEK [29].

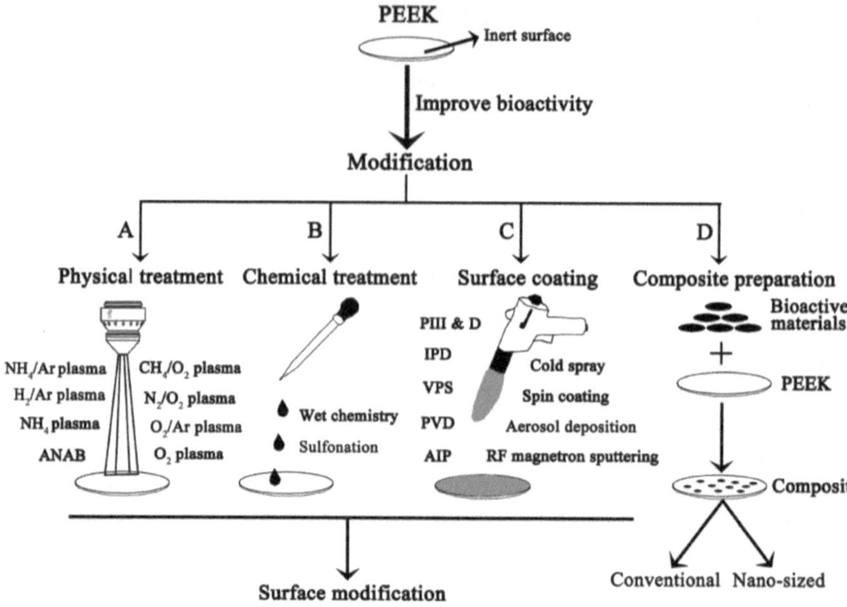

FIGURE 7.6 Scheme of current strategies to improve the bioactivity of PEEK [28]. (Under CC 4.0 Attribution)

Bioactive coatings based on hydroxyapatite or bioglass are applied to metallic implants, including those made of titanium. Metals like titanium are known to be highly biocompatible with good mechanical strength but lack inherent bioactivity, and therefore osseointegration is restricted. Coating such implants with bioactive materials encourages a stronger bone–implant interface, allowing for faster and more effective integration. Many of the coatings are porous as well, similar in nature to natural bone, which is ideal for scaffold bone ingrowth [30].

Osseointegration is highly supported in elderly or osteoporotic patients, where the potential for bone healing and regeneration would be a challenge. Bioactive materials create a more favorable environment for better activity from bone cells. The reduced healing time after surgery and improved long-term performance are expected [31].

7.3.2 Antibacterial and Anti-inflammatory Properties

Antibacterial and anti-inflammatory properties are some of the key aspects that biomedical implant designs need to consider, especially toward infection reduction after the implantation and the response toward inflammation that compromises the implanted device functions. Both infections and inflammation have been considered as major causes that lead to the failure of an implanted device, necessitating revisions or even replacement. Overcoming such challenges can be achieved by using smart materials that have inherent or engineered antibacterial and anti-inflammatory properties. Such materials can form a defensive barrier against pathogens, acting to also modify the host's immune response for healing and long-term implant success [32].

Antibacterial properties may prevent bacterial colonization and biofilm formation on implant surfaces. Once the bacteria adhere to an implant, they can form a protective matrix called a biofilm that protects them from antibiotics and the host's immune system. Bacterial infections around implants are typically due to *Staphylococcus aureus*, *Escherichia coli*, or *Pseudomonas aeruginosa*; they are challenging to treat and, in most cases, become a complication leading to failure of the implant or sepsis if left unmanaged. Smart coatings or antibacterial-materials infusion could be the way either by preventing bacteria from attaching or by killing bacteria upon contact [33].

Concepts for multifunctional surfaces in total hip replacement that are intended to react to different biological and mechanical activities either concurrently or sequentially are shown in **Figure 7.7**. The unique capabilities of the coatings obtained throughout the manufacturing process determine the response. The response depends on the specific abilities of the coatings acquired during the manufacturing process.

Commonly used materials in local antibiotic delivery are silver nanoparticles, copper, and zinc oxide and other specific types of bioactive ceramics like bioglass. Silver nanoparticles have particularly broad-spectrum effects against bacteria because they can disrupt cell membranes, inhibit DNA replication, and create ROS that lead to bacterial death. The other incorporated application of these nanoparticles is in the coating of implants to provide a sustained antibacterial effect. This, in turn,

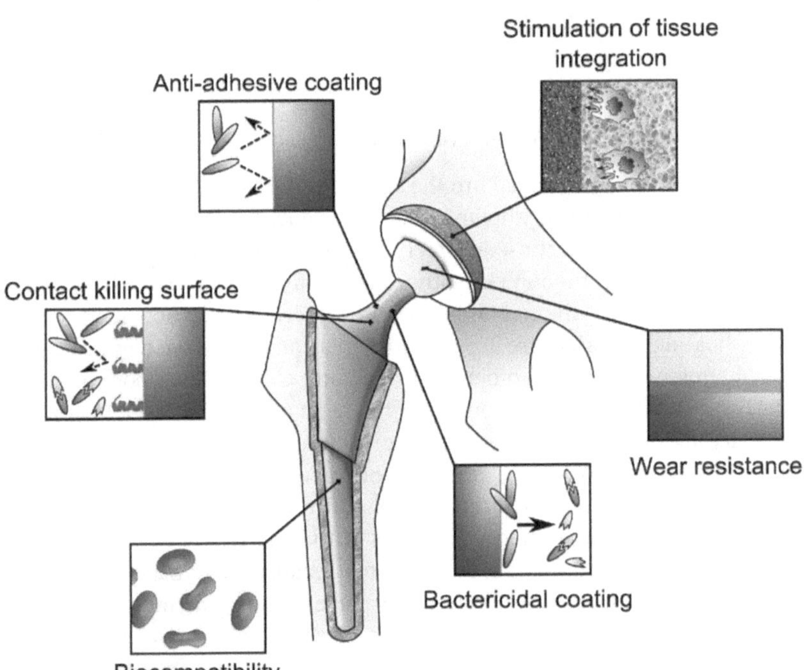

FIGURE 7.7 Ideas of multifunctional surfaces in total hip arthroplasty designed to simultaneously or successively respond to various biological and mechanical tasks [34]. (Under CC 4.0 Attribution)

reduces the possibility of biofilm formation and further infection. In addition to this, there is the release of ions, specifically calcium and phosphate, by bioactive glasses, which promotes antibacterial activity in the environment by inhibiting the growth of bacteria [35].

Different smart materials have been designed to release anti-inflammatory agents or alter the mode of action of the immune response. Some coatings embedded with corticosteroids or NSAIDs can locally suppress inflammation at the site of the implant. Furthermore, materials like Mg alloys, which have a lot of research potential with respect to their application in biodegradable implants, show some degree of inflammatory response attenuation. The ionic effect of Mg can modulate the functioning of immune cells, thus keeping the background clear from inflammation, which is helpful for healing and tissue regeneration. Hydrogels and polymer coatings can be prepared as drug delivery systems that will self-release anti-inflammatory agents specifically in the presence of certain stimuli, for example, in the case of inflamed tissues following a drop in pH, with targeted and controlled delivery without systemic side effects [36].

Moreover, the inherent antibacterial and anti-inflammatory activities of natural polymers like chitosan and hyaluronic acid are also very commonly utilized. Chitosan is a type of biopolymer based on chitin; it works as a bacterium cell wall-disrupting agent and therefore, shows anti-inflammatory activity through the modulation of the immune cells. Hyaluronic acid, one of the important structures within the cell's ground substance, can decrease inflammation due to the regulation of the immune cells' activity and diminished production of pro-inflammatory mediators [37].

7.3.3 Self-Recovery and Wear Resistance

Self-recovery and wear resistance are the most dominating features in the development of advanced biomedical implants that experience mechanical wear and stress over time. These two properties, self-recovery and wear, significantly improve the implant's robustness and functionality, thus increasing the chances of better patients' recovery and minimizing the rate of revisional surgeries or replacements [38].

The self-healing materials are great entities that can restore the damage caused by mechanical stresses, wear, and other environmental elements autonomously. This is particularly advantageous in the context of biomedical implants, as it restores structural integrity and functionality without surgical intervention. A self-healing mechanism typically would involve the injection of microcapsules or vascular networks with healing agents into the material matrix. Once released within the material at the site of damage, these healing agents can aid in the repair of the material. For instance, in polymer-based implant coatings, microcapsules with a healing agent, for example, a monomer or adhesive, may be dispersed within the matrix. If and when this material breaks or fractures, the microcapsules crack and release the healing agent; it polymerizes and fills up the damage region, making the properties of this material original again. This self-healing feature also makes the service life of the implanted device longer and increases the safety of the patient, as complications arising from material degradation are highly reduced [39]. **Figure 7.8** shows the applications of self-healing graphene/polymer composites [40].

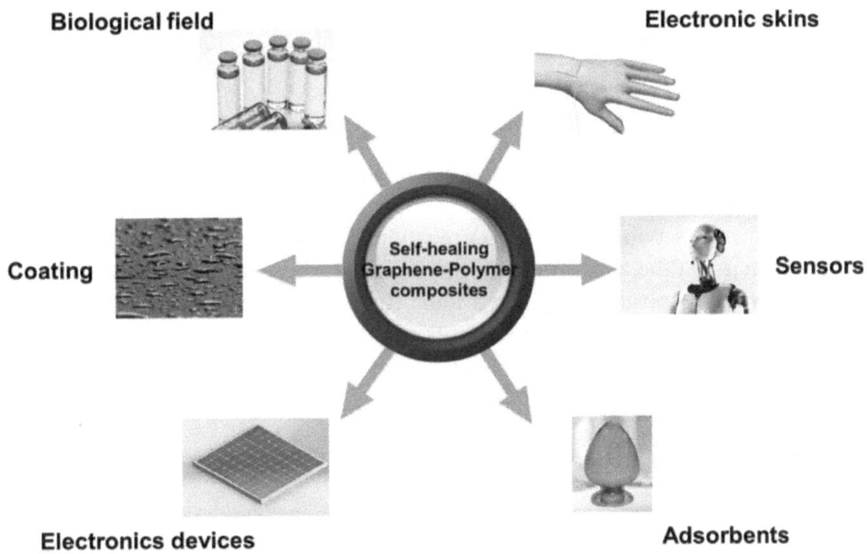

FIGURE 7.8 Applications of self-healing graphene/polymer composites [40]. (Under CC 4.0 Attribution)

Other strategies for self-healing materials involve dynamic covalent bonds or supramolecular interactions that can reform on damage. Such materials would be able to recover their original properties after deformation or crack formation, making them uniquely suitable for load-bearing implants, where mechanical integrity is crucial.

Another important property of biomedical implants is wearing resistance, since many of them need to be repeatedly subjected to loading and movements. Wear can lead to emission of particles into the surrounding tissues, bringing on inflammations and degraded performance of the implant. Therefore, research focuses on developing materials with high wear resistance for assurance of the longevity and reliability of implants. The increase in wear resistance can be achieved by several approaches. Among these techniques for the enhancement of metallic implant, wear resistance is the use of coatings on the metallic implants, like TiN, DLC, and other ceramic-based coatings. The protective layers formed by these coatings give way to friction and wear decrease, increasing the longevity of the material beneath the coatings. Surface modification techniques, such as micro-structuring or the application of gradient layers, may provide further improvements in wear performance and produce surface morphologies that are less sensitive to abrasion and deformation [41].

7.4 CORROSION RESISTANCE

Corrosion is the natural processes in which materials, particularly metals, deteriorate due to the reaction between the material and its environmental surroundings. The highest concern with biomedical implants involves corrosion, which can cause the loss of integrity, functionality, and biocompatibility of the implants. The study of the corrosion mechanisms requires research to lead to more abundant materials resisting degradation and increasing the lifetime of biomedical devices [42].

7.4.1 Mechanism of Corrosion

Electrochemical Reactions: Electrochemical reactions are the major causes of corrosion; they are in the form of electron transfer from the metal to its surroundings. This most often involves two simultaneous reactions, namely oxidation and reduction. Oxidation occurs at the anode in metallic implants, where the metal loses electrons and hence provides positively charged ions. Reduction takes place in the cathode, where electrons are gained, in most cases with the involvement of oxygen or the available reducing agent in the environment [43].

The overall reaction can be written as:

Oxidation (anodic reaction):

$$M \rightarrow M^{n+} + ne^-$$

(where M is the metal, and n is the number of electrons lost.)

Reduction (cathodic reaction):

$$O_2 + 2H_2O + 4e^- \rightarrow 4OH^-$$

Definition of a Corrosion Cell: A corrosion cell is the electrochemical reactions that occur within an anode wherein actual dissolution (corrosion) takes place, cathode wherein the reduction occurs, an electrolyte, which is an ionic solution normally an aqueous, and a conductive path (which could either be the implant material itself or introduced in its surface). These cells are formed because of non-uniformity in metal composition, microstructural difference, and environmental conditions, thus forming various phenomena such as pitting, galvanic corrosion, and crevice corrosion [44].

Pitting corrosion is a type of localized corrosion that is characterized by the existence of very small pits or holes on the metal. In this type of corrosion, material loss is fairly high in time. Pitting occurs because of oxide layer breakdowns on the surface of the metal. Some causes of pitting corrosion involve chlorides in bodily fluids [45].

Corrosion that appears when two dissimilar metals come into contact in the presence of an electrolyte is known as galvanic corrosion. In this type of corrosion, the more active metal is placed at the anode position where it corrodes preferentially. On the contrary, if the other metal is less active, its position is placed at the cathode, where it is protected. This kind of corrosion is specifically relevant to biomedical implants that consist of multiple metallic components [46].

Crevice corrosion occurs in confined geometries, such as joints or gaps between the implant and tissues. The stagnant solution in crevices may evolve to be more acidic or deoxygenated and could become a more favorable medium for corrosion [47].

7.4.2 Smart Materials in Corrosion Prevention

The integration of smart materials into corrosion prevention strategies marks a giant step in the biomedical implants. Smart materials exhibit responsiveness to environmental stimuli, and their active, dynamic, and adaptive approach provides immense possibilities for overcoming corrosion risks, enhancing material longevity, and achieving better performance of an implant. Such materials turn out to be extremely effective in a complex physiological environment threateningly riddled with corrosion risks [48].

7.4.2.1 Self-Healing Materials

Self-healing coatings are one of the first and most promising applications of smart materials in corrosion protection. Such materials are conceived to repair autonomously any damage due to wear or impact as well as corrosion. Self-healing mechanisms may be integrated into coatings by microcapsules or vascular networks containing healing agents, such as polymers or corrosion inhibitors. When the coating is damaged, the healing agents are released, and the gaps and cracks can be filled again, restoring the protective layer. This does not only make the coated piece more resistant to damage but also lowers the dangers of corrosion because it leaves no gap between the metal substrate underneath and the protective layer maintaining continuity over the protective layer [49]. **Figure 7.9** presents the self-healing techniques.

They can be formulated to respond precisely to certain environmental conditions that might point to corrosive environments. Some of the environmental conditions are pH, temperature, or ionic concentration. Temperature-sensitive polymers could be utilized in coatings whose properties change with changes in body temperature, thereby improving their protection features under changing physiological conditions. This adaptive ability therefore guarantees the active performance of corrosion-protection methods depending on the immediate surroundings of an implant [51].

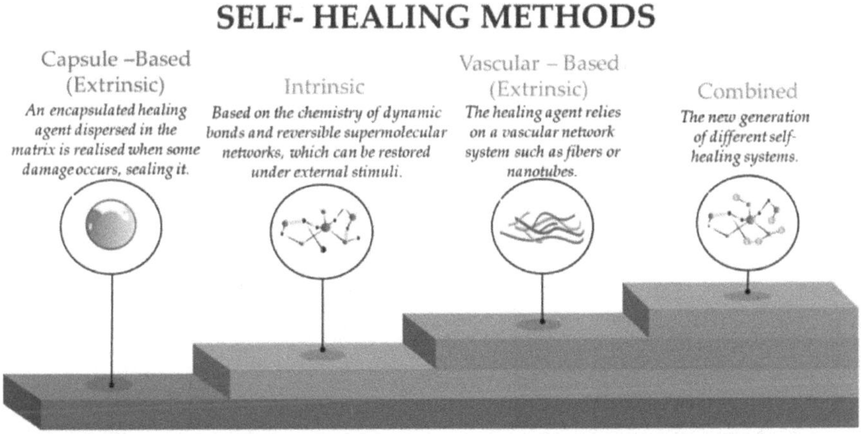

FIGURE 7.9 Self-healing methods [50]. (Under CC 4.0 Attribution)

7.4.2.2 Nanomaterials for Enhanced Protection

The inclusion of nanomaterials in smart coatings has great promise to improve their corrosion protection properties. In polymer matrices, nanoparticles such as zinc oxide and titanium dioxide or graphene may be incorporated to enhance the mechanical properties and provide additional protective benefits through added nanoparticles. Such additives can significantly contribute to providing increased barrier properties against corrosive agents. Moisture and ion permeation film responsible for corrosion are reduced [52].

7.4.2.3 Smart Coatings containing Corrosion Inhibitors

Smart coatings containing corrosion inhibitors comprise another method for preventing corrosion. They can be devised to be released progressively upon corroding factors. A good example would be a coating designed to release a certain inhibitor if it senses high concentrations of chloride ions, commonly present in corrosive environments. The targeted release facilitates protective measures when they are most needed and, therefore, can increase the efficiency of a corrosion prevention strategy [53]. A variety of stimulus-responsive micro/nanocontainer coatings are shown in **Figure 7.10**, along with their different applications in materials science,

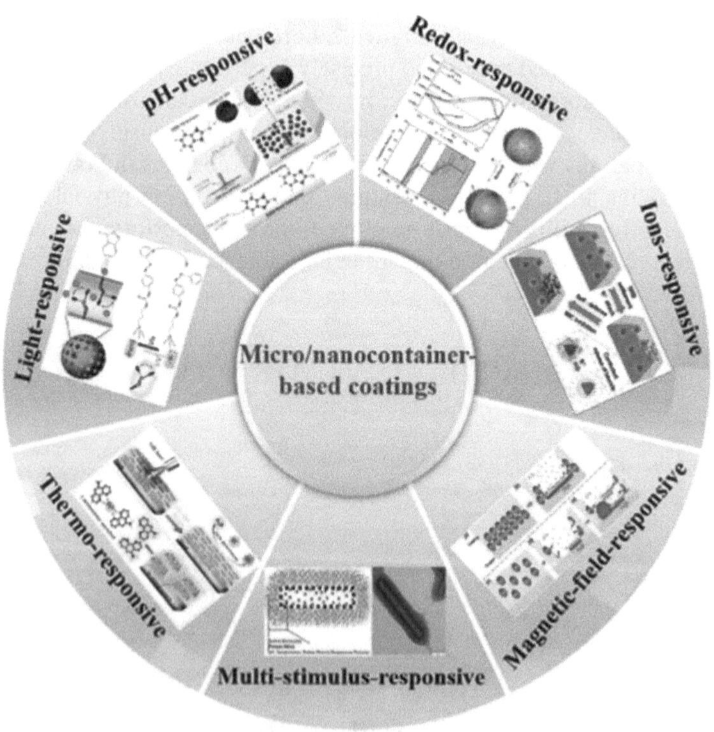

FIGURE 7.10 Various stimulus-responsive micro/nanocontainer coatings and their uses across fields, illustrating how they adapt to environmental changes like temperature or pH for applications in medicine, materials science, and environmental protection [54]. (Under CC 4.0 Attribution)

environmental protection, and medicine. The coatings are shown to adjust to changes in temperature or pH.

7.5 CHALLENGES IN CLINICAL TRANSLATION

Smart materials have the potential for application in clinics as biomedical implants. However, their achievements in healthcare settings depend on numerous challenges to be overcome. The possible benefits of these materials are great advantages, but complications in developing, approvals, and later use in the clinical field pose real difficulties.

One of the main challenges in terms of translating smart materials for clinical application is consistent performance with high reliability over time. In the biomedical application, implants are subjected to very complex mechanical and physiological environments, thus affecting the behavior of smart materials significantly. For instance, average mechanical loading experienced by implants like the joint replacements can cause material's fatigue or failure. Interactions between the smart material and biological tissues are very patient-to-patient variable based on differences in physiology, age, and health status. Smart materials should be robustly tested and validated under simulated physiological conditions to ensure long-term functionality. This may require broad-scale mechanical, chemical, and biological tests to evaluate the functionality of materials under extended in vitro exposure and varied loading conditions [55].

Safety and biocompatibility are the most critical considerations in the clinical translation of smart materials. For an implant, adverse biological response—here considered to be a sustainable but not necessarily severe inflammation, toxicity, or immunogenicity—must not be present. Although most of these smart materials are designed to be biocompatible, compatibility could be highly dependent on the material interaction with surrounding tissues. For example, it may degrade or release its active agents in such a manner as to cause an inflammatory effect or have adverse effects on cellular responses. Extensive in vitro and in vivo studies must be conducted before such smart materials are allowed to be used clinically. These studies must include long-term studies of how it may happen in the body over longer periods [56].

Manufacturing processes of smart materials generally employ sophisticated techniques that are not easily scalable to large-scale production for commerce. Methods such as 3D printing, electrospinning, or nano-coating are relatively sensitive to parameters and may require sophisticated control to produce consistent materials of reproducible quality. In addition, the inclusion of responsive agents like self-healing compounds or corrosion inhibitors in the manufacturing process makes things even more complicated. To facilitate clinical translation, scalable and low-cost manufacturing techniques need to be established that can produce good-quality smart materials [57].

7.6 FUTURE DIRECTIONS

The near future for biomedical implants with smart materials will be marked with immense breakthroughs based on innovative contributions from material sciences, nanotechnology, and personalized medicine. Smart sensors integrated into the implant will allow real-time evaluation and monitoring of the condition of the implant itself, as well as its biological environment, and enable proactive management of any potential complications. Next-generation nanotechnology and biomimicry will continue to inform the development of new smart materials with ever-closer forms and functions to biological tissues, thereby achieving better biocompatibility and osseointegration capabilities [58–61]. Advanced manufacturing techniques—additive manufacturing, in particular—can make complex implants tailored with smart functionalities [62–65]. This will also facilitate some regulatory frameworks and standards for the clinical translation of these new materials. Such interdisciplinary collaboration of researchers, industry, and providers of healthcare will then enable novel solutions that guarantee a high level of safety, efficacy, and long-term stability of biomedical implants. The embracing of such future directions would revolutionize patient care and significantly alter clinical outcomes in biomedical engineering [66, 67].

7.7 CONCLUSION

Smart materials represent a groundbreaking breakthrough for biomedical implants and introduce an innovative solution to critical challenges about biocompatibility, life, and functionality. Realizing such responses through smart mechanisms, like self-healing properties, pH responsiveness, or magnetic actuation, would significantly improve an implant's performance and related outcomes for the patient. Improving osseointegration, effects at reducing bacteria and inflammation, and potential dynamic responses to physiological conditions make smart materials capable, versatile, and clinically relevant.

Despite such immense potential, clinical translation of these smart materials poses challenges in achieving reproducible performance, biocompatibility, and regulatory compliance. Future directions for the field would thus involve advanced functionalization and smart sensors with assessments of new materials to extend further functionality improvements in implants. Ideally, the successful clinical translation in such cases would depend on interdisciplinarity with well-defined frameworks for regulations. With improved research, smart materials for biomedical implants under current development promise patient care with better longevity of the implants and, thus, the quality of life associated with patients requiring surgical interventions. In a nutshell, the future looks bright for these groundbreaking solutions in the field of biomedical engineering.

REFERENCES

1. Amirtharaj Mosas KK, Chandrasekar AR, Dasan A, Pakseresht A, Galusek D. Recent advancements in materials and coatings for biomedical implants. *Gels*. 2022;8(5):323.
2. Cai Z, Du P, Li K, Chen L, Xie G. A review of the development of titanium-based and magnesium-based metallic glasses in the field of biomedical materials. *Materials*. 2024;17(18):4587.
3. Joshi MU, Kulkarni SP, Choppadandi M, Keerthana M, Kapusetti G. Current state of art smart coatings for orthopedic implants: A comprehensive review. *Smart Materials in Medicine*. 2023;4:661–79.
4. Todros S, Todesco M, Bagno A. Biomaterials and their biomedical applications: From replacement to regeneration. *Processes*. 2021;9(11):1949.

5. Tibbitt MW, Rodell CB, Burdick JA, Anseth KS. Progress in material design for biomedical applications. *Proceedings of the National Academy of Sciences.* 2015;112(47):14444–51.
6. Kazanci M. A review of polymeric smart materials for biomedical applications. *Materials Technology.* 2003;18(2):87–93.
7. Wu H, Chen X, Kong L, Liu P. Mechanical and biological properties of titanium and its alloys for oral implant with preparation techniques: A review. *Materials.* 2023;16(21):6860.
8. Tanzi MC, Bozzini S, Candiani G, Cigada A, De Nardo L, Fare S, Ganazzoli F, Gastaldi D, Levi M, Metrangolo P, Migliavacca F. Trends in biomedical engineering: Focus on smart bio-materials and drug delivery. *Journal of Applied Biomaterials and Biomechanics.* 2011;9(2):87–97.
9. Holzapfel BM, Reichert JC, Schantz JT, Gbureck U, Rackwitz L, Nöth U, Jakob F, Rudert M, Groll J, Hutmacher DW. How smart do biomaterials need to be? A translational science and clinical point of view. *Advanced Drug Delivery Reviews.* 2013;65(4):581–603.
10. Montemor MF. Functional and smart coatings for corrosion protection: A review of recent advances. *Surface and Coatings Technology.* 2014;258:17–37.
11. Smith JR, Lamprou DA, Larson C, Upson SJ. Biomedical applications of polymer and ceramic coatings: A review of recent developments. *Transactions of the IMF.* 2022;100(1):25–35.
12. Zwawi M. Recent advances in bio-medical implants; mechanical properties, surface modifications and applications. *Engineering Research Express.* 2022;4(3):032003.
13. Ponmozhi J, Frias C, Marques T, Frazão O. Smart sensors/actuators for biomedical applications. *Measurement.* 2012;45(7):1675–88.
14. Yoshida M, Langer R, Lendlein A, Lahann J. From advanced biomedical coatings to multi-functionalized biomaterials. *Journal of Macromolecular Science, Part C: Polymer Reviews.* 2006;46:347–75.
15. Thakur A, Srivastava R, Bahadur PS, Rana A. Exploring the various biomedical applications of smart materials. In *Discovery, Disruption, and Future Implications of Nanomaterials* (pp. 249–74). IGI Global; 2024.
16. Roy RK, Lee KR. Biomedical applications of diamond-like carbon coatings: A review. *Journal of Biomedical Materials Research Part B: Applied Biomaterials: An Official Journal of The Society for Biomaterials, The Japanese Society for Biomaterials, and The Australian Society for Biomaterials and the Korean Society for Biomaterials.* 2007;83(1):72–84.
17. El Feninat F, Laroche G, Fiset M, Mantovani D. Shape memory materials for biomedical applications. *Advanced Engineering Materials.* 2002;4(3):91–104.
18. Vasić K, Knez Ž, Leitgeb M. Multifunctional iron oxide nanoparticles as promising magnetic biomaterials in drug delivery: A review. *Journal of Functional Biomaterials.* 2024;15(8):227.
19. Bagherifard S. Mediating bone regeneration by means of drug eluting implants: From passive to smart strategies. *Materials Science and Engineering: C.* 2017;71:1241–52.
20. Dobrzański LA, Dobrzańska-Danikiewicz AD, Dobrzański LB. Effect of biomedical materials in the implementation of a long and healthy life policy. *Processes.* 2021;9(5):865.
21. Montoya C, Du Y, Gianforcaro AL, Orrego S, Yang M, Lelkes PI. On the road to smart biomaterials for bone research: Definitions, concepts, advances, and outlook. *Bone Research.* 2021;9(1):12.
22. Ghimire A, Song J. Anti-periprosthetic infection strategies: From implant surface topographical engineering to smart drug-releasing coatings. *ACS Applied Materials & Interfaces.* 2021;13(18):20921–37.
23. Tan RY, Lee CS, Pichika MR, Cheng SF, Lam KY. PH responsive polyurethane for the advancement of biomedical and drug delivery. *Polymers.* 2022;14(9):1672.

24. Nathanael AJ, Oh TH. Biopolymer coatings for biomedical applications. *Polymers.* 2020;12(12):3061.
25. Ahmady AR, Ekhlasi A, Nouri A, Nazarpak MH, Gong P, Solouk A. High entropy alloy coatings for biomedical applications: A review. *Smart Materials in Manufacturing.* 2023;1:100009.
26. Sarraf M, Rezvani Ghomi E, Alipour S, Ramakrishna S, Liana Sukiman N. A state-of-the-art review of the fabrication and characteristics of titanium and its alloys for biomedical applications. *Bio-design and Manufacturing.* 2021:1–25.
27. Pandey A, Sahoo S. Progress on medical implant: A review and prospects. *Journal of Bionic Engineering.* 2023;20(2):470–94.
28. Ma R, Tang T. Current strategies to improve the bioactivity of PEEK. *International Journal of Molecular Sciences.* 2014;15(4):5426–45.
29. Prodana M, Stoian AB, Burnei C, Ionita D. Innovative coatings of metallic alloys used as bioactive surfaces in implantology: A review. *Coatings.* 2021;11(6):649.
30. Arsiwala A, Desai P, Patravale V. Recent advances in micro/nanoscale biomedical implants. *Journal of Controlled Release.* 2014;189:25–45.
31. Talebian S, Mendes B, Conniot J, Farajikhah S, Dehghani F, Li Z, Bitoque D, Silva G, Naficy S, Conde J, Wallace GG. Biopolymeric coatings for local release of therapeutics from biomedical implants. *Advanced Science.* 2023;10(12):2207603.
32. Yuan Z, He Y, Lin C, Liu P, Cai K. Antibacterial surface design of biomedical titanium materials for orthopedic applications. *Journal of Materials Science & Technology.* 2021;78:51–67.
33. Losic D. Advancing of titanium medical implants by surface engineering: Recent progress and challenges. *Expert Opinion on Drug Delivery.* 2021;18(10):1355–78.
34. Gallo J, Holinka M, Moucha CS. Antibacterial surface treatment for orthopaedic implants. *International Journal of Molecular Sciences.* 2014;15(8):13849–80.
35. Chen X, Zhou J, Qian Y, Zhao L. Antibacterial coatings on orthopedic implants. *Materials Today Bio.* 2023;19:100586.
36. Mejía-Manzano LA, Vázquez-Villegas P, Prado-Cervantes LV, Franco-Gómez KX, Carbajal-Ocaña S, Sotelo-Cortés DL, Atehortúa-Benítez V, Delgado-Rodríguez M, Membrillo-Hernández J. Advances in material modification with smart functional polymers for combating biofilms in biomedical applications. *Polymers.* 2023;15(14):3021.
37. Festas AJ, Ramos A, Davim JP. Medical devices biomaterials–A review. *Proceedings of the Institution of Mechanical Engineers, Part L: Journal of Materials: Design and Applications.* 2020;234(1):218–28.
38. Su M, Song Y. Printable smart materials and devices: Strategies and applications. *Chemical Reviews.* 2021;122(5):5144–64.
39. Parvizi J, Antoci V, Hickok NJ, Shapiro IM. Selfprotective smart orthopedic implants. *Expert Review of Medical Devices.* 2007;4(1):55–64.
40. Du Y, Li D, Liu L, Gai G. Recent achievements of self-healing graphene/polymer composites. *Polymers.* 2018;10(2):114.
41. Kaliaraj GS, Siva T, Ramadoss A. Surface functionalized bioceramics coated on metallic implants for biomedical and anticorrosion performance–a review. *Journal of Materials Chemistry B.* 2021;9(46):9433–60.
42. Todros S, Todesco M, Bagno A. Biomaterials and their biomedical applications: From replacement to regeneration. *Processes.* 2021;9(11):1949.
43. Levi DS, Kusnezov N, Carman GP. Smart materials applications for pediatric cardiovascular devices. *Pediatric Research.* 2008;63(5):552–8.
44. Singh SP, Verma PK, Singh S, Kapoor M, Balu R. Microstructural characterization and electrochemical behaviour of HVOF sprayed WC-Co-Cr coatings on 316L boiler steel stainless steel. *Results in Surfaces and Interfaces.* 2024;16:100248.

45. Nikolova MP, Apostolova MD. Advances in multifunctional bioactive coatings for metallic bone implants. *Materials*. 2022;16(1):183.
46. Chen X, Gao Y, Wang Y, Pan G. Mussel-inspired peptide mimicking: An emerging strategy for surface bioengineering of medical implants. *Smart Materials in Medicine*. 2021;2:26–37.
47. Jiang P, Zhang Y, Hu R, Shi B, Zhang L, Huang Q, Yang Y, Tang P, Lin C. Advanced surface engineering of titanium materials for biomedical applications: From static modification to dynamic responsive regulation. *Bioactive Materials*. 2023;27:15–57.
48. Santos-Coquillat A, Martinez-Campos E, Sánchez HM, Moreno L, Arrabal R, Mohedano M, Gallardo A, Rodriguez-Hernandez J, Matykina E. Hybrid functionalized coatings on metallic biomaterials for tissue engineering. *Surface and Coatings Technology*. 2021;422:127508.
49. Lacour SP, Courtine G, Guck J. Materials and technologies for soft implantable neuroprostheses. *Nature Reviews Materials*. 2016;1(10):1–4.
50. Kontiza A, Kartsonakis IA. Smart composite materials with self-healing properties: A review on design and applications. *Polymers*. 2024;16(15):2115.
51. Kumar P, Suryavanshi P, Dwivedy SK, Banerjee S. Stimuli-responsive materials for 4D printing: Mechanical, manufacturing, and biomedical applications. *Journal of Molecular Liquids*. 2024:125553.
52. Oladapo BI, Zahedi SA, Omigbodun FT. A systematic review of polymer composite in biomedical engineering. *European Polymer Journal*. 2021;154:110534.
53. Zhang BG, Myers DE, Wallace GG, Brandt M, Choong PF. Bioactive coatings for orthopaedic implants—recent trends in development of implant coatings. *International Journal of Molecular Sciences*. 2014;15(7):11878–921.
54. Sanyal S, Park S, Chelliah R, Yeon SJ, Barathikannan K, Vijayalakshmi S, Jeong YJ, Rubab M, Oh DH. Emerging trends in smart self-healing coatings: A focus on micro/nanocontainer technologies for enhanced corrosion protection. *Coatings*. 2024;14(3):324.
55. Filip N, Radu I, Veliceasa B, Filip C, Pertea M, Clim A, Pinzariu AC, Drochioi IC, Hilitanu RL, Serban IL. Biomaterials in orthopedic devices: Current issues and future perspectives. *Coatings*. 2022;12(10):1544.
56. Verma PK, Singh S, Kapoor M, Singh S. A review on the surface topography and corrosion behavior of Mg-alloy coatings for biomedical implants. *Results in Surfaces and Interfaces*. 2024:100227.
57. Sánchez-Bodón J, Diaz-Galbarriatu M, Pérez-Álvarez L, Moreno-Benítez I, Vilas-Vilela JL. Strategies to enhance biomedical device performance and safety: A comprehensive review. *Coatings*. 2023;13(12):1981.
58. Verma PK, Vasudev H, Singh G, Singh S. A review on the microstructural and biomedical properties of implants manufactured using additive manufacturing. *Journal of The Institution of Engineers (India): Series D*. 2024:1–5.
59. Singh J, Singh S, Verma A. Artificial intelligence in use of ZrO2 material in biomedical science. *Journal of Electrochemical Science and Engineering* [Internet]. 2022;13:83–97. Available from: https://pub.iapchem.org/ojs/index.php/JESE/article/view/1498.
60. Singh J, Hashmi AW, Behra A, et al. Review of Mg alloys for bio-implants protected by the deposition of chemical conversion coatings. *AIP Conference Proceedings*. AIP Publishing; 2024.
61. Singh J, Singh S, Gill R. Applications of biopolymer coatings in biomedical engineering. *Journal of Electrochemical Science and Engineering*. 2022;13:63–81.
62. Singh CJ, Ram B, Singh J, et al. Experimental investigation on characterization of friction stir processed AZ31-based composite. *Scientific Reports*. 2024;14:15453.

63. Singh J, Hashmi AW, Ahmad S, et al. Critical review on biodegradable and biocompatibility magnesium alloys: Progress and prospects in bio-implant applications. *Inorganic Chemistry Communications.* 2024;169:113111.
64. Hashmi AW, Singh J, Ahmad S. Future perspective of self-healing nano-coatings for corrosion protection. *Discov Disruption, Futur Implic Nanomater.* 2024;597–624.
65. Singh J, Hashmi AW, Kumar A, et al. Review on protection of Mg alloys bioimplants by deposition of micro-arc oxidation coatings. *AIP Conference Proceedings.* AIP Publishing; 2024.
66. Kumar S, Nehra M, Kedia D, Dilbaghi N, Tankeshwar K, Kim KH. Nanotechnology-based biomaterials for orthopaedic applications: Recent advances and future prospects. *Materials Science and Engineering: C.* 2020;106:110154.
67. Sam S, Joseph B, Thomas S. Exploring the antimicrobial features of biomaterials for biomedical applications. *Results in Engineering.* 2023;17:100979.

8 Plasma Spray Coatings for Biomedical Applications Emerging with Additive Manufacturing

Praveen Kumar Verma and Hitesh Vasudev

CONTENTS

8.1 INTRODUCTION

The demand for biomedical implants is highly increased by the increasing incidence of orthopedic, dental, and cardiovascular diseases, as well as advanced surgical practices. In addition to replacing damaged tissues, these implants need to have surface to ensure biocompatibility, durability, and functionality. For instance, the successes of an orthopedic implant depends not only on its bulk mechanical properties but also on its ability to integrate with the surrounding bone tissue, resist wear, and prevent bacterial

DOI: 10.1201/9781003516064-8

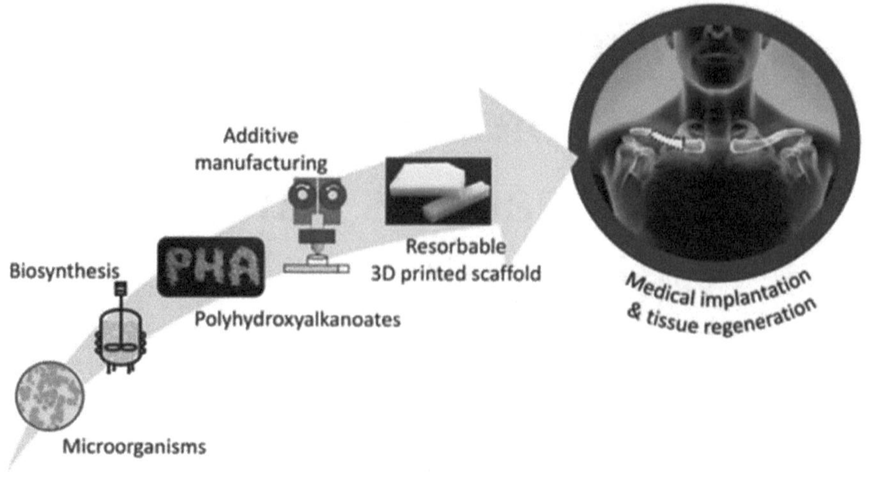

FIGURE 8.1 Biomedical applications of polyhydroxyalkanoate (PHA)-based devices [4]. (CC By 4.0 Attribution)

colonization. Therefore, surface modification is necessary to tailor the implant for its intended biological environment. Among the many techniques applied in the modification of implant surface, plasma spray coating appears to be a versatile effective technique. Plasma spray can create coatings that enhance functional properties as it uses a high-temperature plasma jet to melt and deposit feedstock materials. Bioactive HA is the primary choice in plasma spray coatings, one of the ceramics with super biocompatibility. HA mimics the mineral component of bone, enhancing osteointegration while minimizing implant rejection. More common materials include titanium oxides for better wear and corrosion resistance. Composite coatings are also widely used, for example, HA-based coatings containing zirconia or alumina for greater mechanical strength and longer endurance. The purpose is not only to protect the implant from the hostile biological environment but also to interact beneficially with the host tissues and enhance healing and integration [1–3]. **Figure 8.1** shows the schematic diagram of medical implantation and tissue regeneration.

Meanwhile, additive manufacturing (AM) technology has revolutionized the area of biomedical implant fabrication. Unlike traditional subtractive manufacture, AM fabricates components layer by layer in a virtually limitless manner from the perspective of design freedom. This can result in rather complex geometries as in the case of producing porous structures similar to bone and in the more general sense of producing individualized implants for each unique anatomical need. Beyond this, graded structures become possible that are optimized in relation to varying mechanical and biological properties across an implant [5].

The integration of plasma spraying with AM processes is widely considered a paradigm shift in biomedical implant technology. While the former supports the creation of complex geometries for implants, the latter provides means for surface functionalization during plasma spraying, thereby enhancing its performance in biological environments. For example, plasma spray coatings can be deposited with high precision onto intricate surfaces of AM-fabricated implants to ensure uniform coverage and strong adhesion. This integration addresses critical limitations in both standalone techniques. Traditional plasma spray methods often face challenges in coating irregular geometries, while AM-fabricated implants may lack the necessary surface properties for direct biological application. Combining these technologies will enable scientists to develop implants with mechanical, biological, and functional superiority. Plasma spraying synergistically promotes advanced implant design when coupled with AM. Advanced coatings changing gradually in composition from the bulk material of the implant toward its surface are possible today. The stress concentrations at the interface are minimized, and the properties transition without abrupt changes, thus more closely representing a tissue. In addition to this, plasma-sprayed coatings could be doped with bioactive and therapeutic agents, opening up avenues for implants that do not just replace damaged tissue but actively promote healing or deliver localized therapy [6–7]. Although these benefits abound, a number of drawbacks still persist in combining plasma spray coatings with AM technologies.

The consistent adhesion of the coating to the AM surfaces, especially those produced with high porosity and complex geometries, requires optimization of both processes. The thermal properties of substrates fabricated using AM also create a challenge in plasma spraying since the difference in thermal expansion may lead to peeling off of the coating or cracking of a substrate. Of all these factors, scalability and cost-effectiveness combine while adopting in clinical settings hold their importance [8]. While combining plasma spray coating along with AM, it is therefore poised to revolutionize this biomedical implant technology significantly, as researchers can exploit each technique's best to deliver implants that fulfill the increasingly diverse and demanding requirements for modern medicine by merging such technologies. This chapter focuses on the applications, advantages, and challenges of the convergence of these technologies in biomedical engineering. This synergy is also of special interest for the development of bioactive coatings, functionally graded materials, and innovative designs toward a future of patient-specific high-performance medical devices [9].

8.2 PLASMA SPRAY COATINGS IN BIOMEDICAL APPLICATIONS

Plasma spray technology is one of the most applied thermal spray methods. This technology uses a high-temperature plasma jet to deposit coatings on a variety of substrates. The thermal-sprayed coating material melts through contact with an ionized gas, such as plasma, from feedstock materials that may be metals and ceramics to composite powders. The molten or partially molten particles are accelerated toward the substrate by the plasma jet where they solidify upon impact forming thin films or thick coatings. This rapid solidification imparts some unique microstructural characteristics, in this case, in dense coatings with lamellar structures enhancing material performance in numerous applications [10]. The versatility of plasma spray technology lies in its ability to process a wide range of materials under controlled

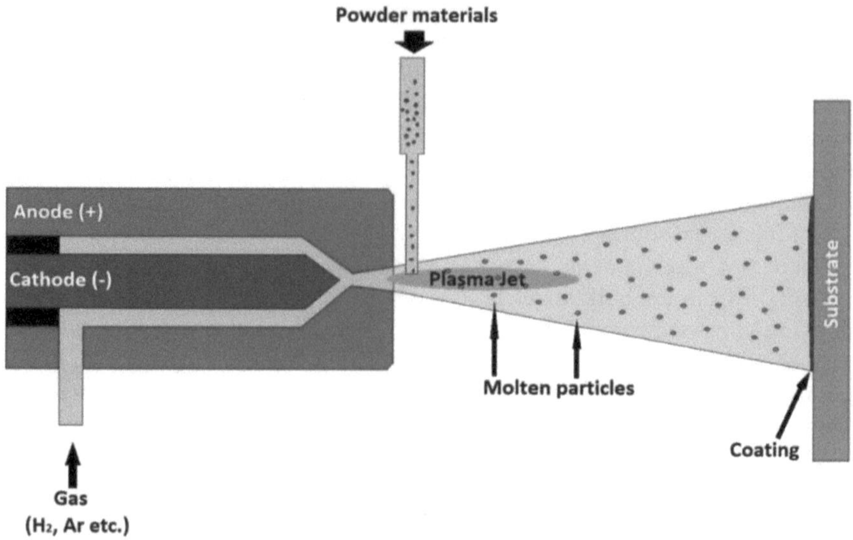

FIGURE 8.2 Plasma spray coating process. [12] (CC By 4.0 Attribution)

conditions. It is particularly useful for biomedical applications, wherein most biomaterials used as coatings for metallic implants are bioactive, such as hydroxyapatite (HA). HA-coated implants display enhanced biocompatibility and osseointegration due to their resemblance in composition to the mineral phase of natural bone. Plasma spraying also provides good control of coating thickness and microstructure to optimize the biological and mechanical properties of implants [11]. **Figure 8.2** illustrates the plasma spraying process.

The process involves several key parameters influencing coating quality, including plasma gas composition, feedstock particle size, and substrate temperature. Proper optimization of these parameters ensures high adhesion strength, low porosity, and controlled crystallinity, which are essential for achieving long-term functionality in biomedical applications. The compatibility of plasma spray technology with AM techniques further adds to its suitability for applying bioactive coatings. Plasma sprays integrated with AM open the potential of creating complex geometries with tailored surface properties to evolve in personalized medicine. For example, the use of plasma-sprayed HA coatings on titanium or stainless steel implants increases their bioactivity and corrosion resistance, which is crucial for the long-term success of implants in vivo [13].

8.3 MATERIAL CHOICES FOR BIOMEDICAL IMPLANTS

Material selection for plasma spray coatings of biomedical implants is critical because the selected materials would directly influence the performance, durability, and compatibility of the implant with biological tissues. The material choice is considered in terms of the application, the body's mechanical and chemical environment, and the specific functional requirements set by the implant. Some of the key materials adopted in plasma spray coatings are hydroxyapatite (HA), titanium oxides, and composite coatings, each of which has its distinct advantages [14].

8.3.1 Hydroxyapatite (HA)

Hydroxyapatite is one of the most extensively used materials in plasma spray coatings and biomedical implants because it closely resembles the mineral phase of the human bone. Its chemical formula, $Ca_{10}(PO_4)_6(OH)_2$, and crystalline configuration make this material highly biocompatible and osteoconductive, as it allows the attachment, growth, and proliferation of bone cells. HA coatings significantly enhance osseointegration, which ensures strong fixation of orthopedic screws, plates, and even dental implants. Plasma spraying offers control over the crystallinity of HA and thickness of the coatings, both being parameters critical to the attainment of optimal bioactivity and long-term stability. Semi-crystalline HA coatings, for instance, degrade in a controlled fashion, releasing calcium and phosphate ions, which enhance the regeneration of bones [15]. **Figure 8.3** shows the use of HA for dental application.

8.3.2 Titanium Oxides

Titanium-based implants are the most prevalent in orthopedic and dental applications due to their high strength-to-weight ratio and excellent corrosion resistance. Coating these implants with titanium oxides by plasma spray enhances their wear and corrosion resistance further. Titanium oxide coatings offer a dense, inert barrier

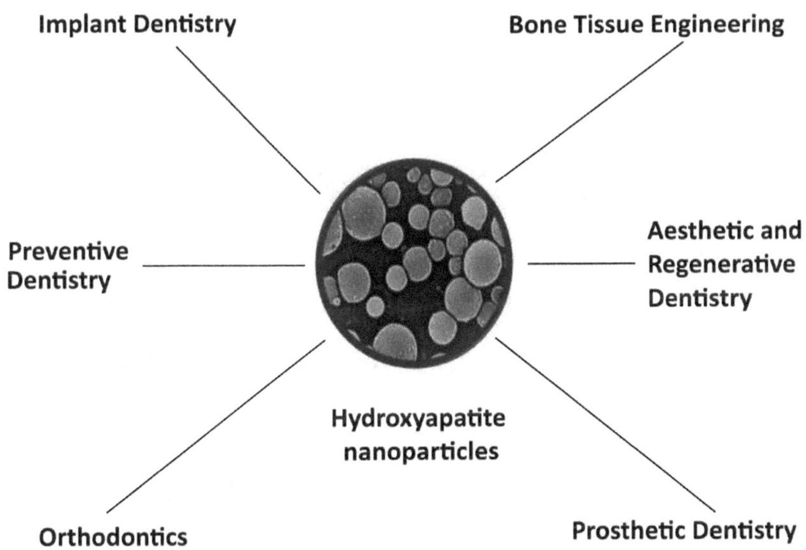

FIGURE 8.3 The use of HA nanoparticles in different fields of dentistry [16]. (CC By 4.0 Attribution)

to aggressive bodily fluids on the underlying substrate, which reduces the chance of ion leaching and potential implant degradation. Moreover, titanium oxides, having bioinert character, along with excellent adhesion properties, are desired for durable long-term implants of high strength [17].

8.3.3 Composite Coatings

Composite coatings are gaining prominence in biomedical applications to address the limitations of single-material coatings. These coatings combine materials like HA with reinforcements such as zirconia (ZrO_2), alumina (Al_2O_3), or bioactive glass to enhance mechanical properties, bioactivity, and wear resistance [18].

HA–zirconia composite coatings exhibit improved toughness and resistance to cracking while retaining bioactivity. Similarly, HA–alumina composites offer higher wear resistance and hardness, making them suitable for load-bearing applications. Bioactive glass provides for bonding to bone and accelerates tissue regeneration. Composite coatings can also provide for the development of functionally graded materials, where bioactive surfaces are gradually transitioned into mechanically robust interiors. Thus, FGMs can be tailored for matching adjacent tissues in terms of mechanical properties, allowing stress concentrations to be minimized and improving implant longevity [19].

8.3.4 Performance Advantages

Plasma-sprayed coatings make a significant contribution to the improvement in the performance of biomedical implants, significantly extending durability, wear resistance, and biological compatibility. Engineered to provide a protective and functional interface between the implant and host tissue, coatings ensure lasting reliability and efficacy in clinical applications. The high-temperature plasma spray process produces very dense and well-adhered coatings that protect the substrate from the onset of mechanical stresses and environmental degradation. Coatings of titanium oxides and composite materials also improve the implant's ability to wear and corrosion resistance under the aggressive physiological environment. This is particularly important for load-bearing implants such as hip and knee replacements where sustained mechanical forces can lead to the degradation of the materials. Plasma-sprayed coatings act as a physical barrier that minimizes the release of ions and wear debris, which could otherwise provoke an inflammatory response and lead to implant failure [20].

Hydroxyapatite (HA) coatings, applied by plasma spray, duplicating the mineral nature of bone, allow for effective rapid bonding between an implant and its host tissue. In case of these examples, such as HA-coated titanium implants, they have demonstrated improved osseointegration relative to the uncoated implant, thereby reducing recovery time and enhancing the implant overall stability. Controlled porosity and crystallinity created using plasma-sprayed HA coating makes it one surface of attachment, proliferation, and regeneration of bone cells ideal to a greater extent. Stronger bone–implant interfaces as a result increase the lessening of loosening failure at the time of long-term implantation. Plasma-sprayed coatings also enable tailoring surface properties to specific clinical requirements. For instance, composite coatings combining HA with zirconia or alumina improve the mechanical properties without sacrificing biocompatibility. Such layers provide a balance of both bioactivity and structural integrity, thereby being useful for implants meant for high mechanical loading [21].

Clinical studies emphasize the advantages of plasma-sprayed coatings. HA-coated dental and orthopedic implants have shown less failure when compared to uncoated implants with each subsequent clinical study. Patients obtained quicker recovery, fewer revisions, and enhanced quality of life. The performance advantages of plasma-sprayed coatings stem from the ability to enhance implant durability, reduce wear, and promote effective bonding with host tissues. By combining mechanical protection with biological functionality, these coatings provide better clinical outcomes and pave the way for advancements in implant technology, especially when combined with AM innovations [22].

8.4 ADDITIVE MANUFACTURING FOR BIOMEDICAL IMPLANTS

8.4.1 AM Techniques in Implant Fabrication

Additive manufacturing, or 3D printing, has dramatically changed the fabrication process of biomedical implants and their production in the form of patient-specific devices, owing to their intricately geometrical forms with mechanical properties tailored appropriately. Among all the AM techniques, SLM and EBM have impressed by offering accuracy and flexibility toward any possible biocompatible metal and its alloy. SLM is a technique whereby a high-power laser is employed to selectively melt and fuse layers of metal powder according to a digital model. This method is well-suited for the manufacture of implants that contain complex geometries, including lattice structures and porous designs that cannot be easily produced by traditional manufacturing methods. The porous architectures also improve osseointegration and tissue ingrowth. Thus, SLM is specifically well-suited for orthopedic and dental implants. In addition, SLM also enables vast processing capabilities for varied materials, such as titanium and cobalt-chrome alloys, as well as stainless steel, which are widely used in biomedical applications [23].

In EBM, the method uses an electron beam as its source of heat to melt metal powders in the sequential layer-by-layer process in a vacuum environment. It is highly efficient in the processing of high-melting-point materials like titanium and its alloys. Porosity control of implants is a noted advantage of EBM for vascularization and the eventual integration with surrounding tissues. The vacuum environment minimizes oxidation, thus ensuring better mechanical properties and biocompatibility in the resulting implants. Both SLM and EBM possess major benefits for manufacturing in comparison with traditional methodologies. They make it possible to provide customized implants with patient-specific demands according to anatomical needs, enhancing both the functionality and comfort of implants. In addition, AM techniques offer design freedom through the ability to implement gradient porosity and complex surface textures that are advantageous in enhancing biological interactions [24].

Beyond the creation of an implant, AM techniques also play an important role in the development of regenerative medicine. Porous scaffolds created by AM support cell proliferation and subsequent tissue regeneration, acting as templates for developing new bone and soft tissues. Since combined with bioactive materials such as HA, these scaffolds mimic the structure and function of native tissues and could provide a solution for critical-size bone defects [25].

8.4.2 Synergies with Plasma Spray Coating

Additive manufacturing in conjunction with plasma spray coating represents a revolutionary approach in the manufacturing of biomedical implants combining design flexibility of AM with the functional benefits of plasma-sprayed surfaces. Such synergy results in the fabrication of advanced implants with superior mechanical stability, improved performance, and durability. Using AM techniques such as SLM and EBM, it is possible to create specific surface features during implant fabrication, including controlled porosity and complex geometries. These provide an optimized basis for plasma spray coatings and enhance the uniformity and adhesion of those coatings. For example, micro-porous surfaces formed using AM methodologies offer mechanical interlocking points for plasma-sprayed materials, with bond strengths between the coating and substrate being considerably improved. Strong adhesion is thus essential for the long-term stability of the coating, especially in load-bearing implants [26].

Plasma spray coating complements AM by providing additional functionalities to the surface of the implant. Coatings such as HA provide osseointegration, mimicking the normal structure of the bone mineral, while composite coatings with alumina and zirconia materials increase the toughness and resistance to wear. Through their combined integration, these technologies allow the creation of functionally graded implants in which the core is made from the AM process, giving structural support, and the plasma-sprayed surface ensures biological compatibility. This type of integration is preferred especially because it facilitates patient-specific customization of implants. While AM allows for the realization of anatomical features identical to those of the individual, plasma spraying provides the surface properties suited best for their biological performance. To illustrate, a plasma-sprayed HA coating on an otherwise AM-fabricated titanium implant may provide a unique combination of strength, corrosion resistance, and bioactivity [27]. **Figure 8.4** shows the implant surface modifications.

Another advantage of the hybrid approach is addressing various challenges that come with traditional implant manufacturing. Careful control over AM and plasma spray parameters ensures the consistency of the quality of coatings developed, even on complex geometries. This is especially important for implants possessing intricate lattice structures for tissue ingrowth and vascularization. The amalgamation of AM and plasma spraying is already promising to take tissue engineering further ahead: Porous AM scaffolds surfaced with bioactive materials may support cell proliferation and differentiation, thus opening new avenues for next-generation implants and regenerative therapies [29].

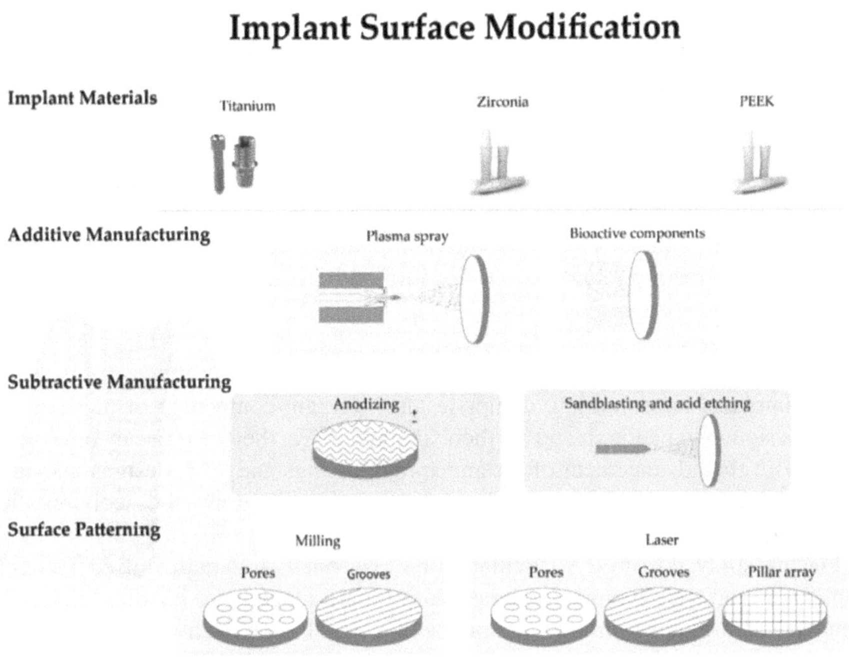

FIGURE 8.4 Schematic image of the most relevant biomimetic surface modification strategies [28]. (CC By 4.0 Attribution)

8.5 APPLICATIONS IN BIOMEDICAL ENGINEERING

8.5.1 Orthopedic Implants

Orthopedic implants such as hip and knee replacements have become indispensable in restoring mobility and alleviating pain for patients suffering from joint disorders or injuries. Plasma spray coatings, together with AM, have revolutionized the design and performance of such implants, significantly enhancing their durability, functionality, and patient outcomes [30].

Plasma spray coatings play a very important role in orthopedic implants, enhancing wear resistance, corrosion protection, and biological compatibility. For example, HA coatings on titanium implants allow for osseointegration, which is stable fixation with the surrounding bone. This is crucial in load-bearing applications where mechanical stability is critical. The bioactivity of HA supports the attachment and growth of bone cells, leading to quicker healing and reduced likelihood of implant failure. Integration with plasma spray technology adds additional benefits to orthopedic implants. SLM and EBM are two techniques using which implants can be built using patient-specific designs, such that the anatomy of the patient is perfectly represented. This customization improves fit and function over time, minimizing further wear and pain. In addition, AM enables implants to be designed with controlled porosity, promoting ingrowth and vascularization necessary for long-term implant success [31].

One of the main benefits of AM with plasma spraying is that implants can be designed with functionally graded structures. For instance, an implant may have a dense core for mechanical strength and a porous surface coated with HA to facilitate bone integration. Such designs avoid stress shielding, which occurs when the implant absorbs mechanical loads, resulting in bone resorption and weakening. The impact of these advancements is evident in clinical outcomes. AM-fabricated and plasma-coated orthopedic implants demonstrate superior longevity and reduced failure rates compared to traditionally manufactured implants. Patients experience improved mobility, faster recovery, and a lower need for revision surgeries [32].

8.5.2 Dental Implants

Dental implants have come to comprise an important component of modern dentistry. Designed to be tough and aesthetically attractive, they help in substituting lost teeth. With the advancement of plasma spray coatings and AM, designs and functionalities in dental implants have improved significantly toward osseointegration, durability, and patient satisfaction [33].

Plasma spray coatings, particularly the HA ones, are mainly used in dental implants to enhance biological compatibility and induce bone bonding. Since HA simulates natural bone mineral composition, its resulting bioactive surface is said to enhance osseointegration. This would be particularly significant in a dental implant situation because stable anchorage to the jawbone can ensure long-term success. The findings of several studies concluded that HA-coated titanium implants significantly reduce healing times and result in higher success rates for dental procedures [34]. **Figure 8.5** shows the processes of producing dental implants.

AM processing, such as SLM and EBM, has further expanded the fabrication of dental implants. In such techniques, customized implants are achieved based on

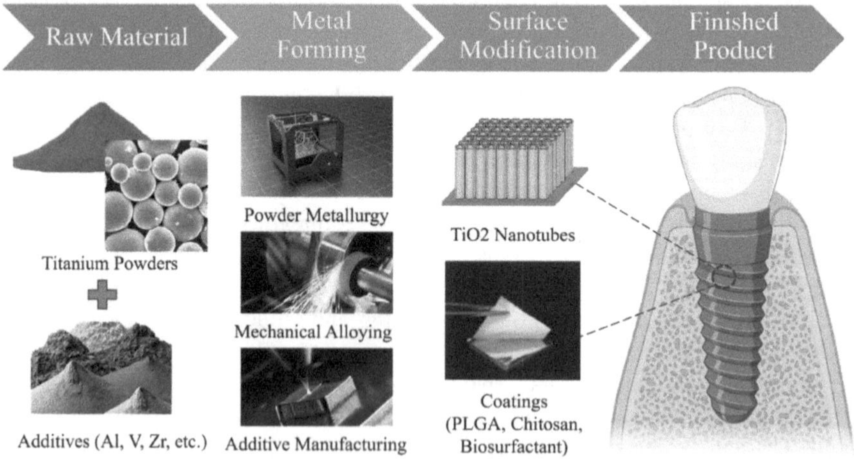

FIGURE 8.5 Scheme demonstrating the processes of producing dental implants [35]. (CC By 4.0 Attribution)

patient-specific anatomy. AM enables the high-precision reproduction of complex forms and features, including threads and grooves, for improved implant stability and load distribution. Furthermore, AM offers the possibility to design porous implant structures to enhance vascularization and tissue integration. The clinical impact of the developments is significant. Dental implants produced with AM that have HA coating were proven to be better than conventionally produced ones with, for example, fewer incidents of peri-implantitis and other adverse effects. Patients benefit from shorter recovery periods, improved implant longevity, and natural feel and function [36].

8.5.3 Bioactive Scaffolds

Bioactive scaffolds represent a new frontier in tissue engineering: designed to support cell proliferation, differentiation, and regeneration of functional tissue, their development has been boosted by the combined use of AM and plasma spray coating for the definition of tailored solutions for critical-sized defects and complex tissue repair. Techniques of AM include SLS and SLA, which allow for the creation of scaffolds with controlled porosity, geometry, and mechanical properties. The scaffolds resemble the extracellular matrix of tissues, providing a structural template for the cells to attach, migrate, and proliferate. AM-synthesized scaffolds possess elaborate architectures, such as interconnected pores and gradient structures, that allow for nutrient and oxygen delivery and vascularization. These scaffolds are complemented by plasma spray coatings, which enhance the surface properties. The coatings, such as HA, mimic the mineral composition of bone and therefore increase bioactivity by encouraging cells [37]. **Figure 8.6** shows the bioactive ceramic scaffolds.

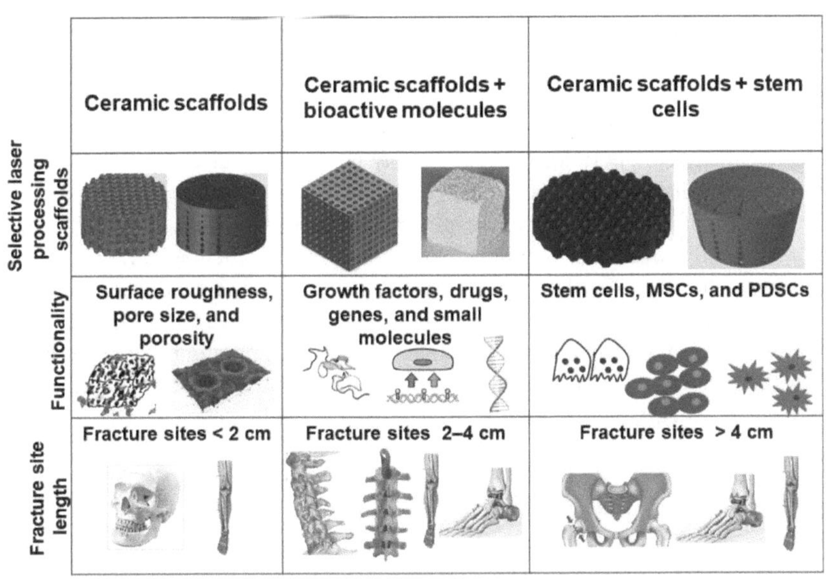

FIGURE 8.6 Three major categories of synthetic bioactive ceramic scaffolds processed by PBSLP used for bone repair [38]. (CC By 4.0 Attribution)

8.6 CHALLENGES IN PLASMA SPRAY–AM INTEGRATION

The integration of plasma spray coating into AM holds transformative potential for biomedical implants but is not without its challenges. The areas in which it presents challenges are mainly adhesion and uniformity, material compatibility, and cost and scalability. The strong and consistent adhesion of plasma-sprayed coatings onto surfaces fabricated by AM is a challenging task. These AM parts inherently contain complicated geometries and surface roughness, which hinder the uniform deposition process during plasma spraying of the coating. Although surface roughness can improve mechanical interlocking, excessive irregularities may form gaps or stress concentrations that result in poor adhesion. Thermal mismatches between the AM substrate and plasma-sprayed material also represent a significant challenge. During the high-temperature spray process, differential expansion and contraction can result in residual stresses at the interface, potentially degrading the integrity of the coating. Tailoring AM surface designs and optimizing spray parameters is critical in mitigating this problem. However, it requires considerable experimentation and control, adding complexity to the process [39].

Feedstock materials used for plasma spraying are incompatible with many AM substrates. Plasma spray coatings, such as HA or composite materials, should seamlessly bond to AM-fabricated implants, generally made of titanium and its alloys. Coatings may fail due to differences in thermal properties, chemical reactivity, or bonding mechanisms between the coating and substrate materials. For example, poor compatibility may lead to delamination or reduced bioactivity. The development of feedstock materials tailored to the properties of the AM-fabricated surface is critical for optimal adhesion and functionality of coatings. The addition of functionally graded materials could also tackle compatibility problems between substrate and coating layers, but this increases the technical complexity of manufacture [40].

High costs associated with the processes on both sides, AM and plasma spray, pose a serious hindrance to extensive use in biomedicine. Methods of AM, including SLM and EBM, are technology-intensive, requiring expensive equipment, materials, and energy-intensive operations. Plasma spray methods require expensive operation due to the specialized equipment, inert gases, and energy used in plasma generation. A combination of such technologies increases overall costs, resulting in implants that are not so readily available for more extensive clinical practices. Another issue is scalability. Typically, it's often very limited to small-batch or custom production for integrating the AM and plasma spray processes. Cost-effective ways to mass produce without sacrificing quality or functionality are very challenging to achieve. Barriers such as these may be mitigated through innovations such as hybrid manufacturing setups, advancements in automation, and more affordable materials [41].

8.7 FUTURE DIRECTIONS

The integration of AM and plasma spray technologies is poised to cause significant jumps in biomedical implants, mainly by the development of functionally graded and smart coatings, as well as the integration of advanced diagnostics and artificial intelligence (AI). Functionally graded coatings, created by combining AM with plasma spraying, offer a unique advantage of mimicking the natural gradient of biological tissues. These coatings progress from a dense, mechanically strong core to a bioactive, porous surface, thus enhancing the mechanical stability of the implant and inducing better integration with the surrounding tissues. For instance, titanium alloy implants can be coated with hydroxyapatite for osseointegration; intermediate layers of materials like alumina or zirconia may be interposed to enhance wear resistance [42, 43].

In addition to functional gradients, the smart coatings also address major challenges in implant longevity and infection control [44, 45]. Smart coatings with embedded responsive materials that include pH-sensitive or antimicrobial agents introduce adaptive functionalities into the coating [46]. An example is a pH-sensitive coating that releases antimicrobial agents in response to the acidic environment that most infections produce; thus, localized protection against microbial growth is provided without systemic antibiotics. This will enhance the overall implantability of the device, further reducing the possible complications. In addition, adding antimicrobial nanoparticles such as silver or zinc into the coating provides long-term protection to the implant, leading to better patient outcomes with reduced infection risk [47–50]. This is also because integrating modern diagnostic means and AI within plasma spraying and AM has streamlined the fabrication of implants. The plasma spray parameters can be tuned in AI algorithms, like distance and feed rate. Hence, the coatings will have an optimum performance with uniform coating. Real-time data obtained from sensors will be analyzed continuously by AI. Due to this, AI algorithms will detect problems and real-time prediction of coating quality, which will result in higher-quality production. It makes significant impacts in simulating various compositions of coating to design specific implants exactly with the requirement of a patient, especially during the phase of designing [51, 52]. The connection between such advanced diagnostics and smart materials-AI therefore promises to significantly better biomedical implants performance while further pushing toward the development that ensures this new generation of very-high functionality, exactly well-complied personalized implants, and would thus come competitively over others [53, 54].

8.8 CONCLUSION

Plasma spray coatings and AM therefore mark a new exciting step in the evolution of biomedical implants, an opportunity to produce implants that are highly functional as well as personalized to the needs of individual patients. With the versatility and precision of AM and the established performance-enhancing capabilities of plasma spray coatings, a new class of implants can be developed that feature optimized mechanical properties, enhanced bioactivity, and superior long-term stability. The key advantage of combining these two is the design of complex geometries and customized shapes essential for improving patient outcomes in various clinical applications, including orthopedic, dental, and tissue-engineering implants.

The most significant benefit of this synergy is that it enables the production of implants with functionally graded coatings. These coatings can thus transform from a mechanically strong and wear-resistant layer to a bioactive layer that supports tissue integration, similar to the natural gradation seen in biological tissues. Another approach would be to coat the AM-fabricated implants with materials like HA, zirconia, or composite materials, so that the bonds of the implant to bone and soft tissues are strengthened, hence an improved overall performance and longer lifespan of the implant. The level of control provided by AM enables the modification of these coatings to meet specific anatomical needs in a patient, with mismatched mechanical properties being but one concern, and with recovery time reduced and longer-term performance improved. While integration of plasma sprayed coatings with AM provides exciting opportunities for biomedical applications, there are still several significant challenges remaining in reaching their full potential. These issues concern adhesion between the coating and the substrate of an AM, thermal mismatches, and material compatibility and must be addressed with care. Surface roughness of parts manufactured via AM may result in a non-uniform and likely less integral plasma-sprayed coating which may create weak points or delamination. Additionally, the high costs associated with both AM and plasma spray technologies may limit their widespread adoption, particularly in resource-constrained clinical settings.

REFERENCES

1. Li Y, Wang Y, Li Z, et al. Biomaterials for orthopedic implants: Surface modifications for enhanced functionality. *J Biomed Mater Res B Appl Biomater.* 2021;109(1):16–28.
2. Zheng Y, Guo Y, Wang Q, et al. Recent advances in the fabrication of biodegradable magnesium alloy-based coatings for orthopedic applications. *Acta Biomater.* 2020;106:81–91.
3. Xie Z, Zhang Y, Cheng S, et al. Bioactive coatings for orthopedic implants: Plasma spraying of hydroxyapatite and biocompatible ceramics. *J Mater Sci Mater Med.* 2021;32(3):47.
4. Giubilini A, Bondioli F, Messori M, Nyström G, Siqueira G. Advantages of additive manufacturing for biomedical applications of polyhydroxyalkanoates. *Bioengineering.* 2021;8(2):29.
5. Chen L, Li X, Zhang L, et al. Plasma-sprayed hydroxyapatite coatings for orthopedic applications: Mechanical properties and biological interactions. *J Biomed Mater Res A.* 2019;107(2):367–77.
6. Verma PK, Vasudev H, Singh G, Singh S. A review on the microstructural and biomedical properties of implants manufactured using additive manufacturing. *J Inst Eng (India): Series D.* 2024:1–5.
7. Kumar A, O'Neill M, Zhang Z, et al. Plasma spray coatings in additive manufacturing: Bridging technology for biomedical implants. *Mater Sci Eng C.* 2022;125:112085.
8. Zhou W, He D, Zhang Z, et al. Bioactive coatings and their therapeutic potentials in biomedical implants. *Acta Biomater.* 2021;124:74–85.
9. Liu C, Li Z, Liu Q, et al. Hybrid additive manufacturing and plasma spray coating for patient-specific implants. *J Manuf Sci Eng.* 2021;143(4):041016.
10. Wang C, Gao Y, Zhang Z, et al. Challenges in combining plasma spray with additive manufacturing for biomedical implants. *Biomaterials Sci.* 2020;8(10):2897–909.
11. Lee W, Kim S, Chung J, et al. Synergy of plasma spray coating and additive manufacturing for personalized biomedical implants. *J Biomater Sci Polym Ed.* 2022;33(8):976–89.
12. Maximov M, Maximov OC, Craciun L, Ficai D, Ficai A, Andronescu E. Bioactive glass—an extensive study of the preparation and coating methods. Coatings. 2021;11(11):1386.
13. Shankar T, Bhagat R, Rao P, et al. Plasma spray coating for biomedical implants: Principles, materials, and applications. *J Therm Spray Technol.* 2020;29(3):671–90.

14. Thakare D, Gupta A, Sharma A, et al. Surface modification of titanium implants with hydroxyapatite coatings for biomedical applications. *J Biomater Appl.* 2021;36(4):560–73.
15. Yang Z, Huang J, Zhang Y, et al. Role of plasma-sprayed hydroxyapatite coatings on titanium and stainless steel implants for improved corrosion resistance and bioactivity. *Biomaterials.* 2020;258:120265.
16. Balhuc S, Campian R, Labunet A, Negucioiu M, Buduru S, Kui A. Dental applications of systems based on hydroxyapatite nanoparticles—an evidence-based update. Crystals. 2021;11(6):674.
17. Kumar R, Singh P, Jang Y, et al. Materials used in plasma spray coatings for biomedical implants: A review. *J Mater Sci Technol.* 2021;62:107–20.
18. Deshmukh R, Kalpande A, Patil S, et al. Plasma sprayed hydroxyapatite coatings for bone repair: Process optimization and biological performance. *Ceram Int.* 2020;46(7):9678–91.
19. Zhang W, Zhu W, Li H, et al. Titanium oxide coatings on implants: Synthesis, properties, and biomedical applications. *Biomater Sci.* 2020;8(3):627–40.
20. Alvarado M, Lopez R, Romero M, et al. Composite coatings of hydroxyapatite and zirconia for improved mechanical properties in biomedical implants. *Mater Sci Eng C.* 2021;118:111487.
21. Singh A, Verma N, Mehta P, et al. Functionally graded hydroxyapatite-alumina coatings for biomedical applications: Design, fabrication, and characterization. *J Biomed Mater Res B Appl Biomater.* 2020;108(6):2324–36.
22. Jain P, Khatri A, Garg H, et al. Wear and corrosion resistance of plasma-sprayed titanium oxide coatings for biomedical implants. *J Mater Sci Mater Med.* 2020;31(9):89.
23. Wang J, Zhang L, Zhuang J, et al. Plasma-sprayed hydroxyapatite and composite coatings: Enhancing mechanical properties and bioactivity for biomedical implants. *J Mater Sci Technol.* 2021;76:143–55.
24. Kim Y, Lee K, Hwang H, et al. Clinical outcomes of plasma-sprayed hydroxyapatite coatings for orthopedic and dental implants. *J Biomed Mater Res A.* 2021;109(7):1335–44.
25. Zhang X, Li X, Chen G, et al. Selective laser melting (SLM) in the fabrication of patient-specific biomedical implants. *J Manuf Process.* 2021;64:264–72.
26. Sun Z, Wu Z, Xu S, et al. Electron beam melting of titanium implants: A review on process, properties, and applications. *Mater Des.* 2020;192:108707.
27. Li Y, Wang H, Zeng Y, et al. Additive manufacturing in regenerative medicine: Development of bioactive scaffolds for bone tissue engineering. *Biomaterials.* 2021;276:121013.
28. Cruz MB, Silva N, Marques JF, Mata A, Silva FS, Caramês J. Biomimetic implant surfaces and their role in biological integration—A concise review. *Biomimetics.* 2022;7(2):74.
29. Santos M, Silva E, Silva F, et al. Additive manufacturing and plasma spray coating integration for advanced biomedical implants. *Mater Sci Eng C.* 2023;136:112759.
30. Verma PK, Singh S, Kapoor M, Singh S. A review on the surface topography and corrosion behavior of Mg-alloy coatings for biomedical implants. *Results Surf Interfaces.* 2024:100227.
31. Gupta S, Subramaniam A, Kumar S, et al. Functionally graded coatings in orthopedic implants: A review. *J Mech Behav Biomed Mater.* 2022;118:104476.
32. Khan M, Choudhary S, Singh R, et al. Plasma spray coating in dental implants: A review of hydroxyapatite and composite coatings. *J Dent Res.* 2023;102(3):297–308.
33. Zhang Z, Wang L, Luo H, et al. Biomaterial coatings for dental implants: Insights into bioactivity, adhesion, and osseointegration. *J Mater Sci Mater Med.* 2023;34(9):58.
34. Sharma M, Singh B, Agarwal S, et al. Hybrid manufacturing of bioactive scaffolds using AM and plasma spray coating for tissue engineering. *J Biomater Appl.* 2023;38(4):493–506.

35. Wu H, Chen X, Kong L, Liu P. Mechanical and biological properties of titanium and its alloys for oral implant with preparation techniques: A review. *Materials*. 2023;16(21):6860.
36. Zhang J, Yang Y, Zhou J, et al. Additive manufacturing and plasma spray for orthopedic implants: An overview of current technologies and future directions. *J Orthop Surg Res*. 2024;19(1):132.
37. Wu X, Liu S, Wei Y, et al. Plasma spray-coated hydroxyapatite on titanium implants: Impact on osseointegration and clinical outcomes. *J Biomed Mater Res Part B Appl Biomater*. 2023;111(8):1694–703.
38. Kamboj N, Ressler A, Hussainova I. Bioactive ceramic scaffolds for bone tissue engineering by powder bed selective laser processing: A review. *Materials*. 2021;14(18):5338.
39. Ahuja A, Patel R, Natarajan P, et al. Titanium-based dental implants: The impact of additive manufacturing and plasma spray coatings on surface properties. *J Biomed Mater Res Part A*. 2023;111(9):2565–73.
40. Shao H, Chen W, Zheng Z, et al. Smart coatings for biomedical applications: Integration of plasma spraying and additive manufacturing technologies. *J Mater Chem B*. 2024;12(10):2402–15.
41. Miller P, Zhang Y, Luo G, et al. Challenges in additive manufacturing and plasma spray integration: Implications for implant development. *Mater Today Commun*. 2024;35:103042.
42. Zheng L, Guo Z, Xu X, et al. Hybrid manufacturing of functionally graded implants: Techniques and applications in bone regeneration. *J Mech Behav Biomed Mater*. 2023;118:104467.
43. Subramanian R, Smith K, Chen L, et al. Future directions in the hybridization of plasma spray and additive manufacturing for next-generation implants. *J Mater Sci Technol*. 2024;47:1823–34.
44. Singh J, Singh S, Verma A. Artificial intelligence in use of ZrO2 material in biomedical science. *J Electrochem Sci Eng* [Internet]. 2022;13:83–97. Available from: https://pub.iapchem.org/ojs/index.php/JESE/article/view/1498.
45. Singh J, Hashmi AW, Behra A, et al. Review of Mg alloys for bio-implants protected by the deposition of chemical conversion coatings. In *AIP Conference Proceedings*. AIP Publishing; 2024.
46. Singh J, Singh S, Gill R. Applications of biopolymer coatings in biomedical engineering. *J Electrochem Sci Eng*. 2022;13:63–81.
47. Singh CJ, Ram B, Singh J, et al. Experimental investigation on characterization of friction stir processed AZ31-based composite. *Sci Rep*. 2024;14:15453.
48. Singh J, Hashmi AW, Ahmad S, et al. Critical review on biodegradable and biocompatibility magnesium alloys: Progress and prospects in bio-implant applications. *Inorg Chem Commun*. 2024;169:113111.
49. Hashmi AW, Singh J, Ahmad S. Future perspective of self-healing nano-coatings for corrosion protection. *Discov Disruption, Futur Implic Nanomater*. 2024;597–624.
50. Singh J, Hashmi AW, Kumar A, et al. Review on protection of Mg alloys bioimplants by deposition of micro-arc oxidation coatings. *AIP Conference Proceedings*. AIP Publishing; 2024.
51. Wu Z, Zhang F, Lin L, et al. Advances in plasma spray coating technologies for biomedical applications. *Mater Sci Eng C*. 2023;137:112785.
52. Xie H, Zhang Q, Yu X, et al. Cost-effective integration of additive manufacturing and plasma spray for biomedical applications: A review. *J Manuf Processes*. 2023;82:163–77.
53. Wang X, Lu B, Liu Y, et al. Smart biomaterials: The role of AI in optimizing plasma spray coating and AM integration. *Smart Mater Struct*. 2023;32(5):055014.
54. Zhang H, Li Z, Zhuang M, et al. Role of advanced diagnostics and AI in improving the performance of additive manufacturing and plasma spray processes for biomedical implants. *J Biomech*. 2024;42(1):3–16.

9 Nanotechnology in Biomedical Manufacturing

Jeet Shah and Saraswathy Nagendran

CONTENTS

DOI: 10.1201/9781003516064-9

9.1 INTRODUCTION

Nanotechnology encompasses materials and products that measure between 1 nanometer and 100 nanometers (**Figure 9.1**) and applies special properties derived from enhanced reactivity, surface-to-volume ratios, and quantum effects, which are relevant to biomedical applications in altering drug delivery, diagnostics, and therapeutics (Mazzola, 2003; Roco, 2003; McNeil, 2005). Nanoparticles refined for targeted drug delivery functions attach to specific cells or tissues for the maximization of the effectiveness of treatment while minimizing side effects (Ferrari, 2005). Diagnostic improvements include nanosensors and nanoprobe systems capable of detecting levels below the ultra-low level of disease markers (Parak et al., 2005). On the imaging side, techniques like MRI have enjoyed improved resolution and contrast with the incorporation of nanoparticle-based contrast agents (Parak et al., 2005). A few examples of the same are shown in **Figure 9.2.**

Nanomaterials in regenerative medicine facilitate tissue engineering by means of scaffolds that provide support for growth and differentiation (Dvir et al., 2011). Nanoparticles can combine therapy and diagnostics into one step as theranostics, hence making disease management much easier (Shi et al., 2010). Nanotechnology has been greatly improving medical treatments; targeted therapies are achieved that deliver drugs to only the cells that are diseased, hence damaging less healthy tissues to achieve better health outcomes for patients (Ferrari, 2005; Jain, 2012). High-sensitivity nanosensors and nanoprobes aid in the early detection of diseases, hence increasing the chances of surviving diseases like cancer (Zhang et al., 2008). Nanoparticles also increase the sensitivity of an imaging modality like MRI to help in accurate diagnosis and treatment planning (Kipp, 2004). In regenerative medicine, nanomaterials play the role of influencing the extracellular matrix to enhance cell adhesion, proliferation, and differentiation for tissue or organ regeneration (Petros & DeSimone, 2010; Roszek et al., 2005). Nanotechnology supports personalized medicine by providing treatment according to individual genetic and molecular profiles that build up perfect therapeutic

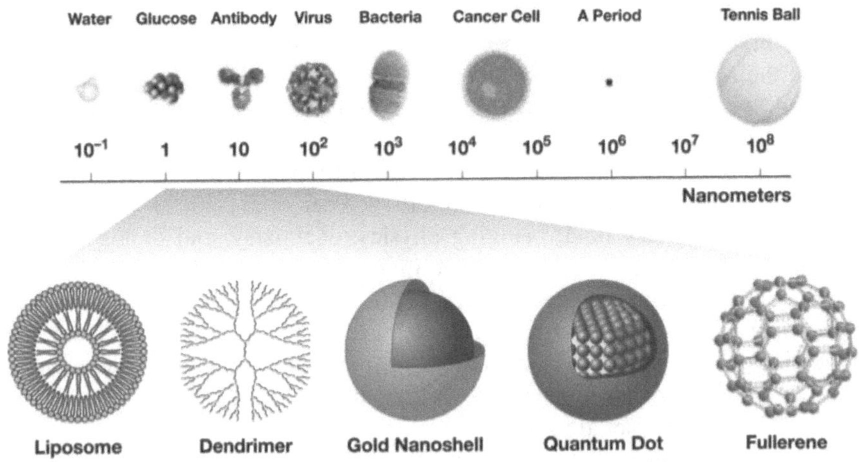

FIGURE 9.1 Relative size of nanoparticles with regard to familiar everyday objects (McNeil, S. E., 2005).

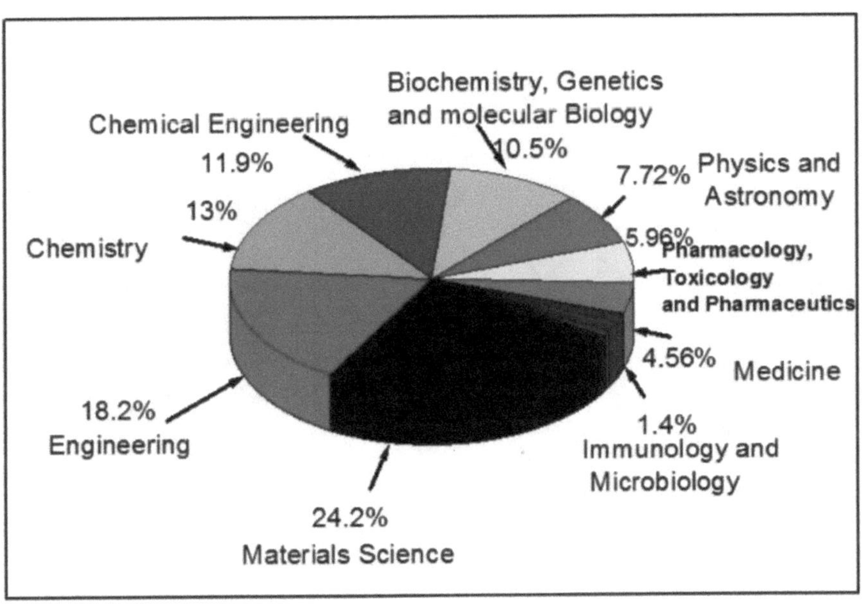

FIGURE 9.2 An analysis of the published documents according to their subject area in Scopus under a keyword search on nanomaterials for biomedical and other applications such as engineering and materials science (Mabrouk, M. et al., 2021).

strategies (Mazzola, 2003). Nanotechnology aids in the improvement of biomedical materials and implants through nanometric surface modifications that increase their biocompatibility and functionality (Shi et al., 2010). It leads toward advanced imaging and diagnostics with the help of nanosensors and nanoprobes used to detect diseases better. It provides ultra-beneficial effects but wants a close check on its biomedical applications to be kept to avoid risks and unsafe conditions of patients concerned (Gref et al., 1995; Peer et al., 2007). And it should be an interdisciplinary field, bringing physics, chemistry, and biology together in association with engineering to drive innovation toward the medical solution (Ferrari, 2005). Nanoscale techniques of manufacturing from electrospinning to chemical vapor deposition will further increase this potential for biomedical applications through methods aimed at the creation of tailored nanomaterials with improved properties for a varied array of medical needs (Ferrari, 2008; Geng et al., 2007; Sakamoto et al., 2010).

As shown in **Figure 9.3**, several types of nanostructures, which are of key importance in drug delivery systems or tissue engineering, can be attained through techniques of self-assembly and top-down fabrication (Shi et al., 2010; Langer & Tirrell, 2004; Zhang et al., 2008). The interdisciplinary nature of nanotechnology drives biomedical manufacturing in innovation for safety and effectiveness in treatments and diagnostics. Tapping into nanoscale properties coupled with state-of-the-art manufacturing techniques, nanotechnology continues to propel healthcare toward a future of precision medicine: tailored interventions (Roszek et al., 2005).

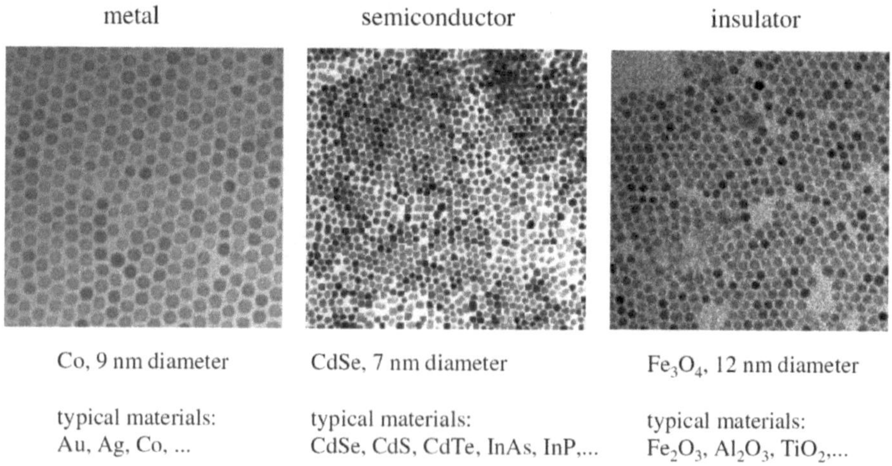

FIGURE 9.3 Colloidal nanocrystals of several substances. Materials that are metallic, semiconductors, or insulators can be used to create colloidal nanocrystals. Co, CdSe, and Fe3O4 nanocrystals placed on a TEM grid are seen in low-resolution TEM images. Every sphere represents a single nanocrystal (Parak et al., 2005).

9.2 CONTROLLED DRUG RELEASE SYSTEMS

9.2.1 Nanoparticles and Nanocarriers in Controlled Drug Delivery

Nanotechnology has given a way to many controlled drug delivery systems in the sense that it allows the delivery of these therapeutic agents to targeted sites in the body (Geng et al., 2007). It ensures effectiveness in the treatment and thus reduces side effects associated with the drugs (Shi et al., 2010). Nanoparticles can help in the encapsulation of therapeutic drugs (Langer & Tirrell, 2004). Separation of therapeutic drugs will save them from different types of degradations with the help of nanoparticles, and it will provide the required controlled release as desired (Zhang et al., 2008). For example, liposomes have vesicles that are spherical in shape and self-assembled by the lipid bilayers; hence, they may embed both hydrophilic and hydrophobic drugs (Shi et al., 2015), providing controlled release and enhanced bioavailability (Langer & Tirrell, 2004). Nanoparticles could potentially bear specificity against the cell or tissues. One of the basic attributes responsible for making this property achievable is basically the nanoparticles being surface-modifiable (Shi et al., 2010). Particularly, the nanoparticle surface is included with targeting ligands such as several antibodies or peptides or small molecules that direct the nanoparticle toward the receptors expressed on some cells (Ferrari, 2008). All this leads to increased specificity in treatment, which is upgraded to a great extent in each case (Shi et al., 2015). Depending to the device being used, there are three types of nanocarriers, viz. polymeric nanoparticles, dendrimers, and micelles for controlled drug delivery (Azzazy et al., 2007). A schematic representation of the preparation process of nanospheres which are a type of nanocarrier is shown in **Figure 9.4.**

Examples involve polymeric nanoparticles, like PLGA, and display controllable release based on degradation of the polymer matrix along with dendrimers, which represent very branched macromolecules that offer multiple functionalization sites for drug conjugation and targeting (Lee et al., 2007). The micelles are a result of self-assembly of amphiphilic molecules and offer potential in the encapsulation of hydrophobic drugs in the core, enhancing solubility and bioavailability (Siegel, 1996).

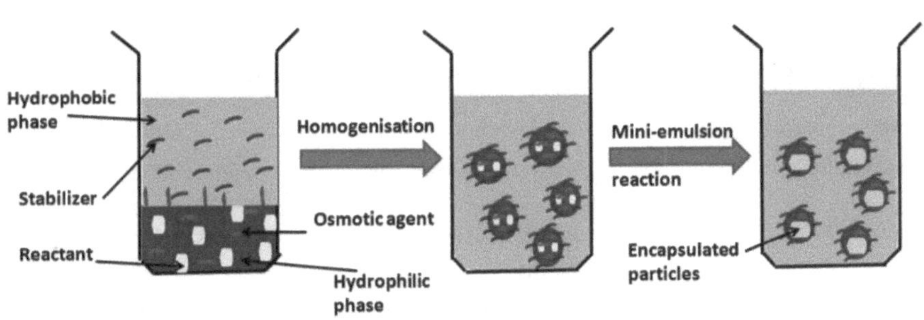

FIGURE 9.4 A schematic of a mini-emulsion process used for the preparation of encapsulated nanospheres (Gharieh, A. et al., 2019).

The surface functionalization of nanoparticles was considered an associate process for achieving targeted drug delivery with enhanced specificity (Zhang et al., 2008). Functionalization using the targeting ligands, such as antibodies, peptides, and more recently the aptamers, confers on the nanoparticles the ability for targeting and binding to specific receptors on the target cells. For instance, nanoparticles that have been functionalized with folic acid have provided a way of targeting cancerous cells that overexpress folate receptors (Kipp, 2004). Following surface engineering with a hydrophilic polymer such as polyethylene glycol, common known as stealth coating, opsonization is minimized, and the circulation time in the bloodstream is maximized (Petros & DeSimone, 2010). This will help avoid being cleared by the host's immune system and allow for the circulation of the nanoparticles in the body long enough to have them reach the target (Roszek et al., 2005). The nanoparticles may be designed to respond to specific stimuli such as pH, temperature, or enzymes in the target tissue. For example, the pH-responsive nanoparticles will release their drug cargo in the acidic environment of tumors to ensure that the drug is delivered at target sites.

9.2.2 Minimizing Off-Target Effects and Side Effects of Drugs

Nanotechnology enhances the therapeutic index of drugs by carrying drugs to the targeted site of action at the appropriate concentration. It helps in reducing the required dosage and magnifying the action of the drug. It directs a drug to deliver at a particular cell or tissue, hence minimizing off-target side effects. This becomes very important during chemotherapy, as it involves standard treatments usually affecting healthy tissue, hence leading to serious side effects (Vasir et al., 2005). Nanoparticles enhance the solubility and stability of hardly water-soluble drugs, thereby increasing bioavailability. This would enable the use of low dosages while continuing to return the therapeutic response (Shi et al., 2010). Besides, nanoparticles protect drugs from enzymatic degradation, ensuring that the unchanged drug is available at the target site (Langer & Tirrell, 2004). The features and functions of nanotechnology in drug delivery is depicted in **Table 9.1.**

TABLE 9.1
Features and Functions of Nanotechnology in Drug Delivery

Feature	Function	Outcome
Targeted Delivery	Directs drugs to specific cells or tissues	Minimizes off-target effects and toxicity
Optimized Dosage	Reduces drug amount required for efficacy	Enhances patient safety and reduces side effects
Improved Bioavailability	Increases solubility and stability of drugs	Enables effective use of poorly soluble drugs
Enhanced Drug Protection	Shields drugs from enzymatic degradation	Ensures active compounds reach the target intact

9.3 NANOTECHNOLOGY IN DIAGNOSTICS AND IMAGING

9.3.1 Development in Imaging Modality

Nanotechnology has opened up and given the breakthrough in modality of the imaging techniques through the use of nanoparticles in the development of an imaging technique that enhances sensitivity, resolution, and detectability in diagnostic techniques with clinical applications which can be a necessary breakthrough to allow the accurate detection and observation of diseases. Contrast agents such as superparamagnetic iron oxide nanoparticles (SPION) are being applied in the MRI system to enhance images' sensitivity and resolution. It enhances contrast between various tissues that enables the image formation of tumors, inflammation, and other abnormal conditions within the body. These can be further functionalized in a manner to reach and bind to specific biomarkers, thus offering diagnostic imaging and therapeutic potential for theranostics. The fact that it is possible to target and thus image accurately the site of the disease by means of MRI with the help of SPION thus remains a significant breakthrough in the process of diagnosis to ensure non-invasive diagnosis (Vasir et al., 2005). The increased absorption of X-rays by gold nanoparticles has been witnessing the fact that it works well as a contrast agent in CT imaging. The contrast of the images gets enhanced, thereby there is clarity in the images generated, and thus the capability of the identification of tumors and even vascular anomalies are pretty high. These gold nanoparticles can be made to target some particular tissues or cells, thereby providing enhanced sensitivity with reduced X-ray radiation dose for the quality images of CT. The improved contrast thus enables an early and accurate diagnosis of pathological changes, which affects the lifespan of the patient significantly (Vasir et al., 2005). Nanoparticles, especially quantum dots and gold, contribute greatly to the current developments in optical imaging, particularly in fluorescence and photoacoustic imaging methods where resolution and sensitivity must be enhanced. Quantum dots are brighter and provide stable fluorescence for labeling and detecting various types of biomolecules and cells. The gold nanoparticles provide enhanced contrast and thus high-resolution images with very fine details, more especially on the image of the tissues and organs. They can be grafted on molecules that are sensitive to targeting the diseases, facilitating real-time tracking and imaging of disease progression at the molecular level (Vasir et al., 2005). In positron emission tomography (PET), nanoparticles can be labeled with isotopes that emit a positron to improve PET resolution and sensitivity. For example, silica nanoparticles are being incorporated with isotopes such as fluorine-18, which has been used to image cancer and neurological diseases. This thus enhances the strength of the signal and is thus detailed imaging of the many processes in the body since there is the availability of these large surface areas that allow attachment of many isotopes.

9.3.2 Nanodevices for the Early Detection of Diseases

Nanosensors, nanoprobes, and other nanodevices make very vital contributions to the early diagnosis of a disease, hence allowing timely interventions that dramatically improve the outcomes for patients (Brigger et al., 2002). Nanosensors illustrate devices capable of specifically detecting selected biological or chemical molecules with high sensitivity and selectivity (Brigger et al., 2002). A simple example is that the glucose nanosensors for level monitoring of the patient with diabetes make it possible to archive real-time data which could be applied in better managing the disease (Brigger et al., 2002). The capability of nanosensors to be interfaced with a wearable device makes continuous monitoring possible and allows the patient to prepare themselves for proactive handling of the monitored disease (Brigger et al., 2002). Additionally, sensors are able to identify biomarkers associated with various diseases such as cancer, cardiovascular, infection among others so as to enable early detection and positive intervention (Alivisatos, 2004). Nanoprobes are particles applied in molecular imaging and provide the possibility of detecting specific diseases biomarkers (Alivisatos, 2004). A very simple example concerns fluorescent nanoprobes which have the ability to bind and attach themselves with the cancer cell, hence making it possible for a tumor to be visualized in its early stage (Alivisatos, 2004). The nanoprobes can also be fabricated to bind to the receptors or the overexpressed protein at the surface of the diseased cells themselves while ensuring no harmless cells have been affected in the process (Nair & Laurencin, 2006). The groups that are best captured for the study include psoriasis, atopic dermatitis, and tinea (Whitesides, 2003). This early diagnosis has implications for the early detection of disease and hence developing more personalized therapy plans earlier on. It is also possible to attach nanoprobes to therapeutic agents, thereby providing a base for theranostic applications (Shi et al., 2015). In that respect, lab-on-a-chip devices integrate several laboratory functions on a single microchip, hence making sensitive diagnoses of diseases within a very short time possible (Azzazy et al., 2007). Nanotechnology is used in these devices while shrinking the size of diagnostic assays to enhance their sensitivity and performance for point-of-care testing and early diagnosis (Lee et al., 2007), and it can handle complicated analysis in the form of DNA sequencing, protein analysis, and cell sorting on a small, portable platform. These are useful, particularly in settings with resource constraints of common laboratory infrastructure (Siegel, 1996). This has been the case as researchers have been developing lab-on-a-chip devices for applications like rapid pathogen detection, personalized medicine, and environmental monitoring (Ferrari, 2008). Nanobiosensors have integration of biological sensing components with a nanoscale transducer and aids in detecting specified biomolecules. For example, very low concentrations of biomarkers of cancer, heart diseases, and infectious diseases can be detected by the nanoparticle biosensor, so it allows for early diagnosis (Geng et al., 2007). Increased sensitivity and specificity of nanobiosensors make them an appropriate technology for monitoring the progression of the disease and treatment response (Sakamoto et al., 2010).

9.3.3 Advancements in Point-of-Care Testing and Real-Time Disease Monitoring

Nanotechnology provides a critical platform for developing portable, user-friendly diagnostics of high sensitivity so that the different stages of a disease, along with the effectiveness of treatment, is continuously monitored with appropriate technology (Shi et al., 2010). In other words, it has become possible to create diagnosis devices at a nanoscale, which would translate into small devices that can be used in remote areas or even in the comfort of one's own home. These can be operated from the point of care, such as the clinic and home (Zhang et al., 2008). Fast responses by the devices result in rapid medical decisions taken (Langer & Tirrell, 2004). Lateral flow assays such as the pregnancy test and the rapid test for COVID-19 make use of gold nanoparticles for visualizing particular markers. Point-of-care testing devices can find applications in venues as much as infectious disease detection and monitoring of cardiovascular risk and chronic conditions (Kipp, 2004). Quick and accurate tests at the point of care bring down the need for the centralized laboratory and increase access to health accordingly (Petros & DeSimone, 2010). Making the sensors wearable devices allows for real-time monitoring of glucose, blood pressure, heart rate, among other physiological parameters (Roszek et al., 2005). The device makes use of in-built nanosensors to allow real-time data and detectable interventions. They have enormous potential for management and control of chronic diseases. Another example where real-time monitoring can be applied is wearable automatic glucose monitors, which are capable of constantly measuring the glucose level and, in real time, transmit the information to a smartphone application for processing and interpretation. It will allow patients and doctors to make decisions from information in real time about proper treatment and lifestyle modifications (Vasir et al., 2005). Wearable technology can also provide monitoring for more vital signs than glucose, such as oxygen saturation or respiratory rates and thus offer a full portrait of the patient's status. Nanotechnology has fostered the development of smart tattoos and patches that considerably improved the system of continuous screening of multiple health parameters and dispensing drugs (Shi et al., 2010). Nanosensors are also applied to contemplate the changes in biomarkers and then transmit this information to mobile devices. For example, smart tattoos change colors depending on changes in the levels of glucose or any other vital biochemical and therefore offer an alternative option in a non-invasive manner for managing diabetes cases (Gref et al., 1995). The same smart patches can be used to obtain skin hydration temperature and pH levels to get an overview of health and disease conditions in the body (Peer et al., 2007). Through nanotechnology, it has been possible to develop implantable devices that would be able to continuously monitor and associate therapies (Torchilin, 2006). For example, nano-scale sensors can be implanted in the body to monitor glucose levels in the blood, identify the presence of cancerous cells, and identify the level of intracranial pressure (Lavan et al., 2003). Such nanosensors could send out data to an external monitor, hence making it quite easy to have real-time health monitoring and hence early detection of a health problem.

9.4 NANOTECHNOLOGY IN TISSUE ENGINEERING

Nanomaterials play an integral part in tissue engineering because they can mimic native extracellular matrices to provide architectural and biochemical support to the native cells (Vasir et al., 2005). Due to their very large surface area and tunable mechanical properties, coupled with the capability to present bioactive molecules at their surfaces, nanomaterials can be considered ideal candidates for scaffolding materials for tissue regeneration. Nanoscale attributes of nanomaterials are able to mimic

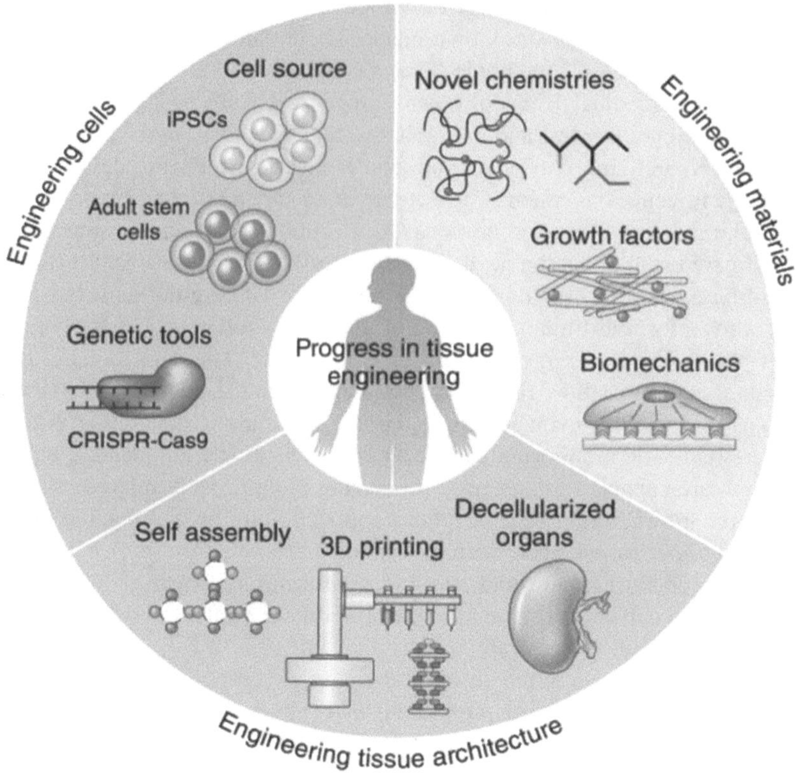

FIGURE 9.5 Summary of tissue engineering progress in the past decade.

the nature of fibrils present in ECM, improving cell adhesion, proliferation, and differentiation (Shi et al., 2010). This is very important in simulating tissue restoration by guiding the management of the organization and functioning of an engineered tissue in detail and integration with the target tissue of the host for regeneration (Gref et al., 1995). The summary of the evolution in this field can be seen in **Figure 9.5**.

Additional cell sources have become available, including iPSCs and adult stem cells, as well as genetic editing tools that enable greater cell manipulation. Improved chemistries and growth factor delivery mechanisms, as well as advances in understanding biophysical cues on cellular behaviors and tissue architecture technologies have contributed to engineering tissues of considerably improved structural, compositional, and functional resemblance to their native counterparts (Langer, R. & Tirrell, D. A., 2004).

The cells can be designed or tailored in their environment within the scaffolds for the incorporation of bioactive molecules as growth factors, peptides, and proteins that facilitate cell-material interaction enhancement (Peer et al., 2007). Applications of this nature will then turn to guide cell migration, differentiation, and ECM formation associated with tissue repair (Langer & Tirrell, 2004). This is because the stiffness and elasticity of the nanomaterials can be determined to be as close to the targeted tissue so that a scaffold can provide the necessary mechanical support for tissue regeneration without interfering with the new tissue formation for complete regeneration (Alivisatos, 2004).

Nanofibers developed through electrospinning are used as scaffolds in tissue engineering because they have a large surface area and porosity to permit cell infiltration but still enable nutrient diffusion within the structure (You et al., 2024). For example, nanofibers produced by biodegradable polymers such as polylactic-co-glycolic acid (PLGA) and polycaprolactone PCL are utilized in the scaffolding of skin, bone, and nerve tissues' regeneration (Meesa et al., 2024). Metallic and semiconducting nanowires have been used in the formation of conductive scaffolds, which provide electrical cues to stimulate cells for growth and differentiation (Nie et al., 2007). Silicon nanoparticles, for example, have been employed in the development of neural interfaces to stimulate the regeneration of nerve tissue in vivo and recover their functionality (Byrne et al., 2008). Due to their superior properties, such as excellent mechanical strength and high electrical conductivity, carbon nanotubes have been embedded to engineering tissue applications (Brigger et al., 2002). Nevertheless, they have been combined into different polymeric matrices through scaffold development resembling composite scaffolds for the regeneration of electrically active tissues like cardiac and neural tissues (Alivisatos, 2004). Also, CNTs can become scaffold matrices by their functionalization with bioactive molecules to enhance biocompatibility and engender specific responses at the cellular level (Nair & Laurencin, 2006).

Tissue engineering is a proper combination of biomaterials, cells, and growth factors in concert to establish and properly modulate the microenvironment required for tissue regeneration (Whitesides, 2003). **Figure 9.6** shows an illustration of a tissue engineering approach that incorporates the seeding of cells within porous biomaterial scaffolds.

In scaffold design, besides biocompatibility and biodegradability, the biomaterials have to be bioactive. Besides having proper mechanical properties, they need to be biocompatible and biodegradable. Commonly used natural materials are collagen, gelatin, and chitosan because of their inherent biocompatibility and bioactivity (Azzazy et al., 2007). Synthetically used polymers are PLGA and PCL because their properties can be modulated and the degradation rates regulated (Langer & Tirrell, 2004; Meesa et al., 2024; Zhang et al., 2008). To regenerate tissue, cells must be present in the scaffold; typically, autologous cells are used to avoid immune rejection (Ferrari, 2008). The applied stem cell types, among many others, are mesenchymal stem cells and induced pluripotent stem cells, which can differentiate into multiple lineages and have demonstrated self-renewal capacity with regenerative potential (Geng et al., 2007). Cellular activities are influenced by growth factors or signaling molecules that control cell proliferation, migration, and differentiation (Sakamoto et al., 2010; Ferrari, 2005). In such aspects, controlled delivery is significant for tissue regeneration by growth factors like bone morphogenetic proteins, vascular endothelial growth factor, and transforming growth factor-beta. Nanomaterials encapsulating growth factors can provide controlled release and sustained bioactivity (Langer & Tirrell, 2004; Zhang et al., 2008).

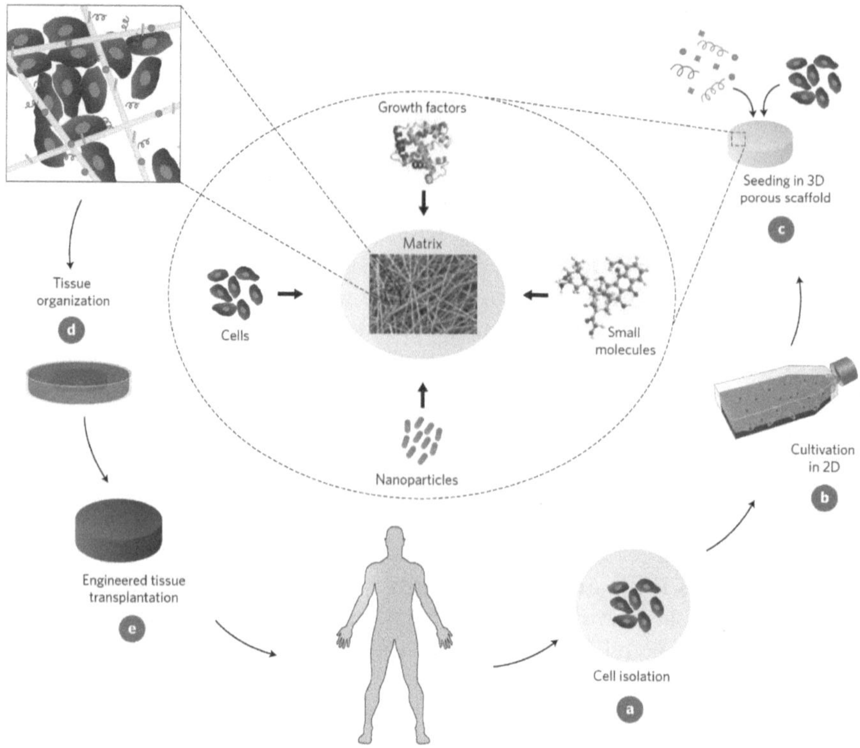

FIGURE 9.6 (a) Cells are obtained from the patient and may be cultured (b) in vitro on two-dimensional surfaces to facilitate efficient expansion. (c) Subsequently, the cells are introduced into porous scaffolds along with growth factors, small molecules, and micro- and/or nanoparticles. These scaffolds provide mechanical support and shape determination while their porous structure enhances mass transfer and waste removal. (d) The cell constructs undergo further cultivation in bioreactors to create optimal conditions for the development of functional tissue. (e) After successfully engineering a functional tissue, the construct is transplanted into the defect site to restore its function (Dvir et al., 2011).

9.5 NANOTECHNOLOGY IN BIOCOMPATIBILITY AND SURFACE MODIFICATIONS

9.5.1 Nanometric Surface Modifications for Material Biocompatibility

Surface modifications at the nanometric scale can enhance the biocompatibility of materials used in the development of medical devices or implants. It can enhance cell adhesion, proliferation, and differentiation while preventing the colonization of bacteria and biofilm formation (Vasir et al., 2005). Nanoscale feature surface modifications, many of which include nanopatterns or nanoroughness, achieve proximity closer to native ECM architecture by interacting with cells at a molecular level to enhance cell adhesion and growth. For example, nanoscale surface roughness on titanium implants has been shown to promote the attachment and proliferation of osteoblasts for enhanced osseointegration (Shi et al., 2010). Nanostructured surfaces are inimical to the adhesion properties of bacterial cells, and therefore, form less biofilm and reduce pathogenicity (Gref et al., 1995). Nanoparticles with well-known broad-spectrum antibacterial properties are embedded into coatings or surfaces of medical devices, hence preventing microbial growth (Peer et al., 2007). Functional coatings by bioactive molecules—for example, peptides, proteins, or polysaccharides—are applied to improve biocompatibility and enhance specific cellular responses (Torchilin, 2006). For instance, heparin coatings reduce the thrombogenicity and enhance the hemocompatibility of blood-contacting devices (Lavan et al., 2003).

9.5.2 Improved Functionality and Lifespan of Implanted Devices

During the last couple of years, nanoparticles have found broad applications in promoting significant improvements in medical implants, ranging from orthopedic devices to dental implants. Nanotechnology is applied in the modification of surface properties of orthopedic implants, primarily for joints and bone screws (Nie et al., 2007). This involves developing nanostructured coatings, including hydroxyapatite, which helps in osseointegration and decreases the wear and corrosion of joints in bones, hence increasing its lifespan (Byrne et al., 2008). It has improved the surface properties in dental implants, hence making them more compatible with the surrounding bone and soft tissues (Vashist & Vashist, 2014). For instance, titanium dental implants that have nanostructured surfaces are associated with better osseointegration with reduced risks of peri-implantitis in dental implantation (Brigger et al., 2002). In cardiovascular implants, advanced coatings for stents and vascular grafts ensure good biocompatibility to reduce restenosis and thrombosis risks (Alivisatos, 2004). Nanostructured surfaces induce endothelialization and resist platelet adhesion, significantly improving the function and durability of cardiovascular implants (Whitesides, 2003).

9.5.3 Modification of Surface Properties for Tissue Adhesion and Vascularization

Nanotechnology-mediated surface modifications have a critical impact on maximizing the potential of tissue adhesion and vascularization of implanted constructs and tissue-engineered success. Nanoscale topography, which results in an increased surface area available for cell attachment and proliferation, thereby enhancing tissue adhesion, allows better interfaces for the same (Shi et al., 2015). Such nanostructured surfaces will, for instance, promote adhesion, differentiation, and bone–implant integration when exposed to osteoblasts (Azzazy et al., 2007; Lee et al., 2007). Vascularization is important for the survival and integration of tissue-engineered constructs. In nanotechnology, angiogenesis or new vessel formation is induced because of the development of all surfaces (Siegel, 1996). For instance, capillary formation is enhanced in angiogenic factor-grafted nanostructured surfaces, for example, VEGF, which is useful in improving implant and scaffold vascularization (Ferrari, 2008).

9.6 THERANOSTICS

9.6.1 Diagnostics and Therapy Integrated

Nanotechnology has been very influential in helping to integrate the diagnostic and therapeutic components into single nanoplatforms for enhanced, personalized management of diseases. Precisely, the synergy of diagnostics and therapy in a single tool improves the precision and efficacy of treatments against various human pathologies, mainly in oncology. In this context, newly developed nanomaterials and nano-drugs have recently been found to improve the potential of theranostic systems by hundreds of times. One example is carbon nanodots, which have recently taken the lead in research interest owing to their unique optical properties coupled with biocompatibility and facile functionalization. CNDs thus permit the diagnosis and treatment of cancer simultaneously; that is, while the fluorescent nature of these dots can provide highly resolved images of tumors, their surfaces can be easily functionalized to carry therapeutic agents. This dual functionality is important in targeted cancer therapy, as it does not only help in the visualization of the tumor sites but also delivers drugs to the cancer cells directly, reducing the damage caused by side effects to healthy tissues (Malhan et al., 2024). Almost parallel to this development in CNDs, there is the development of nano-drugs for neutron capture therapy that added richer functionality and brought huge adaptability when affirming treatment for cancer. These nano-drugs enhance the localization of therapeutic agents at the site of tumors, thus facilitating better neutron capture followed by cancer cell destruction. The combination of nanotechnology and NCT has brought immense hope in treating resistant and deep-seated tumors with very high precision, along with reduced damage to healthy tissues around the areas of tumors (Zhou et al., 2024). Ultrasound-based micro-/nanosystems also reflect the potential of nanotechnology in theranostics. These systems improve the quality of diagnostic imaging and enhance the treatment of various diseases with increased efficacy and precision. Ultrasound-responsive nanoparticles could help surmount limitations to targeted delivery, enhance ultrasound imaging contrast, and provide real-time feedback on therapeutic efficiency by making sure that therapeutic agents are released precisely at the site where needed. This kind of multifunctionality is important when developing an efficient and targeted treatment strategy, thus portraying the huge role played by nanotechnology in advanced therapeutic outcomes.

9.6.2 Advances in Multifunctional Nanocarriers

Nanoparticles have also been excessively probed as drug delivery systems targeted for cardiovascular diseases treatment, such as atherosclerosis. Facilitating both the targeted drug delivery and real-time monitoring, nanoparticles increase the outcome of treatment while minimizing systemic side effects (Pang et al., 2024). Nanocarriers in neuro diseases reveal an example of significant potential of multifunctional nanocarriers for theranostic applications that integrate diagnosis and therapy in a single platform (Rana et al., 2024). Exosome-based nanomedicine has huge progress for the treatment of cancer; for instance, advanced methods including single exosome profiling and exosome barcoding revolutionized cancer theranostics. Such techniques, therefore, personify treatment strategies through effective means in the application. This is done through the delivery of therapeutic agents directly into the cancer cells with simultaneous diagnostic information delivery in view (Mirgh et al., 2024). In tandem with this assertion, theranostic nanoparticles, such as ZIF-8@ICG, have been projected for pH/NIR-responsive drug release and NIR-guided chemo-phototherapy to enhance treatment precision by providing therapy and diagnostics in contemporary single systems for non-small-cell lung cancer. The approach has the advantage of releasing therapeutic agents upon stimulation by specific stimuli, leading to increased efficiency of the treatment while limiting their side effects (Lu et al., 2024). Further, Janus nanoparticles have wide biomedical applications ranging from being drug delivery devices, gene therapy, to theranostics. These dual-functional nanoparticles allow proportioning therapeutic and diagnostic functions simultaneously, increasing the possibility of cancer treatment with comprehensive and targeted interventions (Gharehbaba et al., 2024). Accordingly, theranostic platforms based on polymeric nanomaterials-based innovation have shown much potential in treating triple-negative breast cancer. Such a platform allows for targeting therapy and diagnostic imaging in an attempt to comprehensively manage one of the most challenging types of breast cancer (Baddam et al., 2024). These developments underline the potential of nanotechnology in theranostics by providing all-in-one solutions for diagnostics and treatments.

9.7 DEVELOPMENTS IN CANCER IMMUNOTHERAPY

9.7.1 Next-Generation Nanomaterials Triggering Immune Activation

Nanotechnology has already opened up new avenues for cancer immunotherapy by specifically activating immune cells and targeted delivery of therapeutic reagents. An illustration of the same is shown in **Figure 9.7**.

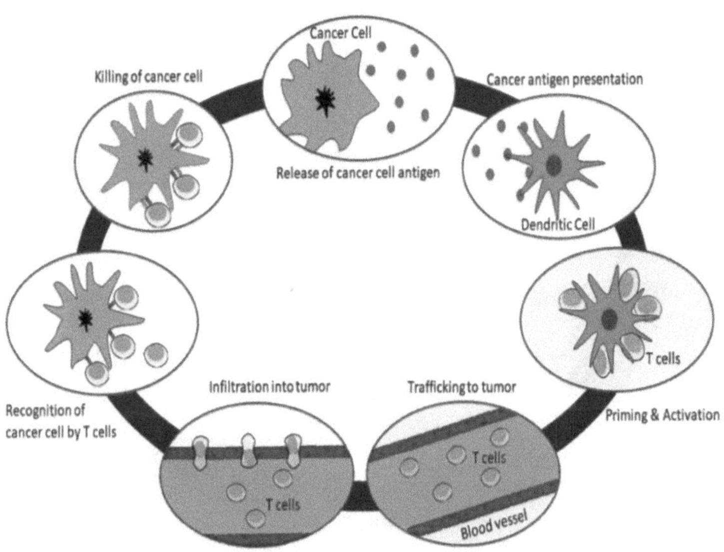

FIGURE 9.7 The cancer immunity cycle. This cycle initiates with the release of antigens from cancer cells and concludes with the establishment of immunity against these cancer cells, involving various types of cells that contribute to this natural process (Akkın, S. et al., 2021).

Improved nanomaterials, such as gold nanoparticles, liposomes, and polymeric nanoparticles, are actively enhancing the effectiveness and specificity of cancer immunotherapy on mechanisms aimed at tumor cells and modulation of immune response (Gonzalez et al., 2024). For instance, gold nanoconjugates demonstrated a huge improvement in miRNA modulation, which significantly impacts the outcome of cancer therapy (Sousa & Conde, 2022).

Recent research has underlined its integration into immunotherapeutic approaches with nanotechnology to improve tumor targeting and immune activation. For instance, melanin-like nanomedicine combined with photothermal therapy has yielded promising results in promoting tumor-specific immune responses (Yue & Zhao, 2021). Moreover, multifunctional chitosan-based nanoparticles developed for targeted drug delivery have significantly enhanced the efficacy of cancer therapy (Tian et al., 2023). Visual representations of various approaches in cancer therapy are shown in **Figure 9.8**.

Furthermore, multifunctional vaccines for cancer immunotherapy have been realized through the participation of nanotechnology. These vaccines make use of nanomaterials, which include gold nanoparticles, liposomes, and polymeric nanoparticles, to improve the delivery capacity and potency of their immunotherapeutic agents (Zhang et al., 2021; Yan et al., 2019). The modulations of immune responses with cancer therapy have been much advanced by progress in applying this RNA nanotechnology (Lin et al., 2020). It has already been demonstrated that melanin-like

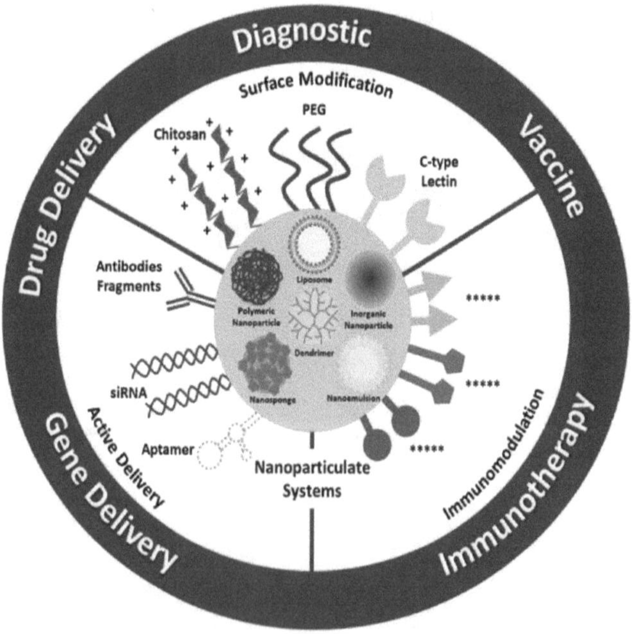

FIGURE 9.8 Various types of nanoparticulate delivery systems and possible approaches in cancer therapy (Akkın, S. et al., 2021).

nanomedicine in photothermal therapy has huge potential for photothermal stimulation to induce tumor-specific immune responses that turn out to increase overall cancer treatment efficacy (Chen, 2023; Gao et al., 2021). It has shown that nanotechnology-based immunotherapy successfully remodels the TME to surmount hurdles against effective cancer immunotherapy (Xie et al., 2022; Bockamp et al., 2020). Nanotechnology-based immunotherapies have been utilized to diminish the immunosuppressive tumor microenvironment, increasing the antitumor immune response (Raza et al., 2021). It has been demonstrated that cell membrane-derived biomimetic nanotechnology is potent against cancer immunotherapy, with superior targeting and reduced side effects (Mahjub et al., 2018).

Nanotechnology has been successfully used in enhancing delivery and efficacy in cancer immunotherapy by developing advanced nanomaterials such as liposomes and polymeric nanoparticles (Asadujjaman et al., 2020). One recent focus has been how to deal with difficulties in cancer immunotherapy by applying nanotechnology to enhance the immune response to enhance treatment outcomes (Cheng et al., 2019; Lou et al., 2019).

9.7.2 Nanoparticle-based Vaccines and Immunomodulators

New ways of cancer treatment have opened up through the development of nanoparticle-based vaccines and immunomodulators. In a way, these nanocarriers increase antigen and adjuvant delivery to mount robust immune responses against tumors (St-Denis-Bissonnette et al., 2022). As cited, RNA-based therapeutics are delivered using nanoparticles, such as liposomes or polymeric carriers, to increase their stability and immunogenicity (Fu et al., 2023).

One such recent development involves peptide-based nanovaccines, which are highly effective in preclinical studies against cervical cancer treatments (Zhang et al., 2022).

Recent research points to the potential of nanotechnology to overcome two traditional limitations of cancer immunotherapy: off-target effects and low immunogenicity (Hong & Dobrovolskaia, 2019). Novel approaches, in particular, cryo-immune engineering and cold-sensitive nanotechnology, have recently shown their potential to enhance the efficiency of immunotherapy by promoting immunogenic death (Li et al., 2019; Ou et al., 2023).

9.8 NANOTECHNOLOGY IN GENE THERAPY

9.8.1 Nanoparticle-Mediated Gene Delivery

Nanotechnology has greatly influenced gene therapy, particularly by facilitating efficient and cell-specific delivery of genetic material. Nanoparticles, such as the lipid-based carriers and polymeric nanoparticles, have been widely applied to enhance the stability and delivery efficiency of siRNA and other nucleic acids (Kim et al., 2019). These carriers not only protect genetic materials from degradation but also enhance their cellular uptake, thereby leading to improved therapeutic outcomes.

For example, lipid nanoparticles have already been efficiently used as siRNA delivery vehicles that provide gene-silencing activity and therefore bear vast potential for the treatment of neurodegenerative and neuromuscular disorders (Gomez Limia et al., 2022). Moreover, nanomedicine strategies have been engineered to improve the delivery of gene-editing tools, including CRISPR-Cas9, and hence offer new perspectives in gene therapy applications for these diseases (Aerts-Kaya & van Til, 2023).

Moreover, recent papers have targeted to overcome the barriers of effective gene therapy by using novel nanocarriers. This includes attempts to optimize nanoparticle formulations for better biocompatibility and targeting efficiency (Tieu et al., 2021). Indeed, it has been shown that vault-derived nanoparticles could be a promising tool for enzyme replacement treatment against *Pseudomonas aeruginosa* biofilm-associated infections (de la Fuente et al., 2021).

9.8.2 Clinical Applications and Challenges

Although promising developments have been made, challenges still exist in translating nanoparticle-mediated gene therapies to clinical practice. One of them can be immunogenicity, off-target effects, and developing effective delivery vehicles. A number of new nanocarriers have been constantly under development by scientists to help move beyond these barriers and provide more functionality at clinical practice for gene therapies.

Recent efforts optimize the formulation of the nanoparticles to improve their biocompatibility and targeting efficiency. For instance, vault-derived nanoparticles were studied as enzyme replacement therapy against *Pseudomonas aeruginosa* biofilm-associated infections (de la Fuente et al., 2021). Finally, the development of smart nanocarriers for the treatment of retinal diseases is one more example of the potential of nanotechnology applied to the cure of genetic disorders.

More recently, nanotechnology approaches have been developed to enhance the delivery and efficacy of cancer immunotherapy, enabling the overcoming of some major barriers to effective treatment (Yang et al., 2020). In this line, approaches have been developed using nanotechnology to promote immunogenic cell death, which really enhances the overall effectiveness of immunotherapy (Fu et al., 2022). There is, therefore, huge potential for nanotechnology having a role in gene therapy and, hence, for the future of personalized medicine and target therapies (Akkın et al., 2021).

9.9 RISKS AND SAFETY CONSIDERATION

9.9.1 Probable Risks and Challenges involved in Application of Nanotechnology in Biomedical Applications

Though it offers a wide range of potential in rendering various biomedical applications, it also has probable risks and challenges associated with it, which have to be addressed to ensure safe and proper use. The major concern about toxicity is that nanoparticles exhibit a higher potential because of their nano size and large surface area, which enhance reactivity (Whitesides, 2003). Nanoparticles might produce unforeseen interactions with biological systems and therefore trigger cytotoxicity, genotoxicity, and inflammatory responses. Risk mitigation may also require that the mechanisms of nanoparticle toxicity be identified, as well as the development of safe exposure limits (Shi et al., 2015). Therefore, it is important to carry out chronic studies to understand the long-term impacts of exposure to single nanoparticles on human health and the environment (Azzazy et al., 2007). Another important consideration for the biocompatibility of nanomaterials is their application in the biomedical field.

Conventionally, a nanomaterial is considered acceptable if it does not show any toxic, immunogenic, or inflammatory reactions and if it gets integrated with the live tissue without opposite reactions. In vitro and in vivo methods of detailed biocompatibility testing with regard to cellular responses, immune reactions, and side effects are necessary (Ferrari, 2008; Loo et al., 2004). Other concerns are raised by the production, use, and disposal of nanomaterials, which could result in environmental implications (Geng et al., 2007). If nanoparticles were disbursed into the environment, an accumulation of these particles in the ecosystems may eventually affect the wildlife and even human health (Sakamoto et al., 2010). The environmental impact assessments and best field practices needed to mitigate the resultant ecological risks of nanotechnology are those related to research on the fate and transport of nanoparticles, their interaction with biological systems, and bioaccumulation processes in the environment (Ferrari, 2005; Shi et al., 2010). Another important aspect that comes with the nanotechnology implementation in health is the ethical and social concerns. An example of these issues is the privacy problem linked to the use of nanosensors or implantable devices. Another major factor is the unequal access of people to developed treatments based on the use of nanotechnology (Langer & Tirrell, 2004). All these concerns require moral guidelines and policies to be set up that regulate the proper use of nanotechnology in health (Zhang et al., 2008). Intensive risk assessments and the initiation of protective protocols for the safe use of nanotechnology in the biomedical sector are highly indispensable (Ferrari, 2005).

An extensive risk assessment has to be made out so as to identify the potential hazards of nanomaterials, the ways of exposure, and the likelihood of adverse effects (Ferrari, 2005). This would involve in vitro and in vivo experimentation to identify the toxicity, biodistribution, and pharmacokinetics of nanomaterials (Ferrari, 2005). Risk assessments are used to identify the potential risk and to formulate safety protocols by determining the hazard assessment right from the production up to the disposal stage of the nanomaterial in its life cycle (Langer & Tirrell, 2004). This includes developing best practices in the handling, application, and disposal of nanomaterials. It includes guidelines on safe laboratory practices, personal protective equipment, and waste management (Zhang et al., 2008). Training needs to be conducted for staff on the perils associated with nanomaterials and measures that can help to reduce the perils. Sustaining a system that is consistent in safety requires regular safety audits and reviews of safety documents (Kipp, 2004).

Compliance with the regulatory bodies' guidelines and standards attains the regulatory compliance for safe nanotechnology usage in biomedical applications. Safe nanotechnology usage is guaranteed through guidelines by various agencies, including FDA, EMA, and ISO, in the safe use of nanotechnology for product development (Petros & DeSimone, 2010; Roszek et al., 2005). These regulations are, therefore, of prime importance to be followed to justify the use of nanotechnology in biomedical applications for safety and efficacy.

9.9.2 Regulatory Guidelines and Standards in the Safe Use of Nanotechnology in Biomedical Fields

The regulatory guidelines and standards should, therefore, mention the safe application of nanotechnology to different biomedical applications. Due to the aforementioned reasons, the regulatory guidelines describe the frame conditions for the development, testing, and commercialization of products based on nanotechnology (Petros & DeSimone, 2010). In this aspect, the regulatory agencies, including the U.S. Food and Drug Administration, the European Medicines Agency, and the International Organization for Standardization, among others, have developed guidance on the assessment and acceptance of products using nanotechnology (Roszek et al., 2005). Guidelines from these agencies also clarify how to characterize, test, and label the nanomaterials under conditions for the safest and most effective results. These guidelines include detailed interactions between the regulatory agencies and researchers to update these guidelines according to the most recent scientific developments.

These testing standards are integrated into the regulatory guidelines, which are specifically formulated to outline the tests needed for evaluating the safety and performance of nanomaterials (Petros & DeSimone, 2010). The testing standards are well-defined in terms of physico-chemical characterization, toxicity, and biocompatibility evaluations (Roszek et al., 2005). It is imperative that such standards are considered in the receipt of regulatory approval for the safe application of nanotechnology in biomedical applications (Roszek et al., 2005). The standards of testing should also consider the unique characteristics of nanomaterials in terms of their size, surface chemistry, and biological interactions. Guidelines on post-market surveillance determine the manner of monitoring information on the long-term safety and effectiveness of nanotechnology-based products (Gref et al., 1995). Such a step will involve the monitoring of adverse events through periodic safety reviews for possible appropriateness of changes in safety measures (Peer et al., 2007). In this regard, post-market surveillance is aimed at promptly and appropriately minimizing the risks arising from nanotechnology products and processes (Torchilin, 2006). Nanotechnology-based products are under continuous surveillance in the everyday environment to determine any possible emerging risk to the patient's long-term safety measure (Lavan et al., 2003).

Standard international harmonization on nanotechnology is very critical in global collaboration and also in building consistency of safety as well as quality across borders. Organizations like the International Council for Harmonisation of Technical Requirements for Pharmaceuticals for Human Use work on unified guidelines that are considered to be safety precautions for implementation in many biomedical fields under nanotechnology.

9.10 FUTURE PERSPECTIVES AND CHALLENGES

9.10.1 Emerging Trends and Future Directions for Nanotechnology in Biomedical Manufacturing

Nanotechnology will be the key driver of progress in biomedical manufacturing, and recent trends and future directions for the same, associated with it, would be related to precision, customization, and interfacing with other technologies. One of the major trends in precision medicine is that nanotechnology facilitates the development of tailored therapeutics based on the genetic and molecular profile of a person (Brigger et al., 2002). It involves the manufacture of nanoparticles or nanocarriers that target certain cells and tissues for the expression of drugs or therapeutic agents. Off-target effects will thus be reduced while the symptoms of deterioration get alleviated (Nair & Laurencin, 2006). For example, nanoparticulates can be made to release the drugs on detection of certain biomarkers, guaranteeing that the unique characteristics of the patient are addressed (Whitesides, 2003).

Another exciting application of nanotechnology is in the development of nanoscale robots, or nanorobots, which will be embedded micro-machines programmed for actions like selective drug delivery, repairing body tissues, or cleaning hazardous substances within an entity. Nanorobots are going to revolutionize minimally invasive surgery and the whole concept of "targeted" therapy (Shi et al., 2015). Nanorobots that can move through the blood to the site of disease are under development, so interventions at the cellular level could be performed by them (Azzazy et al., 2007; Lee et al., 2007). Nano-integration with AI provides enormous development in creating smart diagnostic and therapeutic systems. In this approach, the data from nanodevices and nanosensors gets analyzed by algorithms of AI for the development of procedures pertaining to personal treatment (Siegel, 1996). This integration enhances accuracy and efficiency in medical interventions (Ferrari, 2008). For instance, data patterns from nanosensors can be used in AI-based medical decision-making systems to diagnose diseases or fine-tune treatment protocols (Loo et al., 2004).

Nanotechnology also plays a crucial role in the revolution of 3D bioprinting, an approach involved in designing complex tissue and organ structures (Geng et al., 2007). High-resolution and functional scaffolds have used nanomaterials as bio-inks while printing (Sakamoto et al., 2010). One of the major potential applications is in creating functional tissues and organs suitable for transplantation (Ferrari, 2005). Development in 3D bioprinting with nanomaterials may establish individually tailored tissues and organs with structures and functions similar to those of human tissue (Shi et al., 2010).

9.10.2 Challenges in the Integration of Nanotechnology with Existing Healthcare Systems and Practices

The integration process for nanotechnology within the current healthcare systems and practice is challenged by a number of problems, some of which have to be met for the potential of this technology to be realized. These include the regulatory barriers because the procedures for the regulatory approval of nanotechnology-based products by the regulatory authorities are so rigorous and time-consuming (Petros & DeSimone, 2010). All these products require aggressive testing and validation to meet stringent standards of safety and efficacy (Roszek et al., 2005). In this regard, the streamlining of procedures and guidelines would have to be fine-tuned so that nanotechnology can develop, and its useful application in healthcare is found. At the same time, the issues related to regulations require solutions by regulators, researchers, and experts from the industry who have to work together so that the approval requires less time and effort.

Other important challenges are cost and accessibility. Products comprising nanotechnology are usually very expensive to develop and produce, hence unaffordable for most patients (Petros & DeSimone, 2010). Therefore, the production process needs to be cheaper and more affordable. This would be achieved through scaling up production and enhancing the manufacturing process efficiently (Roszek et al., 2005). Policies and initiatives go on to become very important in the process of making advanced therapies more accessible and affordable to the general public and hence extending the benefits of nanotechnology to a larger section of the population (Roszek et al., 2005).

Public awareness and acceptance of this upcoming technology play an important role in its effective integration into healthcare (Gref et al., 1995). Organizing and propagating awareness among health professionals, patients, and the public about the benefits and risks of nanotechnology is essential to command their trust and acceptance (Peer et al., 2007). An open approach to safety issues and ethical considerations shall be key to attaining public confidence in nanotechnology (Torchilin, 2006). There should be public outreach and educational programs combined with transparent communication about the science and safety of nanotechnology to win the trust of the general public (Lavan et al., 2003).

Nanotechnology in healthcare is an area lending itself well to the practice of interdisciplinarity. It requires interdisciplinary collaboration, as successful integration combines knowledge and skills from disciplines like nanoscience, medicine, engineering, and regulatory affairs. Interdisciplinary research and collaboration between academia, industry, and regulatory agencies are critical steps toward development in this sector. Collaborative efforts can realize innovative breakthroughs through sharing best practices and accelerating technological advancements.

In this scenario, scalability and manufacturability of nanomaterials also become significant challenges. The quality and specified properties are difficult to maintain while scaling up the processes (Byrne et al., 2008). Although some nanoparticle production is possible for research purposes, novel nanotechnological techniques require advanced equipment and often remain limited to small volumes. Items produced through nanotechnology are supposed to be affordable as well as scalable in nature (Siegel, 1996). As such, research and development into nanomanufacturing—including high-throughput synthesis and automation—needs to be increased significantly to meet the increasing demand for nanotechnology-based products (Ferrari, 2008).

9.10.3 Opportunities for Innovation, Collaboration, and Future Research in Nanotechnology for Healthcare Advancement

Being an interdisciplinary area, many opportunities for innovation, collaboration, and further research are connected with this field of nanotechnology in healthcare, propelling advancements in healthcare. According to Nair and Laurencin (2006), research and innovation in the area of nanotechnology are going to generate novel therapies for several diseases, including cancer, neurodegenerative disorders, and infectious diseases. New nano-sized materials, drug delivery systems, and approaches toward therapy could be explored to open up avenues for therapy.

An example of how to achieve improved therapeutic effects is the use of multifunctional nanoparticles that can deliver more than a single type of drug, targeting specific tissues and providing real-time feedback on the effectiveness of the treatment (Shi et al., 2015).

Partnerships between academia, research organizations, and industrial partners are fundamental for generating an impact on nanotechnology in healthcare (Azzazy et al., 2007). Such partnerships can ensure bidirectional flows of ideas and reduce timescales associated with the development of solutions based on nanotechnologies through joint research, funding programs, and knowledge-sharing platforms (Lee et al., 2007). International collaboration also helps in piecing together expertise and resources to pool solutions to global health issues. The gap between transporting ideas from the laboratory to their application in clinics must be bridged so that scientific discoveries intended for nanotechnology applications may indeed improve care solutions for patients (Siegel, 1996). Translational research programs, as mentioned by Ferrari (2008), continue to focus on transferring potential products based on nanotechnology to clinical trials and finally to patients. This calls for satisfying all necessary regulatory requirements and proving clinical utility after thorough testing (Loo et al., 2004). This necessitates the establishment of translational research centers and the extension of collaborative links between researchers, physicians, and industrial partners to expedite the development and commercialization of nanotechnology-based therapies (Geng et al., 2007).

Nanotechnology-based development of tailor-made treatments is directed toward satisfying patient needs that could deliver effective and targeted therapeutics to improve patient healthcare (Sakamoto et al., 2010). Nanotechnology-based diagnostic tools, wearable devices, and the development of non-invasive therapies can provide improved healthcare to patients (Ferrari, 2005). It will be important to develop education and training programs in nanotechnology and its applications within healthcare to develop a competent workforce in this area (Shi et al., 2010). Training healthcare professionals, researchers, and engineers in the newest developments in nanotechnology will be very helpful for integrating these technologies into clinical practice and research (Langer & Tirrell, 2004).

9.11 FUTURE OF NANOTECHNOLOGY IN BIOMEDICAL MANUFACTURING AND ITS POTENTIAL TO REVOLUTIONIZE HEALTHCARE

Nanotechnology has transfigured healthcare via precision medicine, enhanced diagnostics, and advanced treatments will now be assured (Farokhzad & Langer, 2009). The control and alteration of materials at the nano level create chemically targeted drug delivery systems in efficient and safe treatment amid reduced harmful side effects (Peer et al., 2007). For instance, nanoparticles can be synthesized for targeted delivery of drugs to cancer cells, which would cause less harm to the healthy tissue (Bobo et al., 2016). Nanotechnology also supports designing diagnostic tools that are capable of detecting diseases early in their causation, allowing for timely intervention (Alivisatos, 2004). The most recent application of nanotechnology in biosensors that detect viral particles, such as in the case of COVID-19, underlines the potential the field of diagnostics holds (Seo et al., 2020). The nanotechnology and 3D bioprinting techniques have advanced to a stage whereby it has made very precise fabrication of complex tissue structures possible, revolutionizing organ transplantation with these new advances (Murphy & Atala, 2014). In addition, nanotechnology is developing nanoscale sensors and devices that can monitor biological processes in real time, giving unprecedented insight into disease progression and treatment efficacy. Nanorobotics, another growing area of nanotechnology, is also promising in minimally invasive surgeries and drug delivery. Nanorobots, embedded with sensors and nanoscale instruments, are navigated into the human body to perform targeted operations, like drug delivery directly to affected tissues or perform targeted surgeries to treat cancer from body cavities, which is particularly helpful in performing cancer therapy (Mavroidis et al., 2013; Sitti et al., 2015). The robotic approach enables an unprecedented level of precision in medical practice, thereby reducing the complications and enhancing the recovery of patients. With an upward surge in personalization in healthcare, nanoparticles can be designed according to specific genetic and physiological requirements of the patient for a significantly better prognosis from treatment (Venkatesan et al., 2019). Nanotechnology contributes immensely to the field of imaging in terms of improved sensitivity and specificity of diagnostic imaging techniques. It is now possible to optimize or improve imaging modalities like MRI and CT through the use of functionalized gold and magnetic nanoparticles for earlier and more accurate detection of diseases (Bardhan et al., 2011; Huang et al., 2011). All these developments enable clinicians to identify cancers and cardiovascular diseases at their earliest stages so that a better prognosis can be formulated and treatment set up.

Even as these developments are made, the imperfections that surround them have not yet disappeared. Safety issues regarding the toxicity and biocompatibility of nanomaterials have to be addressed with strict care so patients are safe from harm (Nel et al., 2006). The ability of nanoparticles to cross biological barriers such as the blood-brain barrier calls for comprehensive testing and safety evaluations (Silva, 2004). Besides these, the environmental impacts of nanomaterials particularly, their persistence in the environment, are emerging lines of questioning (Karn et al., 2011; Nowack & Bucheli, 2007). Thus, biodegradable and "green" nanoparticles should be developed to minimize the footprints of nanotechnology-based medical applications as much as possible in the environment.

Regulatory challenges are still another added hindrance. The existing regulatory frameworks are least capable of understanding the assessment of safety and efficacy for nanotechnology-based therapies and diagnostics. For example, the regulatory agency of the U.S. Food and Drug Administration (FDA) and the European Medicines Agency (EMA) are putting forward guidelines in this regard for the approval and usage of nanomedicine products (Etheridge et al., 2013; Fadeel et al., 2018). Continuous collaboration between regulatory agencies, scientists, and industry stakeholders can lead to the careful establishment of overall safety protocols for nanomedicines. The integration of nanotechnology with AI, biotechnology, and other next-generation technologies will further bring out its potential to impact healthcare. AI-driven algorithm tools can be helpful in designing nanoparticles with optimized properties for specific applications in medicine and new biological targets identified by biotechnology for nanoparticle-based therapies (Tzounis et al., 2021; Salman et al., 2020). This convergence is poised to speed up the pace of innovations in nanomedicine, leading to more efficient and personalized treatments (Tiwari et al., 2020). Expanding research as well as investment in nanomaterials, nano-engineering techniques, and also across research fields will provide new treatments, along with new diagnostic tools, which will eventually shift healthcare and improve patient outcomes (Huang et al., 2010; Khademhosseini & Langer, 2016).

9.12 CONCLUSION

Nanotechnology made a huge difference in biomedical manufacturing, marking outstanding progress in healthcare. That describes the component of nanomaterials which makes medical diagnostics, therapies, and preventive methods possible on a large scale. Actually, with regard to drug delivery systems, it would be the biggest strides taken in developing nanoparticle construct-based that allowed control over drug release to an unprecedented degree and to deliver it to some specific sites within the body. These have increased the efficiency of therapies while minimizing their side effects. Advanced diagnostic devices using nanotechnology could help in improving the condition at hand, with ways of early diagnosis of diseases invented. Diagnosis tools using nanotechnology are in a position to diagnose a disease in its earliest stages, and this would be easy and more effective for intervention. Nanotechnology has managed to come up with non-invasive treatment methodologies for a myriad of pathologies, from chronic to life-threatening diseases such as cancer and degenerative neurologic disorders. This accrues high precision in the delivery of therapies and therefore low invasiveness in procedures, fast recovery time of patients, and a better quality of life. The challenges in clinic integration are many. Biocompatibility and regulatory rigors are the major concerns, particularly related to long-term safety and environmental impact with its use. Hence, the well-built translational research and international collaboration will act as a gateway for the safe and effective induction of nanotechnology into healthcare. In the near future, research will get directed toward the optimization of functional features of the nanomaterials, university cost procedures for the creation of different nanoplatforms, and reproducibility of results in different settings. Since nanotechnology inherently deals with physics, chemistry, biology, and engineering, it gives promise of continuous innovation and adaption in front of these ever-increasingly complex medical problems. Accordingly, the potentials in this area are huge for biomedical manufacturing with nanotechnology, foretelling advanced health solutions within the next near-to-medium future. Sustained efforts in researching and focused collaborations would yield effective, personalized, and less invasive treatments, totally overhauling patient care worldwide. While nanotechnology holds great promise in manufacturing biomedical devices, the full realization of this potential comes with formidable scientific, regulatory, and ethical barriers. This continuous development can be premised on rigorous research based on international collaboration, safety, and meticulous ethical guidelines developed in tandem. Application of nanotechnology in health ushers a new future in which totally all medical treatments and diagnostics are going to be changed to bring in absolutely a new time for innovative medicine and improved patient outcome.

REFERENCES

Aerts-Kaya, F., & van Til, N. P. (2023). Gene and cellular therapies for leukodystrophies. *Pharmaceutics*, 15(11), 2522.

Akkın, S., Varan, G., & Bilensoy, E. (2021). A review on cancer immunotherapy and applications of nanotechnology to chemoimmunotherapy of different cancers. *Molecules*, 26(11), 3382.

Alivisatos, A. P. (2004). The use of nanocrystals in biological detection. *Nature Biotechnology*, 22(1), 47–52.

Asadujjaman, M., Cho, K. H., Jang, D. J., Kim, J. E., & Jee, J. P. (2020). Nanotechnology in the arena of cancer immunotherapy. *Archives of Pharmacal Research*, 43(1):58–79.

Azzazy, H. M., Mansour, M. M., & Kazmierczak, S. C. (2007). From diagnostics to therapy: Prospects of quantum dots. *Clinical Biochemistry*, 40(13–14), 917–27.

Baddam, S. R., Ganta, S., Nalla, S., Banoth, C., Vudari, B., Akkiraju, P. C., Srinivas, E., & Tade, R. S. (2024). Polymeric nanomaterials-based theranostic platforms for triple-negative breast cancer (TNBC) treatment. *International Journal of Pharmaceutics*, 660, 124346. Elsevier BV.

Bardhan, R., Lal, S., Joshi, A., & Halas, N. J. (2011). Theranostic nanoshells: From probe design to imaging and treatment of cancer. *Accounts of Chemical Research, 44*(10), 936–46. https://doi.org/10.1021/ar200023x

Bobo, D., Robinson, K. J., Islam, J., Thurecht, K. J., & Corrie, S. R. (2016). Nanoparticle-based medicines: A review of FDA-approved materials and clinical trials to date. *Pharmaceutical Research, 33*(10), 2373–87. https://doi.org/10.1007/s11095-016-1958-5

Bockamp, E., Rosigkeit, S., Siegl, D., & Schuppan, D. (2020). Nano-enhanced cancer immunotherapy: Immunology encounters nanotechnology. *Cells*, 9(9), 2102.

Brigger, I., Dubernet, C., & Couvreur, P. (2002). Nanoparticles in cancer therapy and diagnosis. *Advanced Drug Delivery Reviews*, 54(5), 631–51.

Byrne, J. D., Betancourt, T., & Brannon-Peppas, L. (2008). Active targeting schemes for nanoparticle systems in cancer therapeutics. *Advanced Drug Delivery Reviews*, 60(15), 1615–26.

Chen, Y. (2023). Nanotechnology for next-generation cancer immunotherapy: State of the art and future perspectives. *Journal of Controlled Release*, 356, 14–25. Elsevier BV.

Cheng, C. T., Castro, G., Liu, C. H., & Lau, P. (2019). Advanced nanotechnology: An arsenal to enhance immunotherapy in fighting cancer. *Clinica Chimica Acta*, 492, 12–19.

de la Fuente, M., Lombardero, L., Gómez-González, A., Solari, C., Angulo-Barturen, I., Acera, A., Vecino, E., Astigarraga, E., & Barreda-Gómez, G. (2021). Enzyme therapy: Current challenges and future perspectives. *International Journal of Molecular Sciences*. 22(17), 9181.

Dvir, T., Timko, B. P., Kohane, D. S., & Langer, R. (2011). Nanotechnological strategies for engineering complex tissues. *Nature Nanotechnology*, 6(1), 13–22.

Etheridge, M. L., Campbell, S. A., Erdman, A. G., Haynes, C. L., Wolf, S. M., & McCullough, J. (2013). The big picture on nanomedicine: The state of investigational and approved nanomedicine products. *Nanomedicine: Nanotechnology, Biology and Medicine*, 9(1), 1–14. https://doi.org/10.1016/j.nano.2012.09.014

Fadeel, B., Fornara, A., Toprak, M. S., Bhattacharya, K., & Dawson, K. A. (2018). Keeping it real: The importance of material characterization in nanotoxicology. *Biochemical and Biophysical Research Communications*, 503(3), 585–95. https://doi.org/10.1016/j.bbrc.2018.06.103

Farokhzad, O. C., & Langer, R. (2009). Impact of nanotechnology on drug delivery. *ACS Nano*, 3(1), 16–20. https://doi.org/10.1021/nn900002m

Ferrari, M. (2005). Cancer nanotechnology: Opportunities and challenges. *Nature Reviews Cancer*, 5(3), 161–71.

Ferrari, M. (2008). Nanogeometry: Beyond drug delivery. *Nature Nanotechnology*, 3(3), 131–2.

Fu, J., Dong, H., Wu, J., & Jin, Y. (2023). Emerging progress of RNA-based antitumor therapeutics. *International Journal of Biological Sciences*, 19(10):3159–83.

Fu, L., Ma, X., Liu, Y., Xu, Z., & Sun, Z. (2022). Applying nanotechnology to boost cancer immunotherapy by promoting immunogenic cell death. *Chinese Chemical Letters*, 33(4), 1718–28.

Gao, S., Yang, X., Xu, J., Qiu, N., & Zhai, G. (2021). Nanotechnology for boosting cancer immunotherapy and remodeling tumor microenvironment: The horizons in cancer treatment. *ACS Nano*, 15(8), 12567–603. American Chemical Society (ACS).

Geng, Y., Dalhaimer, P., Cai, S., Tsai, R., Tewari, M., Minko, T., & Discher, D. E. (2007). Shape effects of filaments versus spherical particles in flow and drug delivery. *Nature Nanotechnology*, 2(4), 249–55.

Gharehbaba, A. M., Omidi, Y., Barar, J., Eskandani, M., & Adibkia, K. (2024). Innovative horizons in cancer therapy, imaging, and sensing with Janus nanoparticles: A comprehensive review. *Trends in Analytical Chemistry: TRAC*, 178(117822), 117822.

Gharieh, A., Khoee, S., & Mahdavian, A. R. (2019). Emulsion and miniemulsion techniques in preparation of polymer nanoparticles with versatile characteristics. *Advances in Colloid and Interface Science*, 269, 152–86.

Gomez Limia, C., Baird, M., Schwartz, M., Saxena, S., Meyer, K., & Wein, N. (2022). Emerging perspectives on Gene therapy delivery for neurodegenerative and neuromuscular disorders. *Journal of Personalized Medicine*, 12(12), 1979.

Gonzalez, T., Muminovic, M., Nano, O., & Vulfovich, M. (2024). Folate receptor alpha—A novel approach to cancer therapy. *International Journal of Molecular Sciences*, 25(2), 1046.

Gref, R., Minamitake, Y., Peracchia, M. T., Trubetskoy, V., Torchilin, V., & Langer, R. (1995). Biodegradable long-circulating polymeric nanospheres. *Science*, 267(5202), 319–22.

Hong, E., & Dobrovolskaia, M. A. (2019). Addressing barriers to effective cancer immunotherapy with nanotechnology: Achievements, challenges, and roadmap to the next generation of nanoimmunotherapeutics. *Advanced Drug Delivery Reviews*, 141, 3–22. Elsevier BV.

Huang, X., El-Sayed, I. H., Qian, W., & El-Sayed, M. A. (2010). Cancer cell imaging and photothermal therapy in the near-infrared region by using gold nanorods. *Journal of the American Chemical Society*, 128(6), 2115–2120. https://doi.org/10.1021/ja057254a

Huang, X., Jain, P. K., El-Sayed, I. H., & El-Sayed, M. A. (2011). Gold nanoparticles: Interesting optical properties and recent applications in cancer diagnostics and therapy. *Nanomedicine*, 2(5), 681–93. https://doi.org/10.2217/17435889.2.5.681

Jain, K. K. (2012). *The Handbook of Nanomedicine*. Springer Science & Business Media.

Karn, B., Kuiken, T., & Otto, M. (2011). Nanotechnology and in situ remediation: A review of the benefits and potential risks. *Environmental Health Perspectives*, 119(2), 182–9. https://doi.org/10.1289/ehp.1002208

Khademhosseini, A., & Langer, R. (2016). A decade of progress in tissue engineering. *Nature Protocols*, 11(10), 1775–81. https://doi.org/10.1038/nprot.2016.125

Kim, B., Park, J. H., & Sailor, M. J. (2019). Rekindling RNAi therapy: Materials design requirements for in vivo siRNA delivery. *Advanced Materials*. 31(49), e1903637.

Kipp, J. E. (2004). The role of solid nanoparticle technology in the parenteral delivery of poorly water-soluble drugs. *International Journal of Pharmaceutics*, 284(1–2), 109–22.

Langer, R., & Tirrell, D. A. (2004). Designing materials for biology and medicine. *Nature*, 428(6982), 487–92.

Lavan, D. A., McGuire, T., & Langer, R. (2003). Small-scale systems for in vivo drug delivery. *Nature Biotechnology*, 21(10), 1184–91.

Lee, J. H., Yoon, T. J., Cho, Y. S., & Oh, J. K. (2007). In vivo imaging with quantum dots. *Bioconjugate Chemistry*, 18(6), 1559–65.

Li, Y., Ayala-Orozco, C., Rauta, P. R., & Krishnan, S. (2019). The application of nanotechnology in enhancing immunotherapy for cancer treatment: Current effects and perspective. *Nanoscale*, 11(37):17157–78.

Lin, Y. X., Wang, Y., Blake, S., Yu, M., Mei, L., Wang, H., & Shi, J. (2020). RNA nanotechnology-mediated cancer immunotherapy. *Theranostics*, 10(1), 281–99.

Loo, C., Lin, A., Hirsch, L., Lee, M. H., Barton, J., Halas, N., . . . & West, J. (2004). Nanoshell-enabled photonics-based imaging and therapy of cancer. *Technology in Cancer Research & Treatment*, 3(1), 33–40.

Lou, J. W., Zhang, L., & Zheng, G. (2019). Advancing cancer immunotherapies with nanotechnology. *Advanced Therapeutics*, 2.

Lu, K., Pan, X., Zheng, J., Cheng, D., Zheng, L., & Zhang, X. (2024). Theranostic nanoparticles ZIF-8@ICG for pH/NIR-responsive drug-release and NIR-guided chemo-phototherapy against non-small-cell lung cancer. *Journal of Materials Science. Materials in Medicine*, 35(1), 32.

Mabrouk, M., Das, D. B., Salem, Z. A., & Beherei, H. H. (2021). Nanomaterials for biomedical applications: Production, characterisations, recent trends and difficulties. *Molecules*, 26(4), 1077.

Mahjub, R., Jatana, S., Lee, S. E., et al. (2018). Recent advances in applying nanotechnologies for cancer immunotherapy. *Journal of Controlled Release: Official Journal of the Controlled Release Society*, 288, 239–63.

Malhan, A., Guleria, M., Das, U., Singh, S., Prajapati, B. G., Mohite, P., Bhattacharya, S., Chidrawar, V. R., Puri, A., & Datta, D. (2024). Navigating the future of cancer management through carbon nanodots: A review. *Nano-Structures & Nano-Objects*, 39, 101217.

Mavroidis, C., Dubey, A., & Yarmush, M. L. (2013). Molecular machines: Nanorobotics for protein-based cell repair. *IEEE Transactions on Nanobioscience*, 2(1), 51–63. https://doi.org/10.1109/TNB.2003.808581

Mazzola, L. (2003). Commercializing nanotechnology. *Nature Biotechnology*, 21(10), 1137–43.

McNeil, S. E. (2005). Nanotechnology for the biologist. *Journal of Leukocyte Biology*, 78(3), 585–94.

Meesa, B., Surin, P., & Wiwatwongwana, F. (2024). Characterization of nanofibrous scaffolds from blends of gelatin/PCL/CMC for hard tissue engineering application. *Hunan Daxue Xuebao*, 11(5), 45–58.

Mirgh, D., Sonar, S., Nyahatkar, S., Kalele, K., & Adhikari, M. D. (2024). The prospective trajectory of exosomes-based cancer nanomedicine. *Clinical and Translational Discovery*, 4(3).

Murphy, S. V., & Atala, A. (2014). 3D bioprinting of tissues and organs. *Nature Biotechnology*, 32(8), 773–85. https://doi.org/10.1038/nbt.2958

Nair, L. S., & Laurencin, C. T. (2006). Polymers as biomaterials for tissue engineering and controlled drug delivery. *Advanced Biochemical Engineering/Biotechnology*, 102, 47–90.

Nel, A., Xia, T., Madler, L., & Li, N. (2006). Toxic potential of materials at the nanolevel. *Science*, 311(5761), 622–7. https://doi.org/10.1126/science.1114397

Nie, S., Xing, Y., Kim, G. J., & Simons, J. W. (2007). Nanotechnology applications in cancer. *Annual Review of Biomedical Engineering*, 9, 257–88.

Nowack, B., & Bucheli, T. D. (2007). Occurrence, behavior and effects of nanoparticles in the environment. *Environmental Pollution*, 150(1), 5–22. https://doi.org/10.1016/j.envpol.2007.06.006

Ou, W., Stewart, S., White, A., Kwizera, E. A., Xu, J., Fang, Y., Shamul, J. G., Xie, C., Nurudeen, S., Tirada, N. P., Lu, X., Tkaczuk, K. H. R., & He, X. (2023). In-situ cryo-immune engineering of tumor microenvironment with cold-responsive nanotechnology for cancer immunotherapy. *Nature Communications*, 14(1), 392.

Pang, A. S., Dinesh, T., Pang, N. Y., Dinesh, V., Pang, K. Y., Yong, C. L., Lee, S. J. J., Yip, G. W., Bay, B. H., & Srinivasan, D. K. (2024). Nanoparticles as drug delivery systems for the targeted treatment of atherosclerosis. *Molecules/Molecules Online/Molecules Annual*, 29(12), 2873.

Parak, W. J., Gerion, D., Pellegrino, T., Zanchet, D., Micheel, C., Williams, S. C., . . . & Alivisatos, A. P. (2005). Biological applications of colloidal nanocrystals. *Nanotechnology*, 16(10), R9.

Peer, D., Karp, J. M., Hong, S., Farokhzad, O. C., Margalit, R., & Langer, R. (2007). Nanocarriers as an emerging platform for cancer therapy. *Nature Nanotechnology*, 2(12), 751–60.

Petros, R. A., & DeSimone, J. M. (2010). Strategies in the design of nanoparticles for therapeutic applications. *Nature Reviews Drug Discovery*, 9(8), 615–27.

Rana, P., Kaur, G., Chirayimmel, A. J., Rajput, A., Rath, S. K., & Dwibedi, V. (2024). Nanocarriers and nano drug delivery therapy in neuro diseases. In *Nanomaterials for Drug Delivery and Neurological Diseases Management* (pp. 219–51). Springer Nature Singapore.

Raza, F., Zafar, H., Zhang, S., Kamal, Z., Su, J., Yuan, W. E., & Mingfeng, Q. (2021). Recent advances in cell membrane-derived biomimetic nanotechnology for cancer immunotherapy. *Advanced Healthcare Materials*, 10(6), e2002081.

Roco, M. C. (2003). Nanotechnology: Convergence with modern biology and medicine. *Current Opinion in Biotechnology*, 14(3), 337–46.

Roszek, B., De Jong, W. H., Geertsma, R. E., & Riviere, J. E. (2005). *Nanotechnology in Healthcare: QNano Workshop, June 29–30, 2005, St. Louis, MO*. https://catalog.nlm.nih.gov/permalink/01NLM_INST/1o1phhn/alma9912770193406676

Sakamoto, J. H., van de Ven, A. L., Godin, B., Blanco, E., Serda, R. E., Grattoni, A., . . . & Ferrari, M. (2010). Enabling individualized therapy through nanotechnology. *Pharmacological Research*, 62(2), 57–89.

Salman, A., Alafeef, M., & Dweik, M. (2020). Artificial intelligence and nanotechnology integration: Pathways for diagnostics and therapeutics. *Nanotechnology Reviews*, 9(1), 1–11. https://doi.org/10.1515/ntrev-2020-0001

Seo, G., Lee, G., Kim, M. J., Back, S. H., Choi, M., Ku, K. B., . . . & Kim, S. I. (2020). Rapid detection of COVID-19 causative virus (SARS-CoV-2) in human nasopharyngeal swab specimens using field-effect transistor-based biosensor. *ACS Nano*, 14(4), 5135–42. https://doi.org/10.1021/acsnano.0c02823

Shi, J., Kantoff, P. W., Wooster, R., & Farokhzad, O. C. (2015). Cancer nanomedicine: Progress, challenges and opportunities. *Nature Reviews Cancer*, 17(1), 20–37.

Shi, J., Votruba, A. R., Farokhzad, O. C., & Langer, R. (2010). Nanotechnology in drug delivery and tissue engineering: From discovery to applications. *Nano Letters*, 10(9), 3223–30.

Siegel, R. W. (1996). Nanostructured materials: Mind over matter. *Nanostructured Materials*, 7(1–2), 13–17.

Silva, G. A. (2004). Neuroscience nanotechnology: Progress, opportunities, and challenges. *Nature Reviews Neuroscience*, 5(1), 65–72. https://doi.org/10.1038/nrn1533

Sitti, M., Ceylan, H., Hu, W., Giltinan, J., Turan, M., Yim, S., & Diller, E. (2015). Biomedical applications of untethered mobile milli/microrobots. *Proceedings of the IEEE*, 103(2), 205–24. https://doi.org/10.1109/JPROC.2014.2385105

Sousa, D. P., & Conde, J. (2022). Gold nanoconjugates for miRNA modulation in cancer therapy: From miRNA silencing to miRNA mimics. *ACS Materials Au*, 2(6), 626–40.

St-Denis-Bissonnette, F., Khoury, R., Mediratta, K., El-Sahli, S., Wang, L., & Lavoie, J. R. (2022). Applications of extracellular vesicles in triple-negative breast cancer. *Cancers (Basel)*, 14(2), 451.

Tian, B., Hua, S., & Liu, J. (2023). Multi-functional chitosan-based nanoparticles for drug delivery: Recent advanced insight into cancer therapy. *Carbohydrate Polymers*, 315, 120972. https://doi.org/10.1016/j.carbpol.2023.120972

Tieu, T., Wei, Y., Cifuentes-Rius, A., & Voelcker, N. H. (2021). Overcoming barriers: Clinical translation of SiRNA nanomedicines. *Advanced Therapeutics*, 4(9). https://doi.org/10.1002/adtp.202100108

Tiwari, J. N., Tiwari, R. N., & Kim, K. S. (2020). Zero-dimensional, one-dimensional, two-dimensional and three-dimensional nanostructured materials for advanced electrochemical energy devices. *Progress in Materials Science*, 120, 100768. https://doi.org/10.1016/j.pmatsci.2020.100768

Torchilin, V. P. (2006). Multifunctional nanocarriers. *Advanced Drug Delivery Reviews*, 58(14), 1532–55.

Tzounis, L., Missirlis, D., Stergiopoulos, S., & Rudolf, P. (2021). A critical review on the use of nanotechnologies in the fight against SARS-CoV-2: Current trends and future perspectives. *Nanomaterials*, *11*(4), 1004. https://doi.org/10.3390/nano11041004

Vashist, S. K., & Vashist, P. (2014). Recent advances in hydrogel-based drug delivery systems for the human body. *Journal of Materials Chemistry B*, 2(2), 147–66.

Vasir, J. K., Reddy, M. K., & Labhasetwar, V. (2005). Nanosystems in drug targeting: Opportunities and challenges. *Current Nanoscience*, 1(1), 47–64.

Venkatesan, S., Trivedi, R., & Dorairaj, S. (2019). Smart nanocarriers for targeted cancer therapy. *International Journal of Pharmaceutical Sciences and Research*, 10(3), 1051–64. https://doi.org/10.13040/IJPSR.0975–8232.10(3).1051–64

Whitesides, G. M. (2003). The 'right' size in nanobiotechnology. *Nature Biotechnology*, 21(10), 1161–65.

Xie, X., Song, T., Feng, Y., Zhang, H., Yang, G., Wu, C., You, F., Liu, Y., & Yang, H. (2022). Nanotechnology-based multifunctional vaccines for cancer immunotherapy. *Chemical Engineering Journal*, 437, 135505. Elsevier BV.

Yan, S., Zhao, P., Yu, T., & Gu, N. (2019). Current applications and future prospects of nanotechnology in cancer immunotherapy. *Cancer Biology & Medicine*, 16(3), 486–97.

Yang, Z., Ma, Y., Zhao, H., Yuan, Y., & Kim, B. Y. S. (2020). Nanotechnology platforms for cancer immunotherapy. *WIREs Nanomed Nanobiotechnol*. 12, e1590.

You, Y., Xu, F., Liu, L., Chen, S., Ding, Z., & Sun, D. (2024). Construction of thick myocardial tissue through layered seeding in multi-layer nanofiber scaffolds. *Polymers*, 16(18), 2664.

Yue, Y., & Zhao, X. (2021). Melanin-like nanomedicine in photothermal therapy applications. *International Journal of Molecular Sciences*, 22(1), 399.

Zhang, J., Fan, J., Skwarczynski, M., Stephenson, R. J., Toth, I., & Hussein, W. M. (2022). Peptide-based nanovaccines in the treatment of cervical cancer: A review of recent advances. *International Journal of Nanomedicine*, 17, 869–900.

Zhang, L., Gu, F. X., Chan, J. M., Wang, A. Z., Langer, R. S., & Farokhzad, O. C. (2008). Nanoparticles in medicine: Therapeutic applications and developments. *Clinical Pharmacology & Therapeutics*, 83(5), 761–9.

Zhang, P., Meng, J., Li, Y., Yang, C., Hou, Y., Tang, W., McHugh, K. J., & Jing, L. (2021). Nanotechnology-enhanced immunotherapy for metastatic cancer. *The Innovation*, 2(4), 100174. Elsevier BV.

Zhou, Y., Cheng, K., Liu, B., Cao, Y., Fan, J., Liu, Z., & Zhao, Y. (2024). Recent progress of nano-drugs in neutron capture therapy. *Theranostics*, 14(8), 3193–212.

10 Advances in Nanomaterials for Biomedical Healthcare

Applications and Implications

Sachin Gupta, Shivali Gupta, and Gursimran Kaur

CONTENTS

DOI: 10.1201/9781003516064-10

10.1 INTRODUCTION TO NANOSTRUCTURE-BASED TECHNOLOGY IN HEALTHCARE

Nanotechnology is one of the leading fields for transforming materials to their nano scale and molecular scale, which made substantial strides in the healthcare sector, offering transformative potential in diagnostics, drug delivery, and therapeutic applications [1]. Defined by the control of materials sized between 1 nanometre and 100 nanometres, nanostructure-based technology introduces unique properties that arise at this scale, observed increased surface area, enhanced reactivity, and distinct optical behaviour. These properties make nanomaterials particularly suitable for medical applications, where precision and specificity are often critical. Nanotechnology's ability to deliver targeted treatment, improve diagnostic accuracy, and enable personalized medicine makes it an invaluable asset in modern healthcare. In the realm of diagnostics, nanostructure-based technology is leveraged to develop tools that improve the sensitivity and accuracy of disease detection [2]. Quantum dots, a type of nanoparticle, are luminescent and have shown promise in fluorescence-based imaging, facilitating real-time visualization of biological processes. These advances have led to a new generation of diagnostic tools that are not only more accurate but also capable of providing detailed insights at a molecular level. Nanostructure-based technology has also revolutionized drug delivery, addressing one of the most significant challenges in medicine, ensuring that therapeutic agents reach their intended target without causing adverse effects on healthy cells. Conventional drug delivery systems often result in systemic distribution, which can lead to unwanted side effects. Nanostructure-based technology enables the encapsulation of drugs within nanoscale carriers such as liposomes, polymeric nanoparticles, and dendrimers which can travel through the bloodstream and release the medication directly at the site of disease [3].

10.1.1 Overview of Nanostructure-based Technology in Medicine

Nanostructure-based technology has fundamentally reshaped medicine by enabling innovations that rely on the unique properties of materials engineered at the nanoscale, typically between 1 nanometre and 100 nanometres. This scale allows materials to exhibit distinct characteristics, such as enhanced chemical reactivity, improved electrical conductivity, and unique optical properties, which are crucial for diverse medical applications. In diagnostics, for example, nanoparticles act as highly effective contrast agents in imaging techniques like MRI and PET scans, allowing for the visualization of tissues with remarkable detail and aiding in the early detection of diseases [4]. Similarly, in the realm of drug delivery, nanoscale carriers as liposomes and polymeric nanoparticles enable the precise targeting of therapeutic agents, ensuring that medications reach diseased cells with minimal impact on surrounding healthy tissues. This targeted approach is being considered as especially valuable in cancer treatment, where it reduces the toxicity associated with traditional chemotherapy. Moreover, nanostructure-based technology has accelerated progress in personalized medicine by allowing for the delivery of genetic material—DNA or RNA—into specific cells to influence gene expression, opening potential treatments for genetic disorders and some types of cancer [5]. Additionally, in regenerative medicine, nanomaterials serve as scaffolds that support cell growth and tissue regeneration, making them instrumental in wound healing and tissue engineering. Nano-enabled point-of-care diagnostic devices are also transforming healthcare, particularly in resource-limited settings, by facilitating rapid and accurate testing for various diseases. **Figure 10.1** shows the application of nanomaterials which are used in the formulation of medical devices.

Researchers discovered that nanoparticles could enhance contrast in imaging modalities like magnetic resonance imaging (MRI) and computed tomography (CT) scans, enabling physicians to obtain clearer and more detailed images of internal tissues and organs. As nanostructure-based technology continued to advance, its applications expanded beyond imaging. The field of drug delivery began to benefit from nanoscale innovations. Scientists began creating nanoparticles capable of carrying therapeutic agents directly to specific cells or tissues, increasing treatment effectiveness while reducing side effects. This targeted drug delivery was especially revolutionary in oncology, where traditional chemotherapy can harm healthy cells; nanostructure-based technology allowed drugs to be delivered directly to cancerous cells, improving patient outcomes and reducing systemic toxicity [6].

10.1.2 Current State of Biomedical Nanotechnology

The current state of biomedical nanostructure-based technology is marked by significant advancements that are reshaping diagnostics, drug delivery, imaging,

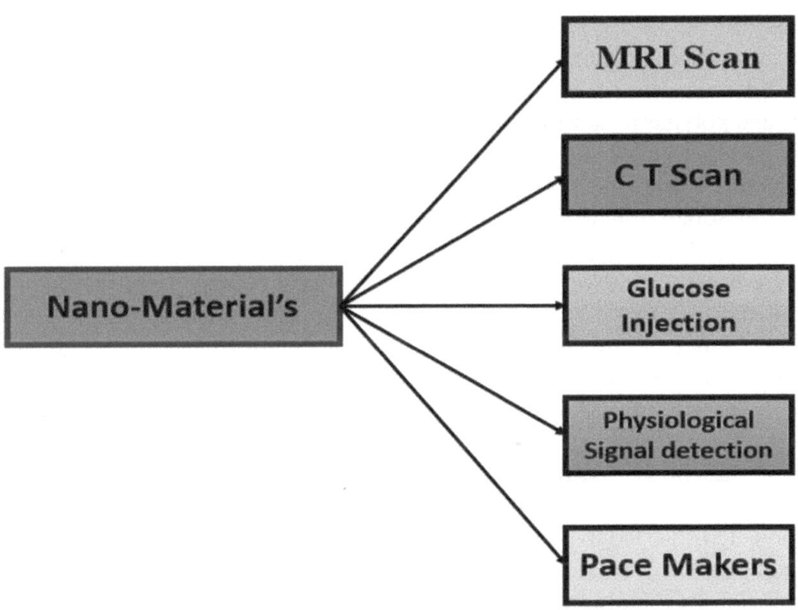

FIGURE 10.1 Applications of nanomaterials in the biomedical sector. (Created by authors)

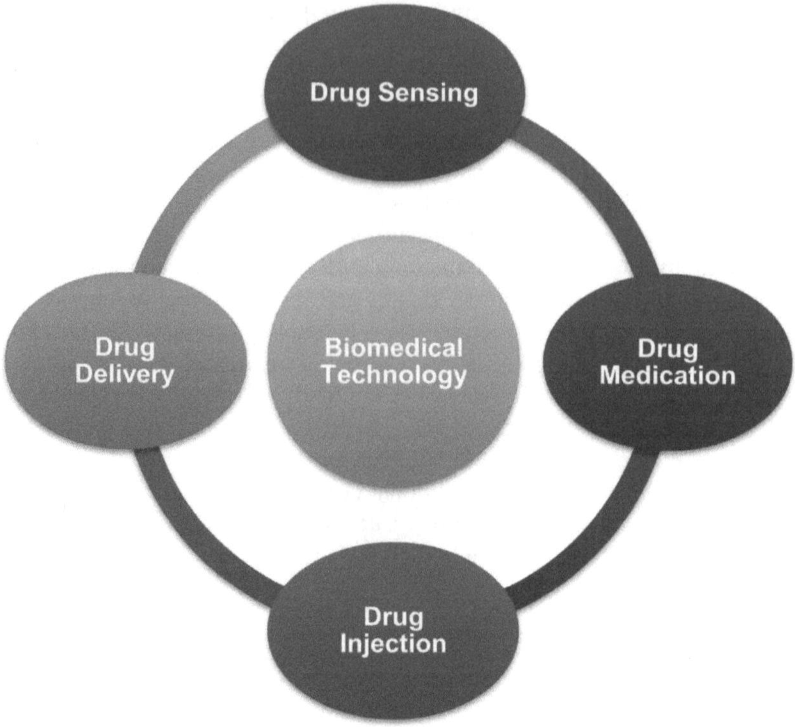

FIGURE 10.2 Advancements in biomedical nano material field. (Created by authors)

and regenerative medicine. This field has made remarkable strides in developing advanced drug delivery systems that utilize nanoscale carriers, observed as liposomes and polymeric nanoparticles, to target specific tissues, enhancing therapeutic efficacy while minimizing side effects. As shown in **Figure 10.2**, this technology is very popular worldwide and has worth millions of dollars in business.

The liposomal formulations like Doxia demonstrate improved outcomes in cancer treatment by delivering chemotherapy directly to tumor cells. In diagnostics, nano structure-based technology has revolutionized early disease detection by employing nanoparticles that bind to disease-specific biomarkers, enhancing the sensitivity of tests like lateral flow assays and improving imaging techniques using magnetic nanoparticles. These nanoparticles serve as contrast agents in modalities observed as MRI, allowing for clearer visualization of tissues and more accurate diagnoses. Additionally, the integration of nanostructure-based technology in regenerative medicine has facilitated the creation of nanofibrous scaffolds that support tissue engineering and repair, providing an optimal environment for cell growth and differentiation. This has led to promising applications in bone and cartilage regeneration, enhancing recovery from injuries [7]. Furthermore, the movement towards personalized medicine is significantly influenced by nanotechnology, as it enables targeted drug delivery tailored to individual patient profiles and the development of diagnostic tools that identify unique disease markers. It has been observed that the researchers continue to explore the integration of artificial intelligence with nanotechnology, the development of autonomous diagnostic and therapeutic systems becomes increasingly feasible, potentially transforming the way healthcare is delivered [8].

10.1.3 Challenges in Nanostructure-based Technology in Healthcare

Integrating nanostructure-based technology into healthcare presents a multitude of challenges that need to be addressed to ensure its safe and effective application. One of the foremost concerns is the safety and biocompatibility of nanomaterials. At the nanoscale, materials can exhibit different properties compared to their bulk counterparts, which may lead to unforeseen biological interactions. Toxicological studies are essential to evaluate the potential adverse effects of nanoparticles on human health and the environment [9]. Ongoing research, regulatory advancements, public education, and interdisciplinary collaboration will play vital roles in overcoming these obstacles, ultimately unlocking the full potential of nanostructure-based technology in improving patient care and outcomes. This high cost can limit accessibility, especially in resource-limited settings where healthcare budgets are constrained. Additionally, the expenses related to research and development, regulatory compliance, and the need for extensive safety testing can further inflate the costs, making it difficult for companies to produce affordable nanotechnology-based solutions. Scalability is another critical issue that researchers and manufacturers face when working with nanotechnology [10]. While many promising applications are demonstrated at the laboratory scale, translating these innovations to a commercial scale presents substantial challenges. The methods used to synthesize nanomaterials in small quantities may not be feasible for large-scale production, and achieving uniformity in size and properties is essential for consistency in clinical applications. For instance, variations in the characteristics of nanoparticles can affect their behaviour in biological systems, which can compromise the efficacy and safety of nanotechnology-based therapies and diagnostics.

10.2 KEY NANOMATERIALS IN BIOMEDICAL HEALTHCARE

Key nanomaterials in biomedical healthcare have emerged as pivotal components driving innovation in diagnostics, therapeutics, and regenerative medicine. These materials not only hold the potential for more effective treatments and diagnostic techniques but also pave the way for personalized medicine, enabling therapies tailored to individual patient needs [11]. Ultimately, the integration of key nanomaterials into clinical practice stands to transform the landscape of healthcare, improving patient outcomes and enhancing the overall quality of medical care.

10.2.1 Classification of Nanomaterials based on Properties

Nanomaterials can be broadly classified into several categories based on their origin, shape, and properties, each exhibiting unique characteristics that contribute to their application in various fields, particularly in biomedicine. One primary classification distinguishes nanomaterials into natural and engineered (or synthetic) types [12]. **Figure 10.3** shows the various properties of nanomaterials in the development of biomedical applications.

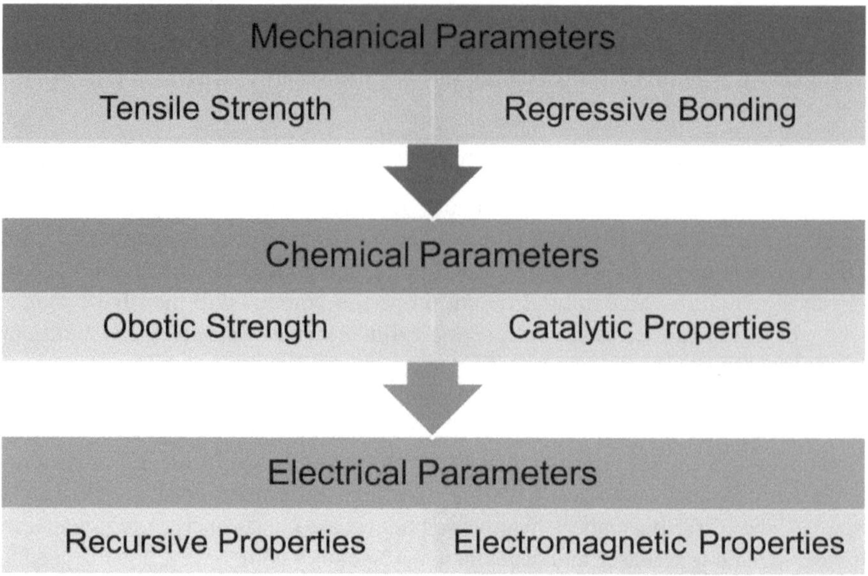

FIGURE 10.3 Various properties of nanomaterial for development of biomedical applications. (Created by authors)

Natural nanomaterials, observed as certain types of clays, proteins, and silica, are derived from biological processes and possess inherent biocompatibility, making them suitable for biomedical applications. In contrast, engineered nanomaterials are specifically designed and synthesized to achieve desired properties and functionalities. Within these categories, nanomaterials can be further classified by their shape, which includes zero-dimensional (0D) nanoparticles, one-dimensional (1D) nanowires, two-dimensional (2D) nanosheets, and three-dimensional (3D) nanostructures [13]. It may be observed that the maximum shapes are able to influence the material parameters as physical and chemical properties. For instance, 0D nanoparticles like quantum dots have unique optical properties and are used in imaging, while 1D nanowires exhibit excellent electrical conductivity and are explored in biosensing applications. Furthermore, the properties of nanomaterials, their high surface area-to-volume ratio, enhanced reactivity, and quantum effects, significantly impact their performance in various applications.

10.2.2 Metal-based Nanomaterials

The material property makes them invaluable in imaging techniques, observed as surface-enhanced Raman scattering (SERS) and in vivo fluorescence imaging, where they serve as contrast agents, enabling the early detection of diseases, including cancer. Silver nanoparticles (AgNPs) are well-known for their antimicrobial properties, making them effective agents in preventing and treating infections. Their high surface area and reactivity allow for rapid interaction with bacterial membranes, leading to the disruption of cellular functions. This characteristic is considered as particularly beneficial in wound dressings, medical devices, and coatings, where AgNPs can reduce the risk of infection and promote healing. Additionally, the incorporation of metal-based nanomaterials into drug delivery systems enhances the targeting and controlled release of therapeutic agents. By modifying the surface chemistry of these nanoparticles, they can be conjugated with targeting ligands that bind specifically to diseased cells, allowing localized treatment while minimizing side effects. **Table 10.1** shows the comparative analysis of various metal-based nanomaterials which are used in biomedical field [14].

10.2.3 Polymeric Nanomaterials

Polymeric nanomaterials have seen to be a crucial category in the realm of nanomedicine, offering remarkable versatility and functionality for a variety of biomedical applications. Their tenable many sizes and kinds of surface properties facilitate the encapsulation of a wide range of therapeutic agents, including small molecules, proteins, and nucleic acids. By adjusting the polymer's composition and structure, researchers can control the release of the encapsulated drugs, achieving sustained or targeted release to enhance therapeutic efficacy. For instance, PLGA nanoparticles can be designed to degrade over time, gradually releasing the drug at a desired rate, which is particularly beneficial for chronic diseases requiring prolonged treatment. Moreover, surface modifications with targeting ligands can enhance the specificity

TABLE 10.1
Properties and Challenges in Metal-based Nanomaterials

Reference	Metal-Nanoparticles	Properties	Applications	Challenges
[15]	Gold	Very high stability	Drug delivery, cancer therapy, design of biosensors	Cost and low biodegradability
[16]	Silver	High antimicrobial properties and conductivity	Antibacterial coat on chips	Potential environmental impact
[17]	Iron Oxide	Biocompatibility in vain system	MRI contrast agents	High oxidation, on physiological limbs
[18]	Zinc Oxide	UV-blocking	Antibacterial coating	Poor stability and toxicity to cells
[19]	Copper	Strong thermal conductivity	Nano-conductive connections	Prone to oxidation
[20]	Titanium Dioxide	High refractive index	Wastewater treatment devices	High toxicity and low environmental persistence
[21]	Platinum	Catalytically active	Cancer treatment and biochemical sensors	Challenge of poor synthesis methods

of drug delivery, ensuring that therapeutic agents are released at the site of action, tumours, or inflamed tissues, thereby reducing systemic side effects [22].

10.2.4 Lipid-based Nanomaterials

SLNs are composed of solid lipids that provide a stable matrix for drug incorporation, resulting in controlled release profiles and improved drug stability. NLCs combine solid lipids with liquid lipids, allowing for higher drug loading capacities and better release characteristics. Both SLNs and NLCs can protect sensitive drugs from degradation, ensuring that therapeutic agents remain effective until they reach their intended site of action. Lipid-based nanomaterials are also utilized in the field of vaccine development. For instance, lipid nanoparticles (LNPs) have been employed in mRNA vaccine formulations, as those used for COVID-19. These lipid nanoparticles encapsulate mRNA, facilitating its delivery into cells where it can be translated into proteins that elicit an immune response [23]. The ability of lipid-based nanomaterials to deliver nucleic acids and other biologics is revolutionizing vaccine technology and enabling rapid responses to emerging infectious diseases. In addition to drug delivery and vaccine applications, lipid-based nanomaterials have potential in imaging and diagnostic applications. They can be functionalized with imaging agents or contrast materials, enabling enhanced visualization in imaging techniques such as magnetic resonance imaging (MRI) or fluorescence imaging. This capability can significantly improve the detection of diseases, including cancer, by allowing real-time monitoring of disease progression and treatment efficacy.

10.2.5 Composite and Hybrid Nanomaterials

Composite and hybrid nanomaterials have emerged as pivotal components in the realm of nanomedicine, providing enhanced functionalities for both therapeutic and diagnostic applications. These multifunctional nanomaterials integrate the properties of different components, allowing for the simultaneous delivery of therapeutic agents and real-time monitoring of treatment responses. By combining various nanomaterials, researchers can exploit their unique characteristics to create materials that outperform their individual constituents, leading to innovative solutions in personalized medicine. One of the key advantages of composite and hybrid nanomaterials is their ability to incorporate multiple therapeutic modalities. For instance, a composite nanomaterial may combine lipids, polymers, and inorganic nanoparticles to create a multifunctional platform capable of targeted drug delivery, imaging, and photothermal therapy.

10.3 DIAGNOSTICS: ROLE OF NANOMATERIALS IN DISEASE DETECTION

Molecular diagnostics also benefit from the integration of nanomaterials, particularly in polymerase chain reaction (PCR) and next-generation sequencing (NGS) applications. Nanoparticles can be used to enhance the efficiency of these techniques by improving the binding of primers and probes, leading to faster and more accurate results. For example, magnetic nanoparticles can be utilized for the rapid isolation of nucleic acids, facilitating the detection of pathogens in infectious disease diagnostics or the identification of genetic mutations in cancer. The development of point-of-care testing devices leveraging nanomaterials has revolutionized disease detection by enabling rapid and accurate testing outside of traditional laboratory settings. These devices can provide immediate results, which are particularly valuable in emergency situations or resource-limited settings. For instance, portable devices using gold nanoparticle-based assays can quickly diagnose conditions like malaria or COVID-19, allowing for timely intervention. Despite the remarkable potential of nanomaterials in diagnostics, challenges remain regarding their standardization, scalability, and regulatory approval. Ensuring consistent quality and reproducibility of nanomaterials is crucial for their effective use in clinical diagnostics [24].

10.3.1 Nanomaterials for Enhanced Imaging Techniques

Nanomaterials have significantly advanced imaging techniques in the biomedical field, enhancing the resolution, sensitivity, and specificity of diagnostic imaging. These materials, due to their unique optical, magnetic, and electronic properties, enable the development of novel contrast agents that improve the visualization of biological structures and disease states [10, 11]. One prominent example is the use of gold nanoparticles (AuNPs) in optical-imaging modalities as surface-enhanced Raman scattering (SERS) and fluorescence imaging. AuNPs enhance the signal of fluorescent markers, allowing for the detection of low-abundance biomarkers, which are particularly valuable in cancer diagnostics. Their tenable many sizes and kind of surface properties enable functionalization with antibodies or other targeting moieties, enhancing specificity for targeted imaging of cancer cells.

10.3.2 Molecular Diagnostics and Biosensors

Nanoparticles, nanowires, and nanosheets are increasingly utilized to create highly sensitive biosensors capable of detecting biomolecules as proteins, nucleic acids, and metabolites associated with specific diseases. For instance, gold nanoparticles (AuNPs) are commonly employed in colorimetric assays; their aggregation leads to visible colour changes, allowing for rapid visual detection without sophisticated equipment. This simplicity facilitates on-site testing, making it accessible for diverse healthcare settings. Additionally, nanomaterials enhance the performance of molecular diagnostics techniques like polymerase chain reaction (PCR) and lateral flow assays. Nanoparticles can improve the binding efficiency of primers and probes, resulting in faster amplification and detection of genetic material [22].

10.3.3 Point-of-Care and Lab-on-Chip Systems

Point-of-care (POC) and lab-on-chip systems contribute a significant role in the enhancement and advancement specifically in medical diagnostics. The rapid advancement in the technology led towards development of the unique properties of nanomaterials, which have the refined sensitivity, specificity, and portability. This makes them ideal for a wide range of applications, from infectious disease detection to chronic disease monitoring. Lab-on-chip devices integrate multiple laboratory functions on a single chip, allowing for the miniaturization of complex analytical processes. By incorporating nanomaterials as nanoparticles, nanowires, and nanosheets, these devices can achieve high-throughput analysis while minimizing sample volumes and reagents [23].

10.4 THERAPEUTIC APPLICATIONS OF NANOMATERIALS

Therapeutic applications of nanomaterials have emerged as a transformative approach in medicine, offering innovative solutions for targeted drug delivery, cancer therapy, regenerative medicine, and gene therapy.

Figure 10.4 shows the growth rate of nanomaterials in the field of biomedical sector over the years. One of the most significant advantages of using nanomaterials in therapeutics is their ability to improve the bioavailability and efficacy of drugs while minimizing side effects. Nanoparticles can be engineered to encapsulate therapeutic agents, allowing for controlled release at specific sites within the body, which is particularly beneficial for treating localized diseases observed as tumours. It has been found that liposomes and polymeric nanoparticles are often used to deliver chemotherapeutic agents directly to cancer cells, enhancing drug concentration in tumour tissues while reducing systemic toxicity [22–28]. Surface modifications of these nanoparticles with ligands or antibodies enable targeted delivery to specific cell types, further increasing the therapeutic index.

10.4.1 Nanomaterials in Drug Delivery and Targeted Treatment

Nanomaterials have significantly advanced the field of drug delivery and targeted treatment, offering innovative strategies to enhance the efficacy and safety

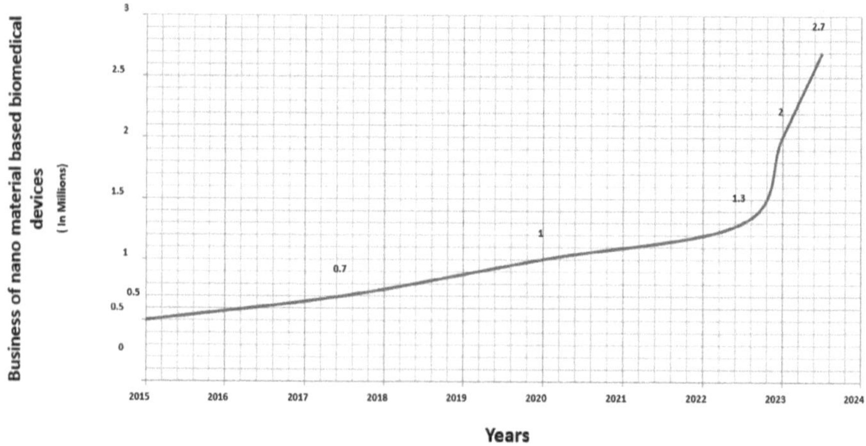

FIGURE 10.4 Exponential growth in the business of nanomaterial-based biomedical devices worldwide [17]. (CC 4.0 Attribution)

of therapeutics. Their unique properties, including high surface area, tenable size, and the ability to be functionalized with various ligands, make them ideal candidates for optimizing drug delivery systems. One of the primary advantages of using nanomaterials in drug delivery is their capacity to encapsulate therapeutic agents, thereby improving their solubility, stability, and bioavailability. For instance, liposomes and polymeric nanoparticles can be engineered to carry hydrophobic drugs, which typically have poor solubility in aqueous environments. By encapsulating these drugs within nanocarriers, their therapeutic potential can be realized, allowing for effective treatment options. Targeted drug delivery is another critical application of nanomaterials that aims to minimize systemic side effects while maximizing drug concentrations at the disease site. This is particularly valuable in cancer therapy, where conventional chemotherapeutics can cause significant harm to healthy tissues. Nanoparticles can be surface-modified with specific ligands or antibodies that recognize and bind to receptors overexpressed on cancer cells [29].

10.4.2 Cancer Treatment: Nanostructure-based Technology in Oncology

Nanostructure-based technology has revolutionized cancer treatment by offering innovative strategies that enhance therapeutic efficacy while minimizing side effects (**Figure 10.5**). One of the most significant advancements in oncology is the use of nanoparticles engineered for targeted drug delivery. These nanoparticles can carry chemotherapeutic agents and are often functionalized with ligands or antibodies that

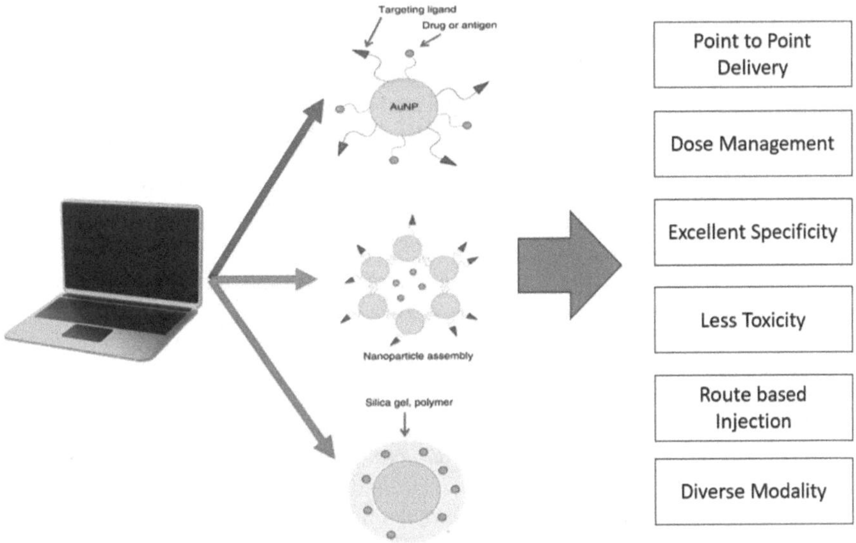

FIGURE 10.5 Treatment of oncology-based tissues using nanomaterial-based biosensors. (Created by authors)

specifically bind to receptors overexpressed on cancer cells, ensuring higher concentrations of the drug accumulate at the tumour site while sparing healthy tissues [30].

10.5 CONCLUSION

The unique properties of nanomaterials, such as their large surface area, tenable size, and the ability to mimic the extracellular matrix, make them particularly suitable for creating scaffolds that support cell growth and tissue regeneration. For instance, nanofibres derived from polymers or natural materials can be electro spun to form three-dimensional scaffolds that facilitate cell attachment, proliferation, and differentiation. These scaffolds can be designed to release growth factors in a controlled manner, further enhancing the regenerative process. Nanomaterials also enable the development of smart scaffolds that respond to specific stimuli, such as pH or temperature changes, allowing for the dynamic regulation of cellular behaviour and tissue development. The integration of nanomaterial with healthcare area leads to important ethical considerations and regulatory challenges that must be addressed to ensure its safe and effective application. The nanostructure-based technology in healthcare applications is rapidly developing and found to be promising in terms of developing the new nanomaterials and delivery systems that enhance therapeutic efficacy and reduce side effects. Innovations in personalized medicine, where treatments are tailored to individual patients based on their unique genetic and biochemical profiles, are likely to be significantly advanced by nanotechnology.

REFERENCES

[1] Mabrouk, M., Das, D. B., Salem, Z. A., & Beherei, H. H. (2021). Nanomaterials for biomedical applications: Production, characterisations, recent trends and difficulties. *Molecules*, *26*(4), 1077.

[2] Bansal, S. A., Kumar, V., Karimi, J., Singh, A. P., & Kumar, S. (2020). Role of gold nanoparticles in advanced biomedical applications. *Nanoscale Advances*, *2*(9), 3764–3787.

[3] Park, W., Shin, H., Choi, B., Rhim, W. K., Na, K., & Han, D. K. (2020). Advanced hybrid nanomaterials for biomedical applications. *Progress in Materials Science*, *114*, 100686.

[4] Modi, S., Prajapati, R., Inwati, G. K., Deepa, N., Tirth, V., Yadav, V. K., . . . & Jeon, B. H. (2021). Recent trends in fascinating applications of nanotechnology in allied health sciences. *Crystals*, *12*(1), 39.

[5] Rahman, M. M., Islam, M. R., Akash, S., Harun-Or-Rashid, M., Ray, T. K., Rahaman, M. S., . . . & Wilairatana, P. (2022). Recent advancements of nanoparticles application in cancer and neurodegenerative disorders: At a glance. *Biomedicine & Pharmacotherapy*, *153*, 113305.

[6] Anjum, S., Ishaque, S., Fatima, H., Farooq, W., Hano, C., Abbasi, B. H., & Anjum, I. (2021). Emerging applications of nanotechnology in healthcare systems: Grand challenges and perspectives. *Pharmaceuticals*, *14*(8), 707.

[7] Nienhaus, K., Wang, H., & Nienhaus, G. U. (2020). Nanoparticles for biomedical applications: Exploring and exploiting molecular interactions at the nano-bio interface. *Materials Today Advances*, *5*, 100036.

[8] Lenders, V., Koutsoumpou, X., Sargsian, A., & Manshian, B. B. (2020). Biomedical nanomaterials for immunological applications: Ongoing research and clinical trials. *Nanoscale Advances*, *2*(11), 5046–5089.

[9] Malik, S., Muhammad, K., & Waheed, Y. (2023). Emerging applications of nanotechnology in healthcare and medicine. *Molecules*, *28*(18), 6624.

[10] Aflori, M. (2021). Smart nanomaterials for biomedical applications—a review. *Nanomaterials*, *11*(2), 396.

[11] Pramanik, P. K. D., Solanki, A., Debnath, A., Nayyar, A., El-Sappagh, S., & Kwak, K. S. (2020). Advancing modern healthcare with nanotechnology, nanobiosensors, and internet of nano things: Taxonomies, applications, architecture, and challenges. *IEEE Access*, *8*, 65230–65266.

[12] Riley, P. R., & Narayan, R. J. (2021). Recent advances in carbon nanomaterials for biomedical applications: A review. *Current Opinion in Biomedical Engineering*, *17*, 100262.

[13] Egbuna, C., Parmar, V. K., Jeevanandam, J., Ezzat, S. M., Patrick-Iwuanyanwu, K. C., Adetunji, C. O., . . . & Ibeabuchi, C. G. (2021). Toxicity of nanoparticles in biomedical application: Nanotoxicology. *Journal of Toxicology*, *2021*(1), 9954443.

[14] Dolai, J., Mandal, K., & Jana, N. R. (2021). Nanoparticle size effects in biomedical applications. *ACS Applied Nano Materials*, *4*(7), 6471–6496.

[15] Ahmed, S. F., Mofijur, M., Rafa, N., Chowdhury, A. T., Chowdhury, S., Nahrin, M., . . . & Ong, H. C. (2022). Green approaches in synthesising nanomaterials for environmental nanobioremediation: Technological advancements, applications, benefits and challenges. *Environmental Research*, *204*, 111967.

[16] Abbasi, R., Shineh, G., Mobaraki, M., Doughty, S., & Tayebi, L. (2023). Structural parameters of nanoparticles affecting their toxicity for biomedical applications: A review. *Journal of Nanoparticle Research*, *25*(3), 43.

[17] Solangi, N. H., Karri, R. R., Mubarak, N. M., & Mazari, S. A. (2024). Mechanism of polymer composite-based nanomaterial for biomedical applications. *Advanced Industrial and Engineering Polymer Research*, *7*(1), 1–19.

[18] Anik, M. I., Hossain, M. K., Hossain, I., Mahfuz, A. M. U. B., Rahman, M. T., & Ahmed, I. (2021). Recent progress of magnetic nanoparticles in biomedical applications: A review. *Nano Select*, *2*(6), 1146–1186.

[19] Murali, A., Lokhande, G., Deo, K. A., Brokesh, A., & Gaharwar, A. K. (2021). Emerging 2D nanomaterials for biomedical applications. *Materials Today*, *50*, 276–302.

[20] Yaqoob, S. B., Adnan, R., Rameez Khan, R. M., & Rashid, M. (2020). Gold, silver, and palladium nanoparticles: A chemical tool for biomedical applications. *Frontiers in Chemistry*, *8*, 376.

[21] Nikolova, M. P., & Chavali, M. S. (2020). Metal oxide nanoparticles as biomedical materials. *Biomimetics*, *5*(2), 27.

[22] Nguyen, E. P., Silva, C. D. C. C., & Merkoçi, A. (2020). Recent advancement in biomedical applications on the surface of two-dimensional materials: From biosensing to tissue engineering. *Nanoscale*, *12*(37), 19043–19067.

[23] Islam, F., Shohag, S., Uddin, M. J., Islam, M. R., Nafady, M. H., Akter, A., . . . & Cavalu, S. (2022). Exploring the journey of zinc oxide nanoparticles (ZnO-NPs) toward biomedical applications. *Materials*, *15*(6), 2160.

[24] Elahi, N., & Rizwan, M. (2021). Progress and prospects of magnetic iron oxide nanoparticles in biomedical applications: A review. *Artificial Organs*, *45*(11), 1272–1299.

[25] Truong, T. T., Mondal, S., Doan, V. H. M., Tak, S., Choi, J., Oh, H., . . . & Oh, J. (2024). Precision-engineered metal and metal-oxide nanoparticles for biomedical imaging and healthcare applications. *Advances in Colloid and Interface Science*, 103263.

[26] Malode, S. J., Pandiaraj, S., Alodhayb, A., & Shetti, N. P. (2024). Carbon nanomaterials for biomedical applications: Progress and outlook. *ACS Applied Bio Materials*, *7*(2), 752–77.

[27] Solangi, N. H., Karri, R. R., Mubarak, N. M., & Mazari, S. A. (2024). Mechanism of polymer composite-based nanomaterial for biomedical applications. *Advanced Industrial and Engineering Polymer Research*, *7*(1), 1–19.

[28] Ghobashy, M. M., Alkhursani, S. A., Alqahtani, H. A., El-damhougy, T. K., & Madani, M. (2024). Gold nanoparticles in microelectronics advancements and biomedical applications. *Materials Science and Engineering: B*, *301*, 117191.

[29] Babu, P. J., Tirkey, A., Paul, A. A., Kristollari, K., Barman, J., Panda, K., . . . & Marks, R. S. (2024). Advances in nano silver-based biomaterials and their biomedical applications. *Engineer Regen*, 5(3), 326–41.

[30] Uniyal, S., Choudhary, K., Sachdev, S., & Kumar, S. (2024). Nano-bio fusion: Advancing biomedical applications and biosensing with functional nanomaterials. *Optics & Laser Technology*, *168*, 109938.

11 Development of Biodegradable Materials

Ruby Celsia Arul Selvaraj, Srinithi Shankar Ganesh, Yokenthira Ramasamy, Vishnu Jayakumar, Esther Titilayo Akinlabi, and Sunday Ayoola OKE

CONTENTS

11.1 ENVIRONMENTAL IMPACT AND LIFE CYCLE OF BIODEGRADABLE PRODUCTS

Pollutants in the environment are on the rise, and plastic is a major cause. Particles of plastic and other pollutants made of plastic are a danger to human health since they are everywhere in the environment and in the food chain. Biodegradable plastics aim to reduce their environmental impact, make the world a better place, and increase sustainability from this perspective. The objectives and priorities for producing different biodegradable polymers are identified in the complete life cycle assessment, which should be taken into account in this chapter. Biodegradable plastics, when handled correctly, can have properties similar to those of traditional plastics and also have additional benefits, such as a reduced carbon dioxide impact on the environment [1].

As an example, composting is a method. There is a growing demand for cost-effective, eco-friendly materials to reduce issues with waste management and pollution. Biodegradable plastics are the focus of this research since their manufacture, uses, sustainability, sourcing, ecological effect, and potential product uses are all important topics. Biodegradable plastics have risen to prominence as a viable option for sustainable packaging in both the academic and commercial sectors in the last several years. By considering biodegradable polymers through the lens of economic

DOI: 10.1201/9781003516064-11

profit, social responsibility, and environmental preservation, researchers were able to assess their sustainability [2].

Pollution, emission of greenhouse gases, and persistence in both aquatic and terrestrial environments are only a few of the environmental problems linked to the lifetime of petroleum-based plastics. As an alternative to plastics made from petroleum, however, many companies now provide bioplastics, a type of polymeric material that is growing in popularity. Because bioplastics are linked to major environmental issues including greenhouse gas emissions and negative land use change, it is crucial to evaluate their true environmental impact [3].

But even then, there aren't many reviews that look at the pros and cons of bioplastics for the environment side by side. In addition, further studies need to examine land use change and the bioplastics life cycle thoroughly to confirm that these new materials are environmentally friendly. These investigations will help policymakers determine if new-generation bioplastics are indeed better for the environment.

Indications that the existing system needs adjustment include the fast depletion of non-renewable resources, the carbon footprint of manufacturing and disposal, and the buildup of plastic trash in oceans and landfills. Exciting possibilities are presented by biodegradable materials as a game-changing tool for combating these environmental crises and driving the industry toward the UN's Sustainable Development Goals (SDGs). The importance of biodegradable materials in this context cannot be justified [4].

Biodegradable materials are an eco-friendly alternative to non-biodegradable ones; they are substances that can be broken down by bacteria or other biological processes. Since these materials offer less waste streams and greenhouse gas emissions, using them is consistent with SDGs 12 (Responsible Consumption and Production) and 13 (Climate Action), among others. The transition to a circular economy, where the end of a product's life cycle is really its regenerative beginning instead of its demise, is reflected in the sustainable life cycle of biodegradable materials, which includes manufacturing, transportation, and disposal [5].

Biodegradable materials are those that, when left to their own devices, can safely decompose and rejoin nature. The ability to decompose into inert substances, mostly as a result of microbes, is what sets them apart from regular plastics. They are fundamentally compatible with the environment since they are biocompatible, nontoxic, and biodegradable (they break down into water, carbon dioxide, and biomass).

Because of these characteristics, there is reason to believe that we can lessen the environmental impact of non-biodegradable trash. The term "biodegradables" is used to describe a broad class of materials that have several uses and distinct characteristics. PLA is a famous example of this. It is made from renewable resources like sugarcane or maize starch and is renowned for its versatility and composability. In a similar vein, several materials offer distinct benefits, such as being biodegradable and durable, flexible, or both [6]. These materials include starch-based bioplastics, cellulose-based biodegradables, and biodegradable polyhydroxyalkanoates (PHAs). With so many choices, we can create tailored solutions for a wide variety of businesses. Naturally, biodegradable materials are better for the environment, which is one of their most appealing features. Biodegradable polymers reduce environmental harm when disposed of properly, in contrast to traditional plastics that persist for millennia. They lessen trash's negative impact and ease the load on landfills.

Creating packaging materials that can be composted or biodegraded presents a chance to lessen the environmental effect of packaging. There may be a significant drop in trash that makes it to landfills and the ocean if these materials are able to supplant conventional plastics. One option to adopt a circular economy is by reusing, recycling, or reusing packaging materials. This offers a great chance for sustainability. Lessening both waste and resource consumption is possible with closed-loop systems [7].

Reduced material use, increased development, and lessened environmental impacts can all contribute to packaging's greener future. Encouraging responsible purchasing can be achieved through promoting sustainable alternatives and educating consumers about the environmental impact of their packaging choices. Sustainable packaging rules and protocols can be more easily established and implemented when numerous parties work together, such as businesses, governments, NGOs, and package manufacturers [8]. Biodegradable materials are those that, when left to their own devices, can safely decompose and rejoin nature. Because conventional packing materials are harmful to the environment, biodegradable alternatives have arisen. We talk about biodegradable packaging materials here [9].

The chapter focuses on the benefits they offer and the most recent developments in environmentally friendly packaging. Also, it includes case studies that show how biodegradable packaging has been successfully implemented. The many unique benefits of biodegradable packaging materials are driving their rising appeal across a variety of package uses. The primary characteristics and advantages of biodegradable packaging are discussed in this section. Because they break down naturally into inert components, biodegradable materials help lessen the long-term environmental effect of packaging waste [10]. **Figure 11.1** shows the environmental impact life cycle of biodegradable products.

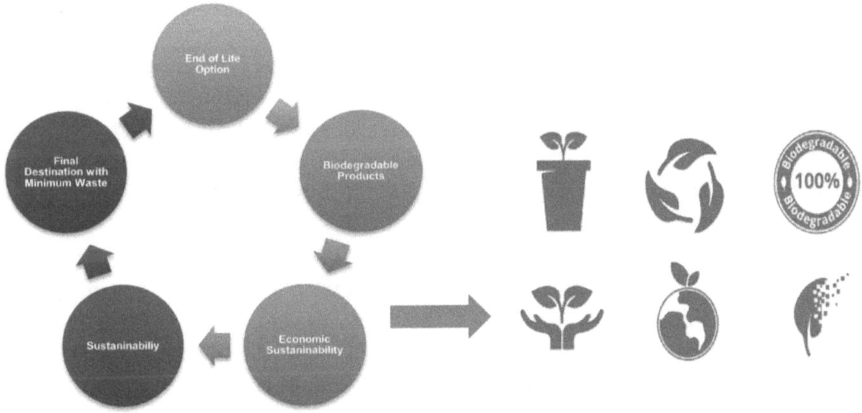

FIGURE 11.1 Environmental impact and life cycle of biodegradable products.

11.2 MATERIALS SCIENCE FOR A SUSTAINABLE FUTURE

After only a short time in the environment, biodegradable polymers decompose into their component parts, making them easy to dispose of. Cellulose and starch are two examples of the many bioresources that producers might use to make them. Other common sources of bioresources include food, animal, and agro-waste. Since bioplastics made from renewable resources tend to be less expensive than those made from microbes, producers are shifting their focus to these materials. Reusing and recycling materials, reducing emissions of greenhouse gases, and promoting biodegradation are just a few of the environmental benefits of using biodegradable polymers. Bacteria, fungus, and other microbes can decompose biodegradable polymers into water, carbon dioxide, and methane [11]. How a substance biodegrades is affected by its chemical makeup. The polymer's structural makeup, molecular weight, and degree of chemical and radiation exposure are all factors that influence biodegradation.

Biodegradable plastics have a bright future in the industry. On the other hand, we need to set up selective biowaste collection, investigate end-of-life treatment options thoroughly, and include it with global organic waste management all at once as the biodegradable plastics industry grows. One benefit of biodegradable plastics is that they can be naturally disposed of once their useful life has ended by means like composting or anaerobic digestion [12].

The use of biodegradable plastic composting has been extensively studied and recognized on a global scale. The biodegradability of a product can be evaluated in both industrial and residential composting facilities. In the absence of oxygen, anaerobic digestion processes organic waste into biogas, a mixture of carbon dioxide and methane. By converting it into heat and power, biogas can be further valorized. Another major challenge to encouraging biopolymer integration into the circular economy is the development of targeted and alternative waste management solutions. Based on their place of origin, biodegradable polymers can be categorized [13].

To better manage nonbiodegradable waste and reduce its accumulation in the environment, biodegradable materials have replaced nonbiodegradable ones in several uses, including packaging and plastic bags. Soft tissue engineering, gene therapy, and other vital human health applications all make use of biodegradable polymers.

Mechanical, thermal, viscoelastic, acoustic, surface morphological, and chemical properties are all part of this category. Using thermal gravimetric analysis, we looked at the materials' thermal characteristics. The study of dynamic mechanical properties revealed the viscoelastic properties. To learn more about the covalent bonding in the composite, Fourier-transform infrared spectroscopy was used to determine the chemical makeup of the material and the functional groups in the natural fibers that were responsible for the reaction [14].

There are now a number of commonplace uses for synthetic polymers. Because they do not break down naturally, these compounds pose a significant threat to ecosystems when they build up over time. An alternative to traditional polymers, biodegradable polymers are currently enjoying a surge in popularity. Naturally occurring microbes can break down biodegradable polymers into beneficial and environmentally favorable compounds, such as carbon dioxide and methane.

Two or more biopolymers are combined with natural fibers to modify their surfaces and improve the physical and mechanical properties of biodegradable polymers.

Plastic bags and components for automobiles and healthcare are just a few examples of the many uses of biopolymers. The benefit of using biodegradable materials is that they can be composted with organic waste or used to generate biomass once they are no longer needed. Beneficial monomers and oligomers can be produced by microbes through the recycling of biodegradable materials. These building blocks are subsequently utilized by microbes to create new goods. With the goal of preventing or minimizing these failures during manufacturing and use, forensic engineers have provided explanations for biopolymer faults [15].

Because of their hydrophilic nature and, in some instances, poor mechanical properties, biodegradable polymers derived from renewable resources degrade rapidly; this is especially an issue in damp conditions. Although they have significant drawbacks, biodegradable polymers—which are made of various plant components—do have some benefits. Because of their potential medicinal applications and biodegradability, bio polyesters have lately acquired popularity [16]. Much emphasis on the particular elements, like processing conditions, biocompatibility, biodegradation technologies, and potential applications in agro-chemistry, medicine, and environmental protection, has received a significant interest. Such sophisticated biodegradable polymers continue to have very low levels of biosafety, as well as very low levels of nano safety in their composites. We center this new viewpoint on anticipating, assessing, and highlighting potential problems related to the use of innovative polymers. **Figure 11.2** demonstrates the sustainability of biodegradable polymers.

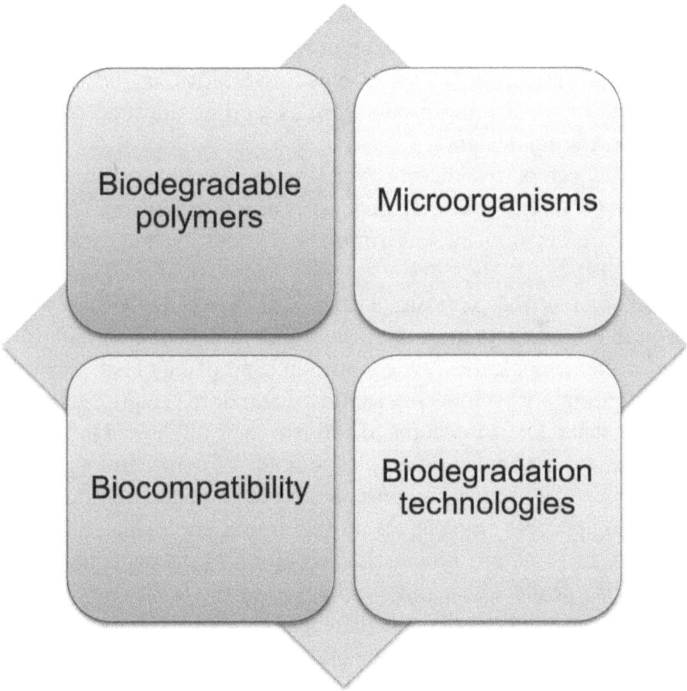

FIGURE 11.2 Sustainability of biodegradable polymers.

11.3 FROM LABORATORY TO MARKET: BIODEGRADABLE MATERIAL INNOVATIONS

Whether it's a pure polymer, a blended product, or a composite, green polymers are biodegradable and made from sustainable resources. Their qualities have attracted a lot of interest because of their possible usage as alternatives to materials made from petrochemicals. The use of biopolymers has several possible advantages, such as the creation of new materials, less reliance on fossil fuels, lower emissions of carbon dioxide, full biodegradability, less need to dispose of these materials in landfills, and the utilization of agricultural resources to create bio/green materials. When making products, it's best to first learn more about these components, including what they are, how they work, and what kinds of natural fibers they interact with [17].

One more thing we can do to protect our communities' and the planet's environments is to cut down on packaging trash. Just in the United Kingdom in 2021, 2.5 million metric tons of unwanted plastic packaging was generated. The most common way we dispose of this plastic waste is by burning it, which releases harmful pollutants into the air or into landfills in the United Kingdom or elsewhere.

Disposing of biodegradable packaging materials, which naturally decompose due to microbial action and return to the natural environment as compost, doesn't create garbage that would otherwise end up in a landfill or worsen environmental contamination. You can add biodegradable materials to your home garden trash or, in certain situations, compost them in an industrial setting. Industrially composted materials typically decompose more quickly [18].

Any substance that makes sustainability claims has a big benefit because it is biodegradable, meaning that it breaks down naturally without being complicated or bad for the environment. Here, we'll look at biodegradability, including its advantages and disadvantages for packaging production, as well as the state of the market for biodegradable packaging design.

Biodegradability refers to something's ability to dissolve and break down organically as a result of fungi, bacteria, and other microorganisms. A biodegradable substance will integrate into the environment without causing any damage to the ecosystem at all [19].

A surprising fact is that certain plastics can break down into smaller parts. Typically, natural by-products like cellulose, starch, algae, and certain proteins serve as the source of these bioplastics. One common kind of bioplastic is PLA, which is created by fermenting cornstarch. International standards require the production of bioplastics under strict control systems to confirm their biodegradability. They are an excellent replacement for conventional plastic made of petroleum.

Plastic no longer truly reflects a sense of luxury in packaging design, especially when the unboxing process emphasizes more durable, ecological, and natural materials. However, a shift toward bioplastics is beginning to occur in the market for hygienic, single-use products, such as packaging in the health and wellness sector. Even though bioplastic may cost more than regular plastic, it's still a cost-effective option for consumer goods like food items [20].

Customers can choose from a variety of eco-friendly and fashionable options when purchasing apparel made from biodegradable materials, such as dresses, tops, and pants. Biodegradable materials offer environmentally beneficial substitutes for conventional shoe materials in the footwear manufacturing process. The environmental effect of frequently used accessories like bags, belts, and hats can be minimized by using biodegradable materials for these goods. Fashion and textile items can match consumer demand for sustainability while also drastically reducing their ecological footprint by utilizing biodegradable fabrics [21].

The medical industry widely uses plastic materials, which have serious environmental effects. Recent developments in biodegradable medicinal materials, however, have the power to completely transform the sector. In this section, we will learn about the cutting-edge biodegradable materials used in packaging, implants, and medical devices. We will examine their rates of deterioration, biocompatibility, and potential to improve patient outcomes while lowering environmental harm [22].

The conventional method of producing cement results in significant carbon emissions and worsens the state of the environment. Scientists and engineers are still making significant strides in the development of biodegradable cement substitutes to lessen the sector's ecological impact. Innovative binders used in biodegradable cement have the ability to decompose over time, reducing their long-term environmental impact. To lessen reliance on non-renewable resources, these binders frequently include organic and waste materials, such as industrial waste or agricultural by-products. Scientific studies have shown that biodegradable cement can match the compressive strength of regular cement, which means it could be a viable alternative for building projects. More than that, it leaves less of a carbon footprint thanks to decreased emissions of greenhouse gases during manufacturing [23]. **Figure 11.3** shows some of the key concepts of biodegradable material innovations.

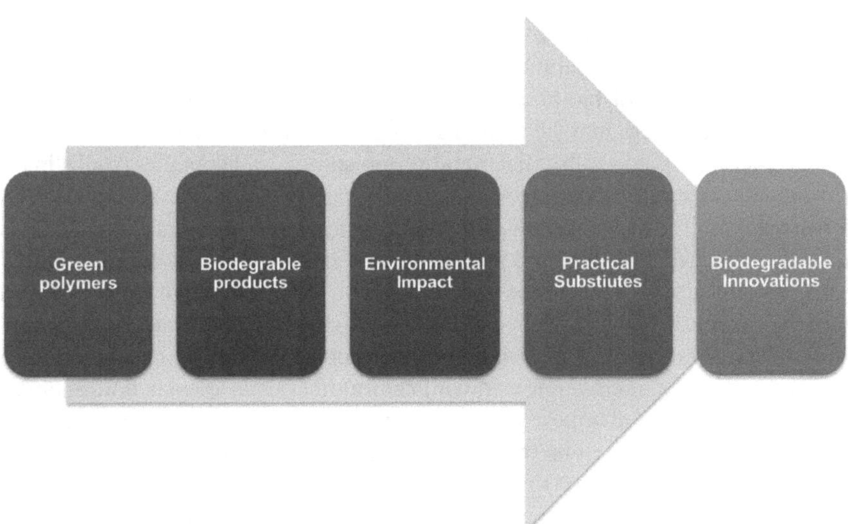

FIGURE 11.3 Biodegradable material innovations: From laboratory to market.

11.4 CHALLENGES AND OPPORTUNITIES IN BIODEGRADABLE MATERIAL ENGINEERING

Many people are interested in bioplastics, natural materials that are biodegradable and/or bio-based because of the positive impact they can have on the environment. Bioplastics make up less than 1 percent of the world's total plastic output each year, despite their extensive application in many different industries, including packaging, food service, agriculture, and transportation. Biodegradability is an often-overlooked quality of a substance that can be put to use when its useful life has ended, provided certain circumstances, a certain disposal environment, and a certain time have passed [24]. This is why biodegradable plastics are being considered as a possible answer to the trash issue. In situations where there needs to be an economical way to dispose of the product once it has fulfilled its function, such as with food packaging, agricultural products, or medical supplies, they should be chosen. In terms of processing, characteristics, and waste management alternatives, the researchers [25] emphasized the potential benefits and upcoming difficulties associated with biodegradable plastics.

Naturally, the best option for achieving sustainable development goals and minimizing environmental effects is to use biodegradable plastics made of renewable resources. Natural processes regenerate natural resources relatively quickly, ensuring that human usage does not deplete their quantity. These comprise biomass, wave, tidal, geothermal, solar, and wind energy. We essentially derive natural resources, including fossil fuels, from deceased species. The problem lies in the fact that the production of fossil fuels spans millions of years, while human use happens over centuries [26]. The raw materials used, the finished product's chemical makeup and structure, the environment in which the product is intended to biodegrade, and other factors all affect how biodegradable plastics are not only on the unprocessed materials that went into making it. Certain bio-based plastics may or may not biodegrade depending on the unique polymer structure of the material. The same processing equipment can be used for both fossil-based biodegradable plastics and bio-based non-biodegradable polymers, making the processes comparable to those of conventional plastics. This also applies to the manufacturing of bio-based, biodegradable polymers, albeit because of their renewable source, there may be some factors that need to be considered [27]. These elements consist of batch-to-batch variability, moisture, flow anomalies (wall slippage), and heat deterioration. Because bio-based biodegradable plastics have a tendency to be hygroscopic, moisture can lead to a number of issues, including an uncontrollably low viscosity, unwanted foaming, and an acceleration of hydrolysis or heat deterioration. As a result, pre-drying is most necessary, along with the proper drying temperature and duration. Chemical blowing agents and other additions that separate water shouldn't be used. The flowability of materials like thermoplastic starch might be affected if they are too dry. Polymers reinforced with natural fibers may display flow anomalies, namely due to the fact that these fibers can have a wide range of geometries and characteristics and their application could lead to wall sliding [28].

Processing bio-based biodegradable polymers with special caution is necessary due to their susceptibility to heat breakdown. Because of the importance of minimizing their exposure to high temperatures, plasticizing units with short residence times are essential for their processing. You can collect organic waste in compostable trash bags and then use them as regular rubbish bags. In addition to increasing the amount of organic waste collected and decreasing the need for landfill space, they can enhance the composting process and the quality of compost. These bags, made mostly of biodegradable materials, represent a sizable market for biodegradable polymers because of their widespread use and high volume of sales. By being able to be plowed back into the field after usage, biodegradable mulch film presents a potential to decrease labor and waste expenses. The biodegradable materials are also used in service packaging for the sale of snack items or meal catering for large groups [29].

Biodegradable trash, particularly polymers, can be turned into useful soil amendment products through composting. Composted organic matter is the result of a regulated aerobic decomposition process involving a diverse community of microbes in a wet environment. You can enrich soil with compost that is rich in nutrients and carbon by using composting facilities or other aerobic waste management methods. However, the European Union is lacking in composting infrastructure. Unfortunately, not all composting sites are equipped to handle compostable packaging; many only handle garden debris. We need major technology advancements, especially in the pre-processing phase, to guarantee a compostable packaging method that works. Separating biodegradable and compostable plastics from regular plastics using near-infrared detection technology is possible but costly to execute [30]. **Figure 11.4** demonstrates the challenges and opportunities in biodegradable material engineering.

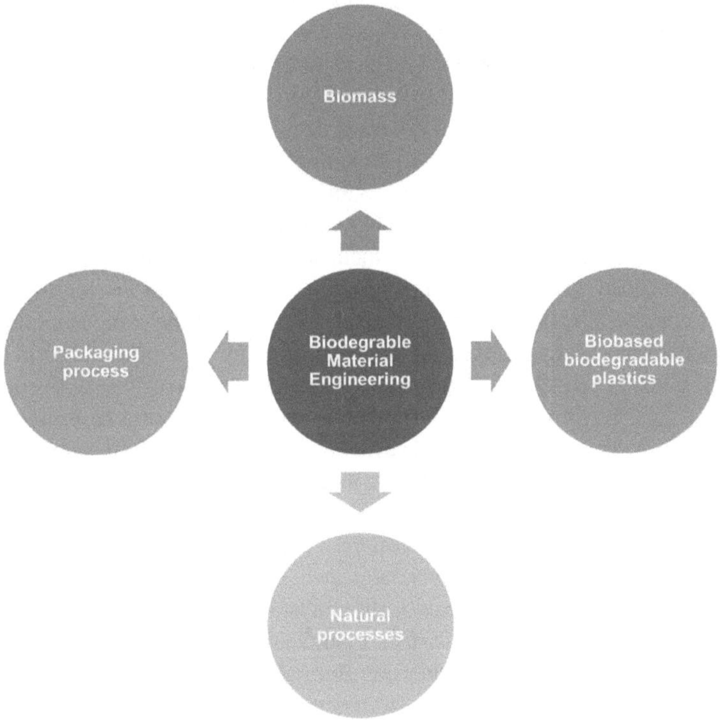

FIGURE 11.4 Challenges and opportunities in biodegradable material engineering.

11.5 BIODEGRADABLE COMPOSITES: TRENDS AND FUTURE DIRECTIONS

Most polymer and composite researchers and manufacturers worldwide are paying more and more attention to biodegradable materials because they fit in nicely with the global sustainable development goal of drastically reducing non-recyclable plastic wastes. In our daily lives, we use non-biodegradable plastics that are not recyclable. As a result, plastic waste has become more commonplace over time, accumulating in landfills and the ocean, posing a serious threat to the ecosystem and ecology everywhere in the world. Consequently, there is a need to employ biodegradable materials in a variety of domains and sectors to get a more environmentally friendly approach to product manufacturing processes and design competencies [31].

At least two components, preferably both, must be derived from biodegradable sources to construct biodegradable composites. The bulk of biodegradable composites are reinforced using fillers, which are a minority phase. Synthetic polymers called biopolymers can be made either by living creatures or by intentionally combining natural components. Bio-based composite materials are being increasingly used as an alternative to conventional, non-renewable synthetic fibers in a variety of end-use applications, such as carbon-reinforced composites and glass, due to rising sustainability and environmental concerns [32].

However, there are certain drawbacks to biocomposite materials. Some of their issues include a lack of resistance to water (hydrophilicity); incompatibility with fibers and matrix; combustibility; lack of thermal stability; subpar electrical properties; difficulty in extraction, processing, surface modification, manufacturing, and characterization; and extremely anisotropic properties. Characteristics, sustainable production, long-term durability, reliability, and serviceability in biocomposites have been the focus of a plethora of recent research efforts, with an eye toward embracing a circular economy [33].

Natural fibers have many advantages, including being inexpensive, abundant, biodegradable, low-density, renewable, and environmentally safe. Compared to aramid, glass, and carbon fibers, plant fibers are noticeably lighter. Plant fibers are beneficial to both the economy and the environment due to their biodegradability and good performance at a low cost. Natural fiber-reinforced composites' characteristics are highly dependent on the fiber content. The properties and surface properties of the composites are heavily affected by the processing parameters. Biocomposites are still mostly used in the automobile and decking industries, nevertheless. Compared to non-renewable composites, green composites are sustainable, biodegradable, and offer a lot of promise [34].

Concerns about the environment and sustainability have led to the development of bio-based composite materials as an alternative to carbon-reinforced composites and glass, two examples of conventional, non-renewable synthetic fibers used in a variety of end-use applications. However, there are several drawbacks to biocomposite materials. Some of their issues include a lack of resistance to water (hydrophilicity), incompatibility with fibers and matrix, combustibility, lack of thermal stability, subpar electrical properties, difficulty in extraction, processing, surface modification, manufacturing, and characterization, and extremely anisotropic properties. Embracing a circular economy, researchers have recently undertaken a plethora of studies to tackle problems with biocomposites' features, sustainable production, long-term durability, reliability, and serviceability [35]. As people become more conscious of the need to address environmental issues and promote sustainability, they are actively seeking for bio-based composite materials to replace conventional, non-renewable synthetic fibers in products like glass and carbon-reinforced composites. Nevertheless, biocomposite materials aren't a perfect substitute due to a few drawbacks. Hydrophilicity, a lack of resistance to moisture, supply chain issues, flammability, poor electrical properties, extraction, processing, surface modification, machining, manufacturing and characterization problems, and highly anisotropic properties are all of these things and more [36].

Characteristics, sustainability, reliability, long-term durability, and sustainable manufacture (via a circular economy in biocomposites) have all been the focus of recent, substantial research. Bioproducts have grown in significance from a commercial perspective throughout the years. Our investigation has led us to chemical processes that may dehydrate ethanol to create "green" ethylene, which in turn can be used to make polyvinyl chloride, "green" polyethylene, and other plastics. The creation of heat-resistant PLA is only one example of how innovation in technology has enhanced the material properties of bio-based polymers, leading to their increased versatility. Plant optimization is gradually producing bio-fibers that are stable [37].

Packaging, biomedical goods, textiles, agriculture, and building are just a few areas that could benefit from these biodegradable biopolymers and biocomposites' eco-friendly alternatives. The area of biofunctional materials encompasses any materials that are either biospecific or biosimulation-based. Function design is the first step in producing biofunctional materials. To build the desired polymer structure, the functionality design must first determine which polymer synthesis, polymer reaction, and polymer modification techniques are most suited to the task at hand [38]. This structure must embody the desired functionality and material property. **Figure 11.5** shows the trends and future directions of biodegradable composites.

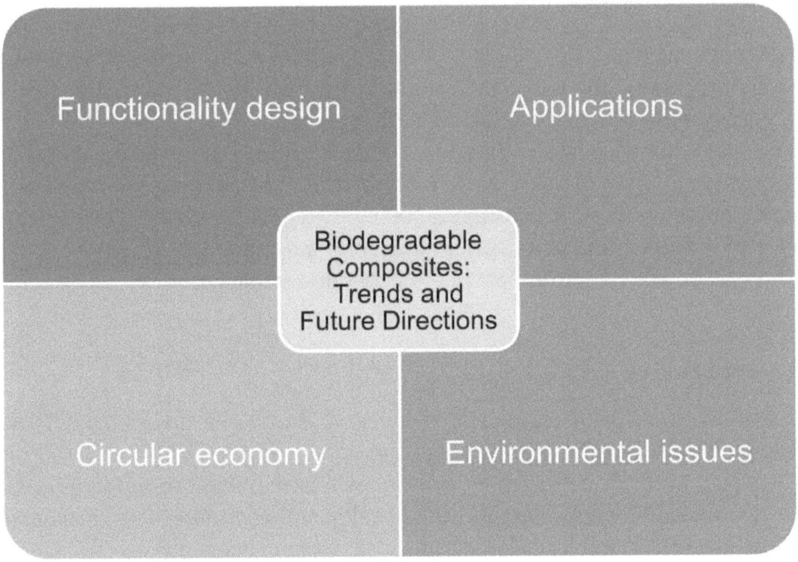

FIGURE 11.5 Biodegradable composites: trends and future directions.

11.6 ENVIRONMENTAL AND ECONOMIC IMPACTS

Sustainability in the environment and economic prosperity are two areas that stand to benefit greatly from the creation and use of biodegradable materials. Because of their indestructibility, conventional plastics mostly made from petroleum have become a major environmental problem. Serious contamination has resulted from this problem, which has an impact on both marine and terrestrial ecosystems and adds to emissions of greenhouse gases during manufacturing and disposal. By organically decomposing through microbial action, biodegradable materials provide a viable option that lessens the buildup of persistent waste in the environment [39].

Materials that break down naturally have a significant positive impact on the environment. Their biodegradability reduces trash in landfills, trash in the ocean, and pollution in both soil and water. Biodegradable materials can lessen our reliance on fossil fuels and our carbon footprints when used in conjunction with renewable resources like starch, cellulose, and PLA. Biodegradable materials improve soil health in agricultural applications like mulch films by breaking down in the field, doing away with the need for time-consuming removal and disposal [40].

The transition to biodegradable materials brings both possibilities and threats to the economy. Because biodegradable alternatives need specialized raw materials and procedures, their initial production cost is typically greater than that of standard plastics. But the market for biodegradable materials has been expanding because of rising customer awareness of the need for sustainable products. Further bolstering their economic viability, governments and organizations throughout the world are promoting their use through subsidies and legislation that aim to reduce plastic waste [41].

Although there are many benefits to using biodegradable materials, there are also certain constraints to their general acceptance. Because biodegradable material production uses maize and sugarcane, which are agricultural resources, there may be conflicts with food supply chains and worries about land usage. Furthermore, not everyone has access to the exact environmental conditions needed for these materials to degrade, such as industrial composting facilities. Optimizing material design, improving processing methods, and establishing strong waste management systems are all necessary to tackle these difficulties.

Their manufacturing, utilization, and disposal must be carefully considered if their potential to revolutionize waste management and decrease pollution is to be fully realized. A sustainable and circular economy can be realized only via the widespread use of biodegradable materials in traditional manufacturing processes [42]. **Figure 11.6** show the environmental and economic impacts.

11.7 APPLICATIONS OF BIODEGRADABLE MATERIALS

Because of their capacity to organically disintegrate and lessen environmental damage, biodegradable materials have varied uses throughout sectors. Their versatility meets the worldwide need for eco-friendly substitutes for traditional materials in a variety of contexts, including packaging, farming, healthcare, and more. The packaging sector is home to one of the most important uses. Sustainable alternatives to single-use products such as bags, food containers, cutlery, and straws are made possible via the

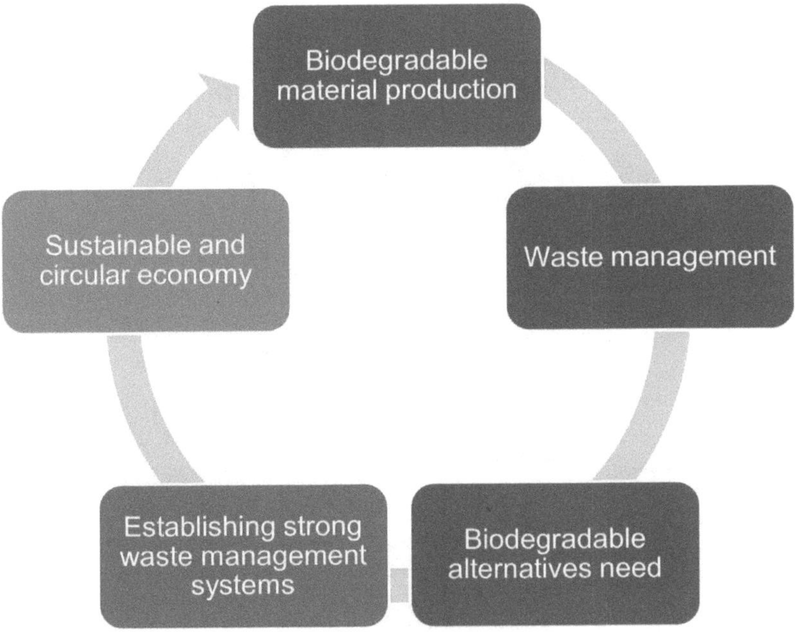

FIGURE 11.6 Environmental and economic impacts.

use of biodegradable films and plastics. These materials are useful in the fight against plastic pollution, particularly in situations where recycling or reusing is not an option. One example is the widespread use of films and starch blends based on PLA in food packaging. These materials are both durable and environment-friendly [43].

Products including mulch films, seed coatings, and plant pots are made from biodegradable materials in the agricultural industry. Because they break down in the soil and add organic matter, these materials don't need to be removed or disposed of. This helps agricultural areas retain more soil over time while cutting down on labor expenses and plastic residue. Biodegradable materials have also been very useful in medicine. Implants, medication delivery systems, and surgical sutures are all made using them. Once they've served their job, they naturally break down in the body. Bioresorbable stents and sutures, made of polylactic-co-glycolic acid and polyglycolic acid for instance, can be removed without further surgical procedures [44].

There has been significant progress in the consumer products sector toward using biodegradable materials. To lessen the ecological footprint of personal hygiene goods, biodegradable polymers are being utilized in the development of items like disposable nappies, sanitary products, and wipes. Similarly, to combat the increasing issue of electronic waste, researchers in the electronics industry are investigating the possibility of using biodegradable components and housings. Clothing and home furnishings made from biodegradable fibers sourced from plants such as bamboo, hemp, and cellulose. In addition to being environmentally beneficial, these materials support circular fashion by making composting possible when they reach the end of their useful life.

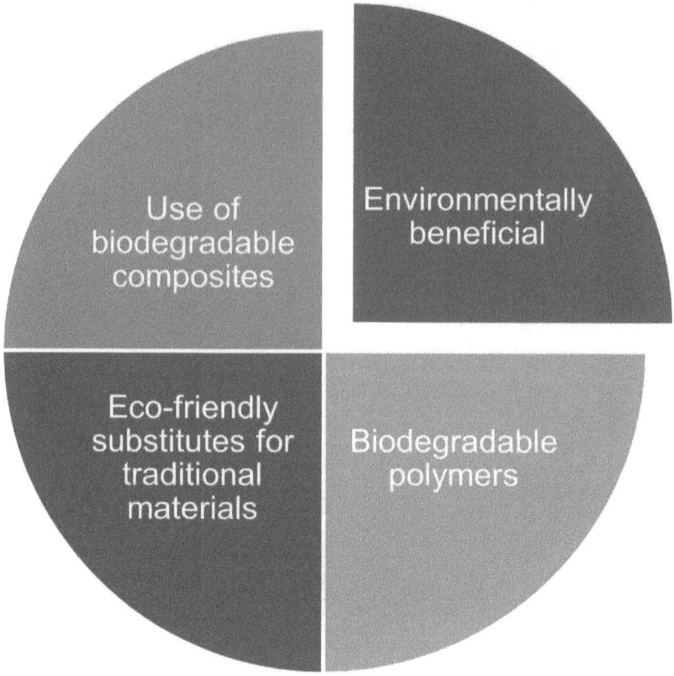

FIGURE 11.7 Applications of biodegradable materials.

Finally, the building and automobile industries are seeing a rise in the use of biodegradable composites. Insulation panels and concrete reinforcements are two examples of building products that include them. These materials provide sustainability without sacrificing performance. The usage of biodegradable polymers in vehicle interior components has reduced the industry's need on conventional plastics without sacrificing durability or attractiveness [45]. **Figure 11.7** illustrates the applications of biodegradable materials.

11.8 MATERIAL DESIGN AND DEVELOPMENT

Biodegradable material development and design calls for a multidisciplinary strategy that brings together chemical, environmental, and material engineering concepts. The main goal is to design materials that can perform their intended functions and then break down naturally into harmless substances. Finding this sweet spot requires thinking about the material's composition, structural qualities, and effect on the surroundings. Choosing the right raw materials is the first step in designing biodegradable products. Natural polymers (such as starch, cellulose, and chitosan) and manufactured biodegradable polymers (such as PLA, polycaprolactone, and polybutylene succinate) are the two main categories into which these fall. Synthetic polymers provide adjustable features including strength, thermal stability, and flexibility, whereas natural polymers are preferred for their inherent biodegradability and renewability [46].

It is common practice to use blending and compounding procedures to improve performance. For instance, PLA may be enhanced for use in films and containers by combining it with plasticizers such as glycerol or other biopolymers, which increase its toughness and flexibility. Nano clays and bioactive compounds are only a couple of the additions and fillers that can improve mechanical qualities, heat resistance, and antibacterial activity. Engineered degradation behavior that matches the application is another aspect of material development. For things to be considered biodegradable, they must be able to break down in particular settings, such as composting facilities, residential composting, or the natural environments of water and soil. Polymer chain length, crystallinity, and hydrophilicity are three variables that may be controlled to accomplish this. For instance, a polymer's disintegration rate is accelerated when the number of its amorphous regions increases, making it more vulnerable to enzymatic attack [47–49].

Making sure the material can be used with the current production methods is another important part of the design process. To enable broad adoption without substantial investment in new infrastructure, biodegradable materials should be processable using traditional processes such as injection molding, extrusion, or thermoforming. When it comes to directing material design, life cycle analysis is crucial. It is important to consider the environmental effect of obtaining, processing, using, and disposing of raw materials. It is important that the biodegradable material has a smaller environmental impact than more conventional options at every stage of its lifespan [50–52].

Finding a content medium between biodegradability and durability, keeping prices in check, and guaranteeing property uniformity are all obstacles in the way of material development. These problems motivate continuous study in fields including additive technology, sophisticated compounding methods, and biopolymer synthesis. In presumption, a comprehensive strategy taking into account practicality, longevity, and financial viability is necessary for the creation of biodegradable materials. These materials are getting smarter all the time thanks to innovation, which means they can be used for more and more things. **Figure 11.8** describes the materials design

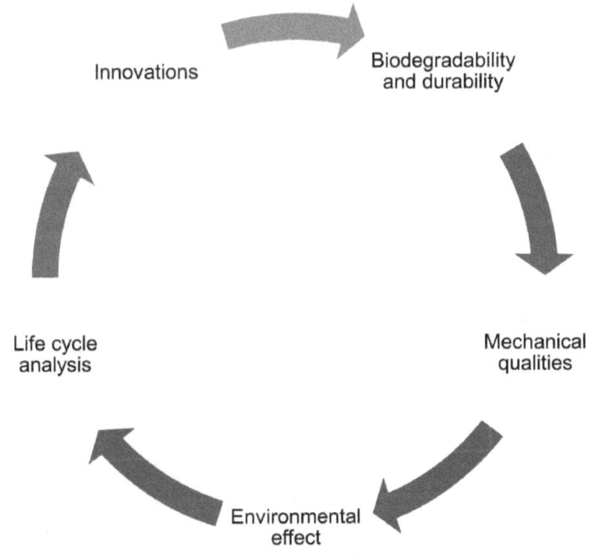

FIGURE 11.8 Materials design and development of biodegradable materials.

TABLE 11.1
Aspects and Details of Materials Design and Development of Biodegradable Materials

Aspects	Facts
Raw Material Selection	• Picking out raw materials, proteins, starch, cellulose, and chitosan are examples of natural polymers. • Man-made polymers, such as polybutylene succinate (PBS), polycaprolactone (PCL), and polylactic acid (PLA).
Material Properties	• Characteristics of materials strength, pliability, and hardness are mechanical qualities. • Stability on a thermal scale: heat resistance. • Capability to break down in particular environments; this is known as biodegradability.
Additives and Fillers	• Plasticizers, such as sorbitol and glycerol, increase the material's pliability. • Examples of nanofillers include silica and nanoclays, both of which improve mechanical and thermal characteristics. • Antimicrobial properties are imparted by bioactive agents.
Blending and Compounding	• To get the right characteristics, mix natural and synthetic polymers. • For instance, a combination of PLA and PCL can increase both the material's flexibility and breakdown rate.
Degradation	• Degradation rate may be controlled by adjusting the crystallinity and length of the polymer chains. • Efficiently biodegrade in natural settings by adjusting hydrophilicity.
Processing Techniques	• Standard production procedures such as injection molding, extrusion, thermoforming, and blow molding are compatible with processing techniques.
Environmental Considerations	• Decompose in certain settings, such as composting facilities, backyard composters, soil, or water. • Reduced environmental impact by utilizing sustainable and renewable resources.
Life Cycle Analysis	• Analyze the effects at each stage of a product's life cycle, from manufacture to use to eventual disposal. • Make sure it leaves less of an environmental impact than regular plastics.
Challenges	• One of the challenges is finding a balance between biodegradability and durability. • Making the product more economically viable by cutting production costs. • Making sure that attributes are consistent from one batch to the next.
Innovations	• Improved bio-based composites developed. • Create new biopolymers with tailorable degrading characteristics. • Application of catalysts derived from microbes or enzymes for specific degradation.

and development of biodegradable materials. **Table 11.1** displays the aspects and details of materials design and development of biodegradable materials.

11.9 CONCLUSION

- The transition to biodegradable items is a major step forward in reducing environmental impact and advancing sustainable practices. Since these items naturally break down through the action of microorganisms, they serve as a good substitute for conventional plastics and other non-biodegradable materials that cause pollution and environmental deterioration.

- To construct a future that is sustainable, materials science must be a driving force behind technologies that minimize environmental impact, boost efficiency, and reduce waste. If we can create better materials, we can revolutionize several sectors, such as the energy, transportation, building, and healthcare industries.
- Significant progress in the field of biodegradable materials research and development has made it possible to create substitutes that function as well as or better than conventional plastics. Applications for these advances are diverse and include consumer items, packaging, agriculture, and medical devices. Increasing customer demand for ecologically friendly products and regulatory challenges are driving the trend toward biodegradable choices. In summary, advances in biodegradable materials have enormous potential to lessen their negative effects on the environment and advance the circular economy.
- A significant advancement in materials research, biodegradable composites offer sustainable alternatives to traditional composites while simultaneously tackling the pressing issue of environmental deterioration. Current trends and projected developments in this area suggest that these materials may have far-reaching effects on many different types of sectors, all while contributing to a greener tomorrow.
- To sum up, sustainable material science is about to have biodegradable composites as a pillar. The persistent patterns of creativity, varied implementation, and emphasis on sustainability establish a robust groundwork for forthcoming progress. Through tackling issues pertaining to efficiency, affordability, and expandability, as well as utilizing regulatory backing, research, and circular economy concepts, the domain of biodegradable composites will persistently progress and make a substantial contribution to a sustainable and eco-friendly future.

REFERENCES

1. Park, D., Lee, H., & Won, W. (2024). Unveiling the environmental gains of biodegradable plastics in the waste treatment phase: A cradle-to-crave life cycle assessment. *Chemical Engineering Journal*, 487, 150540.
2. Hao, L., Ren, S., Li, J., Wang, X., Li, L., & Hao, X. (2024). Feasibility of biodegradable material polylactic acid as a substitute for polypropylene for disposable medical masks production verified by life cycle assessment. *Journal of Cleaner Production*, 141492.
3. de Sadeleer, I., & Woodhouse, A. (2024). Environmental impact of biodegradable and non-biodegradable agricultural mulch film: A case study for Nordic conditions. *The International Journal of Life Cycle Assessment*, 29(2), 275–90.
4. Subramani, R., Mustafa, M. A., Ghadir, G. K., Al-Tmimi, H. M., Alani, Z. K., Rusho, M. A., . . . & Kumar, A. P. (2024). Exploring the use of biodegradable polymer materials in sustainable 3D printing. *Applied Chemical Engineering*, 3870.
5. Riaz, F., Rasul, I., Azeem, F., Zubair, M., Nadeem, H., Imran, M., . . . & Siddique, M. H. (2024). Environmental impact, health implications, and life cycle assessment of bionanocomposites. In *Advances in Bionanocomposites* (pp. 387–406). Elsevier.
6. Thrän, J., Garcia-Garcia, G., Parra-López, C., Ufarte, A., García-García, C., Parra, S., & Sayadi-Gmada, S. (2024). Environmental and economic assessment of biodegradable and compostable alternatives for plastic materials in greenhouses. *Waste Management*, 175, 92–100.

7. Sakib, M. N., Kabir, G., & Ali, S. M. (2024). A life cycle analysis approach to evaluate sustainable strategies in the furniture manufacturing industry. *Science of the Total Environment*, 907, 167611.
8. Saravanan, A., Thamarai, P., Deivayanai, V. C., Karishma, S., Shaji, A., & Yaashikaa, P. R. (2024). Current strategies on bioremediation of personal care products and detergents: Sustainability and life cycle assessment. *Chemosphere*, 354, 141698.
9. Islam, S., Bhat, G., & Mani, S. (2024). Life cycle assessment of thermal insulation materials produced from waste textiles. *Journal of Material Cycles and Waste Management*, 1–15.
10. Zubair, M. U., Ali, M., Khan, M. A., Khan, A., Hassan, M. U., & Tanoli, W. A. (2024). BIM-and GIS-based life-cycle-assessment framework for enhancing eco efficiency and sustainability in the construction sector. *Buildings*, 14(2), 360.
11. Biswal, B. K., Zhang, B., Tran, P. T. M., Zhang, J., & Balasubramanian, R. (2024). Recycling of spent lithium-ion batteries for a sustainable future: Recent advancements. *Chemical Society Reviews*, 53, 5552–92.
12. Karatepe, S., Gözde, M. E. R. T., Karaköse, S., & Akin, F. İ. (2024). Circular economy for a sustainable future: Re-evaluating resources. *Twist*, 19(2), 331–9.
13. GP, J. J. (2024). Exploring titanium dioxide nanotubes: Pioneering advanced applications in efficient water splitting and sustainable hydrogen generation. *International Journal for Multidimensional Research Perspectives*, 2(5), 24–36.
14. Benziane, S. (2024). Innovating prosperity: Intelligent approaches and economic paradigms for sustainable futures. In *Intelligent Methods and Alternative Economic Models for Sustainability* (pp. 194–241). IGI Global.
15. Naik, B., Mishra, R., Kumar, V., Mishra, S., Gupta, U., Rustagi, S., & Rizwanuddin, S. (2024). Micro-algae: Revolutionizing food production for a healthy and sustainable future. *Journal of Agriculture and Food Research*, 15, 100939.
16. Binhazzaa, Z. (2024). *Hydrocarbons Are the Backbone of Sustainable Civilization*. Preprints 2024, 2024030780. https://doi.org/10.20944/preprints202403.0780.v1.
17. Vienken, J., & Boccato, C. (2024). Do medical devices contribute to sustainability? The role of innovative polymers and device design. *The International Journal of Artificial Organs*, 47(4), 240–50.
18. Abatan, A., Lottu, O. A., Ugwuanyi, E. D., Jacks, B. S., Sodiya, E. O., Daraojimba, A. I., & Obaigbena, A. (2024). Sustainable packaging innovations and their impact on HSE practices in the FMCG industry. *Magna Scientia Advanced Research and Reviews*, 10(1), 379–91.
19. Pandit, S., Sharma, P., Prakash, A., Lal, B., Bhuyan, R., Ahmad, I., & Kuila, A. (2024). A comprehensive review on technical lignin, lignin hydrogels, properties, preparation, applications & challenges in lab to market transition. *Industrial Crops and Products*, 211, 118262.
20. Tenuta, L., Testa, S., Antinarelli Freitas, F., & Cappellieri, A. (2024). Sustainable materials for jewelry: Scenarios from a design perspective. *Sustainability*, 16(3), 1309.
21. Erisen, D. E., & Uludag, K. (2024). Estimating biosafety of biodegradable biomedical materials from in vitro ion tolerance parameters and toxicity of nanomaterials in Brain. In *Transformative Approaches to Patient Literacy and Healthcare Innovation* (pp. 201–21). IGI Global.
22. Singh, P., Pandey, V. K., Singh, R., Singh, K., Dash, K. K., & Malik, S. (2024). Unveiling the potential of starch-blended biodegradable polymers for substantializing the eco-friendly innovations. *Journal of Agriculture and Food Research*, 101065.
23. Berkemeier, A., Kühnel, L., Dürigen, D., Hoffmann, H., Zeidler, H., Bullinger, A. C., & Wagenführ, A. (2024). SAMSax—An innovative living lab for the advancement of a circular economy through additive manufacturing technologies. *Sustainability*, 16(2), 823.

24. Jahangiri, F., Mohanty, A. K., & Misra, M. (2024). *Sustainable Biodegradable Coatings for Food Packaging: Challenges and Opportunities*. Green Chemistry.
25. Ghosh, K., & Jones, B. H. (2024). Biodegradable polymers for circular economy transitions—challenges and opportunities. In Nabil Nasr (Ed.), *Technology Innovation for the Circular Economy: Recycling, Remanufacturing, Design, Systems Analysis and Logistics* (pp. 29–41). Wiley.
26. Adeleke, A. K., Montero, D. J. P., Olu-lawal, K. A., & Olajiga, O. K. (2024). Process development in mechanical engineering: Innovations, challenges, and opportunities. *Engineering Science & Technology Journal*, 5(3), 901–12.
27. Alam, F., Ashfaq Ahmed, M., Jalal, A. H., Siddiquee, I., Adury, R. Z., Hossain, G. M., & Pala, N. (2024). Recent progress and challenges of implantable biodegradable biosensors. *Micromachines*, 15(4), 475.
28. Erisen, D. E., & Uludag, K. (2024). Estimating biosafety of biodegradable biomedical materials from in vitro ion tolerance parameters and toxicity of nanomaterials in brain. In *Transformative Approaches to Patient Literacy and Healthcare Innovation* (pp. 201–21). IGI Global.
29. Angolkar, M., Paramshetti, S., Gahtani, R. M., Al Shahrani, M., Hani, U., Talath, S., . . . & Gundawar, R. (2024). Pioneering a paradigm shift in tissue engineering and regeneration with polysaccharides and proteins-based scaffolds: A comprehensive review. *International Journal of Biological Macromolecules*, 130643.
30. Fragassa, C., Vannucchi de Camargo, F., & Santulli, C. (2024). Sustainable biocomposites: Harnessing the potential of waste seed-based fillers in eco-friendly materials. *Sustainability*, 16(4), 1526.
31. Musa, A. A., & Onwualu, A. P. (2024). Potential of lignocellulosic fiber reinforced polymer composites for automobile parts production: Current knowledge, research needs, and future direction. *Heliyon*, 10, e24683.
32. Wang, L., Li, D., Ye, L., Zhi, C., Zhang, T., & Miao, M. (2024). Starch-based biodegradable composites: Effects of in-situ re-extrusion on structure and performance. *International Journal of Biological Macromolecules*, 266, 130869.
33. Yuan, K., Deng, C., Tan, L., Wang, X., Yan, W., Dai, X., . . . & Wang, G. (2024). Structural and temporal dynamics analysis of zinc-based biomaterials: History, research hotspots and emerging trends. *Bioactive Materials*, 35, 306–29.
34. Kim, C. H., Lee, S. Y., Rhee, K. Y., & Park, S. J. (2024). Carbon-based composites in biomedical applications: A comprehensive review of properties, applications, and future directions. *Advanced Composites and Hybrid Materials*, 7(2), 55.
35. Aishwarya, B. K., Revathi, V., Singh, N., Mathew, L., Dhamija, K., Fallah, M. H., & Kalra, R. (2024). Biodegradable polymer biomaterials for tissue engineering applications: A critical review. In *E3S Web of Conferences* (Vol. 529, p. 01051). EDP Sciences.
36. Guleria, J., & Khan, M. A. (2024, February). Biomaterials and biopolymers in circular economy: Latest trends and applications. In *AIP Conference Proceedings* (Vol. 2986, No. 1). AIP Publishing.
37. Arunprasath, K., Vijayakumar, M., Sugumaran, P. J., Amuthakkannan, P., Manikandan, V., & Arumugaprabu, V. (2022). Polymers for structural applications. In *Materials for Lightweight Constructions* (pp. 39–60). CRC Press.
38. Oyiborhoro, G., Anegbe, B., Odiachi, I. J., Atoe, B., & Ifijen, I. H. (2024, February). Environmental impact of multi-component fiber-reinforced composites: Challenges and green solutions. In *TMS Annual Meeting & Exhibition* (pp. 1237–52). Cham: Springer Nature Switzerland.
39. Modrák, M., Trebuňová, M., Balogová, A. F., Hudák, R., & Živčák, J. (2023). Biodegradable materials for tissue engineering: Development, classification and current applications. *Journal of Functional Biomaterials*, 14(3), 159.

40. Guerrero-Martin, C. A., Silva-Marrufo, O., Ortega-Ramírez, A. T., Marín-Tinoco, R. I., Salinas-Silva, R., & Camacho-Galindo, S. (2023). Development of a biodegradable material with oregano stick as a prototype of substitute for wooden agglomerate material. *Sustainability*, 15(19), 14465.
41. Chen, Z., Aziz, T., Sun, H., Ullah, A., Ali, A., Cheng, L., . . . & Khan, F. U. (2023). Advances and applications of cellulose bio-composites in biodegradable materials. *Journal of Polymers and the Environment*, 31(6), 2273–84.
42. Valderrama-Treviño, A. I., Castell-Rodríguez, A. E., Hernández-Muñoz, R., Vázquez-Torres, N. A., Macari-Jorge, A., Barrera-Mera, B., . . . & Montalvo-Javé, E. E. (2024). Development of a biodegradable prosthesis through tissue engineering, for the organ-replacement or substitution of the extrahepatic bile duct. *Annals of Hepatology*, 29(5), 101530.
43. Khan, A. R., Grewal, N. S., Zhou, C., Yuan, K., Zhang, H. J., & Jun, Z. (2023). Recent advances in biodegradable metals for implant applications: Exploring in vivo and in vitro responses. *Results in Engineering*, 20, 101526.
44. Aleksanyan, K. V. (2023). Polysaccharides for biodegradable packaging materials: Past, present, and future (Brief Review). *Polymers*, 15(2), 451.
45. Bhagwat, S. B., & Jaspal, D. (2023). Application of biodegradable materials in oil-spill cleanup: Recent advances and future perspectives. *Advanced Engineering Materials*, 25(20), 2300315.
46. Zhu, J., Wen, H., Zhang, H., Huang, P., Liu, L., & Hu, H. (2023). Recent advances in biodegradable electronics-from fundament to the next-generation multi-functional, medical and environmental device. *Sustainable Materials and Technologies*, 35, e00530.
47. Westlake, J. R., Tran, M. W., Jiang, Y., Zhang, X., Burrows, A. D., & Xie, M. (2023). Biodegradable biopolymers for active packaging: Demand, development and directions. *Sustainable Food Technology*, 1(1), 50–72.
48. Lu, Y., Cheng, D., Niu, B., Wang, X., Wu, X., & Wang, A. (2023). Properties of poly (lactic-co-glycolic acid) and progress of poly (lactic-co-glycolic acid)-based biodegradable materials in biomedical research. *Pharmaceuticals*, 16(3), 454.
49. Sharma, V., Singh, J. P., Hussan, K., et al. (2024). Machine learning approach for predicting the machining characteristics of additive manufactured ABS material. *Proceedings of the Institution of Mechanical Engineers, Part C: Journal of Mechanical Engineering Science*, 09544062241283330.
50. Chohan, J. S., Mittal, N., Kumar, R., et al. (2020). Mechanical strength enhancement of 3D printed acrylonitrile butadiene styrene polymer components using neural network optimization algorithm. *Polymers*, 12(10), 2250.
51. Singh, J. I. P., Sharma, V., Singh, S., et al. (2024). Impact of molding temperature, fiber loading and chemical modifications on the physicomechanical and microstructural morphology properties of woven kenaf fiber/PLA composites for non-structural applications. *Journal of Natural Fibers*, 21, 2326586.
52. Singh, J., Hashmi, A. W., Ahmad, S., et al. (2024). Critical review on biodegradable and biocompatibility magnesium alloys: Progress and prospects in bio-implant applications. *Inorganic Chemistry Communications*, 169, 113111.

12 Additive Manufacturing in Tissue Engineering

Gurpreet Singh and Gaurav Prashar

CONTENTS

12.1 INTRODUCTION

The human body's superior ability to regenerate is restricted by several factors, such as tissue type and the existence of essential hormones. Outside these boundaries, when tissue harm turns into a too-severe condition, we have to take the help of tissue engineering and regenerative medicine by considering these external supports for providing a base for new developing tissue growth and stimulating cellular activity [1]. Scaffolds in both tissue engineering (TE) and regenerative medicine (RM) are vital for backup cell persistence and development. They are infused with progress factors to motivate cell specialism and tissue development, with their physical and chemical composition being key features for effective tissue regeneration [2]. Biomaterials are categorized by their chemical nature and physical properties, degradation behavior, source, and modifications. Material selection is personalized to the specific tissue application. They are commonly divided into ceramics, composites, and polymers. Ceramics, containing components like inorganic materials or calcium salts, are mainly useful in bone regeneration and dental implant purposes because of their biocompatibility and endurance. Polymers and composites

DOI: 10.1201/9781003516064-12

offer adaptability, resulting in various mechanical and biological needs in medical applications [3]. The most common use of these biomaterials is primarily in orthodontics. Polymers, which are significant in binding tissues together, are particularly highly usable in soft tissue engineering applications. Composites made by mixing ceramics and polymers are applicable in orthopedics and dental tissue engineering. Both types of polymers, natural and synthetic, are normally used in TE and RM [4]. Natural forms of biomaterials, like collagen, hyaluronic acid, alginate, and chitosan, are available abundantly and exhibit both biodegradability and biocompatibility properties, which make them widely usable. The degradation of biomaterials stands out as a crucial aspect of natural polymers [5].

Since these biomaterials exist in the extracellular matrix (ECM), cells readily adapt and grow in their presence. Collagen, a widely used natural biomaterial, features prominently in scaffold applications. Recently, biopolymers have gained attention for their potential to create biocomposites with multiple functions and high efficiency. These materials are valued for their low environmental impact, exclusive availability, renewability, eco-friendliness, and lightweight nature [6]. Biopolymeric composites are ready to replace synthetic materials in many areas like optics, biochemistry, and biomedical engineering [7]. Creating architectural designs involves striking a balance between different visions and goals, which can sometimes clash with the integration of new biomaterials [8].

12.2 NECESSITY AND PRODUCTION FOR BIOPRINTED SCAFFOLD

Tissue engineering provides an additional alternative to meet the growing demand for organ transplants. Through TE and RM dealings, we can bridge the gap between patients waiting for organ transplantation and the number of available donors [9]. Organ failure calls for organ replacement from another person as the most effective treatment for degenerative diseases, which are vulnerable to organs like kidneys, pancreas, liver, and heart. Tissue engineering commences with the construction of biomaterials and then scaffolds. These materials undergo chemical and physical changes to meet specific requirements in the production process, such as biodegradability—promotes sustainability, porosity, size, and shape (for fitness)—and bioactivity [10]. The requirements fluctuate based on the biomaterial type, production method, and target tissue. Cells can be cultured on the tissue to create the wanted tissue either inside or outside the body, enabling host cells to replace it. Critical for both methods are growth factors, hormones, and chemical signals, guiding cell differentiation and tissue function [11]. Biomaterials do two jobs: they help cells stick and carry helpful substances like medications and growth factors. Most mammal cells need something to stick to in order to survive. Without it, they often die [12]. Therefore, the surface chemistry and configuration of scrub materials play a vital role in ensuring cell viability and function. Enhancing cell adhesion on biomaterial and scaffold surfaces can be achieved through three strategies: chemical variation, modifications in physical properties, and surface modifications [13]. Primary cells carry out specific functions within organs, while supporting cells contribute to the formation of the organ's structure, matrix, and vasculature.

Differentiating these organizations can involve injecting various types of primary or pluripotent cells [14]. There are different ways to make scaffolds. Once the biomaterials are chosen, they undergo a manufacturing process to become fabrics. These methods involve physical and chemical processes using biomaterials for tissue production. However, not every biomaterial is suitable for each manufacturing method [15]. Biomaterials exist constantly adapted for dissimilar manufacturing methods. These comprise electrospinning, freeze-drying, phase separation, self-assembly, solvent casting, textile techniques, then material injections, and finally the addition of additives. In electrospinning—a fiber production method—an ionic polymer solution is pushed through a small opening with under voltage, resulting in thin fibers as the solvent evaporates, leaving fragmented polymers [16]. While this method can use various polymers, it struggles to create scaffolds with complex shapes. Yet employing a phase separation technique can yield highly porous and intricate 3D scaffolds. This approach involves using a solution with diverse solvent systems for scaffold production [17]. During this process, one phase is separated, either with or without thermal solvents, resulting in the retention of the desired polymer solutions. While this method facilitates the creation of porous products during scaffold production, it is limited by the polymers' inability to achieve high resolution in the final product [18].

Various methods fall under the umbrella of 3D printing; they all share a common approach: layer-by-layer construction. This means that each layer of material is added sequentially until the entire 3D structure is formed. Initially used mainly for prototyping purposes, AM has now expanded its reach into various industries, particularly in mechanical and industrial applications [19]. Hutmacher pioneered the application of AM for TE scaffolds in the year of 2000 [20]. Hutmacher's team spearheaded scaffold designs with multiple filament position orientations. Since then, research has explored different scaffold shapes and their effects on tissue formation. Filament position and orientation can control features like pore volume, pore size [20,21], the shape of pore [20,22], and mechanical properties [23,24] including functional area [21,25] in scaffold geometry [21,26].

12.3 ADDITIVE MANUFACTURING (AM)

The term AM refers to a manufacturing process that builds a single solid object by adding layer over layer in 2D form from 3D model data. In tissue engineering (TE), AM techniques are increasingly popular due to their capabilities to create intricate geometries and microstructures with the application of automation, precision, and reproducibility. Also, they also enable the rapid production of TE constructs tailored to meet specific patient needs, such as defect size and biological features. This chapter offers a detailed overview of various AM techniques used to develop TE constructs from different materials (e.g., polymers, ceramics, composites) with or without bioactive agents, explaining their principles and technological advancements [27, 28]. Various AM techniques for tissue engineering and fabrication are shown in **Figure 12.1**. This manufacturing method offers several pros, including the tendency to produce intricate geometries and to use myriad biomaterials and other materials. Investigators have developed innovative methods for tissue formation, involving multiple cell types and organs, utilizing recyclable polymers and cells [29].

Currently, tissue engineering relies on three chief material extrusion AM machineries for scaffold printing: (a) filament-fed extruders, (b) screw extruders, and (c) syringe extruders. Many marketable bioprinters combine these extrusion methods to print living cells with various biomaterials, facilitating tissue-making technique. Extruders may be classified into the following categories shown in **Figure 12.2**.

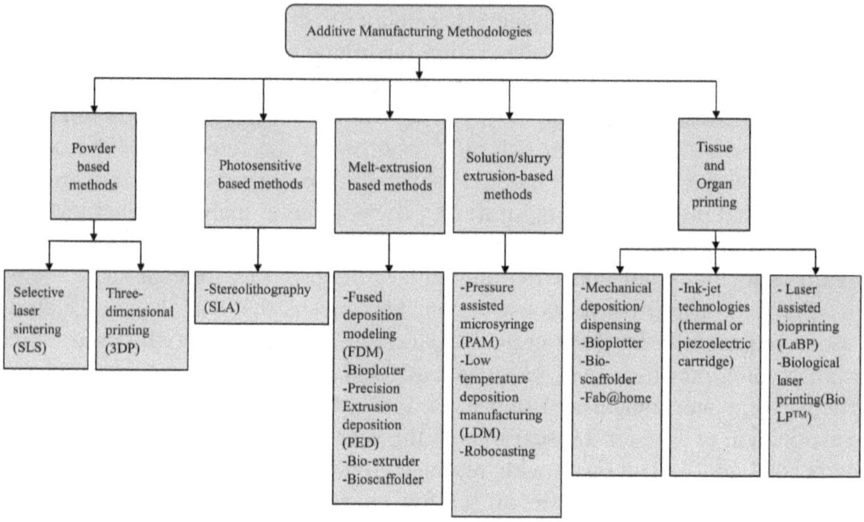

FIGURE 12.1 Proposed categorization of the AM methods typically utilized in tissue engineering.

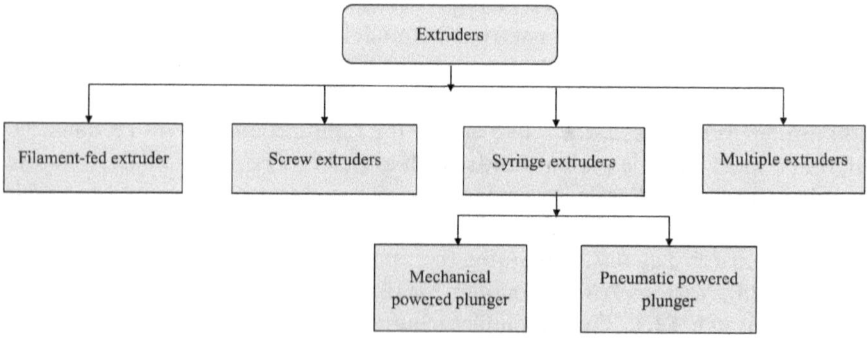

FIGURE 12.2 Classification of extruders employed in AM.

12.3.1 Filament-fed Extruder

In filament-fed AM, polymer filaments with diameters typically ranging from 1.75 mm to 2.85 mm are used. These filaments are supplied into a heater-based melting chamber area, which is attached to the nozzle. The quantity of material extrusion is measured and observed by how quickly the filament is fed into the chamber, following volume protection principles. Additive manufacturing software regulates the extrusion value based on the chosen filament diameter and speed of the nozzle. This method is popular because of its lower hardware incurring costs and suitability for a gradient of polymer melting temperatures. However, a limitation is concerned with material choices that are particularly restricted to those that are available in filament form only.

12.3.2 Screw Extruders

In the aforementioned AM, polymer granules (in small ball form) are usually fed into a screw mechanism covered by a tight-fitting barrel. When the screw starts rotating, it melts the polymer, pushing it toward a nozzle and finally at the barrel's end. Speed of rotation controls how fast the material is extruded. This method's intricate hardware makes it more costly than filament-based printers. Interestingly, screw extruders have the ability to handle materials in paste form.

12.3.3 Syringe Extruders

In syringe-based AM, the material is loaded into a syringe, and the printer controls the plunger to extrude filaments steadily. Syringes typically hold thick substances like hydrogel, but if equipped with a heated jacket, they can handle thermosoftening polymer granules, melted before printing. While polycaprolactone, melting at about 60°C, suits standard syringes, polymers with over 200°C melting points can be used with stainless steel syringes.

In the realm of syringe extrusion systems, two primary methods prevail: pneumatic pressure-driven and mechanically displaced via an electric motor. A striking difference between these methods is how they regulate the speed of extruding material, measured in mm^3/sec. Mechanical displacement factor allows for more straightforward control of this rate, while pneumatic systems rely on various factors like needle shape, material thickness, air pressure, and blockage from previously extruded material to adjust the rate. When considering their potential, the mechanical method shows potential for creating more precise filament shapes and scaffold structures due to its dominant control over extrusion speed. On the other hand, pneumatic systems provide accurate information about the level of forces constituted to the material, which is crucial for managing stress in hydrogels containing cells.

12.3.4 Multi-Extruder System

Bioprinters are commonly equipped with multiple extruders, enabling the printing process of multiple materials in a single operation. This capability proves invaluable for fabricating scaffolds alongside cell-laden hydrogels and assembling tissues comprising a myriad number of cell types and materials. Moreover, the utilization of multiple extruders facilitates the development of gradient structures and seamless transitions between materials [30].

12.4 BIOPOLYMERS AND ITS CATEGORIES

Natural polymers, sourced from living or biological materials like plants, animals, and microorganisms, include carbohydrates and polyhydroxyalkanoates (PHAs). To enhance the properties of resulting composites, these biopolymers are combined one by one or in various combinations during synthesis [31]. A biopolymer's functionality is tied to its composition, especially the behavior of its amorphous or crystalline parts. Cellulose, with its crystalline structure, serves as a prime example of a structural polymer. Meanwhile, chitosan, a notable member of the carbohydrate family, stands out for its versatility. Industries increasingly seek biopolymers that are sustainable, biodegradable, and compatible across various applications [32]. Easily derived from marine life such as lobsters, crabs, and shrimp, this material is valuable for various biopolymer composites. Yet hurdles remain before widespread use of sustainable polymers is possible, including technical and production issues. Despite their eco-friendly nature, these biopolymers often fall short in performance compared to traditional petroleum-based ones, hindering their broader adoption [33,34]. For instance, biopolymer components with single bonds often have weaker mechanical properties than plastics. However, these limitations can be solved in a number of ways, including lubrication, mixing, and reinforcement [35].

Polymers are primarily derived from diverse sources, ranging from polystyrene to natural biopolymers [36]. The three primary forms of polymers can be classified into either biopolymers or bio-based polymer composites, depending on their origin:

1. Biopolymers extracted, separated, and segregated from biomass include starch, keratin, arabinoxylan, and cellulose.
2. Bio-based polymers produced through common chemical processes by using renewable sources involve the fermentation of carbohydrates into monomers.
3. A range of polymers are predominantly sourced from polyhydroxyalkanoates (PHAs) with bacterial cellulose obtained through the digestion of microbial organisms. Biocomposites are materials created from natural or bio-derived polymers such as chitosan, arabinoxylan, PHAs, or PLA [37,38].

Green composites are a type of material composed of biopolymer-natural components along with degradable inorganic fillers. They are notable for their efficiency and sustainable nature, making them an important focus of attention amid increasing environmental concerns and regulatory measures [39]. Biopolymers are resilient molecules sourced from natural resources. Not only are they biodegradable and easily recyclable, but they also contribute to sustainable practices in both trade and the environment. As a result, they are recognized as bio-sustainable products

[40]. Chemically modified biopolymers, such as thiolate arabinoxylan and cellulose acetate, have demonstrated utility in multiple medical applications and other fields. Environmental factors and microbial breakdown facilitate their degradation in suitable conditions. These biopolymers are commonly termed as green organic composites. Many of these compounds incorporate inorganic fillers like titanium, silica, and alumina. Substantial advancements in bioplastic technology have resulted in the availability of numerous viable and environmentally beneficial products on the marketplace [41].

12.5 CHARACTERISTICS OF BIOMATERIALS SUITABLE FOR 3D PRINTING

Bioprinting is a cutting-edge technique that involves using a liquid layer method to shape biomaterials. Essentially, this means that when the biomaterial exits the cranium in a fluid state, it is carefully manipulated into the desired shape. The change from a liquid to a gel or solid form is crucial for bioprinting to work. It lets us create detailed structures like tissue scaffolds by carefully adding layers of biomaterial. This technique helps researchers copy the intricate design of natural tissues, which could be huge for regenerative medicine, tissue engineering, and finding new drugs. In the end, bioprinting could change healthcare by offering personalized fixes for damaged tissues and organs [42]. Polymers and composites are popular choices for 3D printing in the realm of biomaterials because of their flexibility. They can go through different processes to become ready for 3D printing. To make sure the printing goes smoothly, we need to think about things like how easily the material flows (rheological properties) and how it's cross-linked (which affects its stability and structure). These factors determine if the biomaterials are a good fit for 3D printing techniques.

Moreover, the demands for bio inkjet printing contrast with those for extrusion-based bioprinting. In bio inkjet printing, tiny droplets of bio-ink are placed onto a substrate, whereas extrusion-based bioprinting entails layer-by-layer extrusion of bio-ink. Each approach presents unique requirements and attributes, shaping the selection of biomaterials and the printing procedure. Grasping these differences is vital for attaining favorable results in 3D bioprinting endeavors [43].

The 3D bioprinting quality depends upon various key components of polymer biomaterial underuse. While in the developing process, the rheological properties should be considered to produce new polymer or hydrogel bioprinting systems. Four major properties such as viscosity (how thick or thin the material is), Newtonian behavior (how its viscosity changes over different conditions), cross-linking (effects the structure and stability of material), and the Barus effect (how pressure effects the material's viscosity) plays a crucial role in hydrogel bioprinting system. Non-Newtonian systems exhibit distinctive characteristics, showcasing viscosity alterations based on the level of shear pressure exerted upon them. Consequently, they may exhibit a thick consistency under low shear stress, yet thin out and display increased fluidity under higher shear stress. Grasping these unique traits is imperative for refining the printing process and guaranteeing that the biomaterial behaves predictably throughout 3D printing endeavors [44]. There are many problems associated with

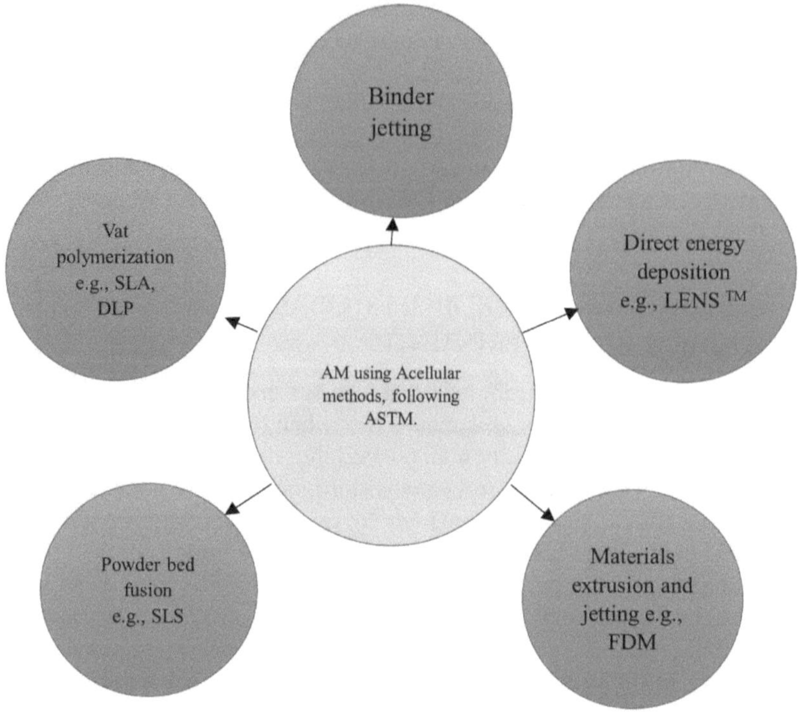

FIGURE 12.3 Cellular methods as per ASTM guidelines.

elevated viscosity levels on polymers such as the risk of nozzle clogging, particularly in fluids that exhibit shear-thickening behavior. Also, the presence of dust particles can disrupt the printing process by expelling polymers in other directions from the print head. This expulsion may lead to polymer expansion, leading to exacerbating printing issues. Proper understanding of these challenges is highly important for the optimization of 3D printing process by mitigating these disruptions [45]. This phenomenon, referred as the Barus effect, holds significant importance in 3D printing process. To minimize the Barus effect, typically, bio-inks are utilized in 3D printing process by which one can identify minimal or no Barus effect in the overall process.

As per the guidelines set out by the American Society for Testing and Materials (ASTM), **Figure 12.3** offers a thorough summary of the several AM techniques for biomaterials. Comprehending and mitigating the Barus effect is imperative for enhancing the functionality and dependability of 3D-printed biomaterials [46].

12.6 POLYMERS CREATED THROUGH 3D PRINTING TECHNIQUE

12.6.1 Natural/Organic Biomaterials

We have explored natural biomaterials employing tissue engineering techniques in our search for more effective ways to overhaul or swap injured human tissue and body part. Scaffolds made of biomaterials have shown potential in this regard [47].

Gelatin, the primary hydrolyzed collagen component, naturally forms within the extracellular matrix (ECM) and can suspend gel cells at lower temperatures. Studies exploring the incorporation of organic starch polymers by means of water-based binders in 3D direct printing have yielded promising outcomes. Additionally, synthetic polymers can be blended with essential biodegradables to achieve the required mechanical properties [48]. Furthermore, starch-based polymers have higher porosity and enhanced cellular integration due to longer degradation time, making them ideal biomaterial for bone TE [49]. In the 3D printing process, many polymer-induced starch granules were examined. Then the quality of processed scaffolds was determined through various optical analysis methodologies such as scanned electron microscopy (SEM) for material topography and composition, differential scanning calorimetry (DSC) for thermal properties, porosity assessment, and compression testing for safety measures [50,51]. Experimentation analysis revealed that novel 3DP material blends can construct 3D porous scaffolds. Furthermore, both composites like starch and cellulose exhibited biocompatibility in polymer-based drug delivery systems [52]. Specimens constructed with larger particles are accessed by mechanical as well as density measurements and exhibited lower mechanical properties caused by minimal sintering and joint limitations. Additionally, smaller-sized particles covered enclosed pores existing in very large volume [53]. Experimental results indicated that by process optimization and by making changes or adjustments to scanning speed and laser power, there is a certain feasibility to fabricate biopolymer scaffolds by using cellulose acetate and starch. The results illustrate that specimens with smaller particle sizes possess sufficient mechanical properties and desired porosities, showcasing potential applications in the designing and fabrication of tissue [54]. The utilization of 3D printing technology in TE has paved the way for the creation of tissue-mimicking geometries through advanced technologies for printing cells and matrix materials. Employing 3D printing for constructing cell-laden structures has demonstrated accurate cell placement and high cell viability within the manufactured constructs [55,56].

12.6.2 Ceramic Scaffolds

Ceramics, categorized as biomaterials, consist of calcium and phosphate, comprising inorganic salts—derived from non-living substances. Due to their osteoconductive and osteoinductive properties, these biomaterials hold substantial promise for both bone and dental tissue engineering [57]. These biomaterials promote the formation of new bone tissues that are consequently termed osteoconductive. Some substances have the ability to induce cell differentiation toward the osteoblast lineage without the aid of growth impacting factors, earning them the designation of osteoinductive [58]. Commonly added polymers include chitosan, poly-lactide-glycolic acid (PLGA), and polyethylene-glycol diacrylate (PEGDA). To enhance mechanical properties resembling bone, materials like zirconium oxide, silica, bioglass, and graphene are incorporated into the configuration of the skin to form composites [59]. Numerous researchers have developed 3D porous materials to promote vascularization within scaffolds. Eventually, various 3D-printed ceramics will undergo sintering and freezing processes to enhance mechanical properties and cytocompatibility [60]. The other mechanical properties, such as the compressive strength of

3D-printed scaffolds incorporating strontium, gahnite, hardystonite, hydroxypropyl methylcellulose (HPMC), and sodium polyacrylate, have been confirmed to match that of 110 MPa bone, with scaffolds having a porosity of 34%. Due to their robust ability to help vascularization, these scaffolds hold tremendous potential in the arena of bone TE [61,62].

12.6.3 Synthetic Biopolymers

Bone, extensively researched among various tissues, is actively investigated due to its crucial role in daily functioning. In cases of disease or injury, surgery is often required to remove the defective portion. However, regeneration is typically limited in terms of shape to a few millimeters from the healthy bone [63]. Renewal is the sole possibility, wherein the excised segment of the bone is substituted with an implant to restore functionality. Polycaprolactone (PCL) is the predominant polymer material utilized as 3D porous scaffold material, renowned for its strong biocompatibility and processability, despite its hydrophobic nature, which restricts cell–scaffold interactions [64]. PCL is also semi-crystalline, leading to extended degradation kinetics, making it a suitable bioresorbable material compatible with both soft and hard tissues. Its hydrophobic nature and low water absorption capacity contribute to these characteristics. Mechanical parameters such as porosity, the compressive modulus, and yield strength of scaffolds fluctuated between the ranges of 40%–85%, 2.74–55.95 MPa, and 1.17–5.03 MPa, respectively. These closely match with the bone in the maxillary region. Furthermore, cytotoxicity testing results indicate the feasibility of the mentioned manufacturing method for PCL scaffolds [65,66]. Apart from PCL, other polymers find applications in tissue engineering through 3D printing. Poly (3-hydroxybutyrate), (PHB) is a natural thermoplastic polyester known for its growth-related properties. It has gained traction in biomedical fields, particularly in the making of tissue engineering scaffolds, owing to its two important properties—biocompatibility and biodegradability [67]. Unlike traditional methods, PHB can be processed via 3D printing without plasticizers [68]. A PCL-based polyester was also synthesized for in vivo evaluation of biodegradation and biocompatibility of 3D PhMgCl scaffolds. 3D plasters utilizing this polymer were produced through fiber filtering, resulting in increased hydrophilicity, accelerated degradation rates, and improved link between the cell material and PCL. Both types of scaffolds, including PhMgCl, exhibited a typical external body response characterized by the existence of fibrosis, macrophages, and lymphocytes [69,70]. The level of tissue within PhMgCl scaffolds has been shown to surpass in terms of scaffolds' interactions and vascularization of PCL. Thus, PhMgCl presents as a capable biomaterial for a bone and cartilage TE, owing to its rapid degradability and proved excellent biocompatibility [71].

12.6.4 Synthetic Biopolymer-based Composites

As the primary components for fabricating multi-materials, two major photo cross-linkable hydrogel biopolymers, namely poly-(ethylene glycol) and poly-(PEG-DA, MW 3400), were utilized as scaffolding materials. Various concentrations of these biopolymers were carefully adjusted to create distinct sectors within the scaffold, resulting in multi-material scaffolds with features such as fluorescence or bioactive PEG markers [72]. The successful demonstration of multi-material spatial control was achieved. Additionally, the swelling behavior balance of these two biopolymers was determined post selective laser sintering (SLS) manufacture, enabling the construction of swollen state structures with the specified sizes [73]. Multi-material SLS is employed, allowing for the relatively simple conjugation of various bioactive ligands or growing features to PEG. This enables the production of customized 3D structures with precise bioactivity that can be spatially controlled [74]. An array of current methods utilize water-insoluble materials, which are not compatible with live cell manufacturing, along with ultraviolet (UV) radiation that can harm cellular DNA. However, recent studies have demonstrated the use of water-soluble dimethacrylate poly(ethyleneglycol)—PEG-DMA harvested stereolithographic designed cells having hydrogel. These scaffolds exhibited higher cell feasibility and movement compared to solid counterparts, most likely due to the increased exchange rate of oxygen and nutrients within the porous internal architecture of the scaffolds [75,76]. The porous hydrogel structures exhibited a clear pore network, restricted pore dispersion, and substantial pore interconnectedness. The resin demonstrated compatibility with cell binding and growth within the scaffold makeups. Human mesenchymal stem cells adhered to the facet of hydrogel assemblies and displayed their proliferative form after seeding. Cell growth was observed after five days of cultivation [77]. These hydrogel structures can find applications in TE, drug transport, cell replacement, and diverse biomedical fields [78,79].

12.7 CONCLUSION AND FUTURE SCOPE

AM is commonly referred to as 3D printing process, which has developed into a significant technology in the field of tissue engineering. It provides precise control over both designing and fabrication of intricate, custom scaffolds that facilitate cell development and tissue regeneration. This chapter examines the capabilities of AM techniques in the fabrication of scaffolds that possess customized mechanical properties and also discusses different polymers fabricated by AM. Through the implementation of layer-by-layer addition and deposition of polymers, AM enables the creation and dimensional accuracy of scaffolds. Additionally, challenges persist in the optimization of material biocompatibility, vascularization, and production scaling. However, the future of AM in TE appears promising, with potential for personalized treatments and advancements in regenerative medicine.

REFERENCES

[1] S. Bose, C. Koski, and A. V. Ashley, "Additive manufacturing of natural biopolymers and composites for bone tissue engineering," *Materials Horizons*, vol. 7, no. 8, pp. 2011–27, 2020.

[2] T. Kuhnt and S. Camarero-Espinosa, "Additive manufacturing of nanocellulose based scaffolds for tissue engineering: Beyond a reinforcement filler," *Carbohydrate Polymers*, vol. 252, article 117159, 2021.

[3] J. Kundu, J.-H. Shim, J. Jang, S.-W. Kim, and D.-W. Cho, "An additive manufacturing–based PCL–alginate–chondrocyte bioprinted scaffold for cartilage tissue engineering," *Journal of Tissue Engineering and Regenerative Medicine*, vol. 9, no. 11, pp. 1286–97, 2015.

[4] S. Pina, J. M. Oliveira, and R. L. Reis, "Natural–based nanocomposites for bone tissue engineering and regenerative medicine: A review," *Advanced Materials*, vol. 27, no. 7, pp. 1143–69, 2015.
[5] B. Dhariwala, E. Hunt, and T. Boland, "Rapid prototyping of tissue-engineering constructs, using photopolymerizable hydrogels and stereolithography," *Tissue Engineering*, vol. 10, no. 9–10, pp. 1316–22, 2004.
[6] S. Pina, V. P. Ribeiro, C. F. Marques, et al., "Scaffolding strategies for tissue engineering and regenerative medicine applications," *Materials*, vol. 12, no. 11, p. 1824, 2019.
[7] N. Di Marzio, D. Eglin, T. Serra, and L. Moroni, "Bio-fabrication: Convergence of 3D bioprinting and nano-biomaterials in tissue engineering and regenerative medicine," *Frontiers in Bioengineering and Biotechnology*, vol. 8, p. 326, 2020.
[8] C. Vyas, R. Pereira, B. Huang, F. Liu, W. Wang, and P. Bartolo, "Engineering the vasculature with additive manufacturing," *Current Opinion in Biomedical Engineering*, vol. 2, pp. 1–13, 2017.
[9] S. Mantha, S. Pillai, P. Khayambashi, et al., "Smart hydrogels in tissue engineering and regenerative medicine," *Materials*, vol. 12, no. 20, p. 3323, 2019.
[10] J. Lee, S.-H. Lee, B. S. Kim, Y.-S. Cho, and Y. Park, "Development and evaluation of hyaluronic acid-based hybrid bio-ink for tissue regeneration," *Tissue Engineering and Regenerative Medicine*, vol. 15, no. 6, pp. 761–9, 2018.
[11] M. Sahranavard, A. Zamanian, F. Ghorbani, and M. H. Shahrezaee, "A critical review on three dimensional-printed chitosan hydrogels for development of tissue engineering," *Bioprinting*, vol. 17, article e00063, 2020.
[12] J. E. Kim, S. H. Kim, and Y. Jung, "Current status of three-dimensional printing inks for soft tissue regeneration," *Tissue Engineering and Regenerative Medicine*, vol. 13, no. 6, pp. 636–46, 2016.
[13] C. R. Lynch, P. P. D. Kondiah, and Y. E. Choonara, "Advanced strategies for tissue engineering in regenerative medicine: A biofabrication and biopolymer perspective," *Molecules*, vol. 26, no. 9, article 2518, 2021.
[14] S. Safinsha and M. Mubarak Ali, "Composite scaffolds in tissue engineering," *Materials Today: Proceedings*, vol. 24, pp. 2318–29, 2020.
[15] S. Kashte and S. Kadam, *Advances and Innovations and Impediments in Tissue Engineering and Regenerative Medicine*, Crimson Publishers, 2019.
[16] S. Gupta and A. Bit, "3D bioprinting in tissue engineering and regenerative medicine," *Cell and Tissue Banking*, pp. 1–14, 2021.
[17] K. Dzobo, N. E. Thomford, D. A. Senthebane, et al., "Advances in regenerative medicine and tissue engineering: Innovation and transformation of medicine," *Stem Cells International*, vol. 2018, Article ID 2495848, 24 pages, 2018.
[18] S. Stratton, O. S. Manoukian, R. Patel, A. Wentworth, S. Rudraiah, and S. G. Kumbar, "Polymeric 3D printed structures for soft–tissue engineering," *Journal of Applied Polymer Science*, vol. 135, no. 24, p. 45569, 2018.
[19] B. J. Tricomi, A. D. Dias, and D. T. Corr, "Stem cell bioprinting for applications in regenerative medicine," *Annals of the New York Academy of Sciences*, vol. 1383, no. 1, pp. 115–24, 2016.
[20] D. W. Hutmacher, "Scaffolds in tissue engineering bone and cartilage," *Biomaterials*, vol. 21, pp. 2529–43, 2000.
[21] T. B. F. Woodfield, J. Malda, J. De Wijn, F. Peters, J. Riesle, and C. A. van Blitterswijk, "Design of porous scaffolds for cartilage tissue engineering using a three-dimensional fiber-deposition technique," *Biomaterials*, vol. 25, pp. 4149–61, 2004.
[22] S. I. Roohani-Esfahani, P. Newman, and H. Zreiqat, "Design and fabrication of 3D printed scaffolds with a mechanical strength comparable to cortical bone to repair large bone defects," *Scientific Reports*, vol. 6, p. 19468, 2016.

[23] J. M. Sobral, S. G. Caridade, R. A. Sousa, J. F. Mano, and R. L. Reis, "Three-dimensional plotted scaffolds with controlled pore size gradients: Effect of scaffold geometry on mechanical performance and cell seeding efficiency," *ActaBiomater*, vol. 7, pp. 1009–18, 2011.
[24] L. Ruiz-Cantu, A. Gleadall, C. Faris, J. Segal, K. Shakesheff, and J. Yang, "Characterisation of the surface structure of 3D printed scaffolds for cell infiltration and surgical suturing," *Biofabrication*, vol. 8, p. 15016, 2016.
[25] D. W. Hutmacher, T. Schantz, I. Zein, K. W. Ng, S. H. Teoh, and K. C. Tan, "Mechanical properties and cell cultural response of polycaprolactone scaffolds designed and fabricated via fused deposition modeling," *Journal of Biomedical Materials Research Part A*, vol. 55, pp. 203–16, 2001.
[26] H. Shao, X. Yang, Y. He, J. Fu, L. Liu, L. Ma, et al., "Bioactive glass-reinforced bioceramic ink writing scaffolds: Sintering, microstructure and mechanical behavior," *Biofabrication*, vol. 7, p. 35010, 2015.
[27] Carlos Mota, Dario Puppi, Federica Chiellini, and Emo Chiellini, "Additive manufacturing techniques for the production of tissue engineering constructs," https://doi.org/10.1002/term.1635.
[28] Andrew Gleadall, Dafydd Visscher, Jing Yang, Daniel Thomas, and Joel Segal, "Review of additive manufactured tissue engineering scaffolds: Relationship between geometry and performance," *Burns & Trauma*, vol. 6, p. 19, 2018. https://doi.org/10.1186/s41038-018-0121-4.
[29] A. Alblawi, A. S. Ranjani, H. Yasmin, S. Gupta, A. Bit, and M. Rahimi-Gorji, "Scaffold-free: A developing technique in field of tissue engineering," *Computer Methods and Programs in Biomedicine*, vol. 185, p. 105148, 2020.
[30] Andrew Gleadall, Dafydd Visscher, Jing Yang, Daniel Thomas, and Joel Segal, "Review of additive manufactured tissue engineering scaffolds: Relationship between geometry and performance," *Burns & Trauma*, vol. 6, p. 19, 2018. https://doi.org/10.1186/s41038-018-0121-4.
[31] M. Mehrpouya, H. Vahabi, M. Barletta, P. Laheurte, and V. Langlois, "Additive manufacturing of polyhydroxyalkanoates (PHAs) biopolymers: Materials, printing techniques, and applications," *Materials Science and Engineering: C*, vol. 127, article 112216, 2021.
[32] L. Chaunier, S. Guessasma, S. Belhabib, G. Della Valle, D. Lourdin, and E. Leroy, "Material extrusion of plant biopolymers: Opportunities & challenges for 3D printing," *Additive Manufacturing*, vol. 21, pp. 220–33, 2018.
[33] R. Velu, D. K. Jayashankar, and K. Subburaj, "Additive processing of biopolymers for medical applications," in *Additive Manufacturing*, pp. 635–59, Elsevier, 2021.
[34] F. Cruz, "Fabrication of HA/PLLA composite scaffolds forbone tissue engineering using additive manufacturing technologies," *Biopolymers*, vol. 11, pp. 227–42, 2010.
[35] V. Dhinakaran, M. Lavanya, K. Vigneswari, M. Ravichandran, and M. Vijayakumar, "Review on exploration of graphene in diverse applications and its future horizon," *Materials Today: Proceedings*, vol. 27, pp. 824–8, 2020.
[36] C.-S. Wu, "Characterization, functionality and application of siliceous sponge spicules additive-based manufacturing biopolymer composites," *Additive Manufacturing*, vol. 22, pp. 13–20, 2018.
[37] J. V. Ecker, M. Kracalik, S. Hild, and A. Haider, "3D-materialextrusion-printing with biopolymers: A review," *Chemical and Materials Engineering*, vol. 5, no. 4, pp. 83–96, 2017.
[38] L. Chaunier, G. D. Valle, D. Lourdin, A.-L. Réguerre, K. Cochet, and E. Leroy, "Viscous sintering kinetics of biopolymer filaments extruded for 3D printing," *Polymer Testing*, vol. 77, article 105873, 2019.
[39] R. A. Ilyas and S. M. Sapuan, "Biopolymers and biocomposites: Chemistry and technology," *Current Analytical Chemistry*, vol. 16, no. 5, pp. 500–3, 2020.

[40] M. D. Sarker, S. Naghieh, N. K. Sharma, L. Ning, and X. Chen, "Bioprinting of vascularized tissue scaffolds: Influence of biopolymer, cells, growth factors, and gene delivery," *Journal of Healthcare Engineering*, vol. 2019, article ID9156921, 20 pages, 2019.

[41] V. Dhinakaran, J. Ajith, A. F. Y. Fahmidha, T. Jagadeesha, T. Sathish, and B. Stalin, "Wire arc additive manufacturing (WAAM) process of nickel based superalloys—a review," *Materials Today: Proceedings*, vol. 21, pp. 920–5, 2020.

[42] P. Zarrintaj, H. Vahabi, T. J. Gutiérrez, M. Mehrpouya, M. R. Ganjali, and M. R. Saeb, "Nanocomposite biomaterials made by 3D printing: Achievements and challenges," in *Handbook of Polymer Nanocomposites for Industrial Applications*, pp. 675–85, Elsevier, 2021.

[43] C. Yu, J. Schimelman, P. Wang, et al., "Photopolymerizable biomaterials and light-based 3D printing strategies for biomedical applications," *Chemical Reviews*, vol. 120, no. 19, pp. 10695–743, 2020.

[44] B. I. Oladapo, S. A. Zahedi, and A. O. M. Adeoye, "3D printing of bone scaffolds with hybrid biomaterials," *Composites Part B: Engineering*, vol. 158, pp. 428–36, 2019.

[45] A. E. Jakus, N. R. Geisendorfer, P. L. Lewis, and R. N. Shah, "3D-printing porosity: A new approach to creating elevated porosity materials and structures," *Acta Biomaterialia*, vol. 72, pp. 94–109, 2018.

[46] M. J. Zafar, D. Zhu, and Z. Zhang, "3D printing of bioceramics for bone tissue engineering," *Materials*, vol. 12, no. 20, p. 3361, 2019.

[47] K. Tappa and U. Jammalamadaka, "Novel biomaterials used in medical 3D printing techniques," *Journal of Functional Biomaterials*, vol. 9, no. 1, p. 17, 2018.

[48] D. J. Richards, Y. Tan, J. Jia, H. Yao, and Y. Mei, "3D printing for tissue engineering," *Israel Journal of Chemistry*, vol. 53, no. 9–10, pp. 805–14, 2013.

[49] M. Guvendiren, J. Molde, R. M. D. Soares, and J. Kohn, "Designing biomaterials for 3D printing," *ACS Biomaterials Science & Engineering*, vol. 2, no. 10, pp. 1679–93, 2016.

[50] H. N. Chia and M. W. Benjamin, "Recent advances in 3D printing of biomaterials," *Journal of Biological Engineering*, vol. 9, no. 1, pp. 1–14, 2015.

[51] D. J. Whyte, R. Rajkhowa, B. Allardyce, and A. Z. Kouzani, "A review on the challenges of 3D printing of organic powders," *Bioprinting*, vol. 16, article e00057, 2019.

[52] Q. Yan, H. Dong, S. Jin, et al., "A review of 3D printing technology for medical applications," *Engineering*, vol. 4, no. 5, pp. 729–42, 2018.

[53] R. J. Mondschein, A. Kanitkar, C. B. Williams, S. S. Verbridge, and T. E. Long, "Polymer structure-property requirements for stereolithographic 3D printing of soft tissue engineering scaffolds," *Biomaterials*, vol. 140, pp. 170–88, 2017.

[54] N. Poomathi, S. Singh, C. Prakash, et al., "3D printing in tissue engineering: A state of the art review of technologies and biomaterials," *Rapid Prototyping Journal*, vol. 26, no. 7, pp. 1313–34, 2020.

[55] D. M. Kirchmajer and R. G. Iii, "An overview of the suitability of hydrogel-forming polymers for extrusion-based 3D-printing," *Journal of Materials Chemistry B*, vol. 3, no. 20, pp. 4105–17, 2015.

[56] A. Skardal and A. Atala, "Biomaterials for integration with 3-D bioprinting," *Annals of Biomedical Engineering*, vol. 43, no. 3, pp. 730–46, 2015.

[57] H. Seitz, W. Rieder, S. Irsen, B. Leukers, and C. Tille, "Three–dimensional printing of porous ceramic scaffolds for bone tissue engineering," *Journal of Biomedical Materials Research Part B: Applied Biomaterials: An Official Journal of The Society for Biomaterials, The Japanese Society for Biomaterials, and The Australian Society for Biomaterials and the Korean Society for Biomaterials*, vol. 74, no. 2, pp. 782–8, 2005.

[58] B. Leukers, H. Gülkan, S. H. Irsen, et al., "Biocompatibility of ceramic scaffolds for bone replacement made by 3D printing," *Materialwissenschaft und Werkstofftechnik*, vol. 36, no. 12, pp. 781–7, 2005.

[59] V. Dhinakaran, B. Stalin, M. S. Sai, J. Vairamuthu, and S. Marichamy, "Recent developments of graphene composites for energy storage devices," *Materials Today: Proceedings*, vol. 45, pp. 1779–82, 2021.

[60] Y. Wen, S. Xun, M. Haoye, et al., "3D printed porous ceramic scaffolds for bone tissue engineering: A review," *Biomaterials Science*, vol. 5, no. 9, pp. 1690–8, 2017.

[61] J.-B. Lee, W.-Y. Maeng, Y.-H. Koh, and H.-E. Kim, "Porous calcium phosphate ceramic scaffolds with tailored pore orientations and mechanical properties using lithography-based ceramic 3D printing technique," *Materials*, vol. 11, no. 9, p. 1711, 2018.

[62] X. Du, F. Shengyang, and Y. Zhu, "3D printing of ceramic-based scaffolds for bone tissue engineering: An overview," *Journal of Materials Chemistry B*, vol. 6, no. 27, pp. 4397–412, 2018.

[63] U. G. Sampath, Y. C. Ching, C. H. Chuah, J. J. Sabariah, and P.-C. Lin, "Fabrication of porous materials from natural/synthetic biopolymers and their composites," *Materials*, vol. 9, no. 12, p. 991, 2016.

[64] M. Hassan, K. Dave, R. Chandrawati, F. Dehghani, and V. G. Gomes, "3D printing of biopolymer nanocomposites for tissue engineering: Nanomaterials, processing and structure function relation," *European Polymer Journal*, vol. 121, p. 109340, 2019.

[65] K. Li, D. Wang, K. Zhao, K. Song, and J. Liang, "Electrohydrodynamic jet 3D printing of PCL/PVP composite scaffold for cell culture," *Talanta*, vol. 211, p. 120750, 2020.

[66] S. Balasubramanian, M.-E. Aubin-Tam, and A. S. Meyer, "3D printing for the fabrication of biofilm-based functional living materials," *ACS Synthetic Biology*, vol. 8, no. 7, pp. 1564–7, 2019.

[67] F. Pati, J.-H. Shim, J.-S. Lee, and D.-W. Cho, "3D printing of cell-laden constructs for heterogeneous tissue regeneration," *Manufacturing Letters*, vol. 1, no. 1, pp. 49–53, 2013.

[68] S. Nagarajan, S. Radhakrishnan, S. N. Kalkura, S. Balme, P. Miele, and M. Bechelany, "Overview of protein–based biopolymers for biomedical application," *Macromolecular Chemistry and Physics*, vol. 220, no. 14, article 1900126, 2019.

[69] W. Xu, X. Wang, N. Sandler, S. Willför, and X. Chunlin, "Three-dimensional printing of wood-derived biopolymers: A review focused on biomedical applications," *ACS Sustainable Chemistry & Engineering*, vol. 6, no. 5, pp. 5663–80, 2018.

[70] J. Saroia, Y. Wang, Q. Wei, K. Zhang, T. Lu, and B. Zhang, "Are view on biocompatibility nature of hydrogels with 3D printing techniques, tissue engineering application and its future prospective," *Bio-Design and Manufacturing*, vol. 1, no. 4, pp. 265–79, 2018.

[71] G. Vozzi, A. Previti, D. De Rossi, and A. R. T. I. Ahluwalia, "Microsyringe-based deposition of two-dimensional and three-dimensional polymer scaffolds with a well-defined geometry for application to tissue engineering," *Tissue Engineering*, vol. 8, no. 6, pp. 1089–98, 2002.

[72] S. Yang, K.-F. Leong, Z. Du, and C.-K. Chua, "The design of scaffolds for use in tissue engineering. Part II. Rapid prototyping techniques," *Tissue Engineering*, vol. 8, no. 1, pp. 1–11, 2002.

[73] T. Rasheed, M. Bilal, Y. Zhao, A. Raza, S. Z. H. Shah, and H. M. N. Iqbal, "Physiochemical characteristics and bone/cartilage tissue engineering potentialities of protein-based macromolecules—a review," *International Journal of Biological Macromolecules*, vol. 121, pp. 13–22, 2019.

[74] Y. Wan, X. Li, and S. Wang, "Recent advances in biohybrid materials for tissue engineering and regenerative medicine," *Journal of Molecular and Engineering Materials*, vol. 4, no. 1, p. 1640001, 2016.

[75] A. George, M. R. Sanjay, R. Srisuk, J. Parameswaranpillai, and S. Siengchin, "A comprehensive review on chemical properties and applications of biopolymers and their composites," *International Journal of Biological Macromolecules*, vol. 154, pp. 329–38, 2020.

[76] E. C. Novosel, C. Kleinhans, and P. J. Kluger, "Vascularization is the key challenge in tissue engineering," *Advanced Drug Delivery Reviews*, vol. 63, no. 4–5, pp. 300–11, 2011.
[77] D. Chouhan, S. Kaushik, and D. Arora, "Trends in bioderived biomaterials in tissue engineering," in *Biomaterials in Tissue Engineering and Regenerative Medicine: From Basic Concepts to State of the Art Approaches*, pp. 163–213, Springer, 2021.
[78] G. P. Udayakumar, S. Muthusamy, B. Selvaganesh, et al., "Biopolymers and composites: Properties, characterization and their applications in food, medical and pharmaceutical industries," *Journal of Environmental Chemical Engineering*, vol. 9, no. 4, article 105322, 2021.
[79] J. Singh, S. Singh, and R. Gill, "Applications of biopolymer coatings in biomedical engineering," *Journal of Electrochemical Science and Engineering*, vol. 13, pp. 63–81, 2022.

13 Bioprinting and Tissue Engineering

Hardeep Kaur, Rimika Thakur, Saksham Singh, Chandra Mohan, Sandeep Singh, and Noushi Zaidi

CONTENTS

13.1 INTRODUCTION

For the last ten years, tissue engineering has been a rapidly evolving field that focuses on the renewal, restoration, or construction of organs or functional tissues closely resembling those present in the human body. Despite this progress, the limited ability of the body's tissues to heal themselves has led to a growing need for organ transplants [1]. Tragically, in early 2024, the United States had approximately 103,000 individuals waiting for organ transplants worldwide, while the number of donor sites does not even account for half of the needy population. Additionally, 17 people lose their lives on average daily while waiting in search of an organ transplant. Despite all these challenges, the overall count of organ transplants carried out in 2023 broke a record by exceeding 46,000 for the first

DOI: 10.1201/9781003516064-13

time. Nevertheless, it is also critical to recognize that there is a sizable worldwide need for organ replacements and transplants due to the organ shortage [2]. On the same note, tissue engineering offers innovative resolutions to the crisis of organ shortage. These technologies use one-by-one layering of bio-inks, a mixture of biomaterials, and live cells to create functioning tissues and organs (**Figure 13.1**). The capacity to generate tissues artificially for an individual patient can drastically minimize the dependency on human donors, minimizing organ rejection risk and enhancing therapeutic results. Tissue engineering is seen as a valuable method of improving life quality and life preservation. The conventional tissue engineering methods involve using scaffolds, isolated cells, or a mixture of cells put inside or within scaffolds that is the same as the natural intercellular matrix (ICM) of the body and simplify tissue regeneration [3,4]. Lately, there has been progress in the creation of scaffolds loaded with cells that replicate the intricate structure of the natural tissues. These scaffolds were synthesized through different bottom-up techniques, including microfluidic, electrohydrodynamic, photo-lithographic methods, and 3D printing procedures. However, 3D bioprinting process, in particular owing to its efficient production capabilities, is popular in this field of tissue engineering applications [2,5]. The technique of three-dimensional bioprinting involves the gradual placement of biomaterials in tiny increments, that may or may not be filled with cells at a later stage, that allows the creation of complex structures that closely resemble natural tissue [1,6]. Regarding bioprinting methods, hydrogels are frequently employed as the primary substance for printing as bio-inks. This is owing to the hydrogel's ability to absorb a considerable amount of water. The cells are protected since hydrogels are water-rich structures that allow the encapsulation of cells in a noninvasive process. This feature of covalent cross-linking of the polymer networks in situ eliminates the necessity of surgical intervention in

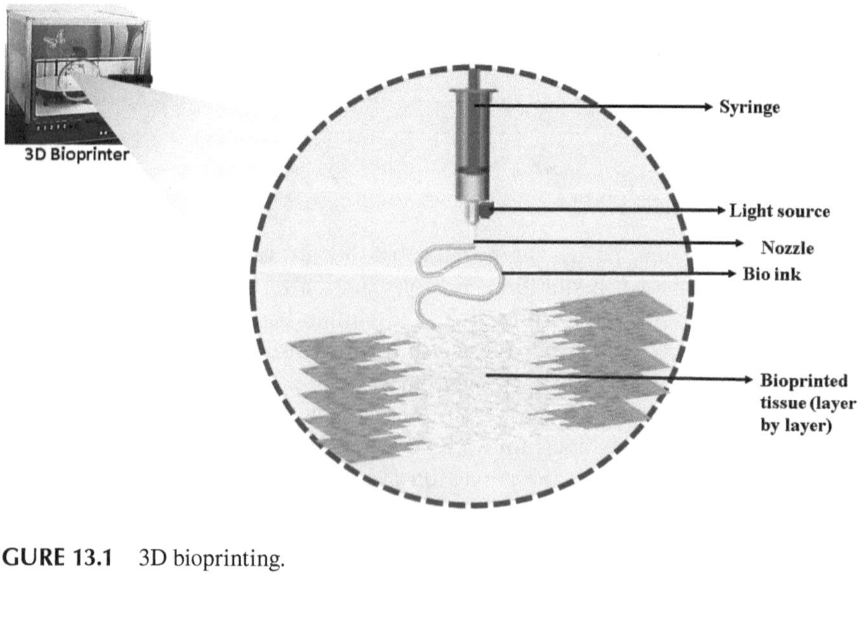

FIGURE 13.1 3D bioprinting.

implantation. After cell encapsulation in hydrogels, the cross-linking of hydrogels can be achieved employing several methods, suitable for maintenance of the viability and cell division of the cells. Hence choosing the right bio-ink is very important to construct a proper cellular micro environment conducive for cell growth and development. In the same way, in bioprinting, the tissue is first modeled numerically or as a scaffold depending on exact medical imaging input.

Subsequently, a mixture known as bio-ink is made containing living cells and biocompatible materials to generate a conducive environment for all the cells. Then the layer-by-layer deposition of the bio-inks is done during bioprinting, utilizing an inkjet, extrusion-based, or laser-assisted bioprinting technique to create the tissue structure. To stabilize their structure after printing, the cross-linking agents are required. Finally, the generated tissues are cultured under controlled conditions to promote cell growth and maturation (**Figure 13.2**). These bioprinted tissues have various applications like organ transplantation, regenerative medicine, disease modeling, and drug testing. This innovative technology has the potential to significantly advance organ generation and improve transplant results, holding great promise in the realm of medical research and treatment development.

This chapter presents current advancements in bioprinting for organ regeneration. Initially, the techniques of 3D bioprinting along with the advantages and disadvantages are introduced. The conditions for the materials that can be printed and cell sources employed in bioprinting are also discussed. Lastly, this chapter explores the existing limitations and future potential opportunities in this rapidly advancing domain.

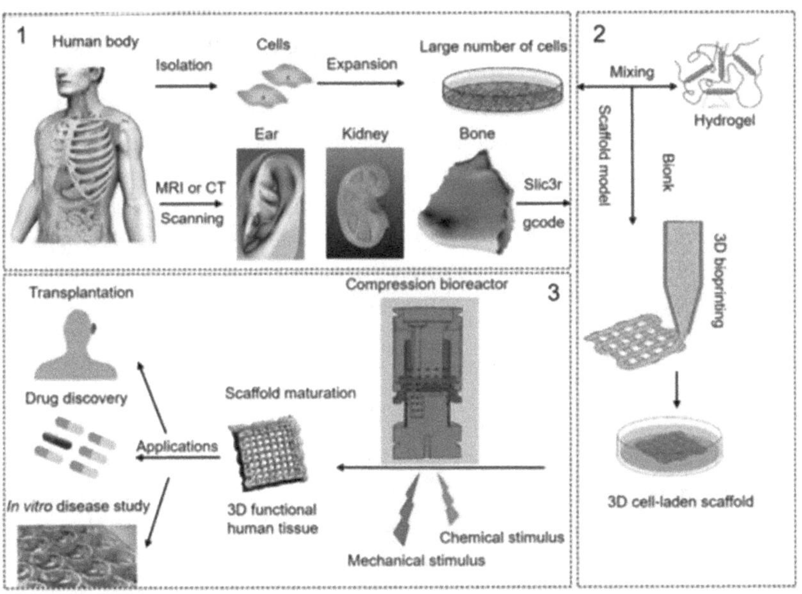

FIGURE 13.2 The processes of 3D bioprinting of human tissues.

13.2 BIOPRINTING TECHNIQUES

13.2.1 Inkjet-based Bioprinting

Originally outlined for printing texts and images with ordinary ink, inkjet printing has presently extended into inkjet bioprinting, which employs bio-inks composed of living cells and biomaterials in its applications of tissue designing and regenerative pharmaceuticals. Inkjet bioprinters generate complex tissue structures layer by layer, giving exact ways to produce biological tissues. Furthermore, inkjet bioprinters can be distinguished into two methods depending on the generation and ejection of bio-ink droplets. These two methods are drop-on-demand (DOD) inkjet printing and continuous inkjet printing (CIJ) [7,8].

CIJ bioprinters can ceaselessly discharge a flow of tiny droplets of ink via the nozzles. The electrostatic field charges and diverts selected droplets to form the wanted pattern, while the uncharged droplets are recycled back into the system. This technology can handle a varied range of ink viscosities and allows for fast printing. However, due to its complexity and the potential for damage to biological cells by constant ink flow and electrical fields, CIJ is not commonly applied in bioprinting. Furthermore, maintaining the viability and sterility of bio-inks also becomes challenging due to the continuous discharge and recycling process [7,8].

On the other hand, in DOD bioprinters, ink droplets can be generated when needed and the placement of the drop in the wanted area is accomplished by placing the drop originator directly above the wanted location before discharging a drop; this provides accurate control over droplet extent and precision. Therefore, DOD is better suited for bioprinting as it helps maintain viability and also helps conserve bio-inks. Thus, DOD bioprinting is favored over CIJ bioprinting because CIJ causes sterility problems with ink recirculation if the undesirable ink is rejected [7–9]. Depending on the actuation mechanism used to produce droplets, DOD bioprinting is divided into the following: (a) thermal inkjet printing and (b) piezoelectric inkjet printing (**Figure 13.3**).

Thermal inkjet bioprinters operate by heating an element that quickly heats the bio-ink, creating a vapor bubble as a result that expels a bio-ink drop from the nozzle. The element used in this method can reach temperatures of about 100–300 degrees Celsius. However, temperatures this high could potentially damage the cells, therefore limiting its use in applications where maintaining the integrity of the cell is paramount. Since thermal DOD is very cost-effective, its applications beyond the bounds of just bioprinting [8,9].

Piezoelectric-based inkjet bioprinters use the concept of acoustic waves to emit bio-ink. This process begins with the piezoelectric crystals in the printhead, which when exposed to an electric field undergo deformation. This deformation is responsible for the formation of acoustic waves that propagate within the ink. These waves are responsible for inducing local pressure fluctuations within the ink chamber. This causes accumulation in the nozzle which results in the expulsion of a minute droplet onto the substrate. This mechanism allows the formation of high degree of accuracy and control in drop formation which renders piezoelectric DOD printing well-suited for applications that require high precision and intricate details such as bioprinting [7,9].

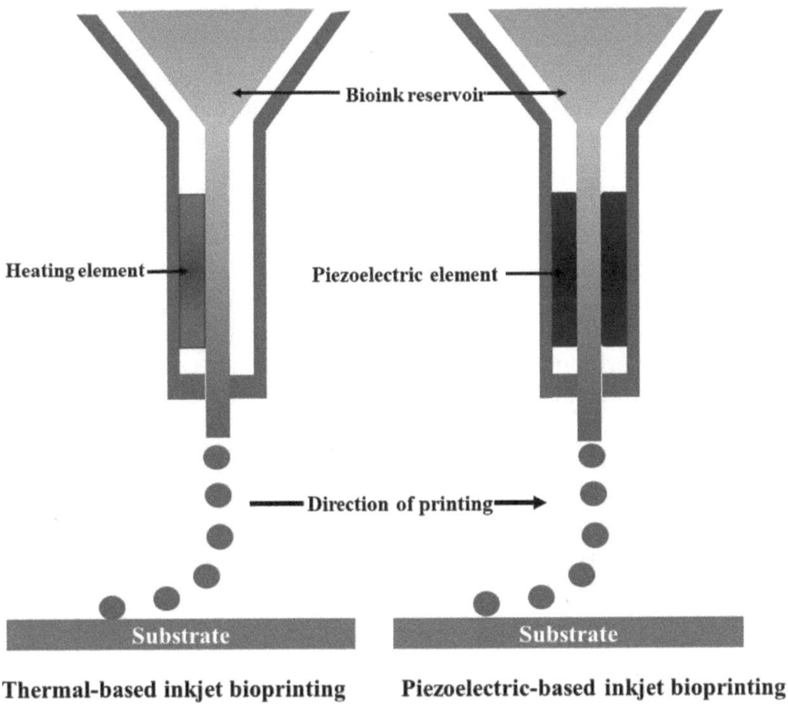

FIGURE 13.3 Inkjet-based bioprinting techniques.

13.2.2 Extrusion-based Bioprinting

Extrusion-based bioprinting is a 3D printing technology that is used in tissue engineering which involves an extrusion system to deposit bio-inks layer upon layer, which ultimately results in the creation of a 3D construct. The extrusion-based bioprinting technique has four essential components that work together to produce customized 3D structures with high accuracy and precision. The prominent parts of this system are a dispensing head containing a syringe loaded with the bio-ink and held at a proper temperature, the positional system that controls movement of the dispensing head in the x, y, and z directions, the printing platform with both positioning and temperature control, and a human interface where individuals can set down the pattern and temperature of deposition, together with other features [10]. Extrusion involves the use of pneumatic, piston, or screwing acting on a syringe to press down the bio-ink to form a 3D scaffold stratum by stratum on the printing platform [11]. Adjustable nozzles allow the creation of the micro-scale structures of different resolutions and complex structures to be achieved. The present method is suitable for constructing human-scale tissues in tissues engineering. The type of the printed substrate is very important as it absolutely determines the conditions that enable cells to grow, proliferate, differentiate, and organize into tissues. It is therefore important to consider the composition of the material in shape to enhance proper tissue engineering. It is evident that extrusion-based bioprinting has several merits; they include the capacity to develop bulk structures within a short time and at a very low cost. Because of that feature, it can be compatible with many forms of bio-inks: with living cells, polymers, and hydrogels [11]. In addition, this method of bioprinting also offers the benefits of a very high cell seeding concentration and an increase in speed of printing to allow scalability, which is very less harmful to the cells than other techniques [10] (**Figure 13.4**). Although extrusion-based bioprinting technology is better studied and established in practice, it has limitations. One of the most important limitations of this technology, as described in the literature, is its inability to create scaffolds using multiple materials. Especially, most of the tissues and organs are usually both heterogeneous and anisotropic, so it is necessary to make an appropriate analog. Another limitation is that the extrusion-based bioprinting technology can print only highly viscous materials to sustain the filament-like structure after deposition. During the printing process, a drop in pressure can cause apoptosis, which can be further minimized by optimization of process parameters, including material concentration, diameter, and nozzle pressure [11]. However, the resolution of the printing process is limited, with a range of approximately 200 μm, which is significantly lower than that of inkjet and laser-based bioprinting techniques. The extrusion-based technique is considered a promising technology in the field of tissue engineering [12].

13.2.3 Laser-based Bioprinting

In this rapidly evolving field of biomedical engineering, few technologies have attracted the interest and potential impact of laser bioprinting. This advanced method is poised to completely revolutionize how we approach the development and

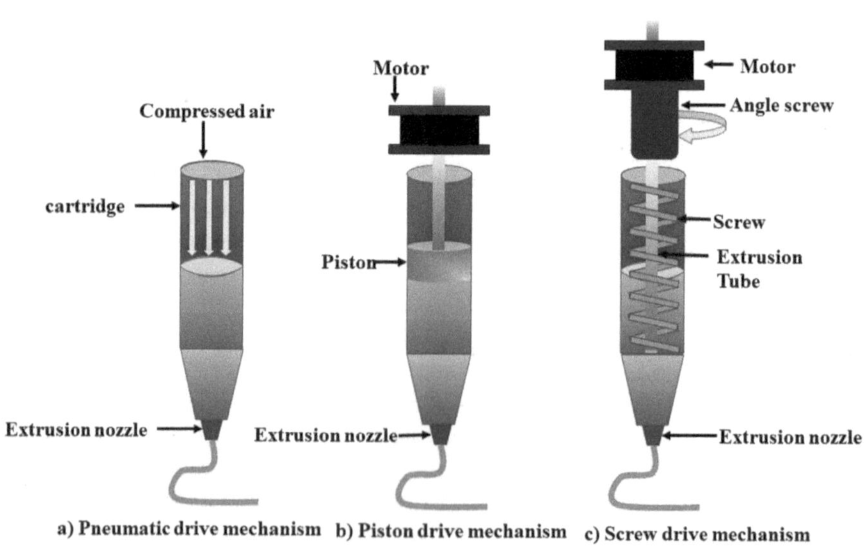

FIGURE 13.4 Extrusion-based bioprinting techniques.

revival of functional tissues and organs and lies at the intersection of advanced laser technology, biomedical sciences, and precision engineering. Laser-assisted bioprinting (LAB) and laser-induced forward transfer (LIFT) are two of the most frequently used techniques in laser-based bioprinting.

In the field of bioprinting, LAB is a sophisticated and accurate technique that uses biomaterials, growth factors, and living cells to deposit bio-inks. This technique is extremely valuable because it can produce very high resolution, complex biological structures with very high precision and detail [13,14].

LAB has three main components:

1. Laser generator
2. Laser path adjusting module
3. Cell transfer module

In the LAB process, the laser generators are the main source of energy. It emits laser light pulses with accurately controlled energy, duration, and wavelength. The range from nanosecond to femtosecond is where the majority of the pulses fall, which is important because it provides the exact amount of energy needed to transfer the bio-ink without heating up and injuring the cells (**Figure 13.5**). The accurate expulsion of bio-ink from the contributor to the acceptor substrate by the laser generator plays a key role in the LAB process [13,14].

The orientation and focusing of the laser ray onto specific areas of the contributor substrate is the responsibility of the laser path adjustment module. The module consists of a number of essential components: focusing optics to focus the laser beam on a specific location, galvanometric systems and mirrors for beam steering, and a computer-controlled positioning system to adhere to a digital model or pre-planned

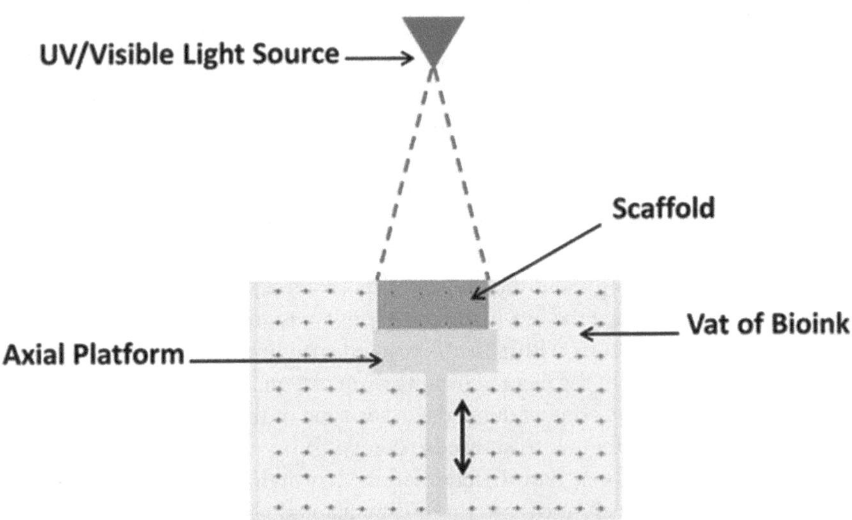

FIGURE 13.5 Laser-based bioprinting technique.

pattern. The precise control of this model is essential to achieve complex three-dimensional structures and high-resolution bioprinting [4,13–15].

Cell transfer modules include elements needed to transfer real bio-ink droplets. It consists of a transparent donor substrate, which has been covered by a thin layer of bio-ink and a layer absorbing laser light. The absorption layer quickly evaporates in contact with the laser pulse and forms a high-pressure bubble that propels the bio-ink drop toward the receiving substrate. These droplets are captured by the receiving substrate placed under the donor substrate. It can be moved or adjusted to help create the desired biological structure layer by layer, which ensures precise and regulated bio-ink deposition [13–15].

Laser bioprinting uses an advanced process known as laser-induced forward transfer (LIFT), which facilitates the precise bio-ink deposition of cells, growth factors, and biomaterials. Originally created for material sciences and microelectronics, LIFT has been adapted for biological applications and provides excellent resolution with less cell damage.

LIFT operates through a meticulously coordinated system comprising three primary components [15].

1. Pulsed Laser Source
2. Donor Substrate or Ribbon
3. Receiving Substrate

To recall, the laser source acts as a heat provider, though it supplies energy with the pulse duration of nanoseconds in most cases. This is important because the difference in temperatures helps to weakly interact and selectively heat the donor substrate while not causing thermal or heat damage to the biological cells and bio-ink. The laser source has to be fine-tuned so that each pulse is capable of initiating the transfer process without at the same time affecting the functionality of the bio-ink components [13–15]. The donor substrate, or ribbon, is a key component of the LIFT process and consists of two main layers: the laser-absorbing layer and the bio-ink layer. The laser absorbing layer, which is a fine polymer film or metal layer absorbs the laser energy, and the material of the layer gets heated and is vaporized at a very high surface area. This process creates a high-pressure bubble, and as was seen before, it offers the pressure needed to dispense the bio-ink. Laser transmitting layer resides in the next place, and it is covered with the layer of bio-ink which contains growth factors, biomaterials, and living cells required for constructing the tissue. The donor substrate design and the choice of its materials as well as their distribution significantly influence the bio-ink droplet transfer together with the viability and full functionality of the cells within the bioprinted structure [4,13–15]. The receiving substrate is used to collect the ejected bio-ink droplets, and it is placed perpendicular to the donor substrate. Its content depends on the type of tissue to be printed, its spatial organization, and function to showcase compatibility with bio-ink in promoting cell adhesion, proliferation, and differentiation. Normally, the receiving substrate is embedded in a relatively movable three-dimensional template which slides in to complement the z-axis of a pre-specified model or follows a pre-designed plan with a fair degree of accuracy. This movement allows for the controlled fabrication of

TABLE 13.1
Bioprinting Techniques—Main Application and Advantages and Disadvantages

3D Bioprinting Techniques	Advantages	Disadvantages	Applications	References
Inkjet-based Bioprinting	High resolution, high viability, and cost-effective	Limited to low-viscosity bio-inks, risk of nozzle clogging, droplet inconsistency, and limited to 2D and simple 3D structures	Tissue and organ printing, drug screening and testing, and cell patterning	[16]
Extrusion-based Bioprinting	Print with very high viscosity bio-inks, can create larger constructs, and is suitable for a wide range of biomaterials	Lower resolution compared to inkjet and laser bioprinting, slower printing speed, and high shear stress may affect cell viability, and risk of nozzle clogging	Organ fabrication, bone and cartilage regeneration, and complex tissue structure regeneration	[17]
Laser-based Bioprinting	High-cell viability, high resolution, and no nozzle clogging	Potential heat damage to cells, limited scalability, limited bio-ink viscosity, and complex setup and maintenance	Skin and nerve regeneration, micro-scale-tissue structures, and high-precision tissue constructs	[18]

multilayered 3D structures. In the LIFT process, the receiving substrate is significant because it has the responsibility for positioning the droplets correctly to form the appropriate biological constructions [13–15]. The main application and advantages and disadvantages of bioprinting techniques are listed in **Table 13.1**.

13.3 MECHANISM FOR GRAFTING ORGANS

The best course of treatment for advanced organ damage and diseases is organ transplantation. However, it has drawbacks such as immunosuppressive medication side effects, immune rejection risks, and a lack of available donors. Thus, 3D bioprinting technology combined with tissue engineering-based organ regeneration and repair offers a promising substitute [19]. Growth and differentiation cues, biomaterials, and cells are used to create new organs (**Figure 13.6**). The mechanism includes cell selection, biomaterial design, bioprinting, in vitro cultivation, pre-transplant assessment, and transplantation.

13.3.1 Cell Selection

The essential step in the tissue engineering procedure is selecting the appropriate cell source when manufacturing an organ transplant. Depending on the organ that needs to be created, one can choose from primary cells, iPSC-derived cells or

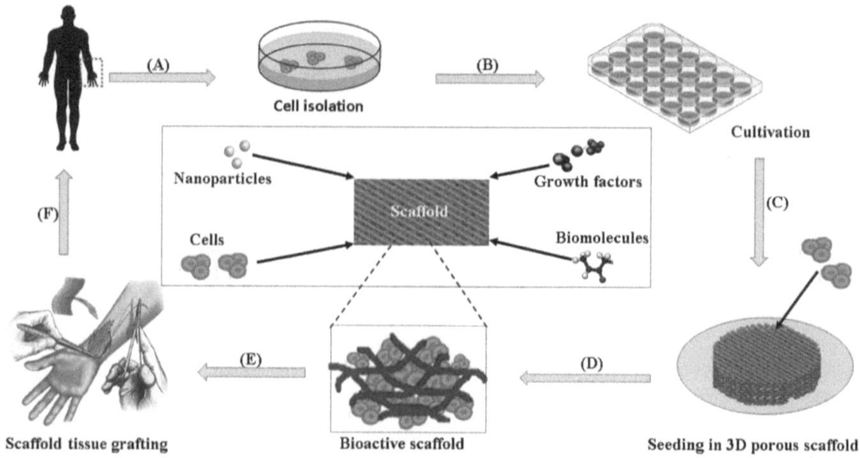

FIGURE 13.6 Mechanism of organ grafting.

embryo-derived cells. The principal goal is to get the necessary number of cells with the required differentiation ability to create the required tissue structure [20,21].

13.3.2 Biomaterial Design

Biomaterials are critical in offering support for the basic framework, biocompatibility, and a suitable environment for the generation of organs that are required in tissue engineering. Therefore, the compatibility of the host is an important criterion when determining biomaterials. Further, they promote cell attachment, proliferation rates, and differentiation of various cells. From the bio-inks, polymers, hydrogels, and ceramic-based materials have been found relevant for fabrication as discussed by researchers [22,23].

13.3.3 Bioprinting

Bioprinting is the process of layering cell and material with precision to develop artificial biological tissues. This process makes it possible to generate the tissues constructed with the actual anatomy that matches the recipient's shape and size depending on the imaging data. Some of the most fundamental strategies of bioprinting are suspension-based bioprinting such as extrusion bioprinting and laser-based bioprinting and inkjet-based bioprinting [12,24,25].

13.3.4 In Vitro Cultivation

Subsequent to bioprinting, the construct is cultured under in vitro conditions to encourage differentiation, integration, and functional maturation. In this stage, the environment of the culture media resembles the physiological conditions of the described organ in the body. There is adherence to stringent physiological and aseptic requirements throughout the cultivation process [26].

13.3.5 Pre-Transplant Assessment

In addition to biophysical assessment, before transplanting the engineered tissue each patient undergoes functional assessment to ensure the quality of the transplanted engineered tissue. Histology, immunological tests, and mechanical tests, among others, are methods that are employed. Mechanical testing determines the organ's structural and mechanical characteristics of under physiological conditions. Histological assessment looks into the distribution of cells and the makeup of the organ tissue, and the immunological test checks the compatibility of the end organ construct with that of the immunophenotype of the recipient [20,27].

13.3.6 Transplantation

The last step of tissue engineering is the implantation of the engineered organ, which on the same lines as organ transplantation is done under aseptic environment in an operating theatre. The use of organ transplantation is promoted by the choice of biomaterials, cells, and bioprinting methods and by optimizing the conditions for in vitro cultures [28].

The outcomes of an organ transplant are based on the nature of the cells to be transplanted, the biomaterials that can be used, and the ability to fabricate the organ. Some of the emerging issues include the following: establishing vasculature, the host immune response, and tissue remodeling [29]. Development of a vascular network is essential for supporting the engineered organ by providing nutrients while throwing out products from the tissues. When properly managed, transplant failure resulting from immune rejection is a preventable aspect. Furthermore, tissue maturation is critical in the long-term success of the organ and effective functional properties of the tissues by enhancing the delivery of nutrients and oxygen to the cultivated tissues [30].

Bioprinting holds great promise for tissue engineering-based organ transplantation, as it can decrease waiting times for grafting, enhance safety, and lessen dependency on organ donors [31]. However, the success of this strategy depends on advancements in biomaterials, bioprinting technology, and safe and effective engraftment of functional tissue in vivo without causing any adverse effects.

13.4 KEY COMPONENTS IN TISSUE ENGINEERING

13.4.1 Scaffolds

A scaffold is a 3D structure that assists as a model or temporary framework to support the cells and guide them to grow and develop into functional tissues and organs. Artificial scaffolds are manufactured and used for the culturing of cells and cell growth domination in repairing injured tissues and organs. The scaffold helps during the process of cell regeneration temporarily and degrades slowly in the progression of the curative process, and a freshly prepared tissue having the desired properties and the desired shape is produced [32]. This property of degradability of the scaffolds allows the prevention of any severe side effects that can develop from the remaining external materials in the body after the whole process (**Figure 13.7**). Thus, the applied scaffold must meet definite mechanical, physical, and chemical

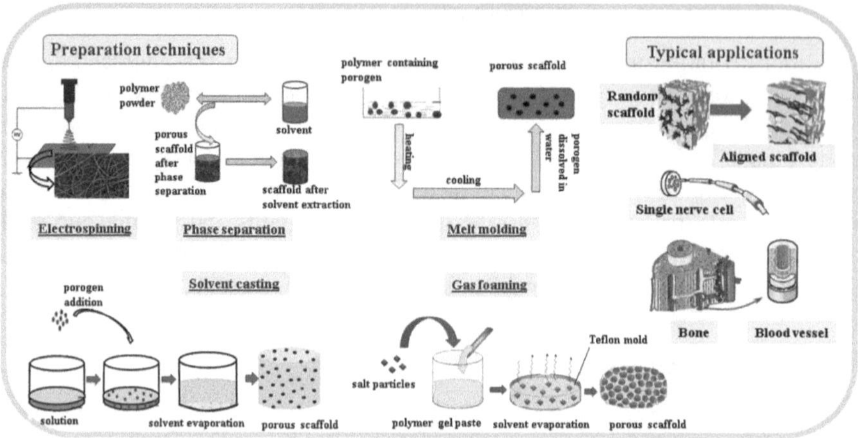

FIGURE 13.7 Preparation technique for scaffolds and their applications.

requirements to facilitate sufficient diffusion of cells and ensure the successful formation of 3D tissue [12]. Scaffold preparation techniques and their advantages, disadvantages, and applications are summarized in **Table 13.2**. Scaffolds are fundamental components used in tissue engineering, and therefore, they must possess certain attributes:

a) They should have interconnected pores with appropriate-sized passageways that support tissue integration and vascularization [33].
b) The scaffold must be biocompatible, which ensures that the implant does not negatively impact the host tissue, and biodegradable to facilitate new tissue formation [34].
c) They should have vigorous mechanical properties to provide an optimal environment for cell growth, support the necessary materials and cell distribution up to the target spot, and generate signals to regulate the composition and functions of the newly formed tissue [32].
d) The scaffold must have the appropriate surface chemistry that promotes cellular attachment, differentiation, and propagation [35].
e) The scaffold should partially resemble the biological role and composition of the extracellular matrix [36].

Various techniques are used to fabricate scaffolds and to enable the engineering of functional tissues and organs with 3D structures. These methods facilitate cell distribution and lead the cell growth to a 3D space (**Figure 13.7**). The chief techniques for the fabrication of these scaffolds are described here.

13.4.1.1 Electrospinning

Electrospinning is a highly popular approach among the various methods used to fabricate scaffolds for creating nano/micro-scale fibrous networks. This technique

TABLE 13.2
caffold Preparation Techniques, and their Advantages, Disadvantages and Applications

Methods	Advantages	Disadvantages	Applications	References
Electro-Spinning	High porosity, great ratio of surface area to its volume	Polymer limited range	Engineering of skin, nerve, and cardiac tissue, bone	[36]
Solvent Casting Method	Moderate porosity, easy method	Small pore size	Engineering of vascular tissues	[40]
Phase-Separation Method	Incorporation of the bioactive agents is possible into the structure	Problems with residual solvents	Drug release and delivery of protein	[41]
Gas Foaming	High porosity, biocompatible, and cost-effective	Closed pore structure, solid polymeric skin	Tissue engineering of bone and cartilage	[32]
Melt Molding	Versatility and inexpensive	Limited control of pore size, weak interconnectivity	Bone, cartilage, and nerve regeneration	[39]

uses electricity to make fibers from a solution [32]. The electrospinning process is controlled by imperiling a polymer solution of very high intensity between two electrodes with opposite charges to an electric field where in the polymer solution onc electrode gets placed, and another electrode is located in the accumulator. Typically, owing to the pumping of the solution, the droplets are formed. Subsequently, a force is induced with the generation of the electric field that allows the drops to overcome the surface tension of the solution, forming a jet of polymer that produces fibers. At the same time, the solvent begins evaporating owing to jet formation, continuing after the release of nanofibers on the collector [37].

13.4.1.2 Solvent Casting

The use of solvent casting for scaffold preparation is a modest, easy, and cost-effective way that does not require large equipment. The process involves evaporation of a solvent to form scaffolds using two methods. The first method is the dipping of mold in a polymeric solution, and a sufficient period of time is provided for the solution to get drawn off, which results in the creation of a film of polymeric sheath. The second method requires the addition of the polymeric solution to the mold and providing enough time for the evaporation of the solvent to create a film of polymeric sheath that sticks to the mold [34,38].

13.4.1.3 Phase Separation

The phase separation method requires a change in the temperature that parts the polymeric solution into two phases. The first phase contains a low concentration of the polymer (polymer-lean phase), while the second phase is a polymer-rich phase. The polymer is mixed with naphthalene or phenol, and molecules that are biologically active are dispersed in the solution. The fluid phase is separated by dropping the temperature down and gets solidified into a two-phase solid. Then the solvent gets detached from the scaffold using abstraction, vanishing, or sublimation, resulting in porous scaffolds containing integrated bioactive molecules [35].

13.4.1.4 Gas Foaming

The gas foaming system utilizes carbon dioxide gas under high pressure to fabricate highly absorbent scaffolds. The porous construction and absorbency of scaffold are directly proportional to the amount of carbon dioxide gas that is liquefied in a polymer. In this process, the highly absorbent polymer is bare to carbon dioxide gas at a very high pressure (800 psi) to soak the polymer along with the carbon dioxide gas [37]. The dissolved carbon dioxide gas becomes uneven under such conditions and splits from the polymer. The result will be the formation of carbon dioxide gas molecule clusters, which diminish free energy and create pore nucleation. These pores generate a substantial expansion in the size of the polymer and a reduction in the density of the polymer. After completion of the foaming process, a 3D porous structure, i.e., scaffold is formed [39].

13.4.1.5 Melt Molding

The melt molding process for scaffold fabrication includes a mixture of PLGA powder and gelation microspheres filled into a Teflon mold of a defined diameter. The mold is heated directly above the glass conversion temperature of PLGA meanwhile smearing pressure onto the mixture, causing the PLGA particles to attach. Afterward, the mold is detached, and the gelatine microspheres are dissolved by submerging the mixture in water, resulting in the formation of a scaffold that is later dried [22].

13.4.2 Bio-Inks

In addition to the advancements in the technologies of 3D bioprinting, printable hydrogels are the bio-inks, playing an essential role in generating functional tissue. Bio-inks are the building blocks of 3D bioprinting, enabling the accurate placement and cell culture within the scaffold [42]. Bio-inks comprise biocompatible hydrogels that provide a 3D microenvironment to the cells for cell growth and cell differentiation. The bio-inks are easy to customize to match the exact requirements of the target tissue like stiffness, porosity, and rate of degradation, to confirm optimal cell growth and function [43] (**Figure 13.8**).

For 3D bioprinting, several factors need to be considered for proper assessment if it will be a good tool for tissue regeneration. Such factors include the ability of bio-ink to bind with cross-linkers and chemical reagents, the capability of subjecting mechanical stresses during the printing process, ability of the post-print culture medium to support cell nutrient requirements, the accuracy of shape reproduction, and printability, respectively [44]. These three aspects affect cell

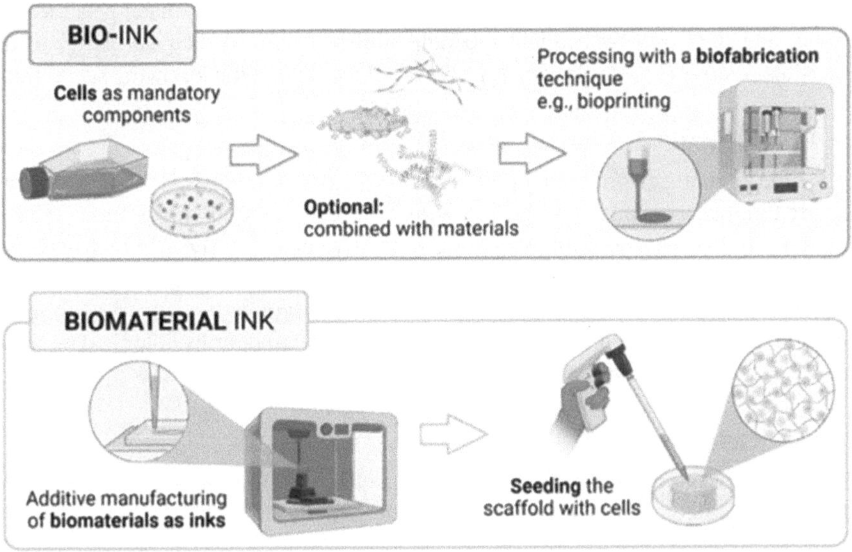

FIGURE 13.8 Bio-ink and biomaterial ink.

behavior and the overall properties of the printed structure as a whole. Specifically, the viscosity and deformability of the bio-ink are especially important for the stability of the shape and structural quality of the printed sample, which is the main determinant of printability. A major challenge of 3D cell printing is to obtain a very good shape fidelity yet applying a minimal injection force to avoid cell death. Also, viscoelastic properties are considered as the basic parameters that define the functional characteristics of bio-inks. Bio-ink viscoelastic properties prevent surface tension from impacting the layers' cohesion and enable adhesion. A storage modulus (G′) that modulates over time is needed to show that the bio-ink is behaving in a more solid-like fashion and capable of storing energy. Consequently, elastic storage modulus, G′, viscoelastic loss modulus, G″, and loss tangent, G″/G′ convey characteristics of the bio-ink, including liquid profile, printability, and cell integration. These rheological properties are important for the successful implementation of bio-inks in bioprinting for tissue engineering [45]. Another important benefit that bio-inks derived from plant sources can constitute is the potential for producing scaffolds with complex shapes and details that have been difficult, or impossible, to accomplish through conventional scaffolding methods. These characteristics make it possible to achieve highly controlled cell positioning and also high-resolution deposition of the biomaterials, thereby enabling the fabrication of highly elaborate final scaffold structures [46]. Bio-inks usually contain diverse biomaterials and growth factors which need to fulfill certain criteria to allow tissue compatibility. These biomaterials should not elicit an undesirable immune response and must be biodegradable to allow for safe degradation and expelling without formation of toxic products. The majority of the standard bio-inks are made from both synthetic and native polymers [42].

Natural polymers are obtained from biological sources, like alginate, gelatine, and chitosan, and they possess brilliant biocompatibility owing to their similarity to the extracellular matrix (ECM). These polymers are elaborated in the following subsections.

13.4.2.1 Alginate

It is a type of natural polymer obtained from brunet seaweeds. It is a polymeric structure that has a negative charge, allowing it to form ionically cross-linked chains by combining it with a solution which has a positive charge. Alginate hydrogels are extensively used in innumerable biomedical submissions owing to their biocompatibility, low toxicity, and cost-effectiveness. However, alginate bio-inks are limited in relation to their ability to maintain long-term constancy under physiological environments because they rely on ionic cross-linking [47].

13.4.2.2 Gelatine

It is a natural polymer obtained from connective tissues of animals, which is classified into two categories based on their processing method:

a) Gelatine obtained through acid treatment and
b) Gelatine produced through alkaline treatment

These types of gelatine exhibit unique properties, such as showing both negative and positive charges, respectively, at a neutral pH and only the gelatine produced through alkaline treatment had lower gel strength and better biocompatibility when compared to the gelatine obtained through acid treatment [46]. Both types of gelatine have various applications in tissue engineering as biomaterials for the manufacturing of bio-inks.

13.4.2.3 Chitosan

Chitosan possesses advantageous properties like biocompatibility, decomposability, and antimicrobial activity, which makes it highly compatible for engineering numerous tissues like the liver, cartilage, bone, and skin [48–50]. The solvability of chitosan varies with pH, and its bio-ink is very easy to get gelled under neutral conditions at a temperature of 40°C, thus making chitosan a suitable material for 3D bioprinting [1].

Synthetic polymers are chemically synthesized and are a valuable resource for creating bio-inks, as they are accurately deposited with excellent mechanical strength and high fidelity.

- **Polycaprolactone:** PCL (polycaprolactone) is a flexible and biocompatible polyester material that cannot be used to encapsulate cells owing to its melting and dissolving when exposed to organic solvents or melted, which are destructive to living cells. However, its stability, comparatively low melting point (~60°C), and long-term deprivation properties have made it a popular choice for applications in the field of tissue engineering using bioprinting technology [46].
- **Polyethylene glycol:** Hydrophilic, non-immunogenic, biocompatible, and protein-resistant PEG is one of the most popular polymers used in 3D

bioprinting. Due to its good water soluble property and hydrophilic nature, it can be used as a sacrificial bio-ink in tissue engineering [51].

13.4.2.4 Polyvinyl Alcohol

Polyvinyl alcohol is a synthetic polymer that is soluble in water and is used predominantly in bio-ink preparation. PVA has certain advantages that are desirable for 3D bioprinting: It has very low cytotoxicity, shows high biocompatibility, and possesses superior mechanical properties, and flexible mechanical properties that make it suitable for 3D bioprinting. Furthermore, regarding procedure, since PVA can be sterilized using various ways, including UV or chemical cross-linking, makes it more suitable and in high demand for tissue engineering [45].

13.4.3 Hydrogels

It is also known that hydrogels have some specific characteristics that are similar to the ECM, and thus it is an element of TE. Hydrogels' mechanical similarity to natural tissues, ease of implantation, and high-water saturation have all contributed to their being one of the most actively researched biomaterials in the field. Due to their unique properties, hydrogels are at the forefront of fostering tissue regeneration, scaffold design, supporting cell attachment, and drug carrier design [52–55]. To ensure biocompatibility and imitate the ECM of native tissues, the use of materials of natural origins has significantly advanced the field, although early natural materials often did not provide adequate indications for cell differentiation toward the formation of new tissues. The first generation of hydrogels of natural origin are no longer relevant and are no longer used due to the integration of technological advances such as nanotechnology [56], 3D printing, and micro fluids. To meet the specific needs of tissues, use cutting-edge methods, and leverage the inherent qualities of natural-based materials, new hydrogels have emerged over the past decade [57–60].

Natural hydrogels made from biological sources have good bioactivity and biocompatibility. Examples of these hydrogels are hyaluronic acid, collagen, gelatine, and alginate. These materials are useful because they naturally have bioactive molecules and cell binding sites that facilitate cell–matrix interactions. On the contrary, specific mechanical and chemical properties can be manufactured into synthetic hydrogels like polyacrylamide (PA), polyethylene glycol (PEG), and polyvinyl alcohol (PVA). This flexibility allows customization to meet the unique needs of different types of tissues, ranging from more rigid structures such as bones to more soft tissues such as cartilage and skin, as shown in **Figure 13.9** [57–60].

The adjustable mechanical properties of hydrogel are the main advantages in the field of tissue engineering. To accurately match the mechanical environment of the target tissue, hydrogels can control their elasticity, stiffness, and degradation rate. It is essential to ensure that the scaffold provides sufficient support during the early stages of tissue formation and degrades at a pace that coincides with the development of new tissue is imperative. For example, hydrogels used for nerve generation can be made more flexible and supportive of cell growth, while hydrogels intended for cartilage repair can be made to withstand compressive forces [57–61].

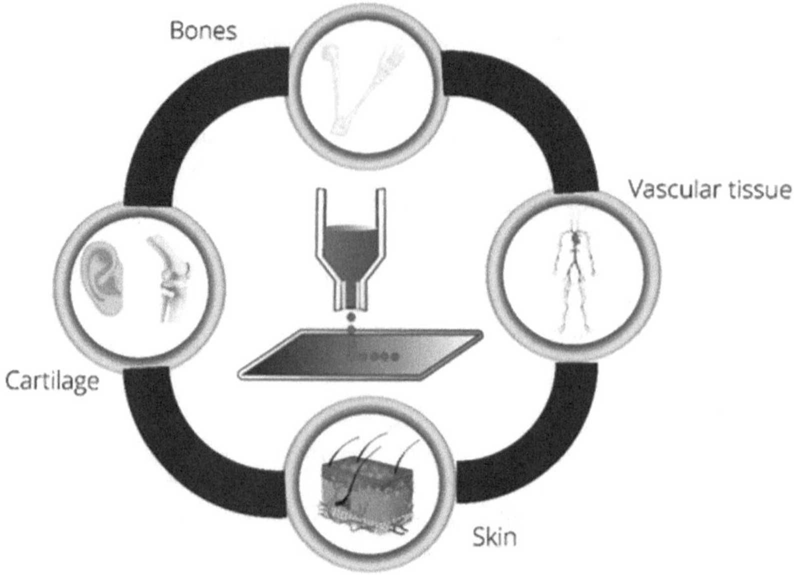

FIGURE 13.9 Hydrogels-based bio-ink applications.

Among the SRFs, hydrogels are particularly suited to cell encapsulation, as the appendages provide a secure environment that can also actively support the health and growth of the cells. By encapsulating cells within hydrogels, we attain equal or better distribution of cells throughout the scaffold as well as a chance to shield the cells from mechanical stress, which is paramount especially when developing sophisticated tissues, where homogenous cell organization of the scaffold is paramount. Hydrogels can also be engineered for the uptake and release of nutrients to the encapsulated cells to feed them and support their roller growth as well as functional nutrients [57–60]. The final benefit of hydrogels is evident also in their ability to encapsulate bioactive molecules like growth factors, cytokines, or signaling proteins to be released in a controlled manner. This specific delivery system is crucial in an organ/tissue repair process due to the possibility of maintaining the constant regeneration process. Thereby, introducing bioactive compounds into the matrix of hydrogel provides a favorable condition for tissue formation and the differentiation of cells [57–60].

Progress in this area has really improved the place of hydrogels in tissue engineering. Current technologies like three-dimensional bioprinting have made it easy to achieve spatial deposition of hydrogel layers and the cells contained therein and flexible tissue constructs. Moreover, the synthesis of intelligent hydrogels capable of reverting to new stimulation modes, including temperature, pH, or specific biomolecules, ensures timely delivery of support needed by the changing tissue. These advances demonstrate the continuous development of hydrogel applications and their growing significance in regenerative medicine [4,57–61].

13.4.4 Cell Source

With its innovative approach to organ replacement and tissue repair, tissue engineering holds tremendous potential for the field of regenerative medicine. Choosing the right cell sources is critical for tissue engineering to be effective because it decides the viability of the tissue engineering techniques since they impact the function, integration, and structure of the engineered tissue. The ongoing innovations in the fields of stem cells, genetic engineering, and cell biology have attributed a basis for modern cell-driven approaches for the tissue regeneration and treatment feasibility. To overcome tissue engineering's inborn challenges such as scalability, immune rejection, and functionality and provide the path for the creation of cutting-edge therapeutic solutions, the cautious selection and applications of diverse cell sources is fundamental [16,17,62–67].

The application of essential cells—both autologous and allogenic—in tissue engineering applications has been explored in recent research. Immunocompatibility and a lower chance of dismissal are two benefits of autologous primary cells. However, troubles with cell sourcing, expansion, and donor cell morbidity emphasize the need for distinctive approaches. Allogenic primary cells provide adaptability when obtained from donors within the same species, in any case, immunomodulation is essential to prevent rejection. Tissue-specific progenitor cells and induced pluripotent stem cells (iPSCs) are two profoundly successful strategies that show promise that tends to these issues and advanced customized regenerative therapies. The integration and usefulness of the engineered tissues can be enhanced by optimizing the cell sources. It is possible to significantly improve tissue regeneration capabilities and cell viability by combining primary cells with modern biomaterial scaffolds. Through the utilization of the inherent characteristics of primary cells in conjunction with inventive biomaterials, analysts can create more effective and dependable tissue engineering approaches. This technique creates new opportunities for the creation of personalized regenerative medicines in addition to addressing the downside of using primary cells [16,17,62–67].

Because of their regeneration capability, stem cells—in particular, iPSCs and mesenchymal stem cells (MSCs) have picked up a lot of attention (**Figure 13.10**). MSCs have immunomodulatory qualities and the capacity to distinction into cell abstractions. They are gained from several sources, such as bone marrow, adipose tissue, and umbilical cord blood. The ability of MSCs to treat various ailments and wounds highlights the need of standardized strategies to ensure the quality and therapeutic efficacy of MSCs in clinical settings. MScs are the imperative cell source used in numerous therapeutic applications due to their capacity to impact immune responses and encourage tissue repair. Conversely, the benefit of patient-specific iPSCs is that the chance of immunological rejection is diminished. Reprogrammed somatic cells are the source of iPSCs, which are viable instrument for tissue engineering since they can distinguish into any kind of cell. The pluripotency and patient-specific characteristics of iPSCs make them tremendously promising, but for clinical translation, problems with their genetic stability and differentiation efficacy need to be resolved. Research into enhancing reprogramming methods and boosting differentiation protocol dependability is vital to ensure the secure and effective use of iPSCs [16,17,62–67].

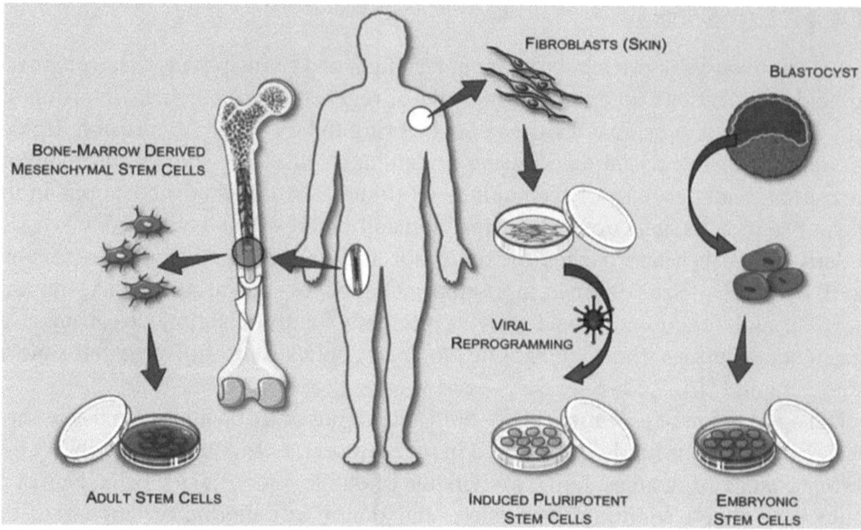

FIGURE 13.10 Stem cells for 3D bioprinting.

Applications for tissue engineering have illustrated a great deal of guarantee for tissue-specific progenitor cells, such as satellite cells in skeletal muscle and neural progenitor cells in the CNS (central nervous system). Since they adhere to particular lineages, these cells function well and integrate more effectively into the target tissues. The commitment of these cells to specific ancestries can rally their integration and usefulness within the intended tissues. Ideally in atherosclerosis, more efficient isolation and expansion techniques play a vital role in boosting therapeutic significance of tissue-specific progenitor cells that have potential utility in muscular dystrophy and neurodegenerative diseases. Altogether, understanding of these cells' properties makes it possible to create individual treatment programs that will yield better results in treating pathological processes in tissues striking patients with damage or degenerative diseases. The growth factors delivery systems, the biomaterial scaffolds, the techniques of isolation have improved the viability of tissue-specific progenitor cells for clinical use as per requirement [68]. These are basic stem cells that have inherent potential for the differentiation into required form of cells within the native tissues, hence their use for accurate and efficient tissue regeneration is the most effective strategy [16,17,62–67].

The availability of gene editing via CRISPR Cas 9 and related systems has opened the door to engineered cell source development with even enhanced attributes. Solutions to problems like immune typical matching or the scarcity of suitable natural cell resources exist through genetically engineered cells. To improve efficiency of tissue engineering, researchers are able to directly manipulate cells to activate certain genes or to activate immunity to immune system. The major challenges that face tissue engineering today include the speed at which natural cells die and issues to do with the immune system. In addition, there is evidence of supplementing engineered cells with artificial cell–cell communication systems with increasing the ability of cells within tissue constructs. By following this strategy, different forms of relationships between cells can be closely controlled—this is known to be of tremendous importance for tissue and organ formation. Therefore, through the establishment of communication channels, researchers can reconstruct tissue-simulating natural environments, resulting in the development of more complex and functional tissue constructs and enhancing the efficiency of the stereotyped tissue engineering therapies [16,17,62–67].

13.5 FUTURE CHALLENGES AND DIRECTIONS

However, for all its potential, there are at least five issues that remain to be discussed and still have no clear solutions. One of the great challenges can be the selection of appropriate biomaterials for the bioprinting process. Such materials have to be biocompatible, in terms of their mechanical properties, as well as to allow the cells to reproduce and grow. Even though existing biomaterials, like hydrogels, have potential, more modern and complicated materials that can imitate human tissue are still required [21]. Analysts in material science, biology, and chemistry must work together to form modern biomaterials [69–71]. Expanding the process's size to produce large structures appropriate for clinical use is another challenge in bioprinting. Small research facilities have found success with bioprinting; but, scaling up to larger structures is troublesome. Innovative print heads and printing strategies will be required to achieve this. Besides, it is required to improve the rationality of cells in tissues that are bioprinted [72]. Less cell reasonability can emerge from the bioprinting handle's complexity, which can harm cells. The advancement of cutting-edge methods that diminish cell damage and increase cell reasonability is vital for the success of bioprinting [73].

A striking challenge in bioprinting is accomplishing the vascularization of bioprinting tissues. Organs and other complex tissues require a variety of blood vessels to supply their cells with nutrients and oxygen. One of the major challenges confronting the tissue-building industry may be connecting blood vessels in bioprinted tissues [27]. Besides, regulatory approval presents another critical obstacle for the bioprinting industry. To enable their interpretation into clinical applications, bioprinted tissues' administrative process, and security considerations must be completely caught on. In spite of these obstacles, bioprinting has critical potential in tissue design, medication testing, and illness modeling [74]. Also, since bioprinting offers tissues and organs for transplantation, it can totally change the field of reformative medicine. Ending the discarding of donor tissue could be a critical advantage of bioprinting over traditional transplantation methods [20]. Individualized bioprinted tissues match the type of tissue in each person, reducing the risk associated with the resistant structure.

Future directions in bioprinting will involve analyzing the opportunities of underutilized blinks, like stem cells and nanomaterials [69]. With developments in mechanical properties, nanomaterials like graphene oxide hold potential for making high-resolution bioprinted structures [73,75]. Moreover, stem cells get distinguished into numerous types of cells, which may give a solution to the constrained accessibility of cell sources for bioprinting. Also, researchers are looking to utilize bioprinted tissues for personalized drug delivery, in which the bioprinted tissue would function as an in vitro model that could expect drug responses exclusive to each patient [20].

Bioprinting complex organs like the liver or heart is another area of future bioprinting research. An essential organ, the liver is accountable for vital functions like manufacturing bile and processing toxins [25]. Due to its intricate structure and need to connect blood vessels, bioprinting a functional liver is troublesome. Another difficult organ to print is the heart, which has an intricate network of blood vessels and sophisticated pumping mechanism. That is why, bioprinting of the functional human heart may help to solve the problem of the lack of donor hearts for transplantation [76].

13.6 CONCLUSION

This chapter focuses on the roles of both the important progresses and the application of 3D bioprinting technology and the corresponding roles in the regenerative medicine field. The use of the bioprinting methods has implications which are discussed here. For tissue bioengineering and to guarantee tissue functionality, there should be control over the process of organ engraftment since the process is complicated and necessitates a well-controlled setting. Achieving tissue engineering success depends on the application of hydrogels, bio-inks, and scaffold architectures. Hydrogels keep cells in a moist condition important for their living state, bio-inks help place cells and other supporting substances into appropriate positions, scaffolds enable structural support and mimic the cells' native ECM (extracellular matrix) [16,17,62–65].

A crucial step in the tissue engineering process is the selection of cell source. The variety of cell sources offer advantages and disadvantages. These sources comprise tissue-specific progenitor cells, engineered cell lines, primary cells, and stem cells. Allogenic cells offer scalability but need to be immunomodulator, whereas primary cells and autologous sources offer immunological compatibility. Substantial regenerative potential is established by stem cells, such as mesenchymal stem cells (MSCs) and induced pluripotent stem cells (iPSCs). Engineered cells provide desired properties for optimized tissue engineering which is enabled by gene editing technologies, while tissue-specific progenitor cells augment functionality and integration [16,17,62–65].

Scalability issues, improving the mechanical and biocompatibility qualities of bioprinted constructs, and navigating ethical and legal issues are some of the field's upcoming challenges. To overcome these obstacles and open the door to more efficient and practically applicable tissue engineering solutions, further developments in bioprinting technologies, cellular biology, and biomaterials are imperative [16,17,62–65].

With its unparalleled potential to create personalized, efficient tissues and organs, 3D bioprinting is at the vanguard of tissue engineering. Regenerative medicine could be completely transformed by combining cutting-edge bioprinting methods, cutting-edge biomaterials, and a thorough grasp of cellular biology. To fully realize the promise of 3D bioprinting's full potential, the transfer of these discoveries from the laboratory to clinical settings, and the renewal of hope for patients suffering from a variety of illnesses depend on ongoing research and bio-disciplinary cooperation [16,17,62–65].

REFERENCES

[1] Fatimi A, Okoro OV, Podstawczyk D, et al. Natural hydrogel-based bio-inks for 3d bioprinting in tissue engineering: A review. *Gels*. 2022;8(3):179.

[2] Derakhshanfar S, Mbeleck R, Xu K, et al. 3D bioprinting for biomedical devices and tissue engineering: A review of recent trends and advances. *Bioact Mater*. 2018:144–56.

[3] Saini G, Segaran N, Mayer JL, et al. Applications of 3d bioprinting in tissue engineering and regenerative medicine. J Clin Med. 2021;10(21):4966.

[4] Zandrini T, Florczak S, Levato R, et al. Breaking the resolution limits of 3D bioprinting: Future opportunities and present challenges. *Trends Biotechnol*. 2023;41:604–14.

[5] Lee JY, Lee H, Jin EJ, et al. 3D bioprinting using a new photo-crosslinking method for muscle tissue restoration. *NPJ Regen Med*. 2023;8.

[6] Sharma S, Kaur H, Thakur M, et al. *Engineering 2D Nanomaterials for Biomedical Applications. 2D Nanomater*. John Wiley & Sons, Ltd; 2024. pp. 333–60.

[7] Saunders RE, Derby B. Inkjet printing biomaterials for tissue engineering: Bioprinting. *Int Mater Rev*. 2014;59(8):430–48.

[8] Wu D, Xu C. Predictive modeling of droplet formation processes in inkjet-based bioprinting. *J Manuf Sci Eng Trans ASME*. 2018;140.

[9] Kačarević ŽP, Rider PM, Alkildani S, et al. An introduction to 3D bioprinting: Possibilities, challenges and future aspects. *Materials (Basel)*. 2018;11(11):2199.

[10] You F, Eames BF, Chen X. Application of extrusion-based hydrogel bioprinting for cartilage tissue engineering. *Int J Mol Sci*. 2017;18:8–14.

[11] Rider P, Kačarević ŽP, Alkildani S, et al. Bioprinting of tissue engineering scaffolds. J Tissue Eng. 2018;9:2041731418802090.

[12] Vaezi M, Zhong G, Kalami H, et al. Extrusion-based 3D printing technologies for 3D scaffold engineering. In *Functional 3D Tissue Engineering Scaffolds Materials, Technologies and Applications*. Elsevier Ltd; 2018.

[13] Dou C, Perez V, Qu J, et al. A state-of-the-art review of laser-assisted bioprinting and its future research trends. *Chem Bio Eng Rev*. 2021;8:517–34.

[14] Ventura RD. An overview of laser-assisted bioprinting (LAB) in tissue engineering applications. *Med Lasers*. 2021;10:76–81.

[15] Chang J, Sun X. Laser-induced forward transfer based laser bioprinting in biomedical applications. *Front Bioeng Biotechnol*. 2023;11:1–11.

[16] Naderi H, Matin MM, Bahrami AR. Review paper: Critical issues in tissue engineering: Biomaterials, cell sources, angiogenesis, and drug delivery systems. *J Biomater Appl*. 2011;26:383–417.

[17] Ullah I, Subbarao RB, Rho GJ. Human mesenchymal stem cells—Current trends and future prospective. *Biosci Rep*. 2015;35.

[18] Wang HM, Hung CH, Lu SN, et al. Liver stiffness measurement as an alternative to fibrotic stage in risk assessment of hepatocellular carcinoma incidence for chronic hepatitis C patients. *Liver Int*. 2013;33:756–61.

[19] Mengel M, Loupy A, Haas M, et al. Banff 2019 meeting report: Molecular diagnostics in solid organ transplantation–Consensus for the Banff Human Organ Transplant (B-HOT) gene panel and open source multicenter validation. *Am J Transplant*. 2020;20:2305–17.

[20] Augustin G, Jeong JH, Kim MK, et al. Stem cell-based therapies and tissue engineering innovations for tendinopathy: A comprehensive review of current strategies and future directions. *Adv Ther*. 2024;2300425:1–23.

[21] Qin L, Yang S, Zhao C, et al. Prospects and challenges for the application of tissue engineering technologies in the treatment of bone infections. *Bone Res*. 2024;12:1–19.

[22] Chimerad M, Barazesh A, Zandi M, et al. Tissue engineered scaffold fabrication methods for medical applications. *Int J Polym Mater Polym Biomater*. 2023;72:1455–79.

[23] Shetty SK, Santhanakrishnan SS, Padurao S, et al. Prioritizing biomaterial driven clinical bioactivity over designing intricacy during bioprinting of trabecular microarchitecture: A clinician's perspective. *ACS Omega.* 2023;9(11):12426–35.
[24] Xie Z, Gao M, Lobo AO, et al. 3D bioprinting in tissue engineering for medical applications: The classic and the hybrid. *Polymers (Basel).* 2020;12(8):1717.
[25] Lewis PL, Shah RN. 3D printing for liver tissue engineering: Current approaches and future challenges. *Curr Transplant Rep.* 2016;3:100–8.
[26] Echeverria Molina MI, Malollari KG, Komvopoulos K. Design challenges in polymeric scaffolds for tissue engineering. *Front Bioeng Biotechnol.* 2021;9:1–29.
[27] Olson JL, Atala A, Yoo JJ. Tissue engineering: Current strategies and future directions. *Chonnam Med J.* 2011;47:1.
[28] Wiles K, Fishman JM, De Coppi P, et al. The host immune response to tissue-engineered organs: Current problems and future directions. *Tissue Eng—Part B Rev.* 2016;22:208–19.
[29] Nelson J, Alvey N, Bowman L, et al. Consensus recommendations for use of maintenance immunosuppression in solid organ transplantation: Endorsed by the American college of clinical pharmacy, American society of transplantation, and international society for heart and lung transplantation. Pharmacotherapy. 2022;42:594–8.
[30] Park C, Jones MM, Kaplan S, et al. A scoping review of inequities in access to organ transplant in the United States. *Int J Equity Health.* 2022;21:1–20.
[31] Wilkinson TM. Living donor organ transplantation. In Richard E. Ashcroft, Angus Dawson, Heather Draper, John R. McMillan (Eds.), *Principles of Health Care Ethics.* Second ed. Hoboken, NJ: John Wiley & Sons; 2007. pp. 483–8.
[32] Eltom A, Zhong G, Muhammad A. Scaffold techniques and designs in tissue engineering functions and purposes: A review. *Adv Mater Sci Eng.* 2019;2019.
[33] Norouzi F, Bagheri F, Hashemi-Najafabadi S. Alendronate releasing silk fibroin 3D bioprinted scaffolds for application in bone tissue engineering: Effects of alginate concentration on printability, mechanical properties and stability. *Results Eng.* 2024;22.
[34] Raeisdasteh Hokmabad V, Davaran S, Ramazani A, et al. Design and fabrication of porous biodegradable scaffolds: A strategy for tissue engineering. *J Biomater Sci Polym Ed.* 2017;28:1797–825.
[35] Capuana E, Lopresti F, Carfì Pavia F, et al. Solution-based processing for scaffold fabrication in tissue engineering applications: A brief review. *Polymers (Basel).* 2021;13.
[36] Zaszczyńska A, Moczulska-Heljak M, Gradys A, et al. Advances in 3D printing for tissue engineering. *Materials (Basel).* 2021;14.
[37] Subia B, Kundu J, Kundu CS. Biomaterial scaffold fabrication techniques for potential tissue engineering applications. In Daniel Eberli (Ed.), *Tissue Engineering.* London: InTech; 2010, pp. 141–57.
[38] Liu T, Wang Y, Kuang T. Oriented porous polymer scaffolds in tissue engineering: A comprehensive review of preparation strategies and applications. *Macromol Mater Eng.* 2024;309:1–20.
[39] Ho MH, Kuo PY, Hsieh HJ, et al. Preparation of porous scaffolds by using freeze-extraction and freeze-gelation methods. *Biomaterials.* 2004;25:129–38.
[40] Collins MN, Ren G, Young K, et al. Scaffold fabrication technologies and structure/function properties in bone tissue engineering. *Adv Funct Mater.* 2021;31.
[41] Lin W, Chen M, Qu T, et al. Three-dimensional electrospun nanofibrous scaffolds for bone tissue engineering. *J Biomed Mater Res—Part B Appl Biomater.* 2020;108:1311–21.
[42] Yu J, Park SA, Kim WD, et al. Current advances in 3D bioprinting technology and its applications for tissue engineering. *Polymers (Basel).* 2020;12:1–30.

[43] Mouser VHM, Levato R, Mensinga A, et al. Bio-ink development for three-dimensional bioprinting of hetero-cellular cartilage constructs. *Connect Tissue Res*. 2020;61:137–51.
[44] Bakhtiary N, Liu C, Ghorbani F. Bioactive inks development for osteochondral tissue engineering: A mini-review. *Gels*. 2021;7.
[45] Colle J, Blondeel P, De Bruyne A, et al. Bioprinting predifferentiated adipose-derived mesenchymal stem cell spheroids with methacrylated gelatin ink for adipose tissue engineering. *J Mater Sci Mater Med*. 2020;31:1–15.
[46] Lee SJ, Lee JH, Park J, et al. Fabrication of 3D printing scaffold with porcine skin decellularized bio-ink for soft tissue engineering. *Materials (Basel)*. 2020;13:1–10.
[47] Neufurth M, Wang S, Schröder HC, et al. 3D bioprinting of tissue units with mesenchymal stem cells, retaining their proliferative and differentiating potential, in polyphosphate-containing bio-ink. *Biofabrication*. 2022;14.
[48] Singh J, Singh S, Verma A. Artificial intelligence in use of ZrO2 material in biomedical science. *J Electrochem Sci Eng* [Internet]. 2022;13:83–97. Available from: https://pub.iapchem.org/ojs/index.php/JESE/article/view/1498.
[49] Singh J, Hashmi AW, Behra A, et al. Review of Mg alloys for bio-implants protected by the deposition of chemical conversion coatings. In *AIP Conference Proceedings*. AIP Publishing; 2024.
[50] Singh J, Singh S, Gill R. Applications of biopolymer coatings in biomedical engineering. *J Electrochem Sci Eng*. 2022;13:63–81.
[51] Kreimendahl F, Kniebs C, Tavares Sobreiro AM, et al. FRESH bioprinting technology for tissue engineering—the influence of printing process and bioink composition on cell behavior and vascularization. *J Appl Biomater Funct Mater*. 2021;19.
[52] Singh CJ, Ram B, Singh J, et al. Experimental investigation on characterization of friction stir processed AZ31-based composite. *Sci Rep*. 2024;14:15453.
[53] Singh J, Hashmi AW, Ahmad S, et al. Critical review on biodegradable and biocompatibility magnesium alloys: Progress and prospects in bio-implant applications. *Inorg Chem Commun*. 2024;169:113111.
[54] Hashmi AW, Singh J, Ahmad S. Future perspective of self-healing nano-coatings for corrosion protection. *Discov Disruption, Futur Implic Nanomater*. 2024;597–624.
[55] Singh J, Hashmi AW, Kumar A, et al. Review on protection of Mg alloys bioimplants by deposition of micro-arc oxidation coatings. In *AIP Conference Proceedings*. AIP Publishing; 2024.
[56] Kaur H, Sharma S, Athwal S, et al. *The Potential Applications of 2D Nanomaterials for Water Purification. 2D Nanomater*. John Wiley & Sons, Ltd; 2024. pp. 361–95.
[57] Mantha S, Pillai S, Khayambashi P, et al. Smart hydrogels in tissue engineering and regenerative medicine. *Materials (Basel)*. 2019;12.
[58] Ruffa AA, Toni B. Engineering applications. *STEAM-H Sci Technol Eng Agric Math Heal*. 2022;299–311.
[59] Manuscript A. 可注射水凝胶作为糖尿病创面修复的动态黏附敷料 *Materials Chemistry B*. 2021;10:4118.
[60] Tan H, Marra KG. Injectable, biodegradable hydrogels for tissue engineering applications. *Materials (Basel)*. 2010;3:1746–67.
[61] Jiang W, Mei H, Zhao S. Applications of 3D bio-printing in tissue engineering and biomedicine. *J Biomed Nanotechnol*. 2021;17:989–1006.
[62] Smith JM, Chowdhry R, Booth MJ. Controlling synthetic cell-cell communication. *Front Mol Biosci*. 2022;8:1–9.
[63] Lavik E, Langer R. Tissue engineering: Current state and perspectives. *Appl Microbiol Biotechnol*. 2004;65:1–8.

[64] Uccelli A, Moretta L, Pistoia V. Mesenchymal stem cells in health and disease. *Nat Rev Immunol.* 2008;8:726–36.
[65] Palakkan AA, Hay DC, Pr AK, et al. Liver tissue engineering and cell sources: Issues and challenges. *Liver Int.* 2013;33:666–76.
[66] Takahashi K, Yamanaka S. Induction of pluripotent stem cells from mouse embryonic and adult fibroblast cultures by defined factors. *Cell.* 2006;126:663–76.
[67] Ogle BM, Bursac N, Domian I, et al. Distilling complexity to advance cardiac tissue engineering. *Sci Transl Med.* 2016;8.
[68] Liu CC. Electrochemical sensors. *Med Devices Syst.* 2006;07:48–1–48–6.
[69] Kaur H, Bhosale A, Shrivastav S. Biosensors: Classification, fundamental characterization and new trends: A review. *Int J Heal Sci Res.* 2018;8:313–33.
[70] Devi G, Kushwaha A, Goswami L, et al. Toxicity assessment of fluoride-contaminated soil and wastewater in solanum tuberosum. *Water Air Soil Pollut.* 2022;233:1–23.
[71] Kaur H, Raveendran A V., Athwal S, et al. Assessment of diabetes biomarker monitoring via novel biosensor activity. *Results Chem.* 2023;5:100777.
[72] Gelain F. Novel opportunities and challenges offered by nanobiomaterials in tissue engineering. *Int J Nanomedicine.* 2008;3:415–24.
[73] Hasan A, Morshed M, Memic A, et al. Nanoparticles in tissue engineering: Applications, challenges and prospects. *Int J Nanomedicine.* 2018;13:5637–55.
[74] Ahmad Oryan AM. An overview on bone tissue engineering and regenerative medicine: Current challenges, future directions and strategies. *J Sports Med Doping Stud.* 2015;5:4–6.
[75] Kaur H, Sareen S, Mutreja V, et al. Spinach-derived carbon dots for the turn-on detection of chromium ions (Cr 3 +). *J Inorg Organomet Polym Mater.* 2023;1–26.
[76] Kieda J, Shakeri A, Landau S, et al. Advances in cardiac tissue engineering and heart-on-a-chip. *J Biomed Mater Res—Part A.* 2024;112:492–511.

14 Advanced Biomaterials as Bioimplants for Load-bearing Applications

Anavadya K. K. and Vijayalakshmi U.

CONTENTS

14.1 INTRODUCTION

The progression made in the biomedical domain has been directly influencing the health and well-being of humankind by acting as a menace to ailments. As the health and lifestyle of humans have evolved significantly in the modern era, associated diseases and injuries have also increased proportionally. Biomaterials therefore find extreme relevance in the present environment. A particular type of biocompatible material that mitigates by replacing or repairing any organ or biological function is

DOI: 10.1201/9781003516064-14

called biomaterials. Each type of material has a specific role to fulfill in biomedicine, with their broad classification as bioinert, bioactive, and bioresorbable materials. Bioinert materials have the ability to be non-reactive to any of the external surroundings inside the body, thus ensuring significance in functions that require a chemically inert environment. Bioactive biomaterials react to the adjoining tissues positively to induce tissue regeneration and promote osteoblast formation. Biomaterials that can break down or degrade on their own, named bioresorbable materials, make up the third group that finds relevance in situations when repeat procedures should be avoided. It is envisaged that an ideal biomaterial will have a high degree of biocompatibility, minimal toxicity, neither carcinogenic nor mutagenic, sufficient mechanical strength and toughness, and not corrosive. Orthopedic applications of biomaterials comprise implants, scaffolds, nanocomposites etc. which partake in load-bearing application, tissue regeneration, bone healing, osseointegration, and many more. This is achieved by materials like ceramics, polymers, metals, and so on. Orthopedic application refers to the utilization of devices, tools, or specific materials for the betterment, recovery, and revitalizing of bone-related injuries and ailments of the musculoskeletal system of living beings. As the applications of biomaterials are a vast domain, we narrow our traverse over to load-bearing applications of biomaterials. Among the biomaterials like ceramics, polymers, metals, and composites that facilitate different functions like osseointegration, tissue regeneration, targeted drug delivery, and so on, we focus on materials that can be used as bioimplants for load bearing. Any dysfunctionality of the spine, skull, joints, pelvis, hip, and knee, which aid in locomotion and provide support to the weight of the human body, is upheld by load-bearing implants. According to WHO statistics from 2023, around 20 million people suffer from injuries due to accidents and approximately 1.19 million people lost their lives resulting from them. Biomaterials functioning as orthopedic implants may become more relevant in the event of accidents, lifestyle diseases, autoimmune disorders, age-related illnesses, and so on. Bioimplants used for orthopedics comprise metals, polymers and ceramic implants, scaffolds, constructs, and many more. While using a bioimplant for a particular purpose, the right materials must be chosen; for example, load-bearing implants need to be of high mechanical strength and least corrosion, dental implants need to be mechanically strong and aesthetically pleasing, and stents and grafts need to be highly biocompatible and biodegradable. The lack of appropriate selection of materials will end up in repercussions like implant failures leading to infections which can be even fatal (**Figure 14.1**).

Implants that bear load are of extreme significance and require numerous specific characteristics combined together including appropriate mechanical strength, fair biocompatibility, minimal cytotoxicity, least corrosion rates, better tribological characteristics, and considerably more. While considering a load-bearing implant, it is essential to look for misalignments if any, implant instability and loosening, bone component damage, soft tissue imbalance, and altered biomechanics which may lead to implant failures (**Figure 14.2**). In this chapter, we delve into those biomaterials that serve as bioimplants that are capable of supporting weight. Biomaterials used as load-bearing implants include metals and metal alloys (cobalt-chromium, nickel-titanium, stainless steel alloys, titanium alloys, etc.), ceramics (alumina, zirconia,

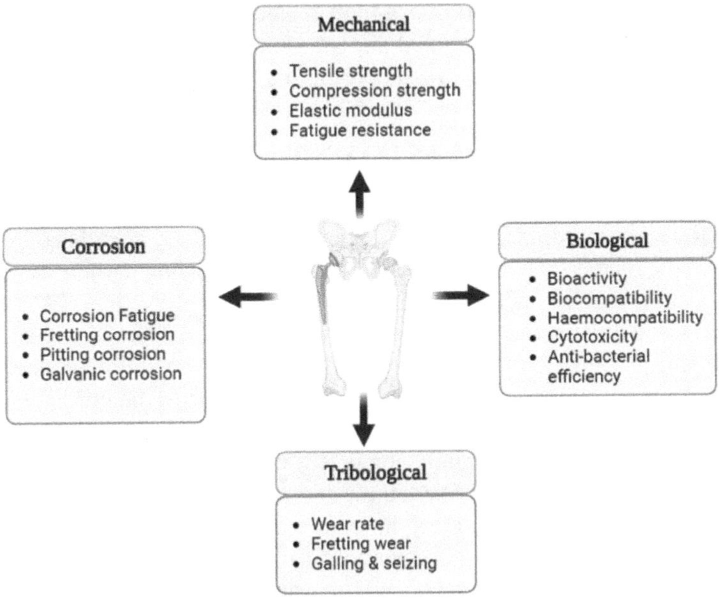

FIGURE 14.1 Properties of a bioimplant for load-bearing application.

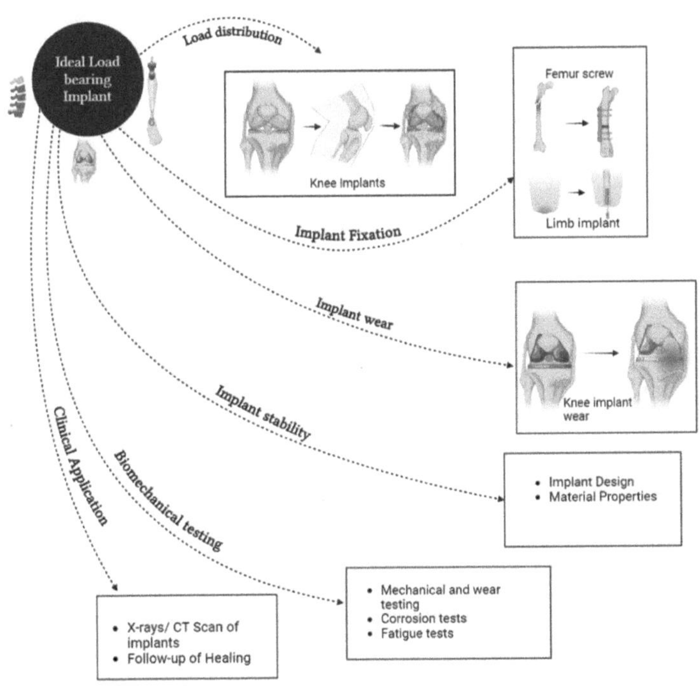

FIGURE 14.2 Representation of various aspects of an ideal load-bearing implant.

pyrolytic carbon), and polymers (ultra-high molecular weight polyethylene). This chapter is pivoted on the conventional and advanced biomaterials that can function as load-bearing implants and endow support to the human system.

14.2 METAL AND ALLOYS AS LOAD-BEARING IMPLANTS

Metals and metal alloys have been a prime requirement in load-bearing applications due to the extraordinary strength, toughness, and elastic modulus they provide. Unlike pristine metals, alloys exhibit distinct properties owing to their varying composition of diverse trace metals. For instance, Titanium alloys like Ti-6Al-4V and Ti-3Al–2.5V have the same set of metals present but in varying compositions and have different properties. Similarly, carbon composition in stainless steel leads to differing properties of the material which ultimately leads to the utilization of similar metal alloys for different biomedical applications. The mechanical attributes of metals and alloys make them greatly competent in load-bearing applications. Apart from the mechanical properties like fatigue resistance, toughness, and lesser elastic modulus, they are also anticipated to have wear resistance and fair biocompatibility. Despite possessing all the aforementioned traits, they nonetheless have drawbacks that increase the risk of infections. The primary obstacle faced by these types of materials is the extremely corrosive environment, which are biological fluids. The bodily fluid's ions have a tendency to erode metal surfaces, which can steer to implant failures. Researchers are coming up with innovative ways to get around this by employing metal alloys and protective coating layers made of materials that are significantly less corrosive and by inducing surface modifications to ameliorate biocompatibility. The corrosive nature of different metals can be arranged as Tantalum < Titanium < Stainless steel < Chromium < Nickel < Cobalt < Copper [1].

14.2.1 Stainless Steel

Stainless steel (SS) was one of the preferred conventional bioimplants for load-bearing applications due to the strength provided by the metal and its inexpensiveness. Subsequently, it was discovered that stainless steel was not as robust as other metals like titanium and its alloys, which also had lower implant failure rates during fracture fixations. Therefore, SS was enhanced with additives like vanadium and platinum to improve its qualities [2]. SS-based implants for load-bearing applications such as screws, nails, bone plates, fracture fixations, prostheses, and many more are being developed lately using additive manufacturing (AM) because of their many advantages over conventionally fabricated alloys. Materials with desired qualities, such as reduced tensile strength and increased biocompatibility, are attainable with the AM method [3]. Coatings and surface alterations were followed up to increase the biocompatibility and adaptability of SS alloys to the hostile environment of bodily fluids, with the goal of lowering the implant failures associated with them. For instance, hydroxyapatite with phase purity was coated over 316L SS to obtain a protective layer of dense coatings with a uniform surface that resists corrosion [4]. Later, the emergence of ultra-graded SS alloys unveiled extensively higher strength comparable to conventional SS alloys, as they do not undergo any phase transformations while processing, generating the idea to change the size and structure of the grains while simultaneously demonstrating increased wear resistance [5]. Improved corrosion resistance with nanostructured SS alloys is another breakthrough. Nanostructured SS alloys offer enhanced resistance to corrosion and are expected to show better tissue adhesion and have a beneficial influence on the biological mechanism involved in tissue repair. With nanostructured implant surfaces having superior structural refinement than microstructure implants, the improvement in corrosion resistance is thought to be mostly due to the change in passive film structure [6].

14.2.2 Cobalt-Chromium Alloys

Co-Cr alloys became a significant material for load-bearing applications due to the passive layer of Cr_2O_3 formation thereby providing corrosion resistance and hence considered one of the safer metals for orthopedics. These alloys usually contain traces of molybdenum and other metals like manganese, nickel, phosphorous, and so on to improve their wear resistance and corrosion resistance as well as biocompatibility which is still less than Ti alloys. In Co-Cr alloys, abrasions, prolonged wear, and the metallic ion release are additional causes for concern [7]. Co-Cr alloys with varying porosities were manufactured additively while taking the microstructure into account as it affects the material's response toward corrosion. Thus concluded that as porosity increased, the mechanical yield and elastic strengths were reduced. Graded metal alloys with different interior microstructures were shown to produce considerably better results than traditional smooth-surfaced implants [8]. They can also enhance the osteoblast adhesion together with proliferation with graded structures imparting better biocompatibility and providing stress distribution in the case of load-bearing implants [9]. The surface modifications in terms of nanostructure aid in imparting better attributes in terms of mechanical and biological aspects to the whole implant system according to the Hall-Petch equation [10].

14.2.3 Titanium and Alloys

Titanium metals and alloys have been used as biomedical implants since the early 1950s attributed to the remarkable corrosion-resistant passivation layer of TiO_2 layer formation atop the metal, which induces better biocompatibility. While pure titanium metal is lightweight and heat-resistant, it is not as mechanically strong as titanium alloys, which can have metal compositions changed to meet specific mechanical requirements. Pristine titanium along with combinations of other metals as alloys finds various applications as load-bearing implants. Titanium implants with an induced specific percentage of porosities have been introduced as a substitute for human cortical bone owing to their similar Young's modulus and strength [11]. Porous titanium metals have demonstrated excellent osseointegration and robust interfacial bonding in in vivo investigations. This is likely due to their irregular surface and rough size, which provide an ideal environment for tissue growth and promote bone–implant adhesion [12]. Osteointegration occurs when the metal fails to form a fibrous tissue encapsulation around the implant surface; as a result, it is fairly biocompatible. Despite their mechanical robustness, in long-term use, they have the potential to cause galling and seizing [13]. Titanium and its alloys have been utilized as tibial components as well as humeral fracture fixation in hip and knee replacements, respectively, as well as acetabular and femoral components. Recently, vanadium containing alloys have been observed to release slightly toxic ions into the body fluid which led to the introduction of Nb-containing alloys like Ti-13Nb-13Zr, Ti-20Nb-13Zr, Ti-20Nb-20Zr, and ultrafine-grained 59Ti-36Nb-2Ta-3Zr, Ti-Nb-Zr-Fe-O, Ti-40Nb, Ti-40Nb–3.5In, and so on. These alloys find various applications as biomedical implants with micro and nanostructures dependent on the fabrication process of the implant allowing nano-porous structures fabricated over the surface of the metals to enhance the tissue growth into the pores [14].

14.2.4 Tantalum

Tantalum metals have gained popularity recently due to their exceptional osteoregeneration and osteoinduction properties and corrosion resistance than titanium metal alloys, which have already been used widely as bioimplants. The increased corrosion resistance, chemical resistance, non-toxic nature, and the bioactivity possessed by these metals made researchers consider their potential applications as load-bearing implants. The two oxides of tantalum, Ta_2O_5 and TaO_2, are formed when exposed to harsh environments and safeguard the implant from being eroded by providing chemical resistance [15]. The finest outcomes to date have come from using this metal in prosthetic covers, acetabular cups, femoral heads, tibia, and patella components. Tantalum and titanium are combined in different proportions to construct the alloy Ti-29Nb-13Ta–4.6Zr, which is used to fabricate knee joints [16]. Improving the Ta surfaces' pore size makes them more conducive to osteoblast cell response and bone tissue attachment and improves cell proliferation [17]. Lately, Ta implants that are openly porous and additively produced have taken dominance because they maintain their mechanical qualities while increasing the adherence of the implant to the bone [18]. Their higher density is a drawback, leading to a lack of pores and low fatigue resistance. Ta metal structures resembling human cortical and trabecular bones can be created by tailoring porosity and pore size, which will aid in bone tissue engineering. With tailored pore size and geometry, the in vivo performance of additively manufactured porous Ta implants showed reduced cytotoxicity, enhanced cell viability, and cell proliferation, with altered macrostructure [19]. The in vivo studies have shown great biocompatibility and interfacial characteristics which lead to proper adhesion of bone–implant surface and mechanical stability.

14.2.5 Magnesium

Magnesium is the most commonly used bioresorbable material as implants attributable to its excellent biocompatibility with the host tissues, ability to avoid the need for revision surgeries, and additional benefit of natural repair of the tissues in the implanted area by Mg ions release. Despite being brittle, they are lighter and weigh less than metals like titanium and have mechanical characteristics comparable to that of natural bones, which leads to their application as lighter implants that can nevertheless withstand adequate strength. When the body can properly metabolize or excrete a material without any buildup in any organs or tissues, that material is successfully degradable inside the body. Magnesium alloy implants have the potential to biodegrade over time, making them a good resorbable metallic material that the body can start to metabolize. The by-products formed in this reactions normally are $Mg(OH)_2$, $MgCO_3$, $Mg_3(PO_4)_2$, $CaCO_3$, and $Ca_3(PO_4)_2$. The matter that needs to be addressed is the possibility that the OH^- ions of the degradation products will leach out and collide with Cl^- ions, raising the pH in the vicinity of the host tissues [20]. To fabricate an implant similar to natural bones, porosity ought to be included to enhance the integration of the implant surface with the bone and lower the yield strength [21]. Although the biological aspects are more dominant, porous micro and nanostructures are crucial for magnesium alloys to overcome existing setbacks such as corrosion in body fluid. Magnesium implants are coated using nanostructured coatings (biodegradable polymeric, silane, calcium phosphate coatings, etc.) to offer greater anti-corrosive properties [22]. The increased strength, fatigue resistance, and corrosion resistance of magnesium matrix nanocomposites (MMNC), as well as the inclusion of nanomaterials into the Mg matrix, have garnered attention. To prevent any negative impacts of the unique composition, the in vivo investigations still need to be thoroughly investigated [23].

14.2.6 Metal Matrix Composites (MMC)

These novel materials are combinations of one particular compound reinforced to a matrix made of metals usually cobalt, titanium, aluminium etc. Very recently, zinc as an MMC has been considered for efficiently biodegradable orthopedic applications owing to its biocompatibility and corrosion resistance. The incorporation of hydroxyapatite tends to tailor the degradation rates and improve osteogenesis [24]. Titanium alloy-based MMCs are also widely used for their corrosion and wear resistance. Si and hydroxyapatite-incorporated Ti-6Al-4V showed greatly enhanced properties including their hardness [25]. Reinforcements of carbon nanotubes (CNT) in MMCs have grabbed attention in the biomedical domain due to the impressive properties exhibited by them despite having practical difficulties in fabricating them. CNTs are tried to be incorporated into various metals like aluminium, magnesium, nickel, titanium, and so on for the purpose of ameliorating mechanical properties for superior performance in load-bearing applications [26]. Iron-based biodegradable bone implants were fabricated by reinforcing calcium silicate into the iron metal matrix, as they were effective for bioactivity, and calcium silicate particularly enhances degradability showing better bioactivity and cell proliferation without not-so-largely reducing the bending strength of iron thereby introducing itself as a potent bone implant [27]. Biodegradable Mg MMCs find very beneficial applications as load-bearing implants due to the prevention of unessential secondary surgeries. Mg metal matrix is reinforced with Zn, Ni-like metals, and also hydroxyapatite-like ceramics to improve the bioactivity [28]. The methods for Mg-MMC fabrication result in improved compressive and tensile strength alongside improved corrosion resistance. Mg-based MMCs are a solution for this by improving the corrosion resistance to a certain extent and offering improved compressive and tensile strength. Such incorporations and reinforcements in metal matrices are highly beneficial as

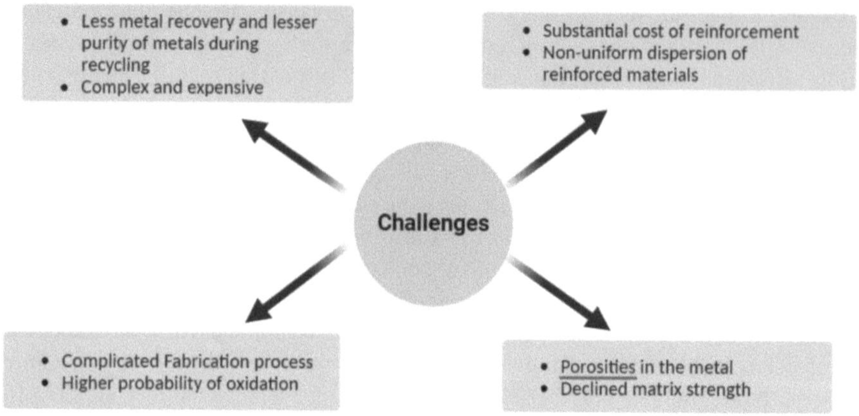

FIGURE 14.3 Challenges posed by metal matrix composites.

load-bearing implants since they provide additional facets to the material by combining properties of the metal and the reinforced component and also by deteriorating the non-desirable characteristics of the material. There are quite a few challenges to overcome to utilize MMCs as a potent and common bioimplant, albeit the favors [29] (**Figure 14.3**).

14.3 NON-METALLIC MATERIALS AS LOAD-BEARING IMPLANTS

14.3.1 Ceramics

Advanced ceramics have always gained attention in the biomedical domain due to their exceptional biocompatibility. Alumina, zirconia, bioactive glass, pyrolytic carbon, and hydroxyapatites have been tried for their application in load-bearing, among which only a few like alumina and zirconia with added stabilizers or dopants showed more strength to take up the role of weight-bearing implants. Yttria-stabilized tetragonal zirconia polycrystal (Y-TZP) and magnesia partially stabilized zirconia (Mg-PSZ) are examples of additions to enhance the mechanical behavior of ZrO_2 implants. A stiffer foundation of the ceramic substrate is an essential factor in preventing implant fracture or failures by decreasing the tensile stress accumulation at the implant [30]. Zirconia-toughened alumina has shown exceptional mechanical attributes to emphasize its use in load-bearing applications. Due to the lower strength and higher fracture rate of alumina, despite having better wear resistance and long-term stability, it was not suggested to use it alone in implants. Later research revealed that ZTA increased the tribological qualities, long-term stability, flexural strength, and toughness of the implants; as a result, it was utilized in hip prostheses and arthroplasty implantations [31]. Pyrolytic carbons are yet another cutting-edge ceramic material used as load-bearing implants due to their mechanical aspects including the optimum structural integrity of the implants, superior wear resistance, remarkable fracture toughness, and biocompatibility [32]. The process of addressing the technical challenges associated with implantation is ongoing. Due to the exhibition of great wear resistance, implant longevity, and other superior attributes in comparison with existing ceramics, pyrolytic carbons gained keen attention very recently for shoulder arthroplasty and hand and wrist joint replacements with more clinical improvements [33]. Ceramics have been used by 3D printing technology for fabricating implants like ceramic scaffolds with improved microstructure, morphology, porosity etc. In addition to serving as the base material for implant construction, ceramics are more prominently used as coatings of these implants as a surface modification technique to exhibit better biological properties and ensure bone–implant bonding.

14.3.2 Polymers

Several polymers have been used in orthopedics, accounting for their tailorable biocompatibility, wide range of mechanical properties, and flexible synthesis for bone defects, bone fracture fixations, segmental bone defects, etc. Ultra-high molecular weight polyethylene (UHMWPE), polyethylene (PE), polymethylmethacrylate (PMMA), high-density polyethylene (HDPE), etc. are some of the advanced polymers used for load-bearing applications. It is necessary to address the debris release, lesser bone-bonding ability, and restricted biological responses [34]. Researchers also noted that when compared to Ti alloys, high-density polymers (HDP) demonstrated no appreciable change in toughness or load-bearing capacity [35]. AM demonstrates its supremacy as the most sophisticated processing approach and offers improved morphology and microstructure depending on the processing parameters, provided there are only a few polymers that could be additively manufactured and used for load-bearing applications. While AM-synthesized polymers may exhibit shrinkage and warping with thermal mismatch, they are still notable for having improved mechanical characteristics and less anisotropy [36]. PLLA, a polymer belonging to the PLA group, is frequently utilized because of its biodegradable nature and its adjustable qualities that allow it to exhibit a high degree of flexibility in load carrying [37]. Significantly ordered thermoplastic fiber that is UHMWPE (**Figure 14.4**) is a highly wear-resistant material that has recently been employed as a sophisticated biomaterial for total ankle and hip replacements with long-term survival. Because they work so well as fracture-fixing devices, polycaprolactones are the type of polymers employed in load-bearing applications. To improve their mechanical resilience, strength, and biological qualities, they could be reinforced with a variety of different materials [38]. Hydroxyapatite combined with PLA was observed to exhibit great in vivo compatibility and better cell differentiation with additional benefits of mechanical stability and acts as bone void fillings in load-bearing implants [39].

14.3.3 Composites

Composites are materials that have been combined to acquire better results without sacrificing their uniqueness. An extensive range of composites has been accessible recently with different characteristics like enhanced biocompatibility, corrosion and wear resistance, mechanical strength, toughness, rigidity, and lightweight qualities. Typically, polymers or ceramics are coupled with metals to provide mechanically robust and biocompatible implants with multiple biological characteristics.

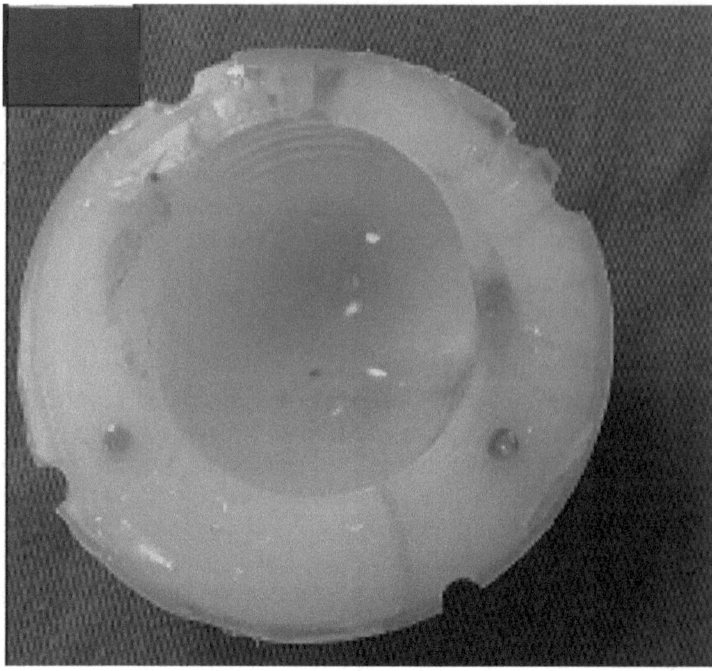

FIGURE 14.4 Acetabular cup made of UHMWPE [40].

Polyetheretherketone (PEEK) is a polymer that is used to reinforce with a lot of other materials since they alone do not impart all the essential qualities required for a load-bearing implant. Likewise, many polymers produce non-toxic breakdown products within the body, allowing for their advantageous in vivo effects while employed as polymerized or cross-linked materials [41]. For segmented bone defects and other injuries, hybrid substrates of polymers and scaffolds have been used as highly potent implant materials. For instance, PLGA-coated β-TCP composites due to their ameliorated properties are observed to show controlled release of biological cues too in addition to the usual characters shown by them [42]. Nanocomposites of ZrO_2-TiO_2 and composites of SiO_2-ZnO were used as coatings over Ti alloy implants to display great adhesion strength along with efficient activity against corrosion and microbial resistance respectively by withholding the discrete properties of partaking ceramics [43, 44]. Fiber and particle composites are the most current and sophisticated materials utilized for load carrying, which accounts for their stability and morphology among which the microstructure and orientation of the fibers determine the tensile strength of the material.

14.3.3.1 Ceramic Matrix Composites (CMC)

These composites have ceramics and other materials or compounds reinforced into a basic ceramic matrix. Attributable to their performance, they are useful in hip prostheses and arthroplasty as implants with better characteristics. Alumina matrix ceramics is one of the first CMCs to be used in orthopedics that provides great biocompatibility, wear resistance, and increased toughness compared to conventional alumina and are used in total joint replacement and as load-bearing implants with satisfactory longevity according to the long-term clinical follow-up [45]. As hydroxyapatites (HAp) have the least mechanical properties compared to other ceramics, using them as HAp matrix and reinforcing with other components imparted better properties. Alumina and chitosan-incorporated HAp were observed to have greater mechanical attributes and hence can be used as potent load-bearing implants. Improved mechanical properties of hydroxyapatite were achieved by decreased elastic modulus and compressive strength along with increased bending strength and fracture toughness, making this composite similar to that of human cancellous and cortical bones [46]. Calcium silicate incorporated in zirconia matrix composite in optimal amounts was observed to have bending strength like human cortical bone and appreciably enhances the biological aspects like osteogenesis and reduced the toughness of zirconia, making the composite to be used as potent load-bearing implants [47]. Fiber-reinforced CMC exhibits unrivaled properties desirable for load-bearing implants like dynamic load capability enhancement and impressive thermal shock resistance in addition to other mechanical attributes along with appreciable corrosion resistance which allows them to be used as effective bone grafts [48].

14.3.3.2 Polymer Matrix Composites (PMC)

Polymers make an ideal matrix for nano reinforcement due to better strength, exceptional bioactivity, and positively modified mechanical behaviors. To improve the properties of other materials like Al_2O_3, TiO_2, hydroxyapatite, and so on, polymers like ultra-high molecular weight polyethylene (UHMWPE) and high-density polyethylene (HDPE) were utilized as matrix reinforcement. A few polymer composites used as load-bearing implants are HA/poly lactic acid, HA/poly ethylene, bioglass/PE, carbon fiber/polyetheretherketone, carbon fiber/UHMWPE, poly glycolic acid/PGA, etc. HDPE with Al_2O_3 and TiO_2 reinforced PMCs show better tensile strength, bending strength, and hardness with the least corrosion behavior [49]. Polyetheretherketone–hydroxyapatite composites were also observed to exhibit exceptionally great fracture toughness and fatigue resistance leading to their application as load-bearing implants due to the mechanical behaviors like ample Young's modulus and tensile strength and adequate porosity aiding in the formation of osteocytes and osteoblast proliferation [50]. Calcium phosphate–polyurethane composites were similarly found to be potent load-bearing implants following the findings that they improve compressive strength. As the reinforcement is calcium phosphate, the bioactivity is not to be worried about [51]. Thus, indicating a large number of polymer matrix composites are available to be used as potent load-bearing implants with enhanced mechanical properties.

14.4 ADVANCED MATERIALS AS IMPLANTS

14.4.1 Hydrogels

After exploring conventional materials as load-bearing implants, researchers are finding novel and futuristic materials that reveal explicit properties and reduce patient suffering to the maximum. Hydrogels are one such material that is gaining popularity in the biomedical field due to the tunable characteristics it can display. Smart hydrogels that have unique distinct internal networking structures are highly suitable for biomedical applications including load bearing. They are classified based on cross-linking as physical, chemical, and dual-network hydrogels. Their applications in bone implants account for the adapting nature of hydrogels in accordance with our human body and their tunable properties by different methods of energy dissipation. The brittle and low mechanical properties of the hydrogels are improved greatly by energy dissipation methods like electrostatic interactions, microphase separation, self-assembly, nanocomposites like nanospheres or nanofibers and thereby fabricating tougher hydrogels [52]. Altering the cross-linking density and addition of layers of interconnected networks of hydrogels will tend to substantial improvement in the mechanical properties due to the dissipation of the load more evenly. Such formed nanocomposite hydrogels are resistant to crack propagation and hence show more mechanical attributes [53]. The biocompatibility of hydrogels is worth mentioning since they have a hydrophilic surface which can reduce the interfacial tension at the implant-tissue barrier and is least toxic to the surrounding host tissues which makes it a biologically compatible material for biomedical applications. A lot of polymers, including PLA (polylactic acid), PLGA (poly lactide-co-glycolide), and PCL (polycaprolactone), as hydrogels find applications as load-bearing implants as temporary and permanent implanted devices [54]. PVA-acrylamide hydrogels were recently found to have high creep resistance, great tribological properties, and increased porosity and pore size and hence used as synthetic cartilages [55].

14.4.2 Shape Memory Materials

Shape memory alloys (SMA) are smart materials comprising ceramics, polymers, and hybrids which are of immense applications in the biomedical field. Due to the exceptional quality of retaining the shape even after plastic deformations, it is very evident that they can be used in load-bearing applications as implants. The shape deformation is regained through phase change which occurs from two stable phases, austenite and martensite. They regain their shape by two methods which are one-way and two-way shape memory effects in which they usually have two different shapes

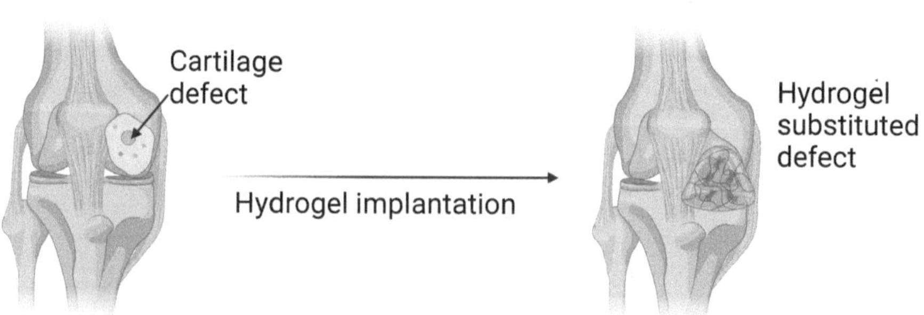

FIGURE 14.5 Hydrogel implantation in cartilage defect of knee bone. (Created in https://BioRender.com)

to memorize with hot and cold temperatures. Ni-Ti alloy (Nitinol) is an SMA with excellent biocompatibility and high corrosion resistance rates which can be tunable in accordance with the grain size. Powder metallurgy yields porous structures that result in lower-density substrates pertinent to implants [56]. In load-bearing applications, SMAs are used as spinal vertebra spacers and healing of bone fractures predominantly. Apart from SMA, shape memory polymers like PEEK and UHMWPE are of foremost importance in arthroplasty and joint replacements due to the high mechanical properties and less wear debris formation of these polymers respectively [57]. Notably, SMPs do not intrinsically have the shape memory effect, and it is induced as a polymerization process. Although their lower density in comparison to SMAs should be noted, they find use as load-bearing implants because of the added biodegradability of certain SMPs, which has led to the development of temporary implants. Porous PCL-based SMPs have been used for load-bearing applications, as they support bone growth and cell proliferation. Shape memory ceramics undergo cracking due to the thermal mismatch and hence have lesser applications as implant materials similar to shape memory hybrids which have difficult fabrication methods but could have better mechanical properties, as they are combinations of desirable materials [58]. The sequence of productivity for shape memory smart materials utilized as load-bearing implants is SMA>SMP>SMH>SMC.

14.4.3 High-Entropy Alloys

High-entropy alloys (HEAs) are that category of materials with nearly equimolar composition of multiple non-toxic elements with superior mechanical and tribological properties, structural stability, corrosion resistance, improved in vitro biocompatibility, longevity, and surface properties that aid in load-bearing applications [60]. A few HEAs for load-bearing applications are $(TiZrNbTa)_{90}Mo_{10}$, TiTaHfNb, TiTaHfNbZr, TiTaHfMoZr, and so on that hold exceptional mechanical properties and surface characteristics. The apatite formation observed with these HEAs

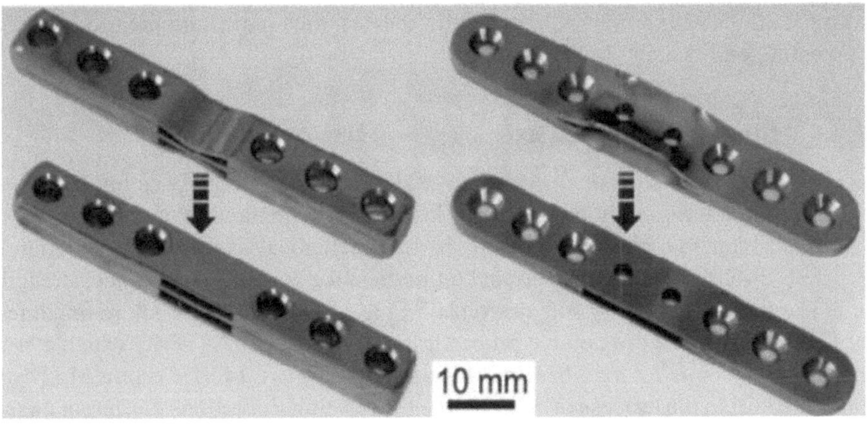

FIGURE 14.6 NiTi shape memory alloys for orthopedic implants [59].

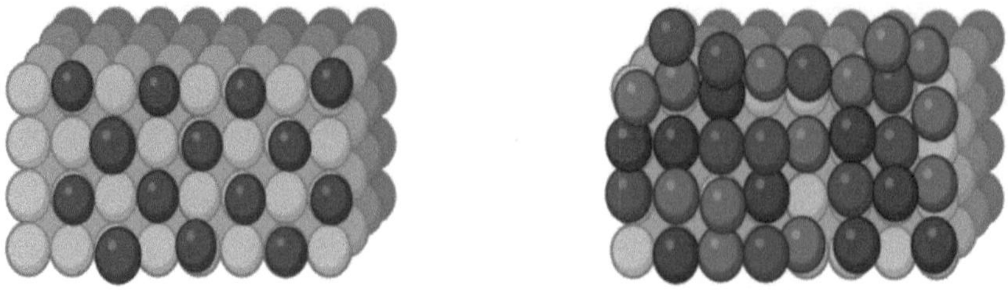

FIGURE 14.7 Crystal lattice structure of (a) conventional bi-metallic alloy (b) high entropy alloy.

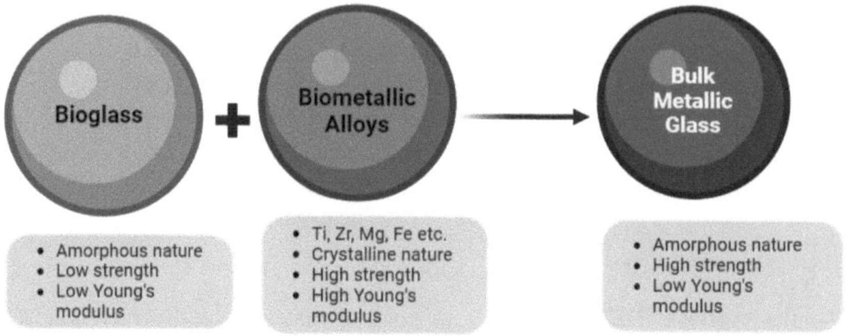

FIGURE 14.8 Diagrammatic representation of BMG comprising qualities of bioglass and metallic alloys [65].

is worth mentioning to showcase their bioactivity [61]. TiZrNbTaMo was observed to provide excellent corrosion resistance in comparison to existing Ti-based and Co-based alloys with remarkable hardening effects, thus indicating the use of HEAs as potential load-bearing implants [62].

14.4.4 Bulk Metallic Glasses

Despite Hench et al. have done countless studies on bioactive glass as implants, it is very brittle and not greatly preferred for load-bearing implants. Porous scaffolds of 3D-printed bioactive glasses can show better mechanical aspects and degradation rates [63]. BMGs showcase exceptional properties like corrosion resistance, strength, toughness, biocompatibility, and desirable Young's modulus. The fracture toughness and fatigue resistance are notable properties of Zr-Cu-Fe-Al-Ag BMG which allows them to be a promising load-bearing implant [64] (**Figure 14.9**). Certain Mg-based BMGs are still in the process of overcoming the existing limitations. Different metal-based BMGS, like Ti-based, Zr-based, and so on, have great mechanical strength and are hence used as implants and serve for the long term inside the human body, whereas Mg-based and Ca-based BMGs act as great fracture repair materials [65]. Among other BMGs, $Zr_{70}Ni_{16}Cu_{6}Al_{8}$ BMG has been identified as a promising novel load-bearing implant for its properties like good mechanical strength, corrosion resistance, osteogenic properties, and hardly cytotoxic nature [66]. The superiority BMGs are showing over current traditional metallic implants makes them a promising candidate for orthopedic application. **Table 14.1** summarizes the popular advanced biomaterials and their applications in a nutshell.

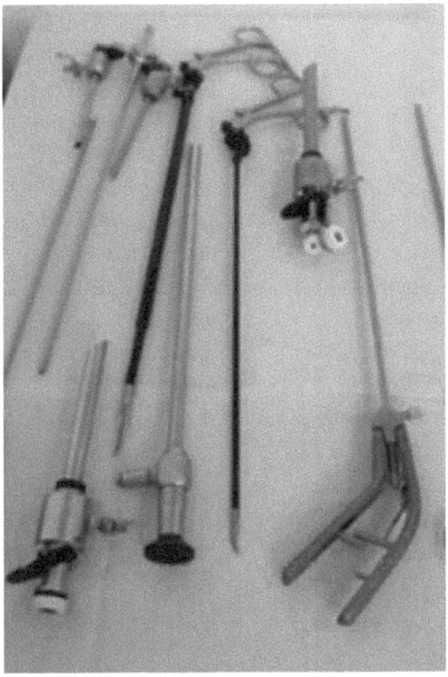

FIGURE 14.9 Bulk metallic glass used as biomedical implants [65].

TABLE 14.1
Various Advanced Biomaterials and their Applications in a Nutshell

Material	Implant	Properties	References
Biodegradable Zinc Alloys	Suitable as femur implants	Significant compression strength and lower modulus value close to natural bone and great biodegradable properties and improves bone healing mechanism	[67]
Polycaprolactone-Polylactic Acid	Bone graft scaffolds	Increased osteoconduction and mechanical properties	[68]
Graphene-Modified Mg Alloys	Potent bone implants	Better cell proliferation	[69]

(Continued)

TABLE 14.1 *(Continued)*
Various Advanced Biomaterials and their Applications in a Nutshell

Material	Implant	Properties	References
Bioactive Polymers	Potential biodegradable implants	Can modulate in vitro biocompatibility by retaining intrinsic mechanical properties of polymers	[70]
Fe-Ag and Fe-Cu-based Smart Nanocomposites	Useful for high-strength implants	Greater mechanical properties including ductility in comparison with conventional nanocomposites. The drug-loading and the slow-release of drugs are worth mentioning for these categories of materials	[71]
CNT-incorporated Zn-based Mg Metal Matrix	Implants like knee prosthesis or bone screws	Great improvement in hardness and greatly helpful in bone tissue regeneration	[72]
Biomineralized Ti_3SiC_2	As lighter load-bearing implants	Improved osteointegration and osteogenic functions. The apatite mineralization also promotes cell differentiation	[73]
Bioresponsive Smart Materials	Spinal interbody cages	Load-sensing capabilities, bone growth assessment, and implant mispositioning can be sensed	[74]
Nanocrystalline Diamond-incorporated Ti-based Alloy	Orthopedic implants	Better osteointegration and bone healing ability and long-term stability of implants	[75]

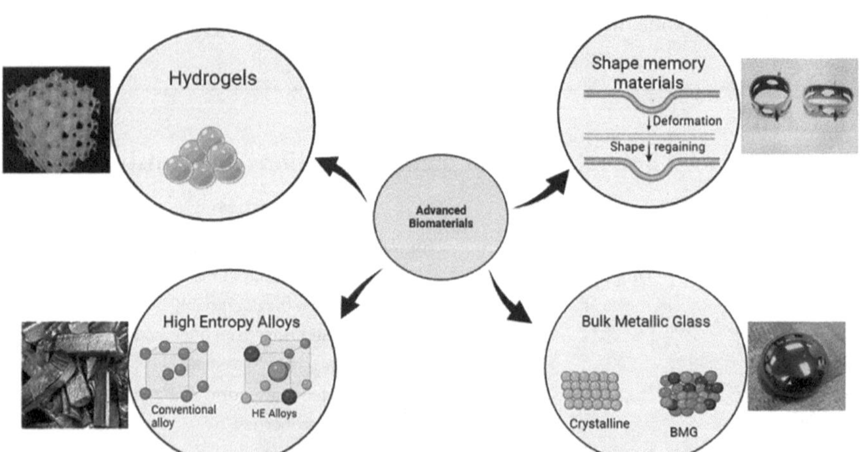

FIGURE 14.10 Advanced biomaterials and their schematic representation in a nutshell.

14.5 ADDITIVE MANUFACTURING IN LOAD-BEARING IMPLANTS

The AM technique or 3D printed technique is a newly emerging prodigiously efficient method for preparing materials for load-bearing applications. The complex geometry and structures that can be fabricated by AM with great precision are useful to the biomedical domain. Metals, ceramics, polymers, and other materials in any shape and size can be fabricated by AM. Laser-based powder bed diffusion has been a very efficient method of fabrication that allows flexible manufacturing and cost-effective synthesis. The structural integrity and rigidity provided by AM-fabricated porous bone scaffolds and implants are worth mentioning. Apart from the mechanical characteristics, the biocompatibility imparted to the material is highly attention-seeking since it also has control over surface roughness and microstructure [76]. Titanium metals have been fabricated using the 3D printing method to use them for total knee replacement surgeries as the stiffness and durability are improved. In AM, even though conventional materials are used for load-bearing applications, the method of fabrication can completely ameliorate the properties and make them distinct. Thus, fabricated smart implants are eminently capable of detecting implant failures in the early stage by neuro-muscular training and postoperative patterns and thereby acting accordingly to impart long-term survival of the implants [77]. Tantalum and copper-incorporated titanium alloys fabricated by AM were proven as a potent next-generation implant owing to their exceptional mechanical strength and in vivo biocompatibility. The modification in the Ti alloy with other incorporations yielded superior biocompatibility and antibacterial efficiency which is attained by nothing aside from AM that could dominate the load-bearing implant category [78]. Ceramic scaffolds were also fabricated with AM to obtain load-bearing components of high biological aspects accounting for the porosity and surface area [79]. At optimized porosity, in vivo results were greatly satisfying with efficient tissue regeneration, all this attained by AM, thus emphasizing AM as a rewarding technique for load-bearing implant fabrication.

14.6 STEM CELL THERAPY

Stem cell therapies are gaining ground accounting for the immense biological aspects that aid in the repair response of tissues or cells attached to the implants and thereby cure a lot of orthopedic diseases like osteoporosis and arthritis. Mesenchymal stem cells (MSC) therapy was observed to be profoundly assisting knee osteoarthritis and deterioration in pain with regrowth of bone cartilage was observed. MSCs, owing to their efficiency in differentiation, result in soothing of musculoskeletal repair of tissues and modulate the cytokines accountable for cartilage degeneration and thereby mitigate knee bone defects [80, 81]. High-strength porous Nitinol alloy scaffolds exhibited great osteogenic properties and cell adherence on treatment with MSC, thereby resulting in an osteoblastic phenotype and load-bearing implant henceforward [82]. TiO_2-ZrO_2 composites reinforced with polycaprolactone reveal fair cell adhesion and proliferation and antibacterial efficiency, along with osteogenic differentiation induced with stem cell therapy. The enhancement in osteogenic properties eventually leads to bone tissue repair [83]. Composites were also explored for their osteogenic properties with the attachment of stem cells to observe the chemotaxis nature of the materials that may later enable them to be used in load-bearing applications. Hydrogel/nanofiber hybrid scaffolds, one of the advanced materials are studied laboriously for human MSC attachment and showed explicit activity in tissue engineering and as load-bearing implant components [84]. Contemporary furtherance shows pronounced studies on stem cell therapy as an advanced technique in load-bearing implant fabrications owing to their extensive biological properties.

14.7 SURFACE MODIFICATION TECHNIQUES

Surface modifications can immensely help in improving the mechanical, biological, and tribological aspects that can be attained by various techniques which are represented in the diagram in **Figure 14.11**. Various surface modifications are applied over load-bearing implants for the purpose of improving specific characteristics like osseointegration, cell attachments, and cell proliferation. Additive and subtractive surface modifications are possible for different requirements. Additive modifications are carried out by methods like electrophoretic deposition, sol-gel, and magnetron-sputtering coating techniques normally over less biocompatible implant surfaces. Subtractive surface modifications like sand-blasting, acid etching, laser peening, and so on can greatly influence the surface microstructures and induce porosity that leads to improved cell adhesion, proliferation, and osteoblast growth into the pores [85]. Different coating methods have been used to improve the properties of conventional biomaterials. Hydroxyapatite with GO and CNT-reinforced composite coatings were used as coatings over SS alloys for the purpose of offering corrosion resistance to the

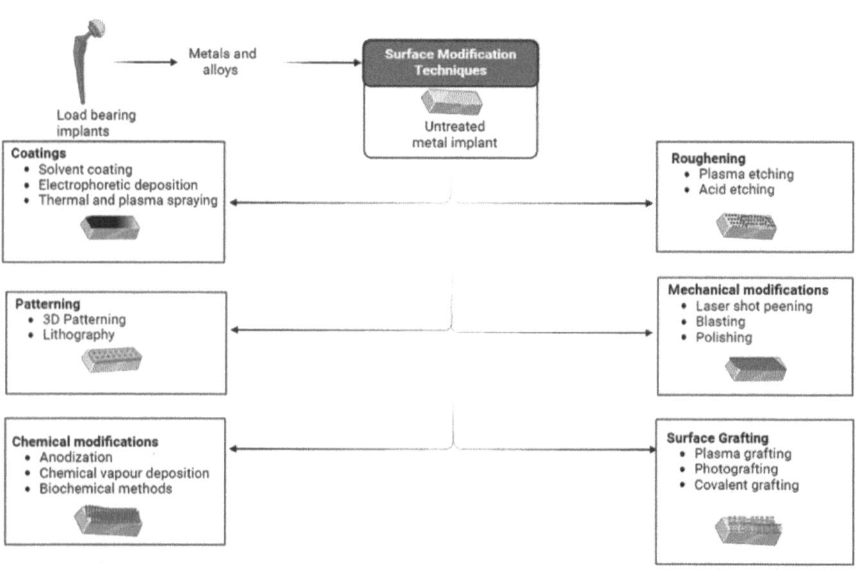

FIGURE 14.11 Different surface modification techniques with the diagrammatic representation of coating surface.

TABLE 14.2
Different Surface Modifications used on Bioimplants

Method	Necessity	Altered Surface Property	References
Mechanical Modifications • Grinding • Blasting • Polishing	Smoothened or roughened surface	The surface topographies will provide better adhesion on implant	[88]
Chemical Modifications • Sol-gel • Chemical vapor deposition	Removes the oxide layer contamination	Improves biocompatibility and adhesion	[88]
Biochemical Modifications	Peptides capable of adhesion on the substrate are used for modification	Improves differentiation of cells and long-term integration	[89]
Electrochemical Methods • Anodization • Electropolishing	Without adding mechanical stress to the substrate, terminates the crystallinity	Improved corrosion resistance and bioactivity owing to the surface topography	[89]
Physical Methods • Thermal and plasma spraying • Sputtering • Glow discharge plasma treatment • Ion implantation	Physical treatment of the substrate surface by kinetic, thermal, or electrical means	Improved corrosion and wear resistance with enhanced biocompatibility	[90]

implant and to induce apatite formation accounting to the chemical moieties present which can enact as nucleating sites [86]. The corrosion resistance provided by the coatings is worth mentioning. Similarly, composites like lanthanide-doped hydroxyapatites as porous coatings over Ti alloys were observed to show great corrosion resistance behavior, better cellular ingrowth due to the porosity, and fair mechanical characteristics [87]. **Table 14.2** tabulates the various surface modifications used for load-bearing implants for improved performances.

14.8 CONCLUSION

Diverse biomaterials have been used as load-bearing implants for a long time to aid patients in reducing the suffering caused by ailments or injuries. Conventional materials like metals, ceramics, polymers, and composites are still being used as fundamental implant bases due to one or the other exceptional attributes provided by them. Recently, numerous advancements have been made in this field on the selection of the materials used, the process of fabrication, and surface modifications even in nanoscale to improve their existing properties and proceed to become a high-potential load-bearing implant with the least shortcomings and more positive attributes. The causes of load-bearing implant failures like misalignments of implants, implant loosening, implant-component damage, and so on need to be taken care of. To overcome these complications, mechanical characteristics like hardness, tensile and compression strength, flexural strength, fatigue resistance, and so on are extremely important while selecting a material as load-bearing implant, along with considering the biological aspects like biocompatibility, non-toxic to the host tissues, promotion of bone cell growth, and corrosion resistance. Corrosion resistance displayed by the implant is extremely vital along with its tribological behavior. To accommodate all these properties, novel and advanced materials are studied for their exceptional properties. After 2000, a lot of improvements have been made in materials like hydrogels, matrix composites, high-entropy alloys, bulk metallic glasses, and so on for using them in load-bearing applications. They make great substitutes for conventional implant substrates owing to their combined, unique, and extraordinary attributes. Our chapter discusses the materials and the advancements made in the biomaterial domain as load-bearing implants briefly.

REFERENCES

1. Priyadarshini, B., Rama, M., Chetan and Vijayalakshmi, U., 2019. Bioactive coating as a surface modification technique for biocompatible metallic implants: A review. *Journal of Asian Ceramic Societies*, *7*(4), pp. 397–406.
2. Barber, C.C., Burnham, M., Ojameruaye, O. and McKee, M.D., 2021. A systematic review of the use of titanium versus stainless steel implants for fracture fixation. *OTA International*, *4*(3).
3. Bandyopadhyay, A., Ciliveri, S. and Bose, S., 2022. Metal additive manufacturing for load-bearing implants. *Journal of the Indian Institute of Science*, *102*(1), pp. 561–84.
4. Stango, A.X. and Vijayalakshmi, U., 2022. Optimization of formation of phase pure hydroxyapatite and fabrication of electrochemically stable HAP coatings on 316L SS for orthopedic applications. *Asia-Pacific Journal of Chemical Engineering*, *17*(5), p. e2801.
5. Muley, S.V., Vidvans, A.N., Chaudhari, G.P. and Udainiya, S., 2016. An assessment of ultra fine grained 316L stainless steel for implant applications. *Acta biomaterialia*, *30*, pp. 408–19.
6. Mahmoudi Hashemi, P., Borhani, E. and Nourbakhsh, M.S., 2016. A review on nanostructured stainless steel implants for biomedical application. *Nanomedicine Journal*, *3*(4), pp. 202–16.
7. Mavrogenis, A.F., Papagelopoulos, P.J. and Babis, G.C., 2011. Osseointegration of cobalt-chrome alloy implants. *Journal of Long-Term Effects of Medical Implants*, *21*(4).
8. Limmahakhun, S., Oloyede, A., Chantarapanich, N., Jiamwatthanachai, P., Sitthiseripratip, K., Xiao, Y. and Yan, C., 2017. Alternative designs of load– sharing cobalt chromium graded femoral stems. *Materials Today Communications*, *12*, pp. 1–10.
9. Pagani, S., Liverani, E., Giavaresi, G., De Luca, A., Belvedere, C., Fortunato, A., Leardini, A., Fini, M., Tomesani, L. and Caravaggi, P., 2021. Mechanical and in vitro biological properties of uniform and graded Cobalt-chrome lattice structures in orthopedic implants. *Journal of Biomedical Materials Research Part B: Applied Biomaterials*, *109*(12), pp. 2091–103.
10. Ghosh, M. and Thirugnanam, A., 2022. Nanostructured biomaterials for load-bearing applications. In *Advanced Materials for Biomechanical Applications* (pp. 187–202). CRC Press.
11. Krishna, B.V., Bose, S. and Bandyopadhyay, A., 2007. Low stiffness porous Ti structures for load-bearing implants. *Acta Biomaterialia*, *3*(6), pp. 997–1006.
12. Bandyopadhyay, A., Shivaram, A., Tarafder, S., Sahasrabudhe, H., Banerjee, D. and Bose, S., 2017. In vivo response of laser processed porous titanium implants for load-bearing implants. *Annals of Biomedical Engineering*, *45*, pp. 249–60.

13. Van Noort, R., 1987. Titanium: The implant material of today. *Journal of Materials Science*, *22*, pp. 3801–11.
14. Kaur, M. and Singh, K., 2019. Review on titanium and titanium based alloys as biomaterials for orthopaedic applications. *Materials Science and Engineering: C*, 102, pp. 844–62.
15. Ying, J., Yu, H., Cheng, L., Li, J., Wu, B., Song, L., Yi, P., Wang, H., Liu, L. and Zhao, D., 2023. Research progress and clinical translation of three-dimensional printed porous tantalum in orthopaedics. *Biomaterials Translational*, *4*(3), p. 166.
16. Putrantyo, I., Anilbhai, N., Vanjani, R. and De Vega, B., 2021. Tantalum as a novel biomaterial for bone implant: A literature review. *Journal of Biomimetics, Biomaterials and Biomedical Engineering*, *52*, pp. 55–65.
17. Huo, W.T., Zhao, L.Z., Yu, S., Yu, Z.T., Zhang, P.X. and Zhang, Y.S., 2017. Significantly enhanced osteoblast response to nano-grained pure tantalum. *Scientific Reports*, *7*(1), p. 40868.
18. Wauthle, R., Van Der Stok, J., Yavari, S.A., Van Humbeeck, J., Kruth, J.P., Zadpoor, A.A., Weinans, H., Mulier, M. and Schrooten, J., 2015. Additively manufactured porous tantalum implants. *Acta Biomaterialia*, *14*, pp. 217–25.
19. Huang, G., Pan, S.T. and Qiu, J.X., 2021. The clinical application of porous tantalum and its new development for bone tissue engineering. *Materials*, *14*(10), p. 2647.
20. Kamrani, S. and Fleck, C., 2019. Biodegradable magnesium alloys as temporary orthopaedic implants: A review. *Biometals*, *32*, pp. 185–93.
21. Staiger, M.P., Pietak, A.M., Huadmai, J. and Dias, G., 2006. Magnesium and its alloys as orthopedic biomaterials: A review. *Biomaterials*, *27*(9), pp. 1728–34.
22. Chakraborty Banerjee, P., Al-Saadi, S., Choudhary, L., Harandi, S.E. and Singh, R., 2019. Magnesium implants: Prospects and challenges. *Materials*, *12*(1), p. 136.
23. Shahin, M., Munir, K., Wen, C. and Li, Y., 2019. Magnesium matrix nanocomposites for orthopedic applications: A review from mechanical, corrosion, and biological perspectives. *Acta Biomaterialia*, *96*, pp. 1–19.
24. Yang, H., Qu, X., Lin, W., Wang, C., Zhu, D., Dai, K. and Zheng, Y., 2018. In vitro and in vivo studies on zinc-hydroxyapatite composites as novel biodegradable metal matrix composite for orthopedic applications. *Acta biomaterialia*, *71*, pp. 200–14.
25. Avila, J.D., Alrawahi, Z., Bose, S. and Bandyopadhyay, A., 2020. Additively Manufactured Ti6Al4V-Si-Hydroxyapatite composites for articulating surfaces of load-bearing implants. *Additive Manufacturing*, *34*, p. 101241.
26. Silvestre, N., 2013. State-of-the-art review on carbon nanotube reinforced metal matrix composites. *International Journal of Composite Materials*, *3*(6), pp. 28–44.
27. Wang, S., Xu, Y., Zhou, J., Li, H., Chang, J. and Huan, Z., 2017. In vitro degradation and surface bioactivity of iron-matrix composites containing silicate-based bioceramic. *Bioactive Materials*, *2*(1), pp. 10–18.
28. Krishnan, R., Pandiaraj, S., Muthusamy, S., Panchal, H., Alsoufi, M.S., Ibrahim, A.M.M. and Elsheikh, A., 2022. Biodegradable magnesium metal matrix composites for biomedical implants: Synthesis, mechanical performance, and corrosion behavior-A review. *Journal of Materials Research and Technology, 20*, 650–70.
29. Arora, G.S., Saxena, K.K., Mohammed, K.A., Prakash, C. and Dixit, S., 2022. Manufacturing techniques for Mg-based metal matrix composite with different reinforcements. *Crystals*, *12*(7), p. 945.
30. Soares, P.M., Cadore-Rodrigues, A.C., Borges, A.L.S., Valandro, L.F., Pereira, G.K.R. and Rippe, M.P., 2021. Load-bearing capacity under fatigue and FEA analysis of simplified ceramic restorations supported by Peek or zirconia polycrystals as foundation substrate for implant purposes. *Journal of the Mechanical Behavior of Biomedical Materials*, *123*, p. 104760.

31. Terrizzi, A.R., Fersini, M., Contaldi, V., Padmanabhan, S.K., Einarsrud, M.A. and Licciulli, A., 2022. Mechanical and tribological properties of injection molded zirconia-alumina for orthopedic implants. *Ceramics International*, *48*(21), pp. 31211–22.
32. Rossa, M., Williamsb, D., Couzensa, G. and Klawittere, J., 2021. Pyrocarbon for joint replacement 5. *Joint Replacement Technology*, p. 145.
33. Franceschetti, E., Gregori, P., Giurazza, G., Papalia, G., Caraffa, A. and Papalia, R., 2023. Short to early-mid term clinical outcomes and survival of pyrocarbon shoulder implants: A systematic review and meta-analysis. *Journal of Shoulder and Elbow Arthroplasty*, *7*, p. 24715492231152143.
34. Shekhawat, D., Singh, A., Bhardwaj, A. and Patnaik, A., 2021. A short review on polymer, metal and ceramic based implant materials. In *IOP Conference Series: Materials Science and Engineering* (Vol. 1017, No. 1, p. 012038). IOP Publishing
35. Batak, B., Cakmak, G., Seidt, J. and Yilmaz, B., 2021. Load to failure of high-density polymers for implant-supported fixed cantilevered prostheses with titanium bases. *International Journal of Prosthodontics*, *34*(5).
36. Nouri, A., Shirvan, A.R., Li, Y. and Wen, C., 2021. Additive manufacturing of metallic and polymeric load-bearing biomaterials using laser powder bed fusion: A review. *Journal of Materials Science & Technology*, *94*, pp. 196–215.
37. Bergström, J.S. and Hayman, D., 2016. An overview of mechanical properties and material modeling of polylactide (PLA) for medical applications. *Annals of Biomedical Engineering*, *44*, pp. 330–40.
38. Bou-Francis, A., Piercey, M., Al-Qatami, O., Mazzanti, G., Khattab, R. and Ghanem, A., 2020. Polycaprolactone blends for fracture fixation in low load-bearing applications. *Journal of Applied Polymer Science*, *137*(32), p. 48940.
39. Stella, S.M., Sridhar, T.M., Ramprasath, R., Gimbun, J. and Vijayalakshmi, U., 2022. Physio-chemical and biological characterization of novel HPC (Hydroxypropylcellulose): HAP (Hydroxyapatite): PLA (Poly Lactic Acid) electrospun nanofibers as implantable material for bone regenerative application. *Polymers*, *15*(1), p. 155.
40. Shahemi, N., Liza, S., Abbas, A.A. and Merican, A.M., 2018. Long-term wear failure analysis of uhmwpe acetabular cup in total hip replacement. *Journal of the Mechanical Behavior of Biomedical Materials*, *87*, pp. 1–9.
41. Evans, S.L. and Gregson, P.J., 1998. Composite technology in load-bearing orthopaedic implants. *Biomaterials*, *19*(15), pp. 1329–42.
42. Kang, Y., Scully, A., Young, D.A., Kim, S., Tsao, H., Sen, M. and Yang, Y., 2011. Enhanced mechanical performance and biological evaluation of a PLGA coated β-TCP composite scaffold for load-bearing applications. *European Polymer Journal*, *47*(8), pp. 1569–77.
43. Chellappa, M. and Vijayalakshmi, U., 2017. In-situ fabrication of zirconium–titanium nano-composite and its coating on Ti-6Al-4V for biomedical applications. *IET Nanobiotechnology*, *11*(1), pp. 83–90.
44. M. Chellappa, U. Anjaneyulu, Geeth Manivasagam and U. Vijayalakshmi, *Synthesis and In-Vitro Electrochemical Study of Composite Coatings on Implant by Electrophoretic Deposition*, International conference on emerging trends in chemical science At: *Journal of Indian Chemical Science, 92*(4), 501–504.
45. Masson, B.A.R.N., 2009. Emergence of the alumina matrix composite in total hip arthroplasty. *International Orthopaedics*, *33*, pp. 359–63.
46. Abere, D.V., Oyatogun, G.M., Oluwasegun, K.M., Ayodele, T.J., Ajayi, S.V., Ohwoekevwo, J.U. and Adejo, O.H., 2018. Synthesis and characterization of alumina-chitosan-hydroxyapatite biocomposites for load bearing application. *European Scientific Journal*, *14*, p. 145.

47. Ding, S.J., Chu, Y.H. and Wang, D.Y., 2017. Enhanced properties of novel zirconia-based osteo-implant systems. *Applied Materials Today*, *9*, pp. 622–32.
48. Behera, A., Swain, B. and Sahoo, D.K., 2020. Fiber-reinforced ceramic matrix nanocomposites. In *Fiber-Reinforced Nanocomposites: Fundamentals and Applications* (pp. 359–68). Elsevier.
49. Haneef, M., Rahman, J.F., Yunus, M., Zameer, S., Patil, S. and Yezdani, T., 2013. Hybrid polymer matrix composites for biomedical applications. *International Journal of Modern Engineering Research*, *3*(2), pp. 970–9.
50. Bakar, M.A., Cheng, M.H.W., Tang, S.M., Yu, S.C., Liao, K., Tan, C.T., Khor, K.A. and Cheang, P., 2003. Tensile properties, tension–tension fatigue and biological response of polyetheretherketone–hydroxyapatite composites for load-bearing orthopedic implants. *Biomaterials*, 24(13), pp. 2245–50.
51. Yoshii, T., Dumas, J.E., Okawa, A., Spengler, D.M. and Guelcher, S.A., 2012. Synthesis, characterization of calcium phosphates/polyurethane composites for weight-bearing implants. *Journal of Biomedical Materials Research Part B: Applied Biomaterials*, 100(1), pp. 32–40.
52. Petelinšek, N. and Mommer, S., 2024. Tough hydrogels for load-bearing applications. *Advanced Science*, p. 2307404.
53. Costa, A.M. and Mano, J.F., 2015. Extremely strong and tough hydrogels as prospective candidates for tissue repair–A review. *European Polymer Journal*, *72*, pp. 344–64.
54. Mehta, P., Sharma, M. and Devi, M., 2023. Hydrogels: An overview of its classifications, properties, and applications. *Journal of the Mechanical Behavior of Biomedical Materials*, p. 106145.
55. Bodugoz-Senturk, H., Macias, C.E., Kung, J.H. and Muratoglu, O.K., 2009. Poly (vinyl alcohol)–acrylamide hydrogels as load-bearing cartilage substitute. *Biomaterials*, *30*(4), pp. 589–96.
56. Patel, S.K., Swain, B., Roshan, R., Sahu, N.K. and Behera, A., 2020. A brief review of shape memory effects and fabrication processes of NiTi shape memory alloys. *Materials Today: Proceedings*, *33*, pp. 5552–6.
57. Abitha, H., Kavitha, V., Gomathi, B. and Ramachandran, B., 2020. A recent investigation on shape memory alloys and polymers based materials on bio artificial implants-hip and knee joint. *Materials Today: Proceedings*, *33*, pp. 4458–66.
58. Behera, A. and Behera, A., 2022. Shape-memory materials. In *Advanced Materials: An Introduction to Modern Materials Science* (pp. 1–42). Springer, Cham.
59. Pfeifer, R., Müller, C.W., Hurschler, C., Kaierle, S., Wesling, V. and Haferkamp, H., 2013. Adaptable orthopedic shape memory implants. *Procedia Cirp*, *5*, pp. 253–8.
60. Shittu, J., Pole, M., Cockerill, I., Sadeghilaridjani, M., Reddy, L.V.K., Manivasagam, G., Singh, H., Grewal, H.S., Arora, H.S. and Mukherjee, S., 2020. Biocompatible high entropy alloys with excellent degradation resistance in a simulated physiological environment. *ACS Applied Bio Materials*, *3*(12), pp. 8890–900.
61. Gurel, S., Nazarahari, A., Canadinc, D., Çabuk, H. and Bal, B., 2021. Assessment of biocompatibility of novel TiTaHf-based high entropy alloys for utility in orthopedic implants. *Materials Chemistry and Physics*, *266*, p. 124573.
62. Wang, S.P. and Xu, J., 2017. TiZrNbTaMo high-entropy alloy designed for orthopedic implants: As-cast microstructure and mechanical properties. *Materials Science and Engineering: C*, *73*, pp. 80–9.
63. Hench, L.L. and Jones, J.R., 2015. Bioactive glasses: Frontiers and challenges. *Frontiers in Bioengineering and Biotechnology*, *3*, p. 194.

64. Khan, M.M., Nemati, A., Rahman, Z.U., Shah, U.H., Asgar, H. and Haider, W., 2018. Recent advancements in bulk metallic glasses and their applications: A review. *Critical Reviews in Solid State and Materials Sciences*, *43*(3), pp. 233–68.
65. Li, H.F. and Zheng, Y.F., 2016. Recent advances in bulk metallic glasses for biomedical applications. *Acta Biomaterialia*, *36*, pp. 1–20.
66. Ida, H., Seiryu, M., Takeshita, N., Iwasaki, M., Yokoyama, Y., Tsutsumi, Y., Ikeda, E., Sasaki, S., Miyashita, S., Sasaki, S. and Fukunaga, T., 2018. Biosafety, stability, and osteogenic activity of novel implants made of Zr70Ni16Cu6Al8 bulk metallic glass for biomedical application. *Acta Biomaterialia*, *74*, pp. 505–17.
67. Yang, H., Jia, B., Zhang, Z., Qu, X., Li, G., Lin, W., Zhu, D., Dai, K. and Zheng, Y., 2020. Alloying design of biodegradable zinc as promising bone implants for load-bearing applications. *Nature Communications*, *11*(1), p. 401.
68. Kim, T., See, C.W., Li, X. and Zhu, D., 2020. Orthopedic implants and devices for bone fractures and defects: Past, present and perspective. *Engineered Regeneration*, *1*, pp. 6–18.
69. Safari, N., Golafshan, N., Kharaziha, M., Reza Toroghinejad, M., Utomo, L., Malda, J. and Castilho, M., 2020. Stable and antibacterial magnesium–graphene nanocomposite-based implants for bone repair. *ACS Biomaterials Science & Engineering*, *6*(11), pp. 6253–62.
70. Kim, S.M., Kang, I.G., Cheon, K.H., Jang, T.S., Kim, H.E., Jung, H.D. and Kang, M.H., 2020. Enhanced bioactivity of micropatterned hydroxyapatite embedded poly (L-lactic) acid for a load-bearing implant. *Polymers*, *12*(10), p. 2390.
71. Sharipova, A.F., Psakhie, S.G., Gotman, I. and Gutmanas, E.Y., 2020. Smart nanocomposites based on Fe–Ag and Fe–Cu nanopowders for biodegradable high-strength implants with slow drug release. *Physical Mesomechanics*, *23*, pp. 128–34.
72. Abazari, S., Shamsipur, A., Bakhsheshi-Rad, H.R. and Berto, F., 2022. Functionalized carbon nanotube-encapsulated magnesium-based nanocomposites with outstanding mechanical and biological properties as load-bearing bone implants. *Materials & Design*, *213*, p. 110354.
73. Xu, Q., Wang, S., Bai, Y., Wang, Q., Yang, R., Wang, X., Li, X. and Zhang, X., 2024. Porous Ti3SiC2 ceramics with improved osteogenic functions via biomineralization as load-bearing bone implants. *Journal of Materials Science & Technology*, *195*, 248–259.
74. Ramakrishna, V.A., Chamoli, U., Rajan, G., Mukhopadhyay, S.C., Prusty, B.G. and Diwan, A.D., 2020. Smart orthopaedic implants: A targeted approach for continuous postoperative evaluation in the spine. *Journal of Biomechanics*, *104*, p. 109690.
75. Nemcakova, I., Litvinec, A., Mandys, V., Potocky, S., Plencner, M., Doubkova, M., Nanka, O., Olejnickova, V., Sankova, B., Bartos, M. and Ukraintsev, E., 2022. Coating Ti6Al4V implants with nanocrystalline diamond functionalized with BMP-7 promotes extracellular matrix mineralization in vitro and faster osseointegration in vivo. *Scientific Reports*, *12*(1), p. 5264.
76. Nouri, A., Shirvan, A.R., Li, Y. and Wen, C., 2021. Additive manufacturing of metallic and polymeric load-bearing biomaterials using laser powder bed fusion: A review. *Journal of Materials Science & Technology*, *94*, pp. 196–215.
77. Yamomo, G., Hossain, N., Towfighian, S. and Willing, R., 2021. Design and analysis of a compliant 3D printed energy harvester housing for knee implants. *Medical Engineering & Physics*, *88*, pp. 59–68.
78. Bandyopadhyay, A., Mitra, I., Ciliveri, S., Avila, J.D., Dernell, W., Goodman, S.B. and Bose, S., 2023. Additively manufactured Ti–Ta–Cu alloys for the next-generation load-bearing implants. *International Journal of Extreme Manufacturing*, *6*(1), p. 015503.

79. Blázquez-Carmona, P., Sanz-Herrera, J.A., Martínez-Vázquez, F.J., Domínguez, J. and Reina-Romo, E., 2021. Structural optimization of 3D-printed patient-specific ceramic scaffolds for in vivo bone regeneration in load-bearing defects. *Journal of the Mechanical Behavior of Biomedical Materials*, *121*, p. 104613.
80. Freitag, J., Wickham, J., Shah, K., Li, D., Norsworthy, C. and Tenen, A., 2020. Mesenchymal stem cell therapy combined with arthroscopic abrasion arthroplasty regenerates cartilage in patients with severe knee osteoarthritis: A case series. *Regenerative Medicine*, *15*(8), pp. 1957–77.
81. Freitag, J., Shah, K., Wickham, J., Li, D., Norsworthy, C. and Tenen, A., 2020. Evaluation of autologous adipose-derived mesenchymal stem cell therapy in focal chondral defects of the knee: A pilot case series. *Regenerative Medicine*, *15*(6), pp. 1703–17.
82. Gotman, I., Ben-David, D., Unger, R.E., Böse, T., Gutmanas, E.Y. and Kirkpatrick, C.J., 2013. Mesenchymal stem cell proliferation and differentiation on load-bearing trabecular Nitinol scaffolds. *Acta Biomaterialia*, *9*(9), pp. 8440–8.
83. Kandel, R., Jang, S.R., Shrestha, S., Ghimire, U., Shrestha, B.K., Park, C.H. and Kim, C.S., 2021. A bimetallic load-bearing bioceramics of TiO2@ ZrO2 integrated polycaprolactone fibrous tissue construct exhibits anti bactericidal effect and induces osteogenesis in MC3T3-E1 cells. *Materials Science and Engineering: C*, *131*, p. 112501.
84. Choi, Y., Park, M.H. and Lee, K., 2020. Injectable thermoresponsive hydrogel/nanofiber hybrid scaffolds inducing human adipose-derived stem cell chemotaxis. *Journal of Industrial and Engineering Chemistry*, *82*, pp. 89–97.
85. Kazimierczak, P. and Przekora, A., 2020. Osteoconductive and osteoinductive surface modifications of biomaterials for bone regeneration: A concise review. *Coatings*, *10*(10), p. 971.
86. Stango, S.A.X. and Vijayalakshmi, U., 2021. Electrochemical deposition of HAP/f-MWCNTs and HAP/GO composite layers on 316L SS implant with excellent corrosion resistance performance. *Materials Letters*, *304*, p. 130666.
87. Priyadarshini, B. and Vijayalakshmi, U., 2021. In Vitro bioactivity, biocompatibility and corrosion resistance of multi-ionic (Ce/Si) co-doped hydroxyapatite porous coating on Ti-6Al-4 V for bone regeneration applications. *Materials Science and Engineering: C*, *119*, p. 111620.
88. Shen, X. and Shukla, P., 2020. A review of titanium based orthopaedic implants (Part-I): Physical characteristics, problems and the need for surface modification. *International Journal of Peening Science & Technology*, *1*(4).
89. Brunette, D.M., Tengvall, P., Textor, M., Thomsen, P., Xiao, S.J., Kenausis, G. and Textor, M., 2001. Biochemical modification of titanium surfaces. In *Titanium in Medicine: Material Science, Surface Science, Engineering, Biological Responses and Medical Applications* (pp. 417–55).
90. Liu, X., Chu, P.K. and Ding, C., 2004. Surface modification of titanium, titanium alloys, and related materials for biomedical applications. *Materials Science and Engineering: R: Reports*, *47*(3–4), pp. 49–121.

15 Wearable Biosensors
IoT-driven Innovations in Healthcare Monitoring and Personalized Medicine

Sachin Gupta, Shivali Gupta, and Gursimran Kaur

CONTENTS

15.1 INTRODUCTION

Wearable biosensors are nowadays considered as an emerging area of research and innovation in modern healthcare. The biosensors are liable to provide continuous, real-time monitoring of various physiological parameters with the use of low power and less resources than conventional methods. With the advancement in Micro Electro Mechanical System (MEMS) technology, these devices are now embedded in various

DOI: 10.1201/9781003516064-15

electronic items, such as wristbands, smartwatches, or various types of adhesive patches for non-invasive measurement of health metrics [1]. Wearable biosensors have the ability to measure and process ongoing health signals and chunk of data outside traditional clinical settings. This facility transforms the biomedical sensor domain from reactive to proactive health management. It has been observed from the latest studies that the integration of wearable biosensors with the Internet of Things (IoT) has further boosted their impact in biomedical sector and healthcare premises. IoT is a versatile framework in which the interconnected devices communicate with each other and exchange the set of data over a wireless network, such as the internet or another ad hoc network. The integration of IoT and biosensors augments the functionality of wearable biosensors by ensuring seamless data transmission and analysis [2,3]. This IoT-based module enables the connectivity of wearable sensors and devices to transmit health data to cloud-based systems in real time which helps healthcare experts and doctors with immediate access to patient information and facilitating timely medical treatments and interventions. There are various studies in which diverse applications and devices are designed to cater to human health under critical situations. There are various medical issues such as Sugar where real-time feedback is required for managing chronic conditions and timely adjustments to treatment, and injection of medical dose can prevent any serious complications and improve patient health outcomes [4,5]. Heart health monitoring is also one of the key research areas where there is need to integrate ECG sensors with IoT to monitor heart activities in real-time phase to alert the medical expert with potential arrhythmias or other cardiovascular issues to take decision before time [6]. The association and compatibility of wearable biosensors and IoT is also encouraging the market of personalized healthcare. In personalized healthcare, the sensor modules enable the chip to collect, treat, and process the signal data on chip and analyse signal so that the medical care team tailors the treatment plans to individual patients. This technology enables the precision of interventions and improving patient engagement in healthcare treatment steps [7]. **Figure 15.1** shows the working mechanism of a bioelectronic sensor.

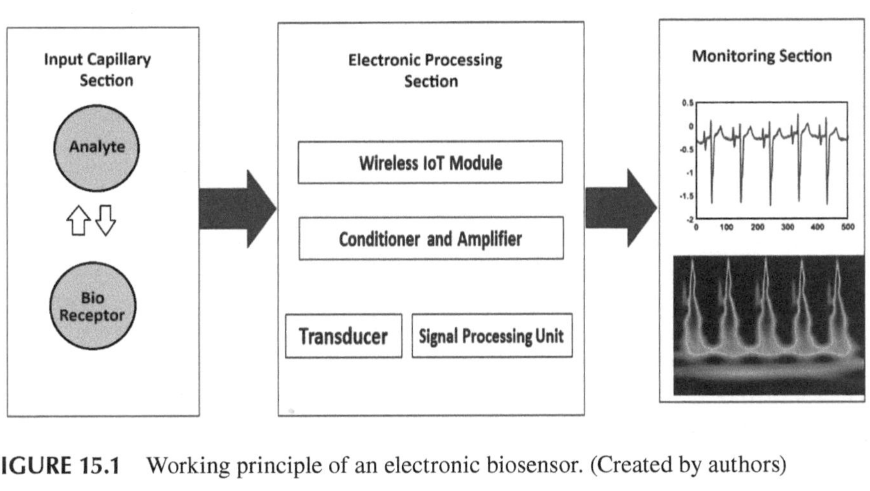

FIGURE 15.1 Working principle of an electronic biosensor. (Created by authors)

As per recent studies, the inclusion of advanced soft computing methods, algorithms, and machine learning models with wearable sensor network can identify health trends and predict potential issues which help the patient to be caseous during recovery period. As per experts, the integration offers more nuanced care in some remote locations and understanding of a patient's health status [8,9]. It has been projected by medical experts and scientific community that the revolution of wearable biosensors and their flexibility to associate with other emerging technologies such as AI and IoT will govern the future of healthcare by providing more comprehensive, real-time insights into health situations. This transformative technology boosts the accuracy and efficiency of health monitoring devices and opens new horizons for personalized and other preventive care of human subjects. There is a need to palpate certain aspects, such as types of wearable biosensors, their association with IoT, and challenges associated with these technologies, for the embedment of a common sight for better understanding at a common platform. Wearable biosensors play a pivotal role in modern health management, as they are capable of continuous and non-invasive monitoring of human health-related physiological parameters. The biosensors are made on certain principal aspects related to material, patch assembly, physical parameter processing, and casing. Due to these properties, the biosensors are embedded in electronic gadgets items like mobile phone, smart bands, smartwatches, and other kind of plastic bands to provide real-time health data.

15.2 CLASSIFICATION OF BIOSENSORS BASED ON PHYSICAL ASPECTS

Wearable biosensors are primarily classified on the basis of certain unique working principles such as electrochemical, optical, and mechanical which are discussed in relation to human healthcare under every phase of their care. **Figure 15.2** shows the broad class of biosensors based on their stimulation principle.

15.2.1 Electrochemical Biosensors

The biosensor typically contains a bioreceptor (such as an enzyme or antibody) that interacts with a target analyte to generate a chemical reaction. This reaction generates motion in the electrons, and as a result an electrical signal is generated in the form of current, voltage, or resistance. The signal is further processed by the electronic sensor and processing unit to quantify the analyte, and then electrochemical biosensors enable the medical expert to scale out the disease or disorder during real-time monitoring. Electrochemical biosensors can detect biochemical reactions by measuring changes in variable electrical signals. As per studies, these sensors are very useful in monitoring specific biochemical markers, such as glucose or cholesterol in the human body. Electrochemical glucose sensors work by employing an enzyme electrode system. When glucose interacts with the enzyme, it produces an electrochemical signal which is proportional to the produced glucose concentration. This signal is further converted into a measurable output [8–11]. As per recent research and development, various non-invasive glucose monitoring devices are developed which use technologies like near-infrared spectroscopy or Raman spectroscopy to

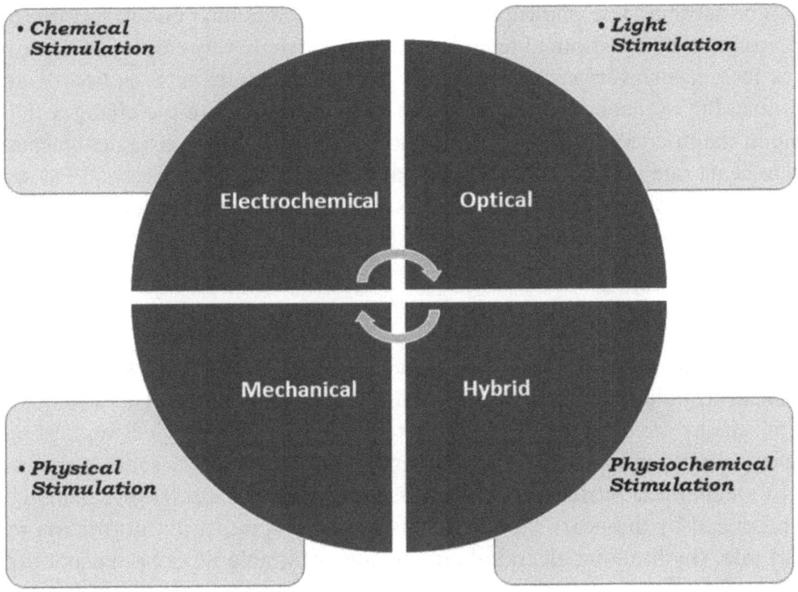

FIGURE 15.2 Classification of biosensors as per their stimulation process (Created by authors).

scale out or estimate glucose levels through the skin by which the excess need for frequent blood samples has been reduced. Another application of electrochemical biosensors is to help athletes and individuals engaged in high-intensity workouts to monitor their physical signals. Lactate sensors measure the concentration of lactate in sweat or interstitial fluid which helps to enhance the insights into physical exertion and recovery status of various body muscles and organs. These sensors use an enzyme-based reaction to detect lactate levels, which can help in optimizing training regimens and preventing overtraining.

15.2.2 Optical Biosensors

Optical biosensors use the principle of light-based physical aspects such as reflection, refraction, coherence, and so on to measure physiological signals of human subjects. These sensors promote the concept of non-invasive monitoring of vital signs, such as heart rate, blood oxygen saturation, and respiratory rate. Pulse oximeters are nowadays available in various hand-held personal healthcare devices which are a type of optical biosensor. Optical biosensors-based devices use the concept of light absorption to scale out the concentration of oxygenated and deoxygenated hemoglobin levels in the blood. Pulse oximeters can calculate blood oxygen saturation level by emitting light through the skin and measuring the intensity of transmitted or reflected light usually on the finger. This application is instrumental in serving individuals for continuous monitoring of oxygen levels and alerts users to potential hypoxemia with severe respiratory conditions, such as chronic obstructive pulmonary disease

(COPD) or asthma. The photo platysma graph (PPG) is also one of the innovative principles in relation to optical technique which is extensively employed in wearable devices to measure various types of health-related signals such as heart rate and blood flow. PPG sensors use the principle of light to measure the changes in blood volume in the microvascular part of the skin. The optical biosensors can accurately estimate heart rate and track cardiovascular health-related parameters. PPG sensors are nowadays very popularly used in fitness trackers and smartwatches for real-time feedback on their heart rate during exercise and other types of hard training [12].

15.2.3 Mechanical Biosensors

Mechanical biosensors are framed to measure physical changes by using core mechanical stimulus such as pressure, strain or deformation, stress, and so on. These types of sensors are used in observing certain types of physiological signals, including heart activity and muscle expansion and contractions. ECG sensors are categorized in mechanical biosensors which are used to detect electrical signals caused to be produced by the heart chamber. This sensor can measure information related to heart rate, rhythm, and electrical conduction. Wearable ECG biosensors use tiny assembly of electrodes which are placed on the skin to capture these variabilities in the signals. The signal is further processed to identify key arrhythmias or other cardiac abnormalities. There are pools of applications and benefits to individuals with certain level of heart conditions or those who have cardiac rehabilitations over the time to indicate early detection of irregularities. Another broad application of mechanical biosensors is to observe and monitor muscle activity and biomechanics. Electromyography (EMG) sensors measure electrical activity in muscles, providing insights into muscle function, fatigue, and rehabilitation progress. EMG sensors are used in rehabilitation settings to assess muscle performance and recovery, helping clinicians to keep record of patient progress [13].

15.2.4 Hybrid Biosensors

The advancement in fabrication technology has resulted in the foundation of hybrid biosensors. These sensors are developed by combining multiple physical and chemical sensing principles to enhance their functionality in various measuring devices. Hybrid sensors integrating electrochemical and optical methods are liable to develop a fusion-based mechanism to simultaneously monitor glucose levels and hydration status of a patient under treatment. These sensors use electrochemical techniques to measure glucose and then the optical sensing module to assess hydration by variability in the produced light absorption or scattering. These kinds of integration leads to the development of comprehensive and advanced health monitoring devices in a single unit. These kinds of sensors may provide the end users with a more holistic and in-depth view of their biological signals [14–18].

Wearable biosensors have transformed various areas of health-related checkups and monitoring by providing real-time data to diagnose diseases in a non-invasive way. There is a pool of applications span in various areas of the healthcare sector in relation to chronic disease management and preventive healthcare sector.

In chronic disease management, wearable biosensors enable continuous monitoring of conditions such as diabetes and cardiovascular diseases, facilitating timely interventions and personalized treatment plans. In preventive healthcare, wearable biosensors play a main role in early detection of health issues and promoting proactive healthcare and management. Wearable biosensors are very flexible to attach with other technologies such as IoT and machine learning methods which are discussed further [19].

15.3 IOT INTEGRATION IN WEARABLE BIOSENSORS

The integration of IoT with wearable biosensors has transformed the health monitoring sector due to its real-time data measurement and collection, resulting in enhanced personalized healthcare for individual. As per studies, the connection and association of wearable devices to a framework of IoT enlarge the power of sensors and contribute to more effective and impactful health management across the world. **Figure 15.3** shows the application modules associated with IoT and biomedical equipment.

15.3.1 Real-Time Data Collection and Transmission

IoT technology is an emerging area in relation to wireless sensor network (WSN) which is used to capture and transmit data from one location to other remote location wirelessly using an ad hoc network. The integration of IoT module in wearable biosensors enables them to collect and transmit health data from the human subjects in real time. Wearable biosensors, such as smartwatches, fitness bands, and medical patches, equipped with IoT capabilities permit the health practitioners to monitor and track various physiological and health-related

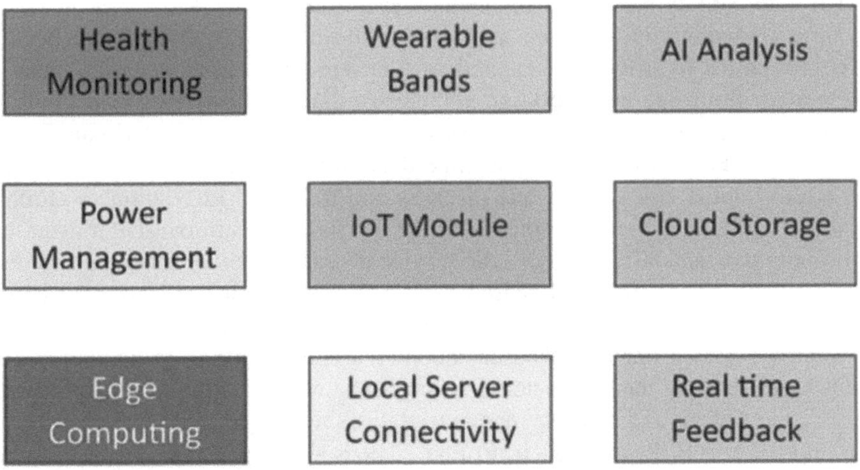

FIGURE 15.3 Current role of IoT in biosensors. (Created by authors)

signals continuously over time. The signals such as stress levels, heartbeat, oxygen level, glucose level, and body temperature are measured and transmitted to user visual interface on time. The collected signal data is transmitted and received wirelessly via latest communication technologies such as Bluetooth, Zig BEE, LoRA, Wi-Fi, or other cellular networks to cloud-based platforms or mobile applications [20–23].

IoT-enabled glucose monitors are one of the best devices of fusion-based sensor network where blood glucose level of subject is regularly traced. Membrane-based sensors are used to measure glucose concentrations inside the interstitial fluid and transmit this informative data to user app-based module in adjunction with cloud server. This kind of fast transmission enables the users to receive alerts for any deviation with respect to its tuned level of normal ranges. By this way, the user can govern the adjustments to insulin dosage or dietary intakes. Similarly, wearable ECG sensors equipped with IoT capabilities transmit real-time data on heart activity to healthcare providers [24]. This continuous monitoring helps the medical practitioners to detect early signs of bradycardia, tachycardia, or arrhythmias or other cardiac abnormalities. Such devices are helpful in timely intervention and reducing the risk of serious cardiovascular shocks. The IoT technology somehow contributes in edge-computing applications where the node processes and formulates the results at a sensor node.

15.3.2 Enhancement in Personalized Healthcare

The association of IoT modules with non-invasive wearable biosensors significantly enhance the power of personalized healthcare by enabling more accurate and personal management of health conditions. The approach of continuous collection and deeply analysing health signals makes IoT-enabled wearable devices a comprehensive understanding of patient's health to serve treatment plans and interventions [25–28].

The adoption of advanced data analytics, fuzzy logic, and other machine learning algorithms is observed as the key innovations in personalized healthcare through IoT to provide the capability of interpret data from wearable sensors. These algorithms can analyse large volumes of data to identify critical kinds of patterns and predict potential health issues. Machine learning models can formulate and process historical and real-time data from wearable devices to predict the health-related risks of various diseases and disorders in relation to chronic conditions such as diabetes, respiratory tract blockage, or cardiovascular diseases. This predictive capability provides the service for early disorder-related symptoms and intervention, making healthcare providers to implement preventive measures before the onset of serious health problems [29].

Wearable biosensors in IoT-based modules are adaptable to individual health needs by calibrating the parameters in accordance with situation, providing health issues-related alerts and possible recommendations to the user. It has been observed from studies that if the patient's heart rate exceeds a set threshold, then the system transmits notifications to both the medical expert and patient under observation and suggests necessary actions such as adjusting medication or seeking medical advice.

The bio sensors not only improve patient health-related care and engagement but also guarantees his health management is aligned with his personal profiles and desires to improve health status. In relation to remote patient monitoring, it has been observed that these sensors have the ability to deliver personalized healthcare through IoT integration at distant locations. These sensor nodes enable patients with chronic conditions to monitor themselves without regular visits to clinics and hospitals. This remote monitoring facility is very valuable for managing long-term conditions, as it allows for ongoing monitoring and timely adjustments to treatment ideas and plans in real-time health signals.

15.3.3 Challenges and Considerations

There are various kinds of benefits for IoT integration with wearable biosensors, but with the advancement there are various challenges and problems which need to be focused by research community, in terms of data privacy and its safety. It has been observed that the continuous communication or transmission of health-related signals and information on a congested network brings issues about potential data breaches and unauthorized access.

There are predefined areas where there is a need of focus by research community such as advancements in cybersecurity to protect data transmitted between wearable devices and remote cloud frame-based platforms. There is need to embed various encryption techniques to protect the data from malpractices during transmission and ensuring that it remains confidential and protected from unauthorized person to access. The blockchain technology can be assumed as a method for enhancing data liability and security. Blockchain mechanism enables a decentralized and protected or immutable ledger of health data. It helps to prevent tampering and ensures the integrity of health devices and sensor nodes in a safe condition. **Table 15.1** shows the comparative analysis of various IoT-based wireless modules in terms of their performance when they are deputed in association with biosensors.

Interoperability of IoT communication frame is also one of the emerging areas of research in relation to wearable biosensors with other health devices and technologies. It has been observed that the biosensor devices must be synchronize with electronic record of health of a patient and enables the management systems to create a health and cohesive observation and watch ecosystem. This integration provides a comprehensive access to patient's health related track of history and real-time data glitches at certain moment of time. It will support more robust a strong decision-making to improve the precision, recall and accuracy of diagnoses and treatment modules.

In areas where there is need of temperament of research experts, the healthcare applications of wearable biosensors are discussed. The main emphasis and elaboration is given on why these technologies are adopted in the biomedical sector for managing diseases history, tracking fitness, and wellness status of patients and enabling remote patient monitoring. Further sections will highlight the practical implications of IoT-enhanced wearable biosensors to impact on improving patient outcomes [28–31].

TABLE 15.1
Comparison of IoT-based Technologies used in Wearable Biosensor Devices for Data Transmission

Module	Latency (ms)	Power Consumption (mW)	Range (metres)	Bandwidth (Mbps)	Application in Biosensors
Bluetooth Low Energy	3–5	0.5–1.2	10–99	1.2	Fitness trackers, heart rate monitors, glucose monitors [11,12]
Wi-Fi	20–52	150–400	120	54–608	Continuous glucose monitoring, smart patches [13,14]
ZigBee	35–110	2–47	10–199	0.29	Long-term patient monitoring, wearable health sensors [15,16]
LoRa	>120	0.12–0.15	3000–12,000	0.0003–0.005	Remote patient monitoring in rural areas, environmental sensors [17,1 8]
NB-IoT	100–118	200–255	1,000–11,000	0.1–0.22	Wearable medical devices for chronic disease management [19,20]
5G	<1.8	300–450	11,000	1000–20,000	Real-time health monitoring, remote surgery assistance [21,22]
RFID	600	0.01–0.03	10,000–50,000	0.0011–0.0056	Periodic health monitoring in remote areas [23,24]

15.4 HEALTHCARE APPLICATIONS OF WEARABLE BIOSENSORS

Wearable biosensors have become very popular in healthcare system because it is able to provide valuable insights and sophisticated management capabilities in relation to a broad class of domains. These devices are capable of bridging the gap in managing chronic diseases, their keeping tracking fitness, and allowing a flexible remote patient monitoring to users. There are certain technical facilities such as real-time data measurement and personalized feedback. Wearable biosensors encourage the effectiveness of healthcare interventions and contribute to patient health improvements in terms of one of the chief outputs [32].

15.4.1 Managing Chronic Diseases

Wearable biosensors are considered as one of the key components in the management of chronic diseases by continuous monitoring of crucial physiological signals and process it to timely data that informs treatment decisions.

15.4.1.1 Diabetes Management

Diabetes measurement and its management is a notable test in medical sector, and it is one of the applications of wearable biosensors. Continuous glucose monitors are the electrochemical sensing mechanism-based device that can scale out glucose levels in the interstitial fluid in a non-invasive way from the skin. These sensors can give real-time glucose readings, which are further communicated to end user's smartphone or other handy monitoring devices. The Dexcom G6 CGM system is one of the latest devices which help the users to monitor their glucose levels in no time and receive alerts for certain health-related episodes. The main key application of this device is to make timely adjustments of certain health-monitoring parameters to their insulin therapy so that the whole mechanism can reduce the situation of risk in association to severe glucose fluctuations. Overall, the system improves glucose control of a patient in a very safe and careful manner [32–34].

15.4.1.2 Cardiovascular Health

As per latest studies and medical health experts, cardiovascular health management is one of the emerging areas where the electronic biosensors are also widely used to take care of the health of human subjects. Today, there are various devices such as Apple products and bands, including ECG, PPG, and oxygen sensors that are able observe and monitor heart rate and its related trends. The Apple Watch Series 5 and 6 are loaded with features like ECG key application that can detect kurtosis and abnormalities. These devices can put an alert to the medical expert in relation to massive heart irregularities. Biosensor-based devices are also associated with heart rate variability measurement system and other facilities which can track autonomic nervous system function. It is useful for managing conditions like hypertension and severe heart failure. The demand for these devices has exponentially increased over the years. **Figure 15.4** shows the demand trend [35].

15.4.2 Fitness Tracking

Fitness tracking is an emerging area of research where the deployment of electronic biosensors has the capability to revolutionize the measurement sector in relation to physical signals, exercise performance, and overall health.

15.4.2.1 Activity Monitors

Biosensors are now being transformed to new levels with the integration of advanced sensing protocols to monitor various kinds of activities of human subjects, such as to measure various metrics like steps taken, calories burned, daily routine, and distance travelled. The IOT-based biosensors provide several comprehensive tracking of daily activities and workouts with feedback to improve the physical fitness and body strength levels and helping to set and achieve fitness goals. These devices need further research and development on other features such as heart rate monitoring, sleep tracking, and position judgement for accurate measurement of exercise level and performance [36].

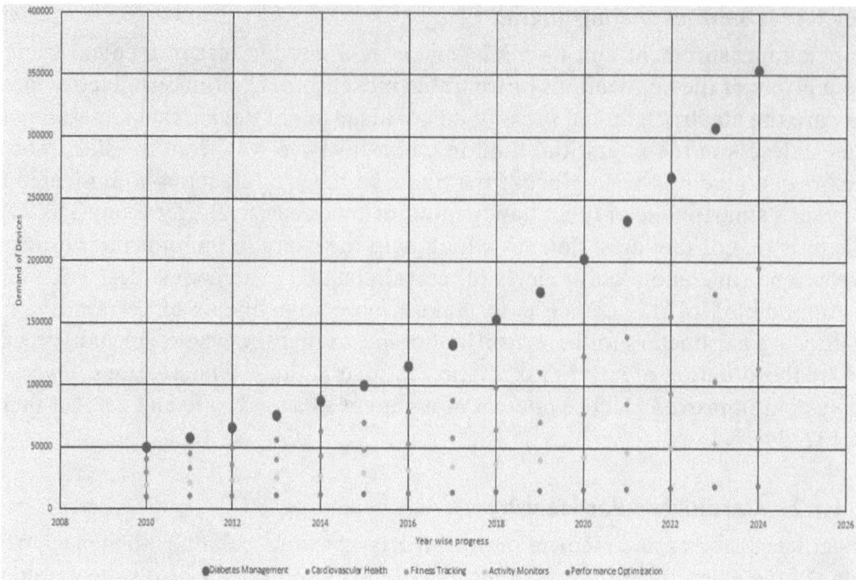

FIGURE 15.4 Demand trend of biosensor-based devices in various application-specific tasks. (Created by authors)

15.4.2.2 Performance Optimization

There are various kinds of human health-related parameters which need an extensive care during the sports and exercise events to scale out the performance and reduce the chances of injury risk. During sports-related events there are certain events and metrics, such as running gait, stride length, and joint angles, which also need to be observed to ensure an optimal performance of athletes. The Catapult Vector machine is a professional device for athletes, as it can scale out and provide data on movement-related classes of patterns and biomechanics, which is liable to help athletes to far improve their training regimens and prevent severe injuries. WHOOP Strap is one of the best examples of IoT-based biosensing devices to measure stress and strain of muscles and their recovery, to emphasize insights into an athlete's training load and recovery status, which can be used to incorporate exercise schedules for improved performance and reduced injury risk [36].

15.4.3 Remote Patient Monitoring

Remote patient monitoring is a facility which is provided by IoT-based modules, and they significantly associate with applications of wearable biosensors for healthcare activities. By this facility the expert can track patients' health status from a remote location with certain clinical tuning parameters. This capability is particularly valuable for managing chronic diseases and supporting long-term care [37].

15.4.3.1 Chronic Disease Management

Wearable biosensors continuously collect health data from human subjects and patients to handle their chronic conditions, such as heart disease, diabetes, and respiratory disorders. Certain devices, such as bioheat-based remote patient-monitoring chips, can measure vital signs, including heartbeats, blood pressure, and oxygen blood saturation. The data is transmitted to healthcare providers in real time. This continuous monitoring allows for timely planning of treatment and early intervention (if there are signs of health deterioration) to improve patient outcomes and reducing hospital readmissions.

15.4.3.2 Post-Surgical Care

After the operation or surgery, it is mandatory to take care of the patient's health and to slate out its recovery. Electronic biosensors are used in post-surgical care to monitor patients' recovery and detect potential complications. The Taction Health application in android is used with a compatible wearable device that tracks post-operative metrics such as heart rate, temperature, and physical activity. This data is shared with the healthcare provider who takes care of the patient's recovery process remotely and informs if any issue arises. This approach not only helps in ensuring a smooth recovery but also reduces the need for frequent in-person follow-up visits [38].

15.4.4 Case Studies for IoT and Biosensors

15.4.4.1 Continuous Glucose Monitoring

As per a research study published in *Diabetes Technology & Therapeutics*, experts and researchers tested and evaluated the impact in terms of accuracy and precision of continuous glucose monitoring on glycaemic control in individuals with Type 1 diabetes in 50 human subjects. The study demonstrated that patients using biosensor-based monitoring system experienced a significant reduction in Hb-Acl levels and a lower incidence of hypoglycaemic episodes as compared to other patients who were using traditional blood glucose monitoring methods. This case study underscores the effectiveness of wearable biosensors in improving diabetes management. This study presents the main highlights and its role in enlarging the patient health care outcomes [39]. **Figure 15.5** shows the related case studies and recent update in the field of biosensors.

15.4.4.2 Wearable ECG Monitoring

A clinical trial published in *Circulation* investigated the use of wearable ECG monitors for detecting atrial fibrillation in patients with a high risk of stroke. The results in the study indicate that wearable ECG devices were very active in identifying fabricator trails and turbulence-based episodes. The observations presume the timely treatment and a reduction in stroke risk. This case study leads the new way of wearable biosensors to enhance cardiovascular care and stop severe complications in early stage of disease in human subjects.

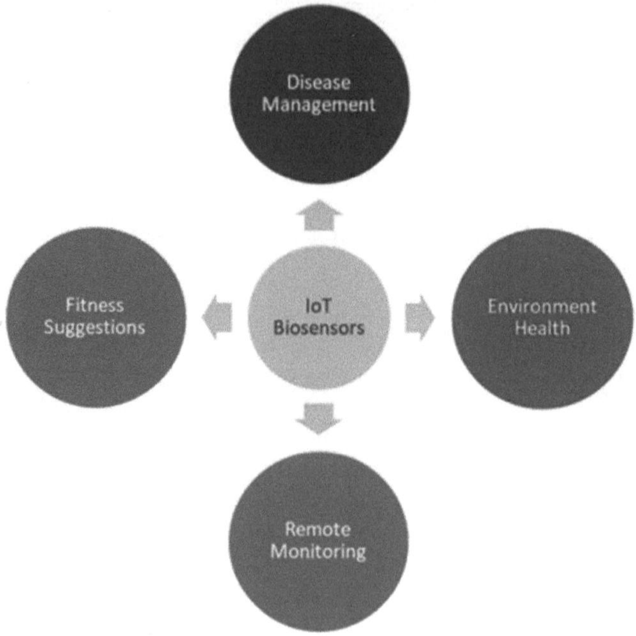

FIGURE 15.5 Recent case studies and progress in IoT-based biosensor gadgets. (Created by authors)

15.5 CHALLENGES IN WEARABLE BIOSENSORS AND IOT INTEGRATION

The association of these electronic biosensors with the IoT devices introduces significant advancements in lab on a chip-based healthcare and monitoring, but there are several key issues and breaches which bring several critical challenges regarding privacy of data and network security, optimal power consumption in terms of current per hour and interoperability [40]. Among these key challenges, the foremost concerns are the data safety and privacy and strong security of sensitive health data which is accumulated by a network of biosensors. The challenges in relation to biosensor and IoT integration are shown in **Figure 15.6**.

The unauthorized access and breaches by some elements can cause issues in these devices, which are deputed to continuously gather and transmit personal health information to end user. Robust encryption methods are the only way to safeguard this data during communication. The end-to-end encryption has various types of security locks by which the health data will be protected during transmission and storage, making it accessible only to authorized persons. The other factors such as multi-factor authentication and biometric verification are also a key solution which can enhance security by adding layers of protection against undesired access. Despite these measures, this is an emerging area of research where constant evolution of cyber threats means that data privacy remains a persistent challenge.

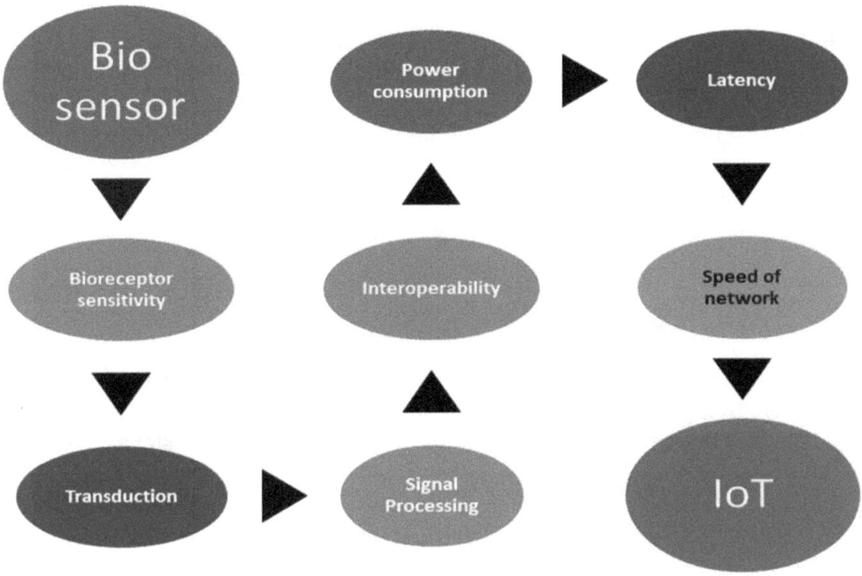

FIGURE 15.6 Research areas related to biosensors and IoT-based modules. (Created by authors)

There is a need for extended studies which will explore advanced technologies to ensure secure health data capturing and transmission over a layered network. Homomorphic encryption is one good application or tool which is used for processing of encrypted data without decryption, hence it will maintain privacy while ensuring analytical and clinical operations. However, the implementation of these technologies on a large scale presents challenges in terms of scalability and latency with existing systems, and their widespread adoption is still emerging [35].

Power consumption and battery drain in relation to assigned load represents another significant issue for IoT-powered electronic biosensors. The sensor nods are continuously trace the signals from the patients due to which the battery rapidly depletes and necessitate frequent recharging or battery replacement is required. The research community is now rigorously focusing on developing energy-efficient sensors unit which will consume low power in relation to optimal communication technologies. Bluetooth low-power devices are designed to minimize energy usage while maintaining functionality of the whole module. Thermoelectric generators and photovoltaic cells are one of the best energy harvesting techniques which are being investigated to convert ambient energy into electrical power. These technologies can extend the life of a battery in relation to its slow drain and reducing the need for frequent recharging. These advancements aim to enhance the practicality and convenience of wearable devices.

Biosensor-based devices regularly use various communication protocols and data formats, which can hinder seamless integration and data exchange. The IEEE 11073 standard provides a framework for health informatics communication, promoting interoperability among medical devices and electronic health records (EHRs). Organizations such as IEEE and ISO are working on developing universal standards and protocols that ensure compatibility and facilitate communication between diverse devices. Furthermore, research is focused on improving semantic interoperability, which involves standardizing data meanings and contexts to ensure consistent interpretation across different systems. Middleware solutions and integration-based platforms are also being developed to support seamless data exchange and integration between various health devices and systems [38].

15.6 FUTURE TRENDS AND ADVANCEMENTS

The future of wearable biosensors is poised to be significantly influenced by emerging technologies, such as AI, Fuzzy logic, and blockchain-based enhanced security and advancements in personalized medicine. AI is set to play a transformative role in wearable biosensors by enabling more sophisticated data analysis and interpretation. With the integration of AI algorithms, biosensing devices can provide more accurate and actionable insights from the vast amounts of data which is collected. Machine learning models can analyse patterns in biometric data to detect early signs of health issues, predict potential problems, and offer personalized recommendations for health management. Advancements in personalized medicine are another significant trend shaping the future of wearable biosensors. Personalized medicine focuses on tailoring healthcare interventions based on individual genetic, environmental, and lifestyle factors. Wearable biosensors are becoming integral to this approach by providing real-time data that can be used to customize treatment plans and optimize health outcomes [26,40].

Blockchain technology is increasingly being explored for its potential to enhance the security and integrity of health data collected by wearable biosensors. The decentralized nature of blockchain in relation to pattern sequence generation provides a secure and tamper-proof ledger for storing health information, which addresses concerns related to data breaches and unauthorized access. By creating an immutable record of health data transactions, blockchain can ensure that data remains accurate and trustworthy throughout its lifecycle. Blockchain can facilitate interoperability among different health systems by providing a standardized framework for data exchange. Certain research groups that are involved into integrating blockchain with wearable biosensors aim to establish secure and efficient methods for managing health data while maintaining privacy and compliance with regulatory standards. As blockchain technology evolves, its application in wearable biosensors is expected to bolster data security and foster greater trust in digital health solutions. Innovations in genomics and proteomics are driving the development of biosensors that can detect specific biomarkers associated with various health conditions. For example, biosensors capable of analysing sweat or saliva for genetic markers can offer insights into individual responses to treatments and enable more precise medication dosing. The convergence of wearable technology with personalized medicine promises to enhance preventive care and treatment efficacy by enabling healthcare providers to deliver more targeted and individualized interventions [38–40].

15.7 CONCLUSION

The integration of wearable biosensors with the IoT represents a profound advancement in healthcare technology, driving significant changes in how health is monitored and managed. Wearable biosensors offer continuous, real-time monitoring of various physiological parameters, such as heart rate, glucose levels, and physical activity, providing invaluable data that supports both preventive and therapeutic interventions. By leveraging IoT connectivity, these devices enable seamless data transmission and communication with other health systems, facilitating a comprehensive approach to health management. This real-time data flow allows for immediate insights and adjustments, enhancing personalized healthcare by tailoring interventions to individual needs.

Artificial intelligence (AI) plays a critical role in amplifying the capabilities of wearable biosensors. AI algorithms can analyse complex data sets collected by these devices, identifying patterns and trends that might not be evident through traditional methods. This advanced data processing enables more accurate health predictions and personalized recommendations. For example, AI-driven analytics can enhance glucose monitoring systems by providing real-time adjustments based on historical and current data, improving the management of diabetes. The integration of AI not only increases the precision of health monitoring but also opens new avenues for personalized treatment strategies and preventive care. Interoperability among different devices and systems is also crucial for effective integration. Standardization efforts are essential to ensure that diverse wearable biosensors and health systems can communicate and exchange data seamlessly. Universal communication protocols and standard data formats are necessary to facilitate this integration and create a cohesive health monitoring ecosystem.

Data privacy and security are foremost among these concerns. As wearable devices collect and transmit sensitive health information, protecting this data from unauthorized access and breaches is paramount. Implementing robust encryption methods and secure authentication protocols is crucial to safeguarding personal health data. The ongoing development of technologies such as blockchain holds promise for enhancing data security by creating decentralized and tamper-proof records, though challenges related to scalability and integration with existing systems remain [13–17].

Power consumption is another significant challenge. Continuous operation of wearable biosensors requires efficient energy use to prolong battery life and reduce the need for frequent recharging. Innovations in low-power technologies and energy harvesting methods are critical to overcoming this issue. Advances in energy-efficient sensors and the integration of energy harvesting solutions, such as thermoelectric generators or photovoltaic cells, are being explored to enhance the practicality and sustainability of wearable devices. AI-based applications are expected to further enhance the capabilities of these devices, making health monitoring even more precise and responsive to individual needs. Blockchain technology offers potential improvements in data security, ensuring that health information remains secure and trustworthy.

ACKNOWLEDGEMENT

Authors are thankful to LPU and research labs for conduction of experiments and exploration of resources.

CONFLICT OF INTEREST

Authors have no conflict of interest.

REFERENCES

[1] Wang, L., et al. "Wearable biosensors in remote healthcare: Current trends and challenges." *Sensors and Actuators B: Chemical*, vol. 303, 2021, p. 127294.

[2] Lin, M., et al. "Advances in flexible electrochemical biosensors for healthcare monitoring." *Biosensors and Bioelectronics*, vol. 155, 2021, p. 112091.

[3] Mishra, S., et al. "IoT-enabled remote health monitoring systems." *IEEE Internet of Things Journal*, vol. 7, no. 3, 2020, pp. 2341–2352.

[4] Kim, J., et al. "Skin-adhesive wearable biosensors for precision health monitoring." *Nature Reviews Bioengineering*, vol. 2, 2023, pp. 13–26.

[5] Zhao, C., et al. "Recent developments in smart wearable biosensors." *IEEE Transactions on Biomedical Engineering*, vol. 68, no. 9, 2021, pp. 2682–2692.

[6] Gupta, M., et al. "Flexible and wearable biosensors: Current status and future perspectives." *Advanced Functional Materials*, vol. 32, no. 12, 2022, p. 2108109.

[7] Lee, S., et al. "Real-time monitoring of health using IoT-enabled wearable sensors." *Journal of Biomedical Materials Research Part A*, vol. 110, no. 8, 2022, pp. 1710–1720.

[8] Fang, Z., et al. "Towards intelligent healthcare monitoring using wearable devices and IoT." *IEEE Access*, vol. 9, 2021, pp. 112792–112804.

[9] Patel, M., et al. "Emerging applications of biosensors in personalized healthcare." *Biosensors*, vol. 12, no. 2, 2022, p. 73.

[10] Zhuang, Y., et al. "Self-powered wearable biosensors for continuous health monitoring." *Nano Energy*, vol. 85, 2021, p. 105941.

[11] Shen, Y., et al. "Review on IoT-enabled wearable biosensors for healthcare applications." *Biomedical Signal Processing and Control*, vol. 63, 2021, p. 102214.

[12] Wei, W., et al. "Applications of flexible wearable biosensors in healthcare monitoring." *Materials Today Advances*, vol. 14, 2022, p. 100208.

[13] Wong, K., et al. "Progress and challenges in wearable biosensors for personalized health monitoring." *ACS Applied Materials & Interfaces*, vol. 12, no. 32, 2020, pp. 35615–35622.

[14] Li, J., et al. "Biosensors for personalized health monitoring." *Sensors*, vol. 20, no. 24, 2020, p. 7178.

[15] Zhou, L., et al. "Wearable biosensors for IoT-based health monitoring." *Journal of Electroanalytical Chemistry*, vol. 906, 2022, p. 115325.

[16] Martin, A., et al. "Wearable biosensors in chronic disease management." *Journal of the American Medical Association*, vol. 324, no. 12, 2020, pp. 1227–1236.

[17] Gupta, D., et al. "Wearable healthcare monitoring systems: Current trends and future directions." *Journal of Materials Chemistry B*, vol. 9, no. 35, 2021, pp. 7633–7647.

[18] Wang, C., et al. "Wireless biosensors for healthcare: Recent advances and future directions." *Biosensors and Bioelectronics*, vol. 162, 2020, p. 112275.

[19] Yao, H., et al. "IoT-integrated wearable biosensors for continuous healthcare monitoring." *IEEE Sensors Journal*, vol. 21, no. 15, 2021, pp. 17128–17138.

[20] Kwon, S., et al. "Multifunctional wearable biosensors for healthcare applications." *Advanced Healthcare Materials*, vol. 9, no. 8, 2020, p. 2001239.

[21] Chen, X., et al. "IoT-enhanced wearable biosensors: Challenges and opportunities." *Journal of Healthcare Engineering*, vol. 2020, 2020, p. 8836736.

[22] Patel, M., et al. "Biosensors for monitoring vital signs in IoT-enabled healthcare systems." *Electrochemistry Communications*, vol. 122, 2021, p. 106906.

[23] Zhao, Z., et al. "Integration of AI and IoT in wearable biosensors for personalized healthcare." *Nature Biomedical Engineering*, vol. 4, no. 6, 2020, pp. 469–80.

[24] Qi, X., et al. "Wearable electrochemical biosensors: Design, challenges, and applications." *Journal of Power Sources*, vol. 499, 2021, p. 229978.

[25] Gao, W., et al. "Wearable biosensors in the Internet of Things: Opportunities and challenges." *IEEE Reviews in Biomedical Engineering*, vol. 14, 2021, pp. 160–72.

[26] Sun, Y., et al. "Advances in AI-driven wearable biosensors for healthcare." *Biosensors*, vol. 13, no. 1, 2023, p. 44.

[27] Jin, Z., et al. "Wearable biochemical sensors for continuous health monitoring." *Journal of Materials Chemistry B*, vol. 8, no. 23, 2020, pp. 5135–5148.

[28] Song, Y., et al. "IoT-based real-time wearable health monitoring systems." *IEEE Transactions on Industrial Electronics*, vol. 68, no. 4, 2021, pp. 3277–3286.

[29] Luo, X., et al. "Flexible wearable biosensors for continuous glucose monitoring." *Biosensors and Bioelectronics*, vol. 151, 2020, p. 111977.

[30] Chen, Y., et al. "AI-enhanced wearable biosensors for precision healthcare." *Journal of Biosensors & Bioelectronics*, vol. 30, no. 6, 2022, pp. 1125–1133.

[31] Rao, P., et al. "Wearable biosensors and IoT: Applications, challenges, and future directions." *Journal of Internet of Things*, vol. 7, 2023, p. 102315.

[32] Liu, Y., et al. "Real-time monitoring with wearable biosensors for healthcare applications." *Nature Communications*, vol. 12, no. 1, 2021, p. 3451.

[33] Yan, X., et al. "Wearable sweat biosensors for precision medicine." *Trends in Biotechnology*, vol. 39, no. 6, 2021, pp. 570–80.

[34] Pan, S., et al. "Recent advancements in flexible wearable biosensors for healthcare." *Advanced Materials Technologies*, vol. 7, no. 4, 2022, p. 2100845.

[35] Zhou, X., et al. "Non-invasive wearable electrochemical biosensors." *ACS Sensors*, vol. 6, no. 2, 2021, pp. 362–9.

[36] Lee, H., et al. "IoT-based wearable biosensors for monitoring physical and physiological signals." *IEEE Sensors Journal*, vol. 20, no. 10, 2020, pp. 4866–4876.

[37] Zhao, Y., et al. "Flexible wearable biosensors for personalized healthcare monitoring." *Sensors and Actuators A: Physical*, vol. 321, 2021, p. 112596.

[38] Kumar, R., et al. "Wireless wearable biosensors for personalized health monitoring." *IEEE Wireless Communications*, vol. 27, no. 1, 2020, pp. 40–46.

[39] Kim, T., et al. "Wearable biosensors for continuous health monitoring." *Biosensors*, vol. 12, no. 3, 2022, p. 190.

[40] Liu, J., et al. "Recent advances in flexible wearable electrochemical biosensors." *Analytical Chemistry*, vol. 94, no. 7, 2022, pp. 3010–3018.

16 Robotics and Automation in Biomedical Manufacturing

State of Art and Challenges

Gaurav Prashar and Hitesh Vasudev

CONTENTS

16.1 INTRODUCTION

The healthcare sector is widely acknowledged as one of the most dynamic and largest sectors worldwide. The goal is to accelerate progress by implementing modernization and innovative strategies. In the past, this industry depended on manual procedures that were time-consuming and susceptible to human mistakes. Indeed, the healthcare system in India is imperfect. The community lacks an adequate number of doctors, nurses, healthcare facilities, and technicians to meet its needs. The quantity of proficient physicians is inadequate to meet the escalating demands of the Indian healthcare system. Simultaneously, these physicians are primarily located in metropolitan regions, resulting in a significant disparity in healthcare professionals between rural and urban communities. Around 74% of the doctors who have completed their graduate studies in India are employed in urban areas, which serve just around one-fourth of the population [1]. Due to the uneven allocation of resources, there is a ratio of one doctor to every 19,000 individuals [2]. By 2030, India will require 2.3 million physicians to achieve the World Health Organization's recommended minimum doctor–patient criteria. The Covid-19 pandemic has demonstrated the un-sustainability of relying heavily on limited manual resources and unworkable congested working conditions of our industrial companies. The manufacture and supply chain of essential products have been closely examined throughout the epidemic, revealing significant

 DOI: 10.1201/9781003516064-16

deficiencies in low-cost manufacturing in distant regions. This has resulted in severe shortages of completed items and raw materials. Consequently, the relocation of manufacturing operations back to domestic shores is unavoidable, as evidenced by numerous governments issuing policy statements urging companies to do so. However, while this development is undoubtedly positive, maintaining cost competitiveness will be of even greater importance. Automation and robotics play a crucial role in achieving and sustaining cost competitiveness. Significant developments in the integration of robotics in manufacturing are depicted in **Figure 16.1.**

The adoption of automation and robotics is expected to become the standard practice, as there is a growing emphasis on minimizing the number of workers in close proximity to each other and ensuring uninterrupted production in the face of any future disruptions to manufacturing and supply chains. Highly responsive and skillful compact collaborative robots will progressively serve as our "Co-Workers." Research will be expedited to cultivate innovative applications for robotics that can be deployed more quickly and are characterized by their adaptability and user-friendliness. Autonomous mobile robotics will become widespread, not just in warehousing and logistics but also in evaluation and sampling. Although the use of automated robotic sanitizing in hospital settings is still in its early stages of development, it may be important to contemplate implementing similar technology in manufacturing facilities.

Even in the field of basic pharmaceutical and biotech manufacturing, there has been a growing recognition of the necessity to use higher levels of automation and robotics [2]. Several companies are exploring ways to free highly compensated chemists and biotechnologists from repetitive duties that do not contribute value, such as environmental and product sampling, as well as to enhance employee safety when working with highly potent, dangerous, and toxic compounds. It is well acknowledged that in biotechnology manufacturing, a significant portion of the operating cost, ranging from 35% to 50%, is attributed to physical labor. The biomedical manufacturing sector, which includes medical devices, diagnostics, and biotechnologies, is experiencing a notable transformation through the incorporation of robotics and automation.

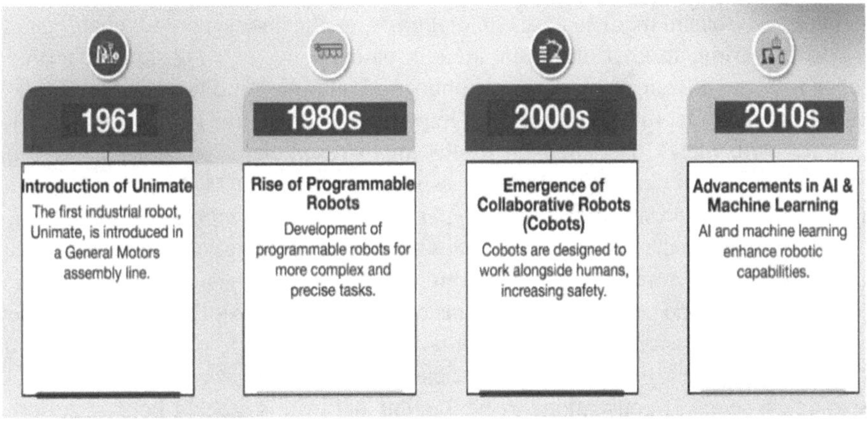

FIGURE 16.1 Significant developments in the integration of robotics in manufacturing.

The implementation of these technologies contributes to the enhancement of production efficiency, the improvement of product quality, and the reduction of human error. Nonetheless, the implementation of these technologies within this highly regulated and intricate industry presents distinct challenges. This chapter examines the present condition of robotics and automation within the biomedical manufacturing sector, along with the challenges encountered by the industry.

16.2 ADVANCEMENTS IN TECHNOLOGY

In the past, robotics was mostly associated with the automotive, fabrication of metal, and consumer goods sectors, and its technology remained relatively unchanged for a long time. However, robotics has now reached a significant milestone in the field of smart manufacturing in the life science manufacturing sector. Compact, agile, robots designed for clean-room environments, with high sensitivity and dexterity. Collaborative robots, autonomous piloted robots, artificial learning, and advanced vision technologies all work together to enable the extensive implementation of automation in both new product development and existing products. Automated and validated manufacturing lines facilitate the management of data and product traceability, making it easier to maintain secure audit trails and comply with regulatory standards. Furthermore, it is important to mention that KUKA not only prioritizes offering robot solutions for the medical device, pharmaceutical, and biotechnology industries but also has a specialized division called the Medical Robotics Division that focuses particularly on medical and operating theatre robotics.

KUKA was been awarded the esteemed "Global Company of the Year" accolade in 2020 for its medical robotics branch. Frost & Sullivan (F&S) a business giant has carried out in-depth analysis of the healthcare robotics market and named KUKA's LBR Med (Medical robot) as one of the versatile robots for its diverse tasks in the healthcare sector. KUKA has been acknowledged as the "Company of the Year" by F&S for its unmatched achievements in the area of medical robots. This medical robot developed by KUKA has become the first certified medical robot to be used in healthcare devices. It is designed and developed to address medical requirements and to be used in different applications in medical care like diagnosis, medical surgery, and rehabilitation.

Rehabilitation, another important area for patients, has seen substantial improvements with the advent of biomedical robots and automation. During rehabilitation, this cutting-edge technology combines important features like robots precision and accuracy with the skill of medical professionals/researchers, resulting in minimal risks and better efficiency [3]. Robotic-assisted rehabilitation (RAR) assists patients in improving muscle strength, flexibility, and limb motor function after stroke [4].

Robotic-assisted therapy (RAT) provides a range of advantages for suffering patients in contrast to other available conventional rehabilitation therapy methods. RAT ensures precise, accurate, and consistent movements resulting in better results. RAT allows medical therapists to customize therapy approaches catering to the patient needs and the progress each patient made leading to efficient rehabilitation process [5]. Hence, RAT expands the scope of conventional rehabilitation and instills a better hope in suffering patients with limited mobility. **Figure 16.2** shows various robotic devices for training.

In the life sciences sector with involvement of machine learning, a significant transformation has taken place during the last decade. The focus of scientists/engineers is

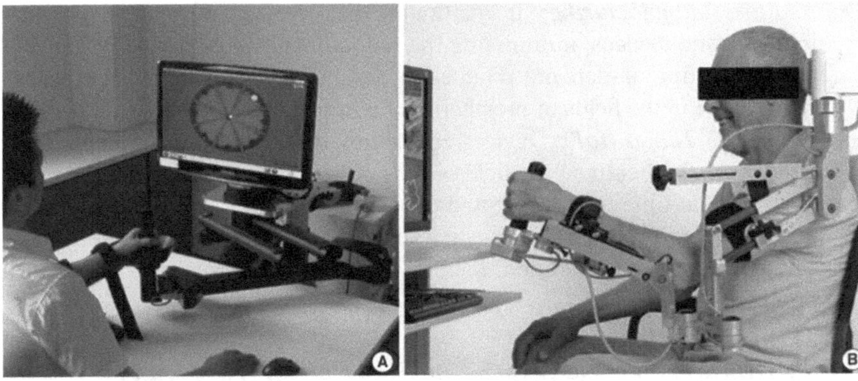

FIGURE 16.2 Different types of robot training equipment: a) For end effectors type, and b) For exoskeleton type [6]. (Open Access article distributed under the terms of the Creative Commons Attribution Non-Commercial License)

on designing and developing smart computers that can mimic human behavior and their responses [7]. Artificial intelligence and robotics (AIR) to medical care industry is still in its initial stages, but with passage of time, with Industrial Revolution 5.0 on the doorstep, there is vast potential for its recognition, adoption, and functionality in the near future [8]. AI no-doubt will revolutionize our work processes in the coming future, especially in the life sciences sector. AI can quickly detect and locate disorders, resulting in faster treatment for patients. The renowned hospitals around the globe have adopted AIR techniques during the crucial time of COVID-19 epidemic for disinfecting and screening COVID-19 patients. During the recent epidemic, several measures such as distantly supervised surgery, distance education, telemedicine, and videoconferencing with doctors were implemented. The pandemic has primarily improved the applicability of robotics in the healthcare industry [9].

In the pharmaceutical manufacturing sector, robots are employed for various tasks, including dispensing, filling, packaging, and labeling of drugs. Robotic arms and automated guided vehicles (AGVs) are utilized for material handling in clean rooms, effectively minimizing contamination risks. In the field of biotechnology, automation plays a critical role, particularly in processes such as cell culture, protein synthesis, and gene editing. Robots facilitate the automation of liquid handling, cell manipulation, and high-throughput screening (HTS), thereby enhancing the efficiency of research and development processes.

16.3 AUTOMATION IN BIOMEDICAL MANUFACTURING

Automation includes a wide range of technologies that extend beyond robotics, with its application in biomedical manufacturing covering multiple domains:

- *Automated Quality Control:* This involves the utilization of advanced machine vision systems and AI-driven analytics for the real-time inspection of medical product quality. These systems guarantee compliance with stringent regulatory standards and minimize the likelihood of defects.

- *Additive Manufacturing:* It facilitates the creation of patient-specific implants and devices, minimizing the requirement for extensive inventory and supporting on-demand production capabilities. This holds significant importance in the fields of prosthetics and implantable devices.
- *Internet of Things (IoT):* Devices enabled by IoT technology are being utilized more frequently in the field of biomedical manufacturing for the purposes of real-time monitoring and data collection. Sensors integrated into machinery and devices monitor parameters including temperature, pressure, humidity, and vibration, thereby maintaining optimal conditions for production processes.

16.4 ADVANTAGES OF IMPLEMENTING ROBOTICS AND AUTOMATION IN BIOMEDICAL MANUFACTURING

- *Enhanced Precision and Accuracy*: Robots provide unmatched precision in manufacturing processes, including assembly, packaging, and testing. This level of accuracy is essential in the biomedical sector, where mistakes can lead to significant repercussions.
- *Enhanced Efficiency*: Automation facilitates uninterrupted production, minimizes downtime, and boosts operational efficiency, thereby addressing increasing demand and lowering costs.
- *Improved Safety and Decreased Human Error*: Automation of hazardous tasks, including the handling of toxic chemicals and operation in sterile environments, reduces risks to human workers and promotes a higher standard of safety.
- *Scalability and Adaptability*: Robots and machinery can be reprogrammed with ease to manufacture various products, thereby allowing for adaptability in response to fluctuations in demand or alterations in product specifications. This holds significant relevance in an industry characterized by varied and continuously evolving product specifications.

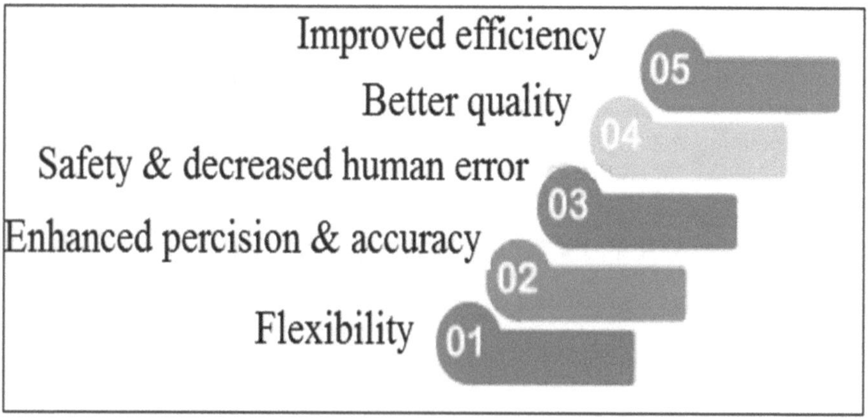

FIGURE 16.3 Advantages of robots in industry.

- *Regulatory compliance* is enhanced through automation, which ensures that products adhere to the stringent requirements set forth by the biomedical industry, including those established by the FDA and EMA. Automated systems are capable of maintaining precise records of manufacturing processes, thereby enhancing traceability and ensuring compliance.
- *Improved Safety and Decreased Human Error*: Automation of hazardous tasks, including the handling of toxic chemicals and operation in sterile environments, reduces risks to human workers and promotes a higher standard of safety.

16.5 CHALLENGES

Various challenges must be addressed in this "New Norm," necessitating collaboration and initiatives from all stakeholders, such as the end user, regulatory authorities, government bodies, research organizations, and automation/robot suppliers.

- Funding research is crucial for the advancement of new technology
- There is now a significant lack of automation and robotics engineers at various skill levels, ranging from apprentices to individuals with a master's degree. This gap is known as the skills gap. This issue requires immediate attention and action in all of our educational institutions, both for the purpose of acquiring new skills and for updating existing ones
- The impact of workplace culture and the willingness of employees to accept and embrace robot technology
- Brownfield plant design may not always be suitable for implementing automation, particularly for the deployment of mobile robotics
- Government initiatives provide financial support to smaller manufacturing enterprises and solution suppliers
- Funding for Agile Innovation
- Loan plans specifically designed to provide funding for working capital needs

Recent developments in smart manufacturing have integrated the use of soft robots to enhance productivity, flexibility, automation, and safety within smart factories. Soft robotics is experiencing a notable increase in popularity, attracting significant interest from both researchers and practitioners. Bionic soft robots, constructed from compliant materials such as silicones, provide effective solutions for manipulating delicate objects, functioning in unstructured environments, and enabling safe interactions between humans and robots. Despite the numerous advantages, fundamental challenges persist, particularly regarding motion precision and stiffness compliance when executing physical tasks that involve external forces. Soft robots present multiple advantages; however, several fundamental challenges must be addressed. **Figure 16.4** illustrates the primary technical challenges identified in the latest literature [10].

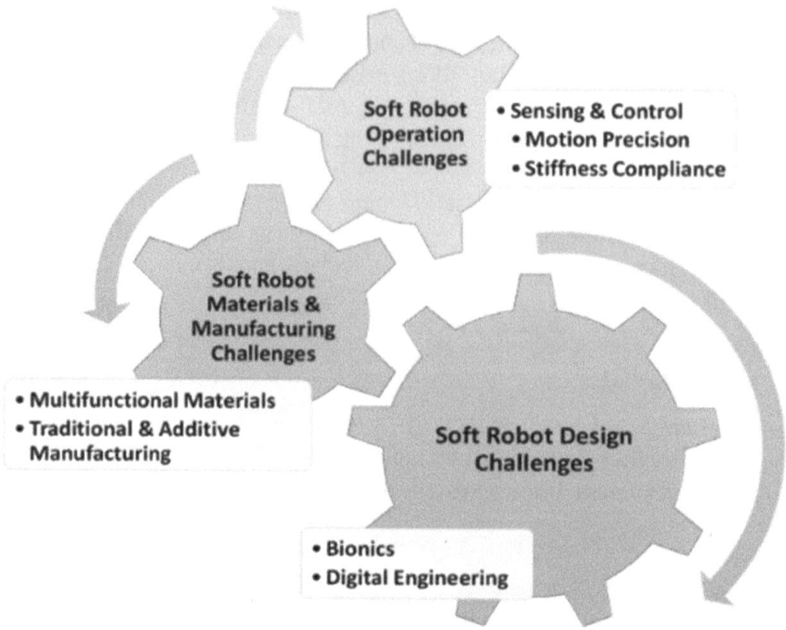

FIGURE 16.4 Key challenges. (Open Access article distributed under the terms of the Creative Commons Attribution License 4.4)

16.6 CONCLUSION

Biomedical robotics and automation have revolutionized healthcare by providing innovative solutions to enhance patient outcomes and streamline medical processes in surgery and rehabilitation. Robotic-assisted surgery has enhanced the ability of surgeons to carry out intricate procedures with more accuracy, decreased invasiveness, and enhanced patient recuperation. Robotic-assisted rehabilitation has improved the efficacy of physical therapy, resulting in improved functional results for patients with different neurological and musculoskeletal disorders. Ongoing research and advancement in the field of biomedical robotics offer the potential for increasingly advanced and easily accessible technology in the future. To assure widespread availability and significant advancements in the healthcare area, it is crucial to tackle the problems associated with cost, training, and integration of these technologies. The synergy of engineers, medical practitioners, and researchers will facilitate the emergence of a novel age in medicine, wherein biomedical robots and automation assume a pivotal position in augmenting human health and well-being. The implementation of these technologies presents various challenges, such as elevated costs, regulatory obstacles, workforce displacement, and cybersecurity vulnerabilities. The ongoing evolution of technology presents substantial opportunities to tackle these challenges via innovation, collaboration, and meticulous planning. The future of biomedical manufacturing is expected to be characterized by the emergence of increasingly autonomous systems that exhibit enhanced adaptability and intelligence. This evolution will facilitate the development of the next generation of medical devices, treatments, and healthcare solutions.

The crucial importance of AI in domains such as pharmaceutical research, disease diagnosis, robotic procedures, remote patient monitoring, and epidemic outbreak prediction is undeniable. Indian society is gradually accepting and recognizing the emerging significance of robotics in the care of old individuals. Currently, it is impractical to consider the deployment and monitoring of health services without the presence of AI and robotics. Several emerging techniques are being developed for the application of robotics in the healthcare industry, which have the potential to become more economically efficient in the future. The role of AI and robotics in revolutionizing healthcare is shown in **Figure 16.5**. However, it is imperative to ensure the quality of robotic treatments by implementing a rigorous and ongoing monitoring system. The utilization of AI and robots in the healthcare industry in India has the potential to be a significant breakthrough in enhancing the current state of healthcare services. It has effectively addressed the shortage of competent health workers and the significant openings in the fields of doctors, nurses, and paramedical staff. The primary obstacle lies in accessing the distant areas of the nation that have inadequate infrastructure and a scarcity of advanced technologies. Based on careful analysis of the facts and feasibility, it is advisable to gradually increase the implementation of robotics and automation in India, starting with well-established and well-equipped institutions.

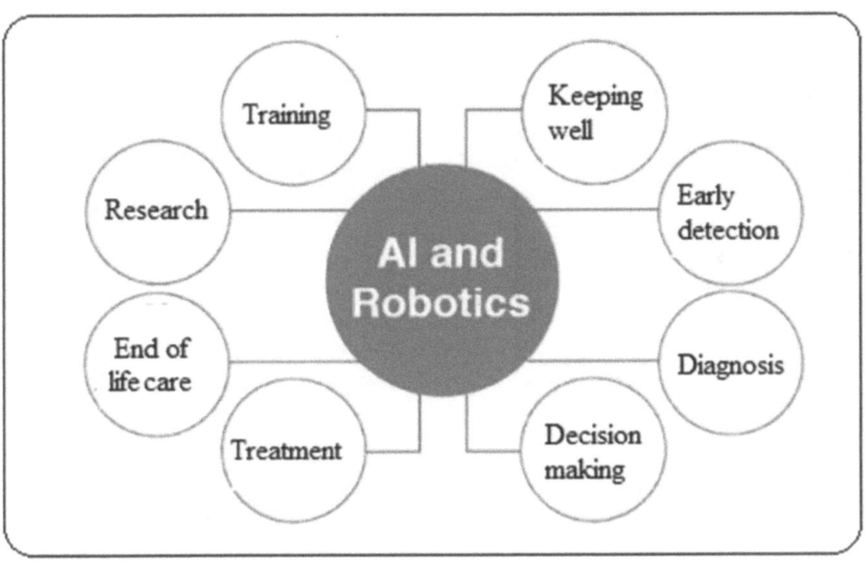

FIGURE 16.5 AI and robotics.

REFERENCES

1. Wani, N.U.H., Taneja, K. and Adlakha, N., 2013. Health system in India: Opportunities and challenges for enhancements. *IOSR Journal of Business and Management (IOSR-JBM)*, *9*(2), pp. 74–82.
2. Ajmera, P. and Jain, V., 2019. Modelling the barriers of Health 4.0–the fourth healthcare industrial revolution in India by TISM. *Operations Management Research*, *12*, pp. 129–45.
3. Chakravarty, S., 2023. Biomedical robotics. In *Advanced Methods in Biomedical Signal Processing and Analysis* (pp. 159–74). Academic Press.
4. Pradhan, B., Bharti, D., Chakravarty, S., Ray, S.S., Voinova, V.V., Bonartsev, A.P. and Pal, K., 2021. Internet of things and robotics in transforming current-day healthcare services. *Journal of Healthcare Engineering*, *2021*, pp. 1–15.
5. Das, A. and Nabi, M., 2019, October. A review on soft robotics: Modeling, control and applications in human-robot interaction. In *2019 International Conference on Computing, Communication, and Intelligent Systems (ICCCIS)* (pp. 306–11). IEEE.
6. Chang, W.H. and Kim, Y.H., 2013. Robot-assisted therapy in stroke rehabilitation. *Journal of Stroke*, *15*(3), p. 174.
7. The Aims of AI. [Jun; 2020], 2018. https://web.colby.edu/st112a2018/2018/04/14/the-aims-of-ai/
8. Ferrucci, D., Levas, A., Bagchi, S., Gondek, D. and Mueller, E.T., 2013. Watson: Beyond jeopardy! *Artificial Intelligence*, *199*, pp. 93–105.
9. Sarker, S., Jamal, L., Ahmed, S.F. and Irtisam, N., 2021. Robotics and artificial intelligence in healthcare during COVID-19 pandemic: A systematic review. *Robotics and Autonomous Systems*, *146*, p. 103902.
10. Ambaye, G., Boldsaikhan, E. and Krishnan, K., 2024. Soft robot design, manufacturing, and operation challenges: A review. *Journal of Manufacturing and Materials Processing*, *8*(2), p. 79.

17 Additive Manufacturing Applications in Biosensors Technologies

Gurmeet Kaur, Jashanpreet Singh, Vikas Sharma, and Rajwinder Singh

CONTENTS

17.1 INTRODUCTION

The use of three-dimensional (3D) printing has made great strides in the fabrication of complicated geometries of functionalised biological structures [1]. With its ability to deposit biomaterials and cells layer by layer with pinpoint accuracy, 3D printing has shown great promise as a tool for tissue engineering. In additive manufacturing, a variety of printing materials called "inks" are used to create three-dimensional things layer by layer. This process is supported by computer-aided design and prototyping. In a similar vein, 3D bioprinting is an AM technique

DOI: 10.1201/9781003516064-17

that builds functional 3D structures with predesigned porous structures by layer-by-layer extruding hydrogel solutions containing live cells or bio-inks [2]. By maximising the mechanical, physical, and biological characteristics of inks and cell distribution, AM allows for fine-grained control over the printed structure's microarchitecture, which is a major benefit [3]. The capacity to print biomaterials and functional entities concurrently, made possible by recent advancements in 3D printing technology, has created new and quickly expanding potential in the biomedical and tissue engineering domains.

Near the levels of sensor prototype and sensing layer organisation, 3D printing technology is expected to have a significant influence on the biosensor community [4,5]. One possible approach to bringing spatiotemporal sensing capabilities to the new 3D cell culturing settings is to realise scaffolds with embedded sensor molecules. Research into the biotechnological uses of 3D printing in the creation of sensors and biosensors is still in its infancy compared to its prevalence in biomedical applications like regenerative medicine and tissue engineering [4,6]. One way to reduce the use and sacrifice of animals in disease research and drug screening is to incorporate sensor or biosensor units into 3D printing processes. This would provide a non-invasive spatiotemporal approach to monitoring cells' microenvironment during culturing and serve as a platform for multiple uses [7].

Starting with a quick overview of the various printing materials and contemporary 3D printing processes, this chapter gets right to the point. Crucially, the study focused on manufacturing processes and printing materials and also examined new research on biosensor uses of 3D printing. By the end of the chapter, readers will have a good grasp of where 3D printing is at in the sensor and biosensor industry, as well as an understanding of the possibilities and threats facing this sector right now.

17.2 EXPLORING THE PAST WITH 3D PRINTING AND SENSORS

Device miniaturisation has contributed to the advancement of several analytical methods, particularly in engineering, biology, and chemistry. The goal is to reduce the size of most systems to a minimum. The same holds true for sensors used to track biological signals both in living organisms and in laboratory settings. Miniaturisation, elastic nature, and design are three categories into which biological sensors fall, and recent advances in microsystems manufacturing have further facilitated their development [8]. This means biosensors need to be compact, elastically modulus-compatible with human tissue, and function-specifically adaptable. On the market today are miniature biomedical sensors such as touch sensors, microfluidic devices, diagnostic tools, disease biomarkers, and electronic probes based on microelectrodes. Etching on glass was the first step in the complicated process of creating micro and nanoscale devices; a Si wafer was eventually used in their stead [9]. The use of Si wafer lithography has expanded because to its stellar reputation when compared to glass. To create devices for different functions, soft lithography employs an elastic polymer known as polydimethylsiloxane (PDMS). With its low elastic modulus (300–500 Kpa), optical transparency, excellent biocompatibility, and tunable gas permeability, PDMS stands out among glass and silicon as an ideal biosensor material [10]. Sophisticated methods (when paired with photolithography) are one of soft lithography's constraints. Other issues include incompatibility with some reagents, several steps, high levels of professional competence, and the possibility of swelling when exposed to organic solvents. Another major drawback of photo-soft lithography is the inability to create 3D structures. One approach may be to construct a 3D device by stacking many 2D devices [11]. That method is tedious and inaccurate, however. Microfluidics, biosensors, and biomedicine are just a few of the many microsystems-related industries that have benefited greatly from the advent of 3D printing. The process of creating an object's three-dimensional structure by adding layers to it is called additive manufacturing (AM) or three-dimensional printing (3D printing) [12]. Materials that are extruded, deposited, or solidified under certain circumstances are used in this procedure to create the desired item. Based on their method of operation, the American Society for Testing and Materials (ASTM) divided AM processes into seven categories: powder bed fusion (PBF), extrusion, material jetting, binder jetting, sheet lamination, and directed energy deposition (DED) [13].

17.3 BASICS OF 3D PRINTING

To create intricate three-dimensional models, AM makes use of CAD and CAM software [14]. The next step is to transform them into STL format, which allows for the slicing and binding of 2D layers. Using a 3D printer to automatically deposit inks onto a substrate, the sliced components may be produced layer by layer [15]. The four main types of 3D printing processes are those that rely on stereolithography, inkjet, extrusion, or laser assistance which have been discussed in previous chapters. Varieties of materials for 3D printing are discussed as follows.

17.3.1 Photopolymerisation in a Vat

One common method of 3D printing, known as vat photopolymerisation, uses ultraviolet (UV) radiation to strengthen the light-curable resin in a liquid state, creating molecular chains and cross-links [16], as shown in **Figure 17.1.** Its capacity to construct intricate constructions with meticulous detailing and excellent surface quality has earned it widespread renown. Here, under certain wavelengths and under controlled printing circumstances, liquid resins are UV polymerised. When compared to other AM methods, this one is quick and precise since the photosensitive resin is cured in a few seconds after being deposited in a vat [17].

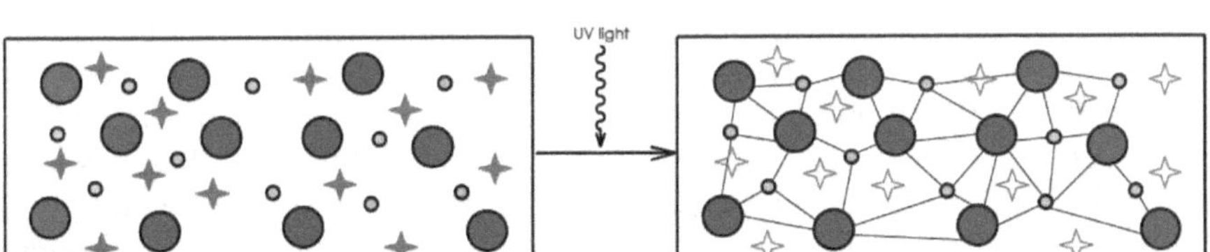

FIGURE 17.1 Liquid photopolymer (left) undergoing light-induced polymerisation [16]. (Permissions under Creative Commons Attribution 4.0 International License)

This method may be categorised as stereolithography (SLA), digital light processing (DLP), and two-photon polymerisation (2PP). Based on the angle of the light source used to cure the resins, SLA subdivides the system into free-surface and confined surface versions. For several uses, the limited surface outperforms the free-surface arrangement. Initial testing shows that the object's height is unconstrained by the vat's dimensions. Second, there is less resin waste and a shorter curing time. A microstereolithography (μSLA) enhancement with a micron-level resolution is a minor change to the SLA [18]. The digital light processing (DLP) printer follows a process that is similar to that of an SLA-constrained surface system; however, instead of ultraviolet (UV) light, a digital projector is used to cure the photo resins. Compared to SLA printers, this method is more quicker, and the resins that have not yet hardened may be reused. To address some issues with SLA and DLP printers, the 2PP system was created. The 2PP system achieves sub-100 nm resolution despite its modest printing speed, providing a better level of precision. Micro stereolithography (SL), which incorporates a digital micromirror device (DMD), was used to create a mobile 3D microfluidic biosensor chip. For routine colorimetric tests, it has a torque-actuated pump and valve, a rotating valve, and a pushing valve. The 3D printed gadget has a cheap production cost, a simple operating procedure, and a quick on-site quantitative detection capability, all of which contribute to a decrease in reagent loss.

The smartphone and its technology were found to conduct a comprehensive and illuminating quantitative study. Using stereolithography printing, a microfluidic device that is completely automated was created. For the purpose of cell cultivation, printed valves and pumps were used. Their device's performance is still below that of PDMS alternatives, despite the fact that overall manufacturing ease was decreased. However, with SL's potential future features, there's hope that their performances will still be outstanding. A strong 3D-printed microfluidic analysis system may be more easily fabricated and characterised with the use of an FDM printer, an SLA printer, and an FDM printer [19]. Continuous monitoring of human tissue metabolite levels is possible with the use of this device in conjunction with clinical microdialysis probes that have been authorised by the FDA

17.3.2 Fusion Powder Bed

Popular for its capacity to generate tiny, precision-demanding, and varied pieces, this process entails layer-by-layer fusing of powdered material to construct three-dimensional structures [20]. This process uses a laser or electron beam to combine powdered materials piece by piece; these materials may be metals, polymers, ceramics, composites, etc. [21–25]. Here, the powder is heated or sinterised while a roller spreads it out across a thin layer. The structure is not complete until this procedure is repeated. Several variables, including laser strength, spot size beam, and powder quality, determine the final 3D structure. Laser power bed fusion (LPBF), electron beam melting (EBM), and selective laser sintering (SLS) are the most frequent forms of PBF. Slow printing time, difficulties in managing porosity, and postprocessing required are major drawbacks of this approach [26,27]. Using metal 3D printing technology, stainless electrodes were created for the electrochemical detection of ascorbic and uric acids. The final product outperforms the gold standard of glassy carbon electrodes in every respect: sensitivity, selectivity, repeatability, and linearity within the concentration range of 0.1–1 mM [28].

17.3.3 Material Flow Control

The process of extruding a liquid mixture of ink and granules is analogous to printing. The printheads are comparable to inkjet printers, but instead of using a continuous filament, microdroplets are used to deposit the ink, creating the 3D structure layer by layer [29]. Printing precisely around curves, edges, and incline surfaces is possible with this non-contact method. Photoresins, hydrogels, and carbon nanotubes are some of the most popular materials. Some examples of printing technologies include inkjet printing (IJP), polyjet printing (PJP), and aerosol jet printing (AJP). The aerosol droplets in AJP are carried by a gas to the nozzle or aperture. They developed an electrochemical detector using a multi-material printer called an Objet Connex 350. A microfluidic platform was 3D printed with a threaded receiving port that can integrate various electrode materials for nitric oxide and dopamine detection. Additionally, a device was designed to measure the release stimulus of decreasing oxygen concentration while collecting adenosine triphosphate (ATP). Neurotransmitters and signaling chemicals might be detected by this sensor. The results prove that 3D printing is a reliable and versatile method for fabricating the electrodes and sensing devices. Using a nano-ink technique, a biosystem that is wireless, stretchy, and implantable was 3D printed. A capacitance flow sensor may be printed in several layers with good performance using this method [30].

17.3.4 System based on Extrusion

Layer-by-layer construction of the build advances along the Z axis by raising or lowering the head in extrusion-based 3D printing, which entails ink deposition onto a stage along the X and Y axes. Processes that use material melting and those that do not are the two main categories of extrusion 3D printing [31]. The fused deposition modeling process is one of the most popular extrusion-based 3D printing methods that relies on melting materials. For FDM printing, an item is created by ejecting plastic or ink via a nozzle. The material melting method relies on maintaining the material temperature slightly above its melting point. This allows for simple extrusion through the nozzle, which in turn allows the filaments to fuse during printing and solidify when cooled. Affordable, fully automated, and compatible with a broad variety of printing materials are just a few of the advantages they provide. Materials such as ceramics, PET, wax blends, TPE, nylon, metals, PLA, ABS, PC, PVA, and COC are all part of the fabrication toolbox [32–37]. The majority of these materials are incompatible with sensor applications due to their low gas permeability and hard plastic nature. Reportedly, a glutamate monitoring implantable biosensor was made using a DIW printer. In this case, thin-film polymer substrates were printed using a nanocomposite ink. This method revealed that the sensor could detect glutamate for in vivo uses, had a low detection limit, and was very sensitive. Using a micro-extrusion 3D printer, microelectrochemical systems with piezoelectric sensors and actuators were created for acoustofluidic applications. These systems are based on microfluidics. The combination of AM with piezoelectric transducers is shown by this device's efficacy [38]. Pneumatic and mechanical extrusion-based processes, which do not involve melting materials, may be categorised according to the use of screws and pistons. Due to its gentle production condition, this method is often used in tissue engineering bioprinting soft hydrogels. You may regulate the printing speed, flow rate, volume, and pressure in pneumatic 3D printing by using air or gas pressure to extrude the ink through the nozzle. The maximum viscosity that may be extruded using this method is determined by the pressure limit. In contrast to its pneumatic cousin, mechanical extrusion makes use of a movable gun and a spinning screw to force ink out of the nozzle across a wider range of viscosities and with more precise spatial control.

17.3.5 Toner-based Printing

The versatility of inkjet-based 3D printing is driving its rising popularity in a number of industries, such as AM, microstructures, textile electronics, and wearable electronics. The adaptable technique has shown potential in printing multi-material structures, practical items, and small-scale 3D objects [39]. The outcome is that it has become an indispensable component of contemporary production methods. 3D printing with ink requires the creation of printable inks that have exact rheological characteristics, including surface tension, shear yield stress, and viscosity. The production of multiple 3D sensors has been made possible by these technical developments in 3D printing, which have opened up new areas in scientific study. Three-dimensional printing using inkjet technology is mainly divided into two categories: thermal and piezoelectric. A heating element doubles as a thin film resistor in thermal inkjet 3D printing. A high-current electrical pulse expands the vapor bubbles in the ink reservoir by vaporising the nearby ink, which causes the ink reservoir to swell. The ink droplets are ejected from the nozzle by the pressure created by this expansion. However, with piezoelectric inkjet 3D printing, the ink chamber's volume is suddenly changed by applying an external voltage to a piezoelectric transducer [40]. By using rotational inkjet printing, a flexible cylindrical enzyme–electrode glucose microsensor was created. This idea proposes fabricating and modifying micro cylindrical substrates in situ using maskless direct writing. According to the clinical requirements, this gadget was able to detect glucose levels in the range of 0–570 mg dL−1. Next, the concept of rotational inkjet printing was advanced as a potential technique for micro-scale fabrication of flexible bioelectronics on substrates of any form. A fully functional enzymatic glucose sensor was manufactured using inkjet technology in conjunction with biodegradable paper. With a unique metal-free construction and a shelf life of 31 days, the printed gadget can detect glucose in saliva. A layer-by-layer assembly was used to print the various components of this sensor, including the conducting polymer [41].

17.4 MATERIALS AND 3D PRINTERS FOR BIOPRINTING

Both the widespread availability of open-source designs and the precipitous decline in the price of 3D printers have contributed to the technology's relative affordability in recent years. Based on their underlying principles, 3D bioprinters may be roughly classified into four categories. Stereolithography, acoustic, microvalve, inkjet, extrusion, laser, and needle array bioprinters are some of the most popular kinds of bioprinters. It is important to choose a bioprinter that is compatible with the intended build and bio-ink. When deciding on a bioprinter, it is common practice to take into account both the target construct's structural qualities and the printing substance (bio-inks) for that application. Size, intricacy, and the kind of printed tissues or organs are three frequently recognised structural attributes of the goal build. On the other hand, while deciding on the best bioprinting method, the viscosity, composition, and cross-linking processes of the bio-inks are often taken into account. Printer resolution, speed, scalability, and compatibility with target biomaterials are other factors to be taken into account [41].

17.4.1 Bio-Ink Technology

Living cells or a supporting hydrogel component make up bio-inks, which are materials utilised for 3D bioprinting. The capacity to customise the printability, mechanical properties, and degrading characteristics of porous hydrogels is crucial for the 3D creation of robust, cellularised structures, and these bio-inks make that possible. The bio-inks used in 3D printing are biomaterials that encapsulate cells; as such, they must be compatible with both the printing process and the culture of 3D cells. Bio-inks that include sensor units, contain growth factors, and have thermo-responsive characteristics are also used in bone regeneration and regenerative medicine [42]. After bioprinting, the active ingredients in bio-inks may operate as an extracellular matrix to facilitate cell adhesion, cell proliferation, and cell differentiation. Bio-inks are made from biomaterials that are bioactive, printable, rheologically stable, mechanically strong, and biocompatible. Biological systems may interact with bio-inks in 3D bioprinting, which can be either natural or synthetic or a combination of the two. The materials used in 3D bioprinting are often transformed into hydrogels, which are three-dimensional insoluble water matrices. The three-dimensional hydrophilic polymers known as hydrogels are able to soak up and hold onto large amounts of water without actually dissolving in the liquid. The formation of hydrogels is caused by the hydration of the hydrophilic domains of polymeric networks in water. The existence of cross-links and the linked structure of the polymer chains are what make up the "network" in this context; these features are essential for keeping the polymer chains or segments from dissolving into the surrounding water phase. Due to their printability-enhancing viscosity, they find extensive use in the fabrication of 3D scaffolds for tissue engineering. The rheological behaviors of the bio-ink, including its storage modulus (G′) and loss modulus (G″), are also important for printability and may be adjusted in many ways to suit printing requirements. In order for hydrogels that have a low viscosity and a high loss modulus to self-support the layer-by-layer deposition that occurs during printing, a cross-linking step is usually required, either before or after printing, or even during printing itself. **Figure 17.2** provides an overview of the formulation process for bio-inks used in 3D bioprinting. To make hydrogels, many methods have been used to produce cross-links. Hydrogels may be produced via either physical or chemical means [43]. Physical cross-linking, in contrast to chemical cross-linking, is accomplished by ionic contact and is often reversible by physical methods; it also establishes a covalent

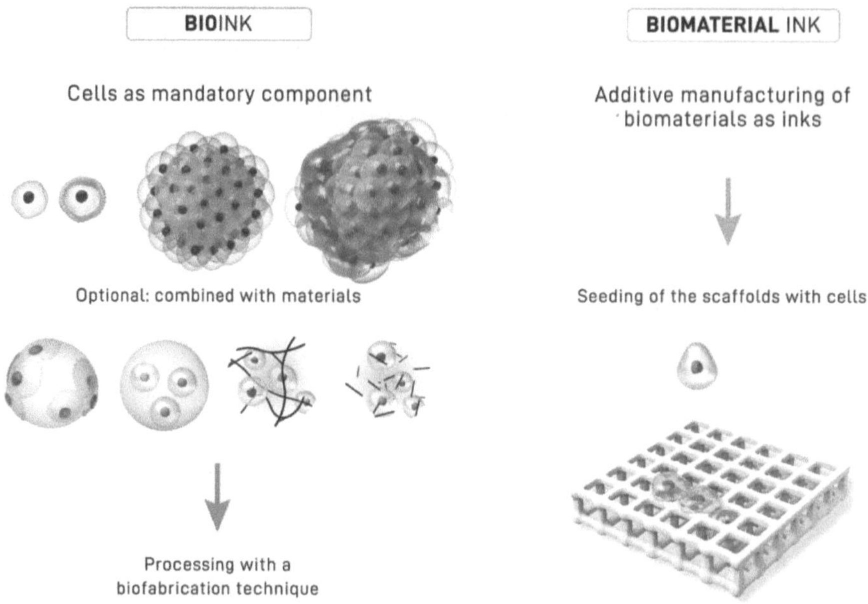

FIGURE 17.2 Formulation process for bio-inks used in 3D bioprinting [45]. (Permissions under Creative Commons Attribution 4.0 International License)

connection between distinct polymer chains. Hennink and Nostrum's paper details the processes and methods of many hydrogel cross-linking techniques in great detail. For bioprinting to work, the printability of the final product depends on the cross-linking techniques used and how well they can be controlled. Developing printing materials with good structural integrity and printing fidelity is an area of intense study. In terms of science, bio-inks may be roughly classified into two groups: biomaterial inks with low viscosity and those with high viscosity. The printing quality is compromised, and processing with low viscosity bio-inks requires technical effort since, after extrusion, they tend to collapse owing to gravity. Many methods are used to handle plotted low viscosity paints after printing. These include in situ cross-linking for ionically cross-link-able inks, UV exposure for inks with photoreactive groups, and printing into sacrificial support baths. Bio-inks with a high viscosity enable the airborne direct production of volumetric structures that are resistant to structural collapse. Bio-inks with both high or low viscosities have their uses in AM and their pros and cons. As an example, 3D printing has made use of a gelatine and alginate composite, with the former serving as the initial structural support and the latter being cross-linked by calcium chloride [44].

17.4.2 3D Printing with a Variety of Biomaterials

Numerous 3D bioprinting uses have been made possible by the advent of novel printing biomaterials and formulations. Although additive printing processes are versatile, not all materials are well-suited for biosensing and other applications. To use any of these methods, one must first create bespoke materials with adaptable characteristics that meet the demands of the specific application. Depending on the intended uses and required physicochemical qualities of the bio-ink, 3D printing may employ either synthetic or naturally occurring polymers or a mix of the two (semi-synthetic). Alginate, gelatin, chitosan, collagen, hyaluronic acid, and fibrinogen/fibrin are some of the naturally occurring polymers used in 3D printing. On the other hand, polyvinyl alcohol is one example of a manufactured substance.

17.5 BIOSENSOR TECHNOLOGY

There is a growing need for efficient and quick sensing device production in the process industries, environmental monitoring, and medical diagnostics. Biosensor technology has come a long way in the last several decades, thanks to the growing variety of clinical and environmental analytes that need more sensitive, faster, and less expensive analytical instruments. Analytical methods, both modern and traditional, can identify clinical and environmental analytes with a high degree of accuracy and sensitivity. Cost, the need for skilled staff, and the impracticality of doing analysis on-site are still obstacles to the widespread use of these methods [46]. Because of their low cost, ease of construction, and, most crucially, their ability to be miniaturised into portable forms, biosensors are seen as the preferred instruments to meet the increasing need for diagnostics and monitoring. Biosensors are small analytical tools that use a biological sensor. By translating a physical or chemical signal into an optical or electrical signal, biosensors may detect biomolecules in complicated samples, as shown in **Figure 17.3**. This signal can then be processed

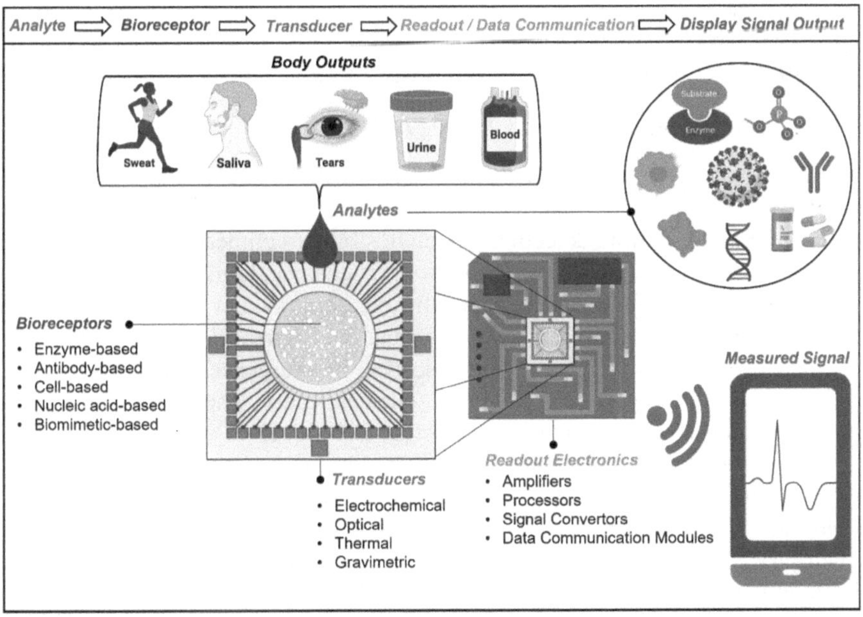

FIGURE 17.3 Schematic representation of biosensing [47]. (Permissions under Creative Commons Attribution 4.0 International License)

to get the analyte concentration, either quantitatively or semi-quantitatively. With its many benefits over traditional analytical techniques, including rapidity, simplicity, affordability, non-destructive characteristics, and on-site detection, biosensors have become crucial in many domains. They are made up of display units, signal transducers, and biological recognition elements (BREs). One way to categorise biosensors is by the biorecognition element type or transducer type that went into their creation. Catalytic biosensors, like enzymes and DNAzymes, and affinity biosensors, like nucleic acid biosensors and immunosensors, are categorised according to the sort of biorecognition they perform. As recognition elements (bioreporters), live cells and microbes may express certain genes (indicator genes) in response to trigger chemicals (inducers) in some whole-cell biosensors. Hormones, receptors, antigens/antibodies, enzymes, live cells, nucleic acids, carbs, and tissues are all examples of BRE. These biological resources may bind to analytes and then be used to measure their concentration in a sample. Enzyme-based biosensors are able to detect molecules with very low detection limits and great selectivity because they combine specialised biochemical identification with high-efficiency catalysis. The formation of stable complexes is the molecular recognition mechanism used by other biorecognition molecules, such as interactions between antigens and antibodies, nucleic acids and complementary sequences, and proteins and receptors. Optical, electrochemical (label-based or label-free), mechanical, and conductometric biosensors are further biosensor classifications. Biosensors may be categorised according to the signal transducers used, such as thermal, electrochemical, piezoelectric, magnetic, optical, mechanical, or radioactive.

17.6 TRIPARTITE CLASSIFICATION OF BIOSENSORS ACCORDING TO TRANSDUCER TYPES

17.6.1 Optical Biosensors for Use in AM Systems

The high sensitivity and selectivity, simplicity of deployment, and cost-effectiveness of optical biosensors make them an analytical approach that has found widespread use in the real-time detection of analytes in both clinical and environmental samples. Biosensor setup uses the absorption, reflectance, luminescence, or fluorescence emissions across the visible, near-infrared, or ultraviolet (UV) portions of the electromagnetic spectrum to transduce information. **Figure 17.4** depicts Jablonski's diagram showing the two kinds of luminescence. Fluorescence, which may be measured in a variety of ways (e.g., intensity, quenching efficiency, anisotropy, decay time), is the most widely used optical detection technique.

Using biorecognition components like enzymes, antibodies, oligonucleotides, or even complete cells and tissues is the simplest approach to get specificity in an optical biosensor [49]. Enzymes catalyze processes very specifically, and if the reactants or their products are colored or glow in the dark, or if optical transducers are used, it is possible to see them directly. That is why the analyte concentration is proportional to the steady-state concentration of detectable species. **Figure 17.5** shows a cross-section of a fiber-optic enzymatic biosensor that includes an enzyme layer, an indicator layer that detects oxygen and pH levels, and a transparent inert support that

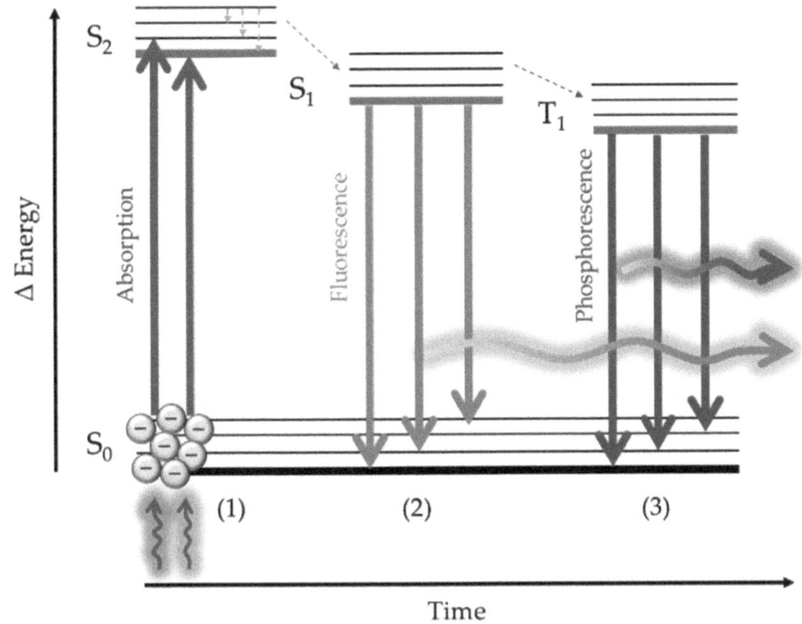

FIGURE 17.4 Jablonski's diagram showing the two kinds of luminescence [48]. (Permissions under Creative Commons Attribution 4.0 International License)

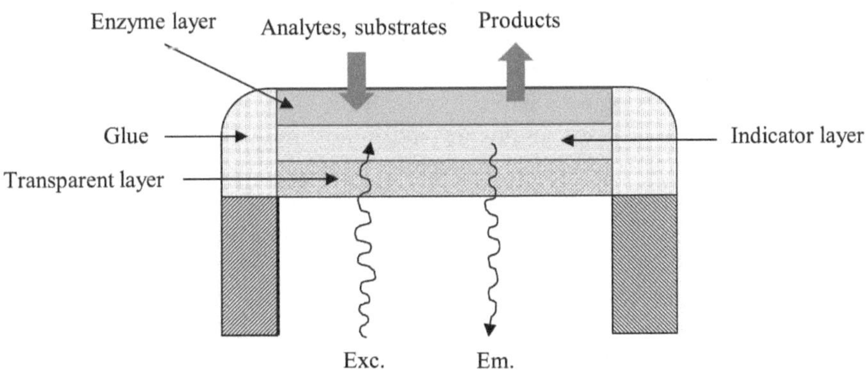

FIGURE 17.5 Schematic diagram representing the cross-sectional view of a typical fiber-optic enzymatic biosensor. (Created by authors)

is attached to an optical fiber. To make the indicator layer, an indicator dye may be dissolved into the polymer matrix or adsorbed onto microbeads physically or covalently; then, the microbeads can be combined with the polymer matrix. During an enzymatic process, the indicator layers detect when the product has consumed the substrate [50]. Enzymes may be chemically or physically immobilised onto polymer membrane surfaces by entrapment in polymer networks like hydrogels. A sandwich

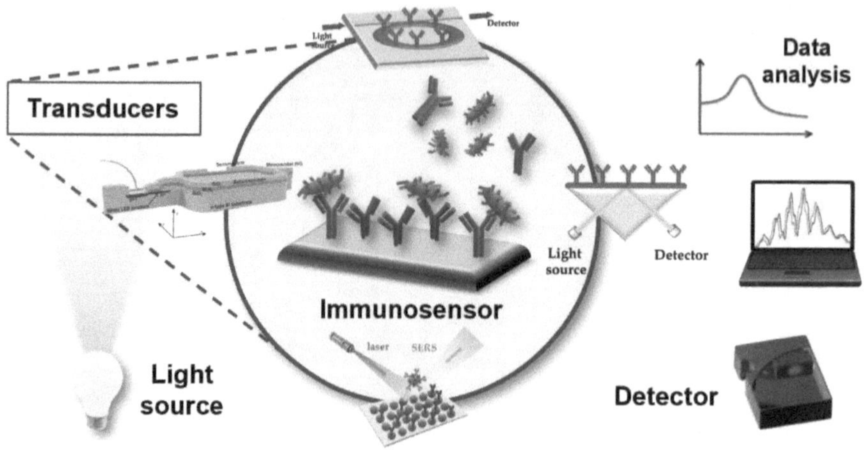

FIGURE 17.6 A sandwich immunosensor attached to an optical fiber [53]. (Permissions under Creative Commons Attribution 4.0 International License)

sensor attached to an optical fiber is shown in **Figure 17.6**. This sensor allows light to be transmitted from an excitation source to the sensor foil, which in turn reflects the light back to a photodetector [51]. Because an indication layer isn't always necessary, a variant of optical sensors that employ chemiluminescent and bioluminescent processes is often easier to implement. Clinical medicine, environmental analysis, and bioprocess monitoring all make extensive use of them to keep tabs on critically important analytes. The format of immunosensors is used to illustrate an optical sensor that is based on affinity (**Figure 17.6**). An antigen–antibody binding event is a non-covalent contact that, in principle, may be reversed. The substantial association constants and very slow dissociation rates make most immunoreactions irreversible in practice [52]. Nevertheless, there has been an emphasis on finding ways to make the immunosensors reusable by rinsing them in solutions with different osmolarities, ionic strengths, or pH levels. This will enable the use of a single sensor for several measurements. Optical sensors are only one of several biosensing applications that have benefited from additive manufacturing's simple operating principle and rapid manufacture of complicated 3D objects. It is now common practice to use 3D printed objects that include sensor components to monitor vital signs such as skin temperature, heart rate, blood pressure, respiration rate, brain activity, and body mobility [52]. It is common practice to print the sensing component separately or include it into the printed base when making 3D printed sensors.

17.6.2 Biosensor for Electrochemistry

By combining the sensitivity of electroanalytical methods with the biological selectivity of the biological component, an electrochemical biosensor can detect specific analytes by converting biological responses into electrical signals. This technology has many potential uses, such as pathogen detection, disease diagnosis, food safety, and environmental monitoring. In electrochemical biosensors, as in other biosensor types, the biorecognition element identifies the analyte, which triggers a binding or catalytic event that, according to the transduction element's monitoring of the analyte concentration, generates an electrical signal proportional to the analyte concentration. Biocatalytic devices and affinity sensors are the two primary types of electrochemical biosensors which are based on the biological recognition mechanisms they use. To identify the analyte of interest and generate electroactive species, biocatalytic devices use enzymes, entire cells, or slices of tissue. An antibody, nucleic acid, or receptor forms a specific binding contact with the analyte in affinity sensors. The detection limits of biocatalytic biosensors are very low since they use the catalytic power of enzymes [54]. As a result of a shortage of suitably selective enzymes, many biochemical analytes cannot be detected by enzymatic methods; hence, affinity biosensors have emerged as a viable alternative. Biomolecules like antibodies (Ab), membrane receptors, or oligonucleotides bind selectively and robustly to a target analyte in affinity sensors, which then generate a quantifiable electrical signal. The conformation and size of the binding site to the target analyte are the primary determinants of molecular recognition in affinity biosensors. These sensors are very sensitive and selective due to the biomolecule's strong affinity and specificity for its ligand. To get the biomolecules as near to the surface of the electrochemical transducer as possible, many physical and chemical methods have been investigated for immobilising them onto the transducer. Stable preservation of the immobilised biological entity's structure and function is an ideal immobilisation strategy. Immobilisation ought to provide improved selectivity, recyclability, and stability. **Figure 17.7** shows the commonly used immobilisation procedures. So far, physically immobilising proteins on electrode surfaces has been the most accessible method. The natural structure of the biomolecules is maintained since physical immobilisation does not include the creation of covalent bonds. When biomolecules with functional groups (NH_2, COOH, OH, or SH) are immobilised chemically, the electrodes and biomolecules traditionally establish covalent bonds. Incorporating the enzyme into a carbon paste, enclosing it in a gel or electropolymerised film, or utilising bio-specific interactions like biotin-avidin binding, adsorption, cross-linking, or covalent attachment are all examples of standard methods for enzyme immobilisation (**Figure 17.7**). The three primary units of measurement in electrochemistry are current, potential, and impedance. Depending on the analytical demands, the following electrochemical detection methods—voltammetry/amperometry, conductometry, electrochemical impedance spectroscopy (EIS) [55], and potentiometry—have been used to varied degrees of popularity. With the tremendous flexibility and comparatively reduced building costs of custom-made, complicated measuring systems, electrochemical methods may greatly benefit from using 3D printing technology. Conductive electrodes with unusual forms or materials may be made using 3D printing technology. A potential way forward for the development of new biosensors is the use of these electrodes in electrochemical sensors for redox and catalytic reactions. To improve the sensor's sensitivity and accuracy, this method allows bioelectronics to be integrated with a 3D environment for biological experiments. This approach's scalability adds to the growing number of biosensors with enhanced capabilities for a wide range of uses. As an example, Cantù and colleagues used aerosol jet

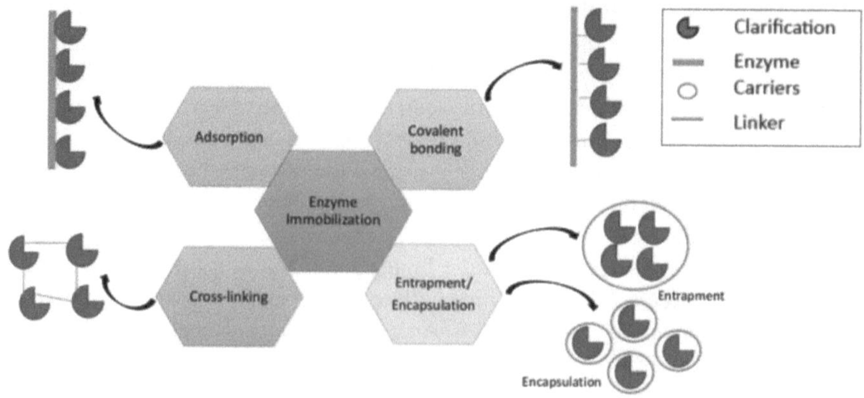

FIGURE 17.7 Schematic diagram for immobilisation procedures [56]. (Permissions under Creative Commons Attribution 4.0 International License)

3D printing to create miniature electrochemical detectors for proteins. The authors demonstrated that 3D printing has the potential to enhance the reproducibility and reliability of measuring methods that may be integrated into various biotechnological applications.

17.6.3 Physical Sensor

The term "physical sensor" refers to any device that can take in physical stimuli and process them either digitally or analogically. Force, heat, light, electricity, magnetism, and sound are just a few of the physical impacts that physical sensors may use to detect physical quantities. The resonant mass sensor from microelectromechanical systems (MEMS) is one kind of physical sensor that applies calorimetry or changes in mass. This sensor can detect changes in mass because it can directly measure the biophysical characteristics, mass, and growth rate of individual adhering cells [57]. For instance, the magnetoelastic sensor is a physical sensor. The sensor community is very interested in magnetoelastic sensors since they provide a great platform for measuring pressure and many other environmental factors. Chemical analyte concentrations, such as pH, ammonia, glucose, and carbon dioxide, may be monitored using magnetoelastic sensors by means of a mass-changing chemically sensitive layer. Chemical sensors may be realised by covering the magnetoelastic sensor with a film that changes mass and is chemically sensitive. Another kind of physical sensor with widespread use in biomedical engineering and health monitoring is the piezoelectric sensor, which is known for its great sensitivity and rapid reaction time. A lot of people are interested in using piezoelectric polymer sensors for self-powered sensing and energy harvesting because of their high piezoelectric constant, low density, and flexibility. This is because piezoelectric sensors work by converting mechanical and electrical energies into one another [58]. With its many sensing and actuation applications, this kind of sensor technology shows great diversity and adaptability when it comes to making self-powered, label-free biosensors to detect biomarkers. Biosensing, medical diagnostics, industrial monitoring, and safety assurance are just a few of the many fields that have found a home for physical sensors like acoustic wave sensors. These sensors detect and analyse physical, chemical, and biological factors by using the principles of sonic wave propagation. Biosensing applications have shown great sensitivity and reliability of surface acoustic wave (SAW) sensors, such as Love-mode acoustic wave sensors. An interdigitated transducer receives an acoustic wave that has been transmitted across a device substrate. The piezoelectric effect then converts this signal back into an electric signal, allowing for the quantification of changes in the surface properties of the device substrate. Any changes to the mechanical wave are reflected in the output electric signal. On the basis of the previous approach, acoustic wave sensors are built, where the SAW may be adjusted by either increasing the surface mass or varying the substrate length and interlayer spacing. The electronics and communications industries have also paid close attention to film bulk acoustic wave resonators (FBARs) for the purpose of sensing biological compounds and physical factors, including humidity, temperature, and pressure.

17.6.4 Biosensor Applications of the Bioprinting Method

The sensor and sensing layer organisation level will soon be affected by 3D printing technologies in the biosensor community. Because of their inherent complexity, many sensors are often grouped into composite designs made of numerous components [59]. So it's important to find new ways to fabricate sensors so that complicated ones may be made quickly. The fast developing area of AM is well appreciated since it allows for the printing of various biomaterials into complex 2D and 3D structures that might be used for sensing. The field of biotechnology engineering has been ushered into a new era by the merging of AM techniques with biomaterials. In fact, new printing materials and a variety of 3D printers have opened new possibilities for most biosensor developers, allowing for the seamless fabrication of complex hydrogel scaffolds with complex geometries and sensing layers integrated in. As a result, 3D bioprinting is now being expanded to encompass important biotechnological applications, such as the incorporation of active biomolecular recognition elements into 3D printed objects for (bio)sensing. The deposition and patterning of printing material loaded with reporter biomolecules may be done precisely and rapidly using several bioprinting processes, including electrodeposition, ink-jet printing, microcontact printing, and extrusion. This allows for the fabrication of biosensors. From individual biomolecules like proteins and enzymes, to larger ones like mammalian cells, algae, and bacteria, the bioprinted library has it all. Rapid screening of numerous analytes is possible with 3D bioprinted biosensors thanks to multiplexing and high-throughput analysis. One potential application of sensing capabilities in 3D printing materials for tissue engineering is the rapid patterning of various sensor molecules across a wide concentration range. This could enable the detection of biomarkers of cellular responses at threshold levels, opening the door to a kind of spatiotemporal monitoring of the cellular environment in parallel experiments.

When using bioprinting for biosensing applications, it is crucial to consider the transduction characteristics of the biomaterials utilised as bio-ink. To create a sensorised 3D model, it is essential to immobilise BRE. Various methods of manufacture have been used up till now.

17.7 CONCLUSION AND FUTURE PERSPECTIVES

Recent trends in AM have shown that it is possible to produce functional materials with the necessary microstructures, complicated 3D topologies, and a great variety of combinations of materials and component parts to have a profound influence on biomedical sciences and biosensor technology. Nanoscale, microscale, and macroscale manufacturing have influenced biosensors development with an augmentation of miniaturisation flexibility, and patient-specificity. Developed trends consist of 3D printing technologies which are able to combine several materials and different biomolecules which improve biosensor activity. Scientists and engineers are working on the creation of multi-nozzle printers to increase the rate of parts production and overcome such issues as layer misalignment and compatibility with subsequent processing. Materials, substrate, and bio-ink, biopolymers microfluidics, and functional bio-inks in 3D printing biosensors are on the rise. The most recent works reveal current advancements in the integration of nanomaterials, imprinted polymers, and higher-resolution approaches enabling related enhancements of sensitivity, selectivity, and reproducibility. In tissue engineering application, non-invasive monitoring is possible with functionalised bio-inks incorporated with biocompatible elements. For instance, chemically modified alginate, which exhibits properties such as cell adhesion, photo, and electric conductivity, has become a promising material in biosensor maturation. New biocompatible printing materials and bio-functionalisation methods are on the verge of drastically changing AM for biosensors, especially in the form of soft hydrogel-based 3D printed devices in biotechnology.

REFERENCES

[1] Munaz A, Vadivelu RK, John JS, et al. Three-dimensional printing of biological matters. *J Sci Adv Mater Devices*. 2016;1:1–17.

[2] Askari M, Naniz MA, Kouhi M, et al. Recent progress in extrusion 3D bioprinting of hydrogel biomaterials for tissue regeneration: A comprehensive review with focus on advanced fabrication techniques. *Biomater Sci*. 2021;9:535–73.

[3] Bose S, Ke D, Sahasrabudhe H, et al. Additive manufacturing of biomaterials. *Prog Mater Sci*. 2018;93:45–111.

[4] Chan HN, Tan MJA, Wu H. Point-of-care testing: Applications of 3D printing. *Lab Chip*. 2017;17:2713–39.

[5] Bhatia D, Paul S, Acharjee T, et al. Biosensors and their widespread impact on human health. *Sensors Int*. 2024;5:100257.

[6] Bounegru AV, Apetrei C. Carbonaceous nanomaterials employed in the development of electrochemical sensors based on screen-printing technique—A review. *Catalysts*. 2020;10:680.

[7] Zaidi M. *Exploring Microenvironmental Heterogeneity in Cancer and Renal Biology Through Spatial Transcriptomics and Multiplexed Immunohistochemistry*. University of Toronto (Canada); 2024.

[8] Hsu T-R. *MEMS and Microsystems: Design, Manufacture, and Nanoscale Engineering.* John Wiley & Sons; 2008.

[9] Luttge R. *Nano-and Microfabrication for Industrial and Biomedical Applications.* William Andrew; 2016.

[10] Liu G, Lv Z, Batool S, et al. Biocompatible material-based flexible biosensors: From materials design to wearable/implantable devices and integrated sensing systems. *Small.* 2023;19:2207879.

[11] Kunwar P, Xiong Z, Zhu Y, et al. Hybrid laser printing of 3D, multiscale, multimaterial hydrogel structures. *Adv Opt Mater.* 2019;7:1900656.

[12] Jadhav A, Jadhav VS. A review on 3D printing: An additive manufacturing technology. *Mater Today Proc.* 2022;62:2094–9.

[13] Koltsaki M, Mavri M. A comprehensive overview of additive manufacturing processes through a time-based classification model. *3D Print Addit Manuf.* 2024;11:363–82.

[14] Bănică C-F, Sover A, Anghel D-C. Printing the future layer by layer: A comprehensive exploration of additive manufacturing in the era of industry 4.0. *Appl Sci.* 2024;14:9919.

[15] Zub K, Hoeppener S, Schubert US. Inkjet printing and 3D printing strategies for biosensing, analytical, and diagnostic applications. *Adv Mater.* 2022;34:2105015.

[16] Pagac M, Hajnys J, Ma Q-P, et al. A review of vat photopolymerization technology: Materials, applications, challenges, and future trends of 3D printing. *Polymers (Basel).* 2021;13:598.

[17] Gibson I, Rosen D, Stucker B, et al. Vat photopolymerization processes. In: *Additive Manufacturing Technologies 3D Printing, Rapid Prototyping, and Direct Digital Manufacturing.* New York, NY: Springer; 2015. pp. 63–106.

[18] Ali MA, Hu C, Yttri EA, et al. Recent advances in 3D printing of biomedical sensing devices. *Adv Funct Mater.* 2022;32:2107671.

[19] Amin R, Knowlton S, Hart A, et al. 3D-printed microfluidic devices. *Biofabrication.* 2016;8:22001.

[20] Paul AA, Aladese AD, Marks RS. Additive manufacturing applications in biosensors technologies. *Biosensors.* 2024;14:60.

[21] Sharma V, Kumar V. Application of Box-Behnken design and response surface methodology for multi-optimization of laser cutting of AA5052/ZrO2 metal– matrix composites. *Proc Inst Mech Eng Part L J Mater Des Appl.* 2018;232:652–68.

[22] Sharma V, Kumar V. Comparison of machining characteristics of metal matrix composites using CO2 laser curve cutting process. *Proc Inst Mech Eng Part E J Process Mech Eng.* 2018;232:349–68.

[23] Sharma V, Kumar V. Investigating the quality characteristics of Al5052/SiC metal matrix composites machined by CO2 laser curve cutting. *Proc Inst Mech Eng Part L J Mater Des Appl.* 2018;232:3–19.

[24] Sharma V, Kumar V, Bist A. Investigations on morphology and material removal rate of various MMCs using CO 2 laser technique. *J Brazilian Soc Mech Sci Eng.* 2020;42:1–14.

[25] Sharma V, Singh JP, Raman R, et al. Machine learning approach for prediction analysis of aluminium alloy on the surface roughness using CO2 laser machining. *Proc Inst Mech Eng Part E J Process Mech Eng.* 2024;09544089241231093.

[26] Sunitha K, Vasudev H. A short note on the various thermal spray coating processes and effect of post-treatment on Ni-based coatings. *Mater Today Proc* [Internet]. 2022;50:1452–7. Available from: https://linkinghub.elsevier.com/retrieve/pii/S2214785321058132.

[27] Singh J. Applications of laser technology for processing and post-treatments of powders and coatings. *Handb Laser-Based Sustain Surf Modif Manuf Tech.* 2023;135–66.

[28] Bambuwu AN. *Detection of Metals Using Bi-Modified Glassy Carbon Electrodes: An Insight into Their Performance.* Newcastle University; 2023.

[29] Wickström H. *Exploring Printed Drug Formulations for Inkjet and Stencil Printing: A study in Pharmaceutical Sciences*. Thesis, Turku, Finland: Åbo Akademi University; 2020. https://urn.fi/URN:ISBN:978-952-12-4009-6

[30] Park S, Kim H, Kim J-H, et al. Advanced nanomaterials, printing processes, and applications for flexible hybrid electronics. *Materials (Basel)*. 2020;13:3587.

[31] Jandyal A, Chaturvedi I, Wazir I, et al. 3D printing–A review of processes, materials and applications in industry 4.0. *Sustain Oper Comput*. 2022;3:33–42.

[32] Chohan JS, Mittal N, Kumar R, et al. Mechanical strength enhancement of 3D printed acrylonitrile butadiene styrene polymer components using neural network optimization algorithm. *Polymers*. 2020;12(10):2250.

[33] Singh R, Toseef M, Kumar J, et al. Benefits and challenges in additive manufacturing and its applications. In: Kaushal S, Singh I, Singh S, et al., editors. *Sustainable Advanced Manufacturing and Materials Processing* [Internet]. 1st ed. Boca Raton: CRC Press; 2022. pp. 137–57. Available from: www.taylorfrancis.com/books/9781003269298/chapters/10.1201/9781003269298-8.

[34] Singh J. Sustainability issues in laser-based additive manufacturing. In *Handbook of Laser-Based Sustainable Surface Modification and Manufacturing Techniques*. CRC Press; 2023. pp. 167–89.

[35] Ahmad S, Hashmi AW, Singh J, et al. Innovations in additive manufacturing of shape memory alloys: Alloys, microstructures, treatments, applications. *J Mater Res Technol*. 2024;32:4136–97.

[36] Sharma V, Singh JP, Hussan K, et al. Machine learning approach for predicting the machining characteristics of additive manufactured ABS material. *Proc Inst Mech Eng Part C J Mech Eng Sci*. 2024;09544062241283330.

[37] Singh JIP, Sharma V, Singh S, et al. Impact of molding temperature, fiber loading and chemical modifications on the physicomechanical, and microstructural morphology properties of woven kenaf fiber/PLA composites for non-structural applications. *J Nat Fibers*. 2024;21:2326586.

[38] Chen C, Wang X, Wang Y, et al. Additive manufacturing of piezoelectric materials. *Adv Funct Mater*. 2020;30:2005141.

[39] Zhu C, Gemeda HB, Duoss EB, et al. Toward multiscale, multimaterial 3D printing. *Adv Mater*. 2024:2314204.

[40] Al-Chami H. *Inkjet Printing of Transducers*. University of British Columbia; 2010.

[41] Rydzek G, Ji Q, Li M, et al. Electrochemical nanoarchitectonics and layer-by-layer assembly: From basics to future. *Nano Today*. 2015;10:138–67.

[42] Sponchioni M, Palmiero UC, Moscatelli D. Thermo-responsive polymers: Applications of smart materials in drug delivery and tissue engineering. *Mater Sci Eng C*. 2019;102:589–605.

[43] Bustamante-Torres M, Romero-Fierro D, Arcentales-Vera B, et al. Hydrogels classification according to the physical or chemical interactions and as stimuli-sensitive materials. *Gels*. 2021;7:182.

[44] Sonaye SY, Ertugral EG, Kothapalli CR, et al. Extrusion 3D (bio) printing of alginate-gelatin-based composite scaffolds for skeletal muscle tissue engineering. *Materials (Basel)*. 2022;15:7945.

[45] Groll J, Burdick JA, Cho D-W, et al. A definition of bioinks and their distinction from biomaterial inks. *Biofabrication* [Internet]. 2019;11:13001. https://doi.org/10.1088/1758-5090/aaec52

[46] Rao AS, Radanovic M, Liu Y, et al. Real-time monitoring of construction sites: Sensors, methods, and applications. *Autom Constr*. 2022;136:104099.

[47] Polat EO, Cetin MM, Tabak AF, et al. *Transducer Technologies for Biosensors and Their Wearable Applications*. Biosensors; 2022.

[48] De Acha N, Socorro-Leránoz AB, Elosúa C, et al. *Trends in the Design of Intensity-Based Optical Fiber Biosensors (2010–2020).* Biosensors; 2021.
[49] Shanbhag MM, Manasa G, Mascarenhas RJ, et al. Fundamentals of bio-electrochemical sensing. *Chem Eng J Adv* [Internet]. 2023;16:100516. Available from: www.sciencedirect.com/science/article/pii/S266682112300073X.
[50] Scheller F, Kirstein D, Kirstein L, et al. Enzyme electrodes and their application. *Philos Trans R Soc London B, Biol Sci.* 1987;316:85–94.
[51] Paul AA, Markus V, Kristollari K, et al. *Alginate-Based Applications in Biotechnology with a Special Mention to Biosensors.* London: IntechOpen; 2023.
[52] Parupelli SK, Desai S. The 3D printing of nanocomposites for wearable biosensors: Recent advances, challenges, and prospects. *Bioengineering.* 2023;11:32.
[53] Kourti D, Angelopoulou M, Petrou P, et al. Optical Immunosensors for Bacteria Detection in Food Matrices. *Chemosensors.* 2023;11(8):430.
[54] Kim J, Jia H, Wang P. Challenges in biocatalysis for enzyme-based biofuel cells. *Biotechnol Adv.* 2006;24:296–308.
[55] Ryu H, Thompson D, Huang Y, et al. Electrochemical sensors for nitrogen species: A review. *Sensor Actuator Rep.* 2020;2:100022.
[56] Mohidem NA, Mohamad M, Rashid MU, et al. Recent advances in enzyme immobilisation strategies: An overview of techniques and composite carriers. *J Compos Sci.* 2023;7(12):488.
[57] Park K, Millet LJ, Kim N, et al. Measurement of adherent cell mass and growth. *Proc Natl Acad Sci.* 2010;107:20691–6.
[58] Yang Z, Zhou S, Zu J, et al. High-performance piezoelectric energy harvesters and their applications. *Joule* [Internet]. 2018;2:642–97. Available from: www.sciencedirect.com/science/article/pii/S2542435118301260.
[59] Hatchett DW, Josowicz M. Composites of intrinsically conducting polymers as sensing nanomaterials. *Chem Rev.* 2008;108:746–69.

18 Quality Control and Regulatory Compliance in Biomedical Manufacturing

Vikas Sharma, Jashanpreet Singh, and Abdul Wahab Hashmi

CONTENTS

DOI: 10.1201/9781003516064-18

18.1 INTRODUCTION

Quality control (QC) and compliance are two essential considerations in biomedical manufacturing especially in the manufacturing of medical devices. Due to the changes that have occurred in the health sector, the patient needs in terms of safe and top quality medical products have been made higher [1]. The quality control and compliance are all about in biomedical manufacturing with focus on quality standards. QC is a complex procedure that is carried out in a specific system for the purpose of monitoring the medical device during its life cycle. It involves the practical measures like strict inspection and testing requirements and confirming with international guideline ISO: 13485 that relates to establishing requirements concerning quality management for the medical devices [2]. The regulatory requirement must be satisfied with a necessity to protect the health of the general public and the quality of the biomedical products.

The quality assurance and compliance are critically essential for the completion of the task. Many medical devices have defects that may cause harm or fatalities among the patients using them. Sound quality control measures need to be put in place to avoid formation of defects which will make the products to perform poorly. Moreover, implementation of QMS support manufacturing operations decrease expenses related to recalls and non-compliance fines. It has been noticed that trust is a vital element within this industry, and quality as well as compliancy is critical in ensuring that the necessary confidence for overall safety.

This chapter also highlights the significance of issues of quality assurance and conformity. The defective medical devices may also cost one's life. As such, comprehensive quality assurance is essential in preventing the generation of product flaws and guaranteeing product performance [3]. Also, efficient quality management systems help organization functional, minimize the expenses related to the product recall or non-adherence penalties, and improve the manufacturer's position within the sphere of healthcare [4,5]. As the interaction between the user and the product entails trust, high levels of quality and compliance need be observed in the industry for convenience of the healthcare service providers and patients.

The main objective of the chapter is to review the important strategies used in quality control in biomedical manufacturing industries, establish the effects of compliance and regulations on manufactured products, and evaluate the practices that improve quality assurance. Moreover, this chapter aims at identifying the manufacturers who can enhance their quality management systems for serving regulatory compliance. To apply a critical review of the existing practices and trends in the literature, this chapter will enhance the ongoing process on enhancing quality assurance across biomedical products.

18.2 REGULATION OF BIOMEDICAL MANUFACTURING

The industry is framed under the biomedical manufacturing regulatory framework reactivity of different national and international bodies [6]. The duty of these bodies is to set standards in the production of these medical products to enhance their safety. In this section, the focus will be towards the key regulatory authorities that exist in the market, regulatory demands placed concerning biomedical products, as well as the variations across different regions of the world.

18.2.1 Overview of Key Regulatory Bodies

The innovation and competitiveness of the medical device business are greatly influenced by national regulatory authorities. These organizations determine whether products are safe and effective enough to be sold to the public [7]. They act as the gatekeepers (**Figure 18.1**). There are several prominent regulatory bodies which govern biomedical manufacturing across different regions such as U.S. Food and Drug Administration (FDA), European Medicines Agency (EMA), and International Organization for Standardization (ISO). The Food and Drugs Administration, also known as the U.S. FDA, is the federal body that oversees the usage of medical devices in the United States. It uses a risk-based system of classifications which divide the devices into Class I: devices that pose low risks, Class II: products that present moderate risks, and Class III: those that pose significant risks [8]. Every class has specific regulatory measures, for instance the 510(k) notification or PMA, the approval depending on the category of the device. In Europe, the EMA coordinates the authorization of medical devices with national competent bodies. The most comprehensive European regulation is the MDR that instructs manufacturers on the recognition of classes depending on the risk such as FDA. Before products can be marketed, the

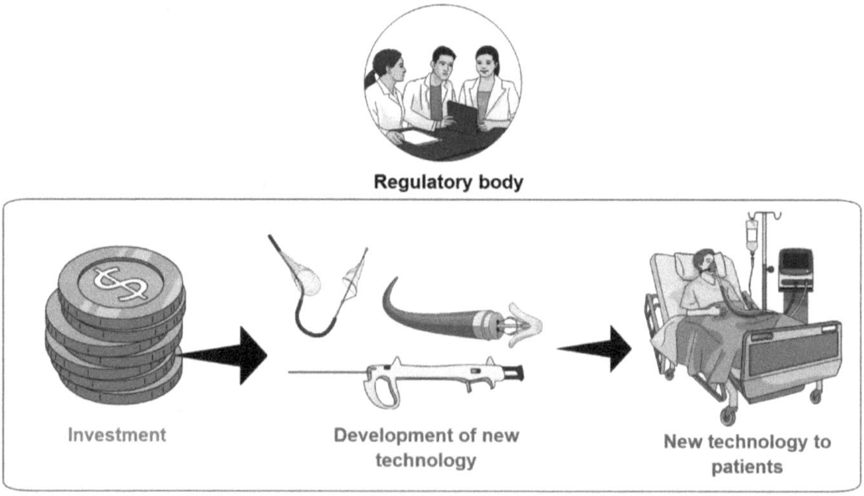

FIGURE 18.1 Regulatory bodies' involvement in the innovation cycle of medical device industry.

devices undergo conformity assessment with regard to essential requirements. ISO establishes the standards used globally for quality management systems with relation to biomedical manufacturing. The ISO 13485 is one of the standards that help in providing requirements for quality management systems which aim at the conformity of an organization's activities, products, and services [9].

18.2.2 Stability Testing and Regulatory Requirement of Biomedical Products

Regulatory requirements for biomedical products encompass several critical areas like Quality Management Systems (QMS), premarket approval processes, and post-market surveillance. The manufacturers follow a QMS that meets a certain regulation like FDA QSR or ISO 13485. Such systems help to guarantee that products are developed and produced to conform to the expected safety and efficacy levels. Depending on the classification device manufacturers are required to provide FDA the 510(k) premarket notification and PMA application containing the data about safety and effectiveness [10] The Class III device is usually more heavily regulated; thus it undergoes more testing and documentation than Class I. Once the devices are commercialized, it becomes the responsibility of the manufacturers to conduct post-market performance surveillance and to report on adverse events. This ongoing oversight is important to keep the product safe of its hazards during its life cycle of a device.

18.3 QUALITY CONTROL TECHNIQUES IN BIOMEDICAL MANUFACTURING

Quality assurance is crucial in biomedical production to guarantee the safety, reliability, and compliance to standard production requirements. This section discusses different critical quality control techniques as shown in **Figure 18.2**.

18.3.1 Sampling and Testing Procedures

Sampling is one of the decisive stages of quality control since the results of tests reflecting the quality of products depend on the sampling. There are various methods employed to ensure representative samples are collected such as the following.

18.3.2 Sampling Methods

Some of the usual methods of sampling are random sampling, stratified sampling, and systematic sampling [11]. Each method is appropriate depending on the circumstances and the kind of product being tested. The systematic sample includes sampling at regular intervals can be helpful in large production batches.

18.3.3 Testing Protocols

The test procedure that is supposed to meet the standard procedures is FDA standard procedure or ISO standard procedures [12]. They specify that the samples must be

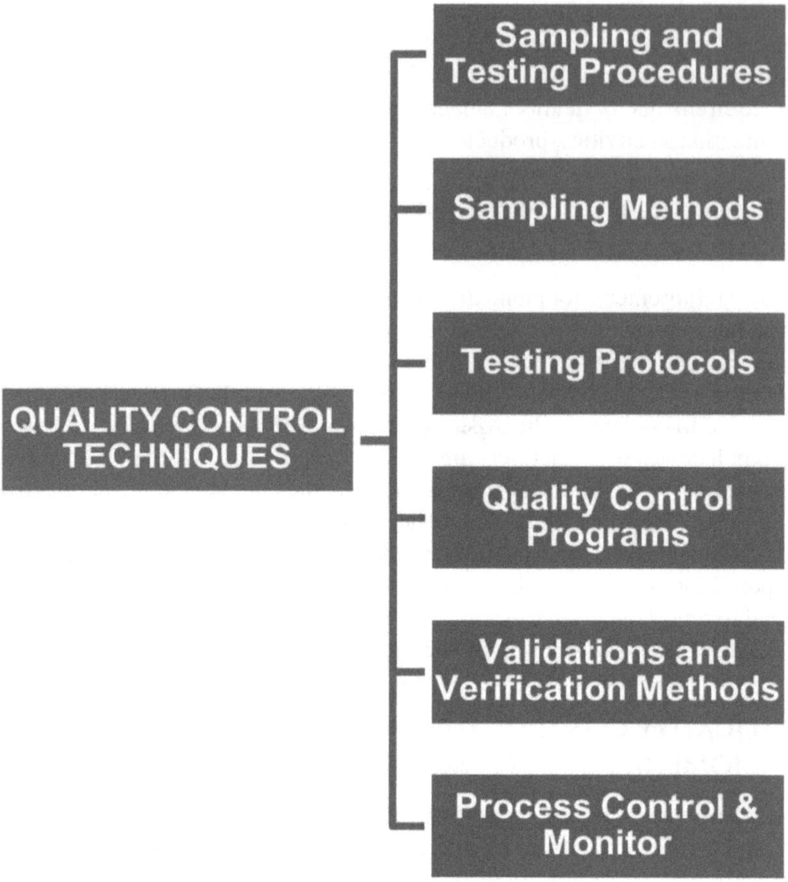

FIGURE 18.2 Various critical quality control techniques.

acquired, managed, and tested to increase the probability of getting accurate results. For instance, the FDA has included elaborate instructions on ways to avoid contamination during sample collection using aseptic practices.

18.3.4 Quality Control Programs

Like the EMA, testing and regulatory agencies in the pharma industry also have annual testing programs for CAP with risk-based sampling to monitor product quality annually [13]. These programs may contain stages as screening and further check-up or other forms of examinations.

18.3.5 Validations and Verification Methods

The validation and verification in manufacturing is an important step to deliver products that meet specific requirements. In the validation process to control the process, the product should meet the required specifications periodically. This may include process validation that seeks to establish that processes run to standard and method validation that seeks to determine that established analytical methods will give satisfactory results [14]. The confirmation can be achieved by executing the process under different circumstances in a view to identifying strengths or weaknesses of the process.

For the verification process it is assured that correct processes are being followed in the production of the validated processes. This can include monitoring equipment for its correctness with SOPs and maintenance record as well as others [15]. Internal verification activities also include the regular audit and inspection, which are important elements of verification activities. Moreover, record keeping is critical to maintain validation and verification activities as a logged record keeping system must be in place for records that support product documentation. These are supposed to capture all test results, any observed variations from expected results, and steps taken to address the variance.

18.3.6 Process Control and Monitor

For the quality to be preserved from one process step to the other, substantial control over the process is required. Sensors and automated devices allow real-time monitoring integral and significant operating parameters used in industrial processes collectively referred to as CPPs [16]. This enables manufacturers to make the necessary correction where necessary before non-conforming items are made. Statistical process control (SPC) techniques depend on probability distributions to measure and control the production processes. From performance data of various stages of production, manufacturers can be able to predict or discover error patterns that point to quality concerns. Among various SPC tools, control charts are the most well-known tools used to plot a process's stability on a time line [17]. Every organization has certain quality issues which need to be solving on urgent basis with the help of Corrective and Preventive Actions (CAPA) system. It includes the identifying causes of such straying, putting measures to address the problem, and or finding ways to avoid a recurrence of such occurrences in future.

18.4 INNOVATION IN THE MEDICAL DEVICES SECTOR

To be classified as an innovation, medical technology must show a therapeutic advantage in a randomized clinical trial, with the status quo as the control group and a clinically meaningful main objective [18]. But this criterion may not be enough to describe medical device advances. That's because, for ethical reasons, most novel medical devices can't go through blind randomized clinical trials. Both the regulatory use of "big data" information derived from electronic health records and expanded patient registries—and the application of randomized clinical trials as the gold standard for evaluating clinical evidence based on medical practice are discussed nowadays [19]. Ciani et al. [20] categorized the current definitions of innovations in medical devices using three criteria—the origin of the invention, the level of disruption it caused, and its effects (**Figure 18.3**). The technology-push perspective holds that innovation is best understood as an entrepreneurial process, including the phases of ideation, invention, development, and commercialization. According to the demand-pull theory, new developments in medicine may help satisfy unmet clinical demands. Nevertheless, mixed or interactive models (coupling models), stage models, networks, and open innovation models have already surpassed both methods, which are part of the linear models of innovation (Davey et al., 2011). The health service is lagging behind other consumer product categories when it comes to introducing novel medical equipment because of the hurdles to innovation [21]. Medical device businesses, on the other hand, may benefit from open innovation models as they facilitate the management of stakeholder ideas and reduce current market entry barriers. Research has shown that when academic

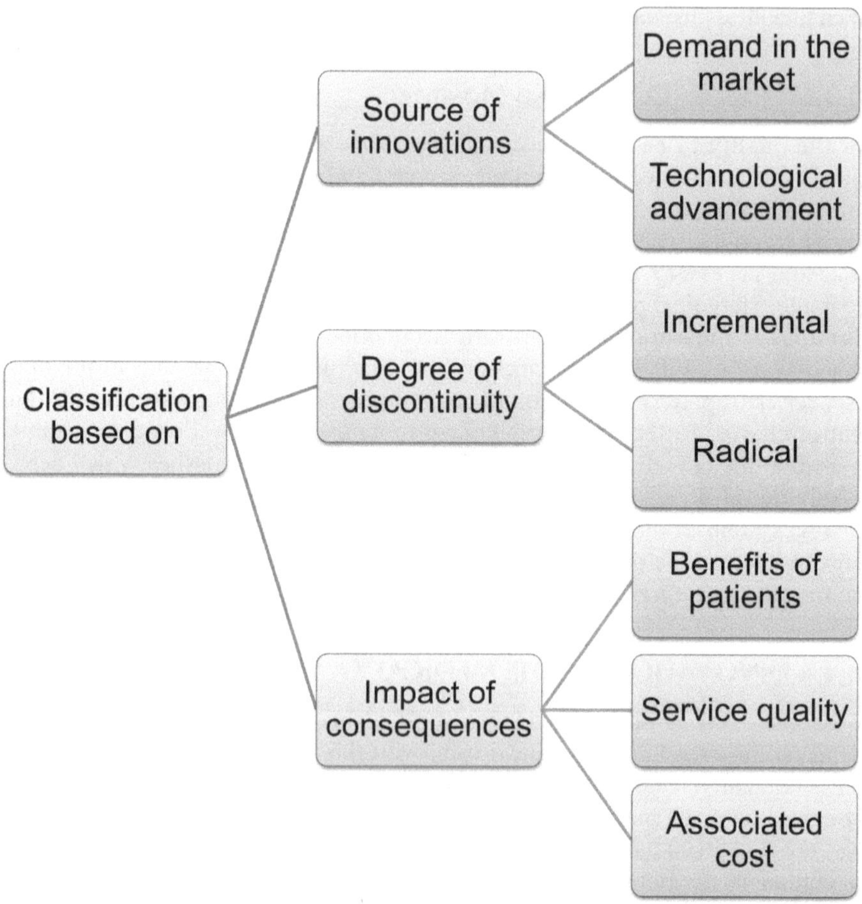

FIGURE 18.3 Criteria used to categorize advances in the medical device sector.

institutions, healthcare providers, businesses, and government agencies work together, they can create groundbreaking medical devices, which emphasizes the importance of the partnerships between medical device developers and key users/clinicians [22]. Participation in a new technology, as well as direct requests and offers, may strengthen these ties. On the other hand, there is a lot of debate over the ethics of doctors having financial ties to medical equipment companies. Although there are specialists who are concerned that these partnerships might impact doctors' choices about patient care and the documentation of results, which could put patients at risk, there are also those who argue that these relationships are necessary for the advancement of medical technology [23].

There are numerous examples in between the two extremes, but generally speaking, innovations in medical equipment may be either incremental or revolutionary, depending on their severity [24]. The third method involves categorizing medical device innovations according to their positive effects, which involves thinking about service quality, costs, and ethical considerations from the perspective of the user/consumer, individual organizations, or the entire health system, in addition to the direct clinically meaningful benefit. Learning curve device optimization also relies on the scholarly events, tasks, seminars, and workshops.

18.5 IMPACT OF REGULATIONS ON INNOVATION IN BIOMEDICAL DEVICES

All stages of the invention life cycle are affected by regulatory problems (**Figure 18.4**). Medical device designers and developers must keep them in mind from the very beginning of the process, all the way through pre- and clinical testing, product regulatory reviews, production, and post-marketing monitoring [25]. Thus, the innovation and competitiveness of the medical device business are dependent on the connection between national regulatory authorities and developers of medical devices. Governmental policies and activities in this area provide the external framework for innovations in medical goods, since they are necessary for regulatory bodies to approve the new product before it can be sold (**Figure 18.5**). Regulatory concerns are a real concern for developers' right from the start of the revolutionary medical device's design and development phases [26]. A manufacturer's quality management system, which has to have suitable risk management, serves as the internal foundation for R&D&I operations pertaining to medical devices (**Figure 18.5**). To prove conformity with the "Essential Principles of Safety and Performance of Medical Devices" (Global Harmonisation Task Force, 2012), quality and risk management strategies must be implemented across the whole medical device life cycle. Medical device and accessory risk management includes hazard identification and description; risk analysis, appraisal, and control; and control effectiveness monitoring. Most nations' harmonized legislative requirements use the procedures outlined in the international standard ISO 14971:2007 for medical device risk management [27]. One of the primary goals of the design controls outlined in the Food and Drug Administration's (FDA) Quality Systems (1997) and the

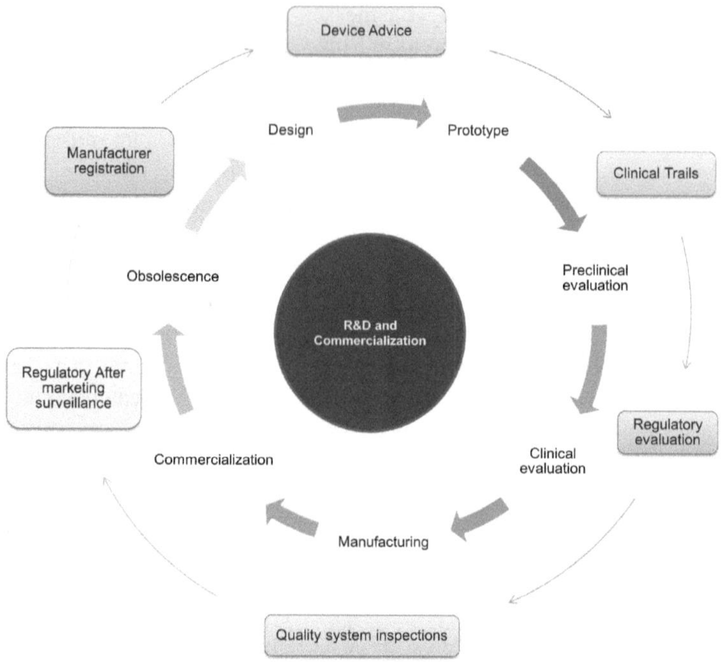

FIGURE 18.4 Relationship between the activities of regulatory bodies and the R&D&I process.

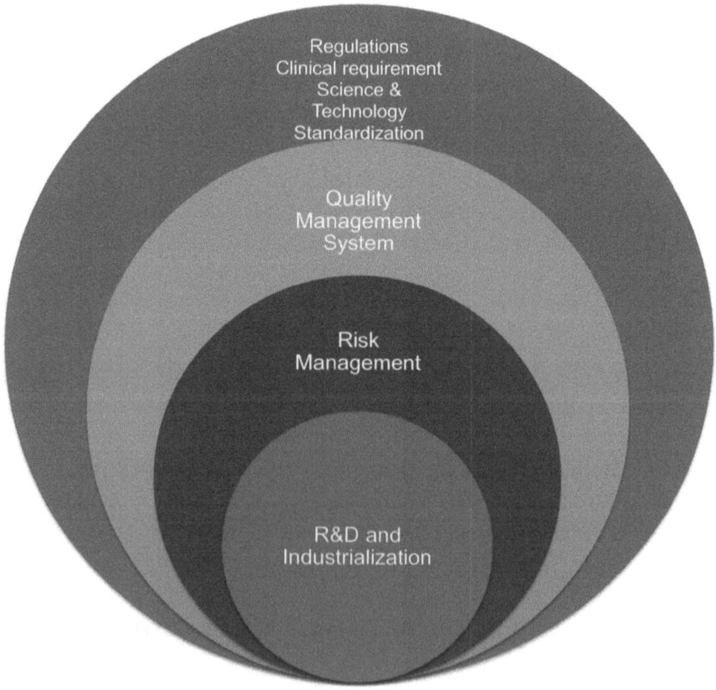

FIGURE 18.5 Internal and external framework for the development of new medical devices.

International Organization for Standardization's (ISO) 13485 quality system standard (2016a) is risk management.

Medical devices designed for human use are covered in both publications, which contain standards for procedures, facilities, and controls for design, manufacture, packing, labelling, storage, installation, and service [28]. As an additional component of their risk management system, device manufacturers are obligated to gather post-market information, which may include clinical data. Uncertainty over the regulatory procedure and high product heterogeneity are hallmarks of newer revolutionary medical devices. Discouragement towards medical device innovation is fuelled by the "regulatory uncertainty" that surrounds the timing and approval of such devices by national regulatory agencies (Fleming, 2015). **Figure 18.6** shows how "technological uncertainty" and "content and format uncertainty" are the two parts of "regulatory uncertainty" that Stern (2017) breaks down. To alleviate any doubts, it is recommended that developers and regulators engage early on in the product development and regulatory approval processes to help identify and resolve important scientific and regulatory concerns pertaining to the novel medical device. Testing techniques may be better studied if developers and regulators met face to face [29].

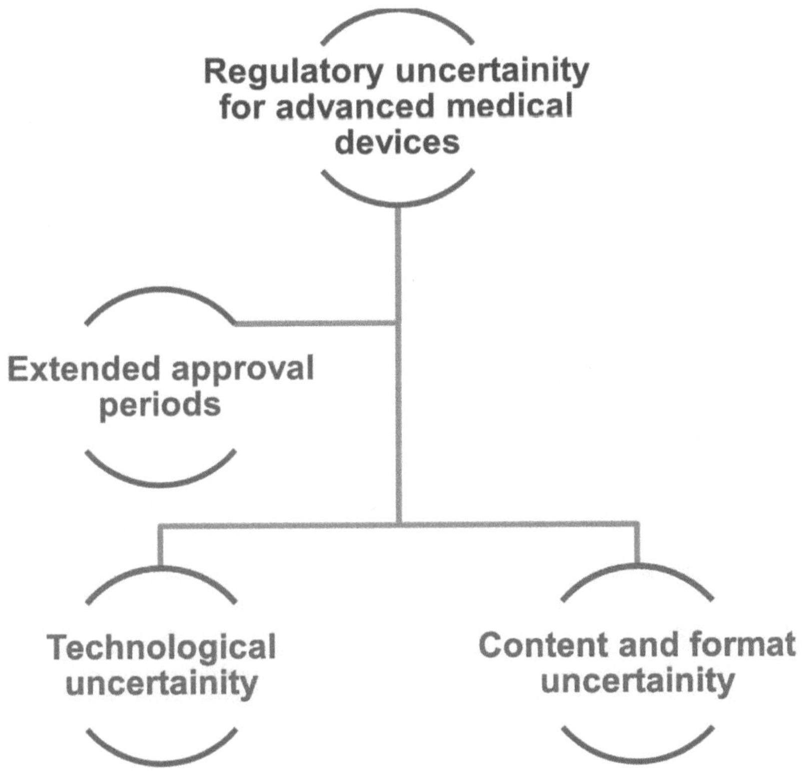

FIGURE 18.6 Regulatory uncertainty for inventive new items to get clearance.

18.6 FUTURE TRENDS IN BIOMEDICAL QUALITY CONTROL AND COMPLIANCE

The biomedical industry is standing on the principal of change as the regulatory environment continues to evolve and as new mechanisms of quality control are developed. The new directions need to be provided for the regulation and guidelines, digital transformation and compliance, and others on improved quality assurance [30].

18.6.1 Emerging Regulatory Standards and Guidelines

With the advancement in the biomedical, the regulatory authorities also have to be updated for the new conditions and innovations. The key trends include the following.

18.6.1.1 Increased Focus on Data Integrity

The regulatory agencies are focusing more on data integrity to get more accurate and reliable data on trials and approvals [31]. This trend is particularly relevant as more data collection and analysis are integrated into digital platforms that require better safeguards against data fabrication or mistakes.

18.6.1.2 Adoption of International Standards

The incorporation of these standards into some national statutes integrates with the ISO 13485. It is from these standards that quality management systems can build to improve product safety and effectiveness across borders. The FDA also encourages product compliance with ISO standards issued internationally to establish uniformity in quality control [32].

18.6.1.3 Regulatory Adaptation to Digital Technologies

With the advancement of the applications of the telemedicine and mobile health, the regulators are also providing the rules and standards that ought to govern the advanced innovations. This involves the development of post-approval risk management of SaMD and the post-market regulation of data, respecting of laws including HIPAA.

18.6.2 Use of Digital Transformation in Compliance

Digital transformation is reshaping compliance processes within the biomedical sector by introducing automation, data analytics, and real-time monitoring.

- *Automation of Compliance Processes*: Various organizations are gradually incorporating automated systems to help address some of the tasks. It provides the automation for the entry and real-time processing of data, which also helps in the preparation and documentation of reports for compliance with regulations [33]. The increased efficiency and automation also reduce human interferences which improve the reliability of compliance.

- *Data Analytics for Predictive Compliance*: There has been the adoption of innovative and sophisticated methods of data analysis that are used to forecast compliance risks. The use of historical data as well as trend analysis helps the organization for non-compliance risk. This predictive approach helps in creating positive organizational culture and tends to sustain a high-level quality control.
- *Enhanced Engagement with Quality Management Systems (QMS)*: Educational technologies are enhancing staff interaction with QMS as more of the processes become streamlined and easy to follow. The user-friendly interfaces and real-time report can be fully promoted which resulted into the quality management which can be improved comprehensively [34].

18.7 FUTURE PERSPECTIVE ON NEW QUALITY CONTROL TECHNIQUES

The future of quality control in biomedical manufacturing is expected for significant advancements through innovative methodologies such as integration of Artificial Intelligence (AI), blockchain for traceability, and continuous quality improvement (CQI) practices [35–37]. Manufacturers are incorporating the use of AI in improving input quality and control. The machine learning systems can learn from large sets of data collected from manufacturing processes to produce early warning signs of a problem with product quality. This capability means that there can be real-time changes of some of the production process parameters, hence minimizing the defects. Blockchain technology is also gradually becoming a best practice, allowing biomedical production to improve traceability [38,39]. In solving issues of trust and to increase the efficiency of supply chain, blockchain has the capability to offer an unalterable record of each operation within the supply chain. It becomes possible for products to be traced from their manufacturing up to the time they were supplied to the market. As it can be seen organizations are not adopting traditional QC and QI approaches focusing on separate periodical assessment. Continuous quality improvement (CQI) practices approach refers to the constant appraisal of processes and results being generated to establish opportunities for change [40,41]. **Figure 18.7** illustrates the detailed role of AI in QA of medical devices.

18.7.1 Advancements in Product Design

By giving manufacturers more leeway to innovate in terms of product design and development, AI encourages innovation and healthy competition in the medical device industry. As a result of AI methods, healthcare items are now more innovative and competitive than ever before [42–44]. The increasing use of AI to improve medical device goods is evidence that the industry recognizes AI's transformational potential [45,46]. AI-powered manufacturing defect detection encourages innovation and continuous progress which demonstrates AI's significance in maintaining and enhancing product quality via incremental breakthroughs [47].

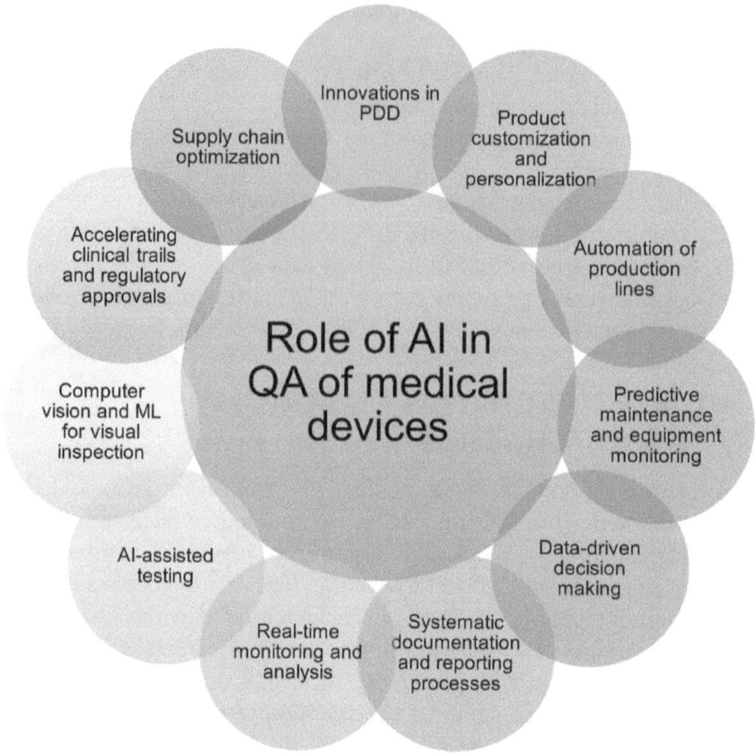

FIGURE 18.7 Role of AI in QA of medical devices.

18.7.2 Enabling Customers to Individualize their Products

To meet the needs of each patient, it is necessary to personalize and customize medical equipment. Artificial intelligence makes this process simpler. Manufacturing technologies powered by artificial intelligence have made it possible to tailor medical equipment to the specific requirements of individual patients [48,49]. Customized solutions that enhance the efficiency and comfort of medical equipment can only be made possible with this level of knowledge.

18.7.3 Lines of Production Automation

In manufacturing lines, AI drastically cuts down on labour-intensive, repetitive tasks, allowing humans to focus on more valuable endeavours like invention and product development [50,51]. Since trained workers would be able to concentrate on the more intricate and imaginative parts of production, this may lead to better product creation in terms of both efficiency and originality.

18.7.4 Monitoring and Predictive Maintenance of Equipment

AI analyses sensor data to optimize equipment maintenance plans, which in turn allow manufacturers to anticipate when their machinery may need repairs or replacement components [52,53]. The uninterrupted functioning of crucial industrial machinery is guaranteed by the predictive modelling abilities of artificial intelligence, which analyse intricate data to foresee any problems [52,54]. Predictive maintenance ensures that equipment runs at its best by reducing the likelihood of expensive failures and unscheduled downtime. An example of AI's adaptive learning capabilities is a production process learner that mimics human operators by analysing device logs for problems and suggesting fixes [55].

18.7.5 Inventory Management

AI enhances the efficiency of the supply chain by monitoring inventory levels, predicting demand changes, and detecting potential disruptions [55]. AI has the potential to streamline the supply chain, enhance manufacturing parameters, and expedite the delivery of medical equipment by processing large data sets [56].

18.7.6 Speeding up of Regulatory Approvals and Clinical Trials

The use of AI may help simplify compliance processes and guarantee that items are safe and up to par before they reach store shelves [57,58]. Because of the profound effect that prompts access to cutting-edge technology has on patient outcomes, the medical device industry places a premium on accelerating time-to-market.

18.7.7 Eye-cracking Computer Vision and ML Systems

AI methods, such as computer vision and machine learning, automate or greatly enhance crucial quality assurance (QA) procedures. There is no longer any need for human inspectors when AI-enabled vision systems can spot irregularities and faults in manufacturing processes. This guarantees top-notch medical equipment production while improving QA's accuracy and consistency [59,60].

18.7.8 Testing using AI

By enhancing the efficiency and accuracy of testing methods, AI technology optimizes them [48]. Medical equipment may be evaluated more precisely and thoroughly with the help of AI, which improves the product's overall quality and dependability.

18.7.9 Analytics and Real-Time Monitoring

To anticipate issues, AI systems may analyse massive data sets in real time for patterns and mistakes [48]. It seems that maintaining high-quality assurance requirements and quickly fixing any production-related problems would benefit from real-time monitoring.

18.7.10 Efficient Reporting and Documentation Procedures

Both accurate documentation and full audit trials are made possible by AI's automation of documentation procedures [61]. All production processes are well-documented and can be readily audited thanks to this automation, which also improves regulatory compliance.

To enhance production and provide useful insights for informed decision-making, AI systems sift through mountains of data. By deriving useful insights from production data, AI-driven analytics improve decision-making processes and aid in the implementation of a thorough quality control plan throughout the manufacturing process [62]. This means that the industry is undergoing a transformation as a result of AI being used for quality control and manufacture of medical devices. This is accomplished by maximizing supply chain efficiency, automating manufacturing lines, optimizing maintenance schedules, and enhancing product customization. Accelerating clinical trials, ensuring stringent quality control, and supporting data-driven decision-making are three ways in which AI is changing the medical device industry.

18.8 QUALITY AND COMPLIANCE IN INDIA'S BIOMEDICAL MANUFACTURING

The manufacturing industry in India has many bodies to oversee its operations to meet set standards aimed at protecting the public health. The Central Drugs Standard Control Organization (CDSCO) is the main controlling authority of the country authorized to issue licence, implement the standard of GMP certification, AUDIT & Compliance for manufacturing of medicines and medical device [63,64]. The enhancement of regulation is continued with Medical Device Rules (MDR) enacted in 2017, which categorizes devices on the basis of risk in use and requires registration and compliance conforming to risk levels [65–67]. The Bureau of Indian Standards (BIS) regulates certification of particular medical devices for safety and performance standards [63,68]. The National Accreditation Board for Testing and Calibration Laboratories (NABL) certifies laboratories to ensure its accuracy, as testing follows the international standards to support data on the quality of products [69,70]. These are groups of bodies that are superimposed to ensure compliance to standard, safety, and efficacy of biomedical products in the country. These organizations work in coordination as the industry expands and fulfils the need to ensure the quality of work being delivered in India. Also, to meet the international benchmarks associated with biomedical industry and thus the ongoing development of India as a biomedical powerhouse in the world.

18.9 CONCLUSION

Quality control and compliance remain essential in manufacturing the biomedical products which meet the standard safety and efficacy. This chapter examines the interaction between regulations and quality management in the manufacturing environment and its impact on the manufacturing environment. The effective methodologies have been presented that meet the demands of both national and international legislations. According to the future trends in compliance, new developments in the field and technologies are improving the compliance regulation and product quality. The emphasis also has been given on data accuracy, digitalization of compliance as well as advances in improved compliance measurement. The application of AI-

and blockchain may help the manufacturers to address challenges towards quality. Moreover, it is important to maintain the culture of quality control in constant manner due to the growing healthcare demands.

REFERENCES

[1] Chassin MR, Galvin RW. The urgent need to improve health care quality: Institute of medicine national roundtable on health care quality. *Jama*. 1998;280:1000–5.

[2] Linck W, Tinoco MAC, Bonato SV, et al. A maturity assessment methodology for ISO 13485 implementation in the medical devices industry. *Int J Qual Reliab Manag*. 2024;42(5):1411–37.

[3] Khinvasara T, Ness S, Shankar A. Leveraging AI for enhanced quality assurance in medical device manufacturing. *Asian J Res Comput Sci*. 2024;17:13–35.

[4] Godman B, Acurcio F, Guerra Junior AA, et al. Initiatives among authorities to improve the quality and efficiency of prescribing and the implications. *J Pharma Care Heal Sys*. 2014;1:1–15.

[5] Stegemann S, Ecker F, Maio M, et al. Geriatric drug therapy: Neglecting the inevitable majority. *Ageing Res Rev*. 2010;9:384–98.

[6] Renn O, Roco MC. Nanotechnology and the need for risk governance. *J Nanoparticle Res*. 2006;8:153–91.

[7] Organization WH. *The Safety of Medicines in Public Health Programmes: Pharmacovigilance, an Essential tool*; 2006. https://www.who.int/publications/i/item/9241593911

[8] Jamshidi A, Rahimi SA, Ait-Kadi D, et al. A comprehensive fuzzy risk-based maintenance framework for prioritization of medical devices. *Appl Soft Comput*. 2015;32:322–34.

[9] Karthika B, Vijayakumar AR. ISO 13485: Medical devices–quality management systems, requirements for regulatory purposes. In *Medical Device Guidelines and Regulations Handbook*. Springer; 2022. pp. 19–29.

[10] Darrow JJ, Avorn J, Kesselheim AS. FDA regulation and approval of medical devices: 1976–2020. *Jama*. 2021;326:420–32.

[11] Cochran WG. Relative accuracy of systematic and stratified random samples for a certain class of populations. *Ann Math Stat*. 1946;17:164–77.

[12] Bas A, Burns N, Gulotta A, et al. Understanding the development, standardization, and validation process of alternative in vitro test methods for regulatory approval from a researcher perspective. *Small*. 2021;17:2006027.

[13] CMM. *CAPA see Corrective and Preventive Actions*; 2023. https://www.fda.gov/inspections-compliance-enforcement-and-criminal-investigations/inspection-guides/corrective-and-preventive-actions-capa

[14] Taverniers I, De Loose M, Van Bockstaele E. Trends in quality in the analytical laboratory. II. Analytical method validation and quality assurance. *TrAC Trends Anal Chem*. 2004;23:535–52.

[15] Akyar I. Standard operating procedures (what are they good for?). *Latest Res into Qual Control*. 2012;12:367–91.

[16] García MV, Irisarri E, Pérez F, et al. An open CPPS automation architecture based on IEC-61499 over OPC-UA for flexible manufacturing in Oil&Gas industry. *IFAC-PapersOnLine*. 2017;50:1231–8.

[17] MacCarthy BL, Wasusri T. A review of non-standard applications of statistical process control (SPC) charts. *Int J Qual Reliab Manag*. 2002;19:295–320.

[18] Berry DA. Emerging innovations in clinical trial design. *Clin Pharmacol Ther.* 2016;99:82–91.
[19] Piantadosi S. *Clinical Trials: A Methodologic Perspective.* John Wiley & Sons; 2024.
[20] Ciani O, Armeni P, Boscolo PR, et al. De innovatione: The concept of innovation for medical technologies and its implications for healthcare policy-making. *Heal Policy Technol* [Internet]. 2016;5:47–64. Available from: www.sciencedirect.com/science/article/pii/S2211883715000805.
[21] West J, Bogers M. Leveraging external sources of innovation: A review of research on open innovation. *J Prod Innov Manag.* 2014;31:814–31.
[22] McShea M, Holl R, Badawi O, et al. The eICU research institute-a collaboration between industry, health-care providers, and academia. *IEEE Eng Med Biol Mag.* 2010;29:18–25.
[23] Kassirer JP. *On the Take: How Medicine's Complicity with Big Business Can Endanger Your Health.* Oxford University Press; 2004.
[24] Blume SS. *Insight and Industry: On the Dynamics of Technological Change in Medicine.* MIT Press; 1992.
[25] Whitmore E. *Development of FDA-Regulated Medical Products.* Quality Press; 2012.
[26] Pietzsch JB, Shluzas LA, Paté-Cornell ME, et al. Stage-gate process for the development of medical devices. *J Med Devices.* 2009;3(2):021004.
[27] van Vroonhoven J. *Risk Management for Medical Devices and the New BS EN ISO 14971.* ASM International; 2020.
[28] Sastri VR. *Plastics in Medical Devices: Properties, Requirements, and Applications.* William Andrew; 2021.
[29] Cole PM, Michel MK, Teti LO. The development of emotion regulation and dysregulation: A clinical perspective. *Monogr Soc Res Child Dev.* 1994:73–100.
[30] De Haes S, Caluwe L, Huygh T, et al. *Governing Digital Transformation.* Dalam Manag Prof.; 2020.
[31] Christie SM. *An Exploratory Study of the Impact of Quality Management Practices on Data Integrity FDA-483 Observations Received by Pharmaceutical Manufacturers in Florida.* Theses and Dissertations; 2023. p. 1312. https://repository.fit.edu/etd/1312.
[32] Rodríguez-Pérez J. *Quality Risk Management in the FDA-Regulated Industry.* Quality Press; 2017.
[33] Boda VVR, Allam H. Automating compliance in healthcare: Tools and techniques you need. *Innov Eng Sci J.* 2021;1.
[34] Eswaran M, Bahubalendruni MVAR. Challenges and opportunities on AR/VR technologies for manufacturing systems in the context of industry 4.0: A state of the art review. *J Manuf Syst.* 2022;65:260–78.
[35] Thangamani R, Kamalam GK, Vimaladevi M. Revolutionizing healthcare processes: The dynamic role of blockchain innovation. In *Blockchain for Biomedical Research and Healthcare Concept, Trends, Future Implications.* Springer; 2024. pp. 229–67.
[36] Alhaj NA, Jamlos MF, Manap SA, et al. Integration of hybrid networks, AI, ultra massive-MIMO, THz frequency, and FBMC modulation towards 6G requirements: A review. *IEEE Access.* 2024 12:483–513.
[37] Sharma A, Singh M, Gupta M, et al. IoT and blockchain technology in 5G smart healthcare. In *Blockchain Applications Healthcare Informatics.* Elsevier; 2022. pp. 137–61.
[38] Liu X, Barenji AV, Li Z, et al. Blockchain-based smart tracking and tracing platform for drug supply chain. *Comput Ind Eng.* 2021;161:107669.
[39] Justinia T. Blockchain technologies: Opportunities for solving real-world problems in healthcare and biomedical sciences. *Acta Inform Med.* 2019;27:284.
[40] Thawesaengskulthai N, Thawesaengskulthai D. *Selecting Quality Management and Improvement Initiatives.* PhD Thesis. University of Nottingham; 2007.

[41] Al Moosa NH. *A Qualitative Study of Change: Implementing Quality Assurance and Continuous Quality Improvement in Health Professions Education During a Period of Transition*. Villanova University; 2014.
[42] Ramesh H. *A Framework for Corporate Innovation Management and Managerial Innovation in Medical Devices Industry*; 2023. https://lutpub.lut.fi/handle/10024/165899
[43] Haleem A, Javaid M, Singh RP, et al. Medical 4.0 technologies for healthcare: Features, capabilities, and applications. *Internet Things Cyber-Physical Syst.* 2022;2:12–30.
[44] Ali Mohamad T, Bastone A, Bernhard F, et al. How artificial intelligence impacts the competitive position of healthcare organizations. *J Organ Chang Manag.* 2023;36:49–70.
[45] Qayyum MU, Sherani AMK, Khan M, et al. Revolutionizing healthcare: The transformative impact of artificial intelligence in medicine. *BIN Bull Informatics.* 2023;1:71–83.
[46] Dwivedi YK, Hughes L, Ismagilova E, et al. Artificial Intelligence (AI): Multidisciplinary perspectives on emerging challenges, opportunities, and agenda for research, practice and policy. *Int J Inf Manage.* 2021;57:101994.
[47] Aldoseri A, Al-Khalifa KN, Hamouda AM. AI-powered innovation in digital transformation: Key pillars and industry impact. *Sustainability.* 2024;16:1790.
[48] Ahmed Z, Mohamed K, Zeeshan S, et al. Artificial intelligence with multi-functional machine learning platform development for better healthcare and precision medicine. *Database.* 2020;2020:baaa010.
[49] Bohr A, Memarzadeh K. The rise of artificial intelligence in healthcare applications. In *Artificial Intelligence in Healthcare*. Elsevier; 2020. pp. 25–60.
[50] Mhlanga D. *Responsible Industry 4.0: A Framework for Human-Centered Artificial Intelligence*. Taylor & Francis; 2023.
[51] Filippucci F, Gal P, Jona-Lasinio C, et al. *The Impact of Artificial Intelligence on Productivity, Distribution and Growth: Key Mechanisms, Initial Evidence and Policy Challenges*; 2024. https://www.oecd.org/en/publications/the-impact-of-artificial-intelligence-on-productivity-distribution-and-growth_8d900037-en.html
[52] Diez-Olivan A, Del Ser J, Galar D, et al. Data fusion and machine learning for industrial prognosis: Trends and perspectives towards Industry 4.0. *Inf Fusion.* 2019;50:92–111.
[53] Lee J, Ni J, Singh J, et al. Intelligent maintenance systems and predictive manufacturing. *J Manuf Sci Eng.* 2020;142:110805.
[54] Kashpruk N, Piskor-Ignatowicz C, Baranowski J. Time series prediction in industry 4.0: A comprehensive review and prospects for future advancements. *Appl Sci.* 2023;13:12374.
[55] Gautam S. *The Learning Code: Designing AI-Driven Adaptive Learning Systems for Social Learning*. The Pennsylvania State University; 2024.
[56] Paramesha M, Rane NL, Rane J. Big data analytics, artificial intelligence, machine learning, internet of things, and blockchain for enhanced business intelligence. *Partners Univers Multidiscip Res J.* 2024;1:110–33.
[57] Miroedova S. *Thesis Study: Analysis of the Implementation of Artificial Intelligence in Warehouses of E-Commerce SMEs Based on Feasibility Study*; 2023. https://www.theseus.fi/handle/10024/812680
[58] Hassija V, Chamola V, Gupta V, et al. A survey on supply chain security: Application areas, security threats, and solution architectures. *IEEE Internet Things J.* 2020;8:6222–46.
[59] Kumar Y, Verma SK, Singh A, et al. *IoT-Enabled Healthcare Systems: Applications, Benefits, and Challenges*. CRC Press; 2024.
[60] Naeem N. Artificial Intelligence based techniques for authenticity of food products in Food fraud. *Int J Electron Crime Investig.* 2024;8.
[61] Fedyk A, Hodson J, Khimich N, et al. Is artificial intelligence improving the audit process? *Rev Account Stud.* 2022;27:938–85.

[62] Soori M, Jough FKG, Dastres R, et al. AI-based decision support systems in industry 4.0, a review. *J Econ Technol.* 2024. https://doi.org/10.1016/j.ject.2024.08.005
[63] Shristi. Class I, Class II. Understanding medical device regulations in India: A guide to regulatory compliance. Legal Service India.com is Copyrighted under the Registrar of Copyright Act (Govt of India) © 2000-2025; ISBN No: 978-81-928510-0-6. https://www.legalserviceindia.com/legal/article-17890-understanding-medical-device-regulations-in-india-a-guide-to-regulatory-compliance.html#google_vignette
[64] Patel V. *Pharmaceutical Science-Quality, Regulations, and Drug Development.* Cipher Publisher; 2024.
[65] Hartikainen M. *Conformity of Medical Device Regulation in Health Technology Company.* Masters Thesis. Metropolia University of Applied Sciences, Metropolia, Finland; 2020. https://urn.fi/URN:NBN:fi:amk-2020052915322
[66] Fearne J. *Establishing a Patient Centred Medical Device Body.* PhD Thesis. University of Malta, Malta; 2024. https://www.um.edu.mt/library/oar/handle/123456789/128817
[67] Umapathi UT, Vijayakumar V, Muthusamy S, et al. Regulatory requirement for medical devices. *Int J Drug Regul Aff.* 2024;12:9–19.
[68] Radhadevi N, Balamuralidhara V, Kumar TMP, et al. Regulatory guidelines for medical devices in India: An overview. *Asian J Pharm.* 2012;6.
[69] Kiran M. Accreditations for biologicals. In *Quality Control and Regulatory Aspects for Biologicals.* CRC Press; 2024. pp. 47–60.
[70] Singh RR, Pallavi K. NABL accreditation—advantages and disadvantages and its process in India. *J Evol Med Dent Sci.* 2023;12:261–7.

19 Social and Economic Aspects of Advanced Manufacturing Processes in Biomedical Sciences

Jashanpreet Singh and Vikas Sharma

CONTENTS

DOI: 10.1201/9781003516064-19

19.1 INTRODUCTION

Advanced manufacturing processes (AMPs) refer to the collection of different techniques and approaches that involve the efficient and optimized production line that is characterized by sophistication, precision, and flexibility in industries [1]. Such techniques in the biomedical field includes additive manufacturing (AM), bioprinting, and automation strategies which are revolutionizing the creation and application of new medical devices and therapies, as well as implants and more [2]. These processes do not only lead to enhancement of the quality of products that are associated with the healthcare system but also facilitates the processes of speed prototyping and also cycling that can enhance the ability of the healthcare system to respond to the needs of the patients.

The importance of these AMPs in biomedical science is immense. These processes help to develop highly specific therapeutic approaches corresponding to the critical client needs, which in turn optimize therapeutic effectiveness [3]. For example, the possibility to manufacture patient-unique instruments increases its compatibility rates and lowers the amount of rejections. Additionally, the role of AMPs is shown in the enhancement of research and development cycles, thereby enhancing the speed of conversion of innovation to practices among clinics. When the focus on molecular medicine is taking shape, the need for AMPs rises significantly higher, as such treatments are aimed at a range of different patients.

19.2 TYPES OF AMPS

19.2.1 Additive Manufacturing (3D Printing)

Additive manufacturing has also transformed the fabrication of prosthetics and implants through the generation of geometry tailored to the specific anatomic detail of the patients [4–6]. The AM works on layer-by-layer technique as shown in **Figure 19.1**. Through it, the integrating technology facilitates production of lightweight but strong and robust products which improve comfort zone and working performance besides shortening surgical duration. Furthermore, for the fabrication of new drug delivery systems that can deliver medicine that is released in predetermined and personalized rate, 3D printing is being applied [7–10]. They can increase the levels of compliance and effectiveness of treatment by providing necessary medication right on time. The role of 3D printing in personalized medicine is discussed in the examples of several successful cases. For example, custom cranial implants have been designed from patient imaging data leading to better surgical results as well as shorter healing times for patients who have suffered traumatic brain injury [5,11,12]. Likewise, 3D printed, bioresorbable scaffolds for tissue engineering have had positive experiences in clinical trials with patients with severe burns or defects [13,14]. These examples demonstrate not only the technical possibility of the technology but also that the potential of AM is not only about the technology itself but also about changing how care is delivered for patients.

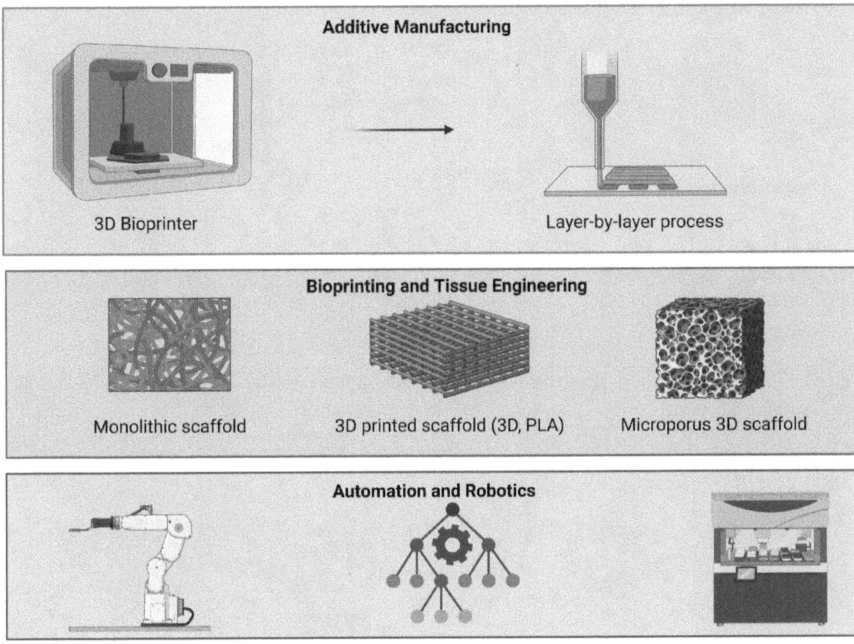

FIGURE 19.1 Various advanced manufacturing processes. (Created in https://BioRender.com)

19.2.2 Bioprinting and Tissue Engineering

Bioprinting is a novel innovation in tissue engineering that helps in layer-upon-layer assembly of living cells that can be used to construct tissues and organs [15–17]. It may be said that this technology has great prospects in the problem of organ deficit and increase in transplant efficiency due to the bioengineered organs not eliciting immune response from the recipient's body. Furthermore, bioprinting enables scientists to construct complicated tissue arrangements and also mimic the original organs of the human body. Bioprinting is on the cusp of reinventing regenerative medicine as being able to build multiple tissue structures required to support the survival and functionality of the cells post transplantation [18,19], as shown in **Figure 19.2**. Greater attention is paid to develop tissue constructs based on bioprinting technologies, which will have a blood supply system required for large tissue constructs viability. The possibility of such tissues can cut short waiting lists for organ transplants while rejecting the dangers otherwise linked to such operations.

19.2.3 Automation and Robotics

The application of automation and robotics in the performance of surgical processes improves on the quality of tools used in surgeries by providing accurate implements for use in operations while at the same time shortening the time required for patients' healing time [20,21]. Robotic surgery is steadily becoming part and parcel of many

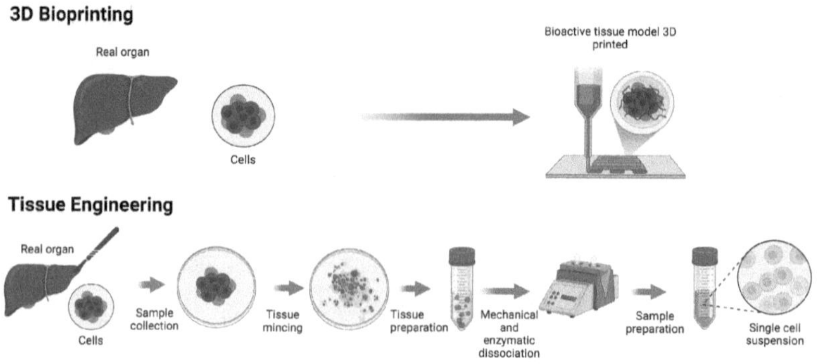

FIGURE 19.2 Schematic diagram for 3D printing and tissue engineering. (Created in https://BioRender.com)

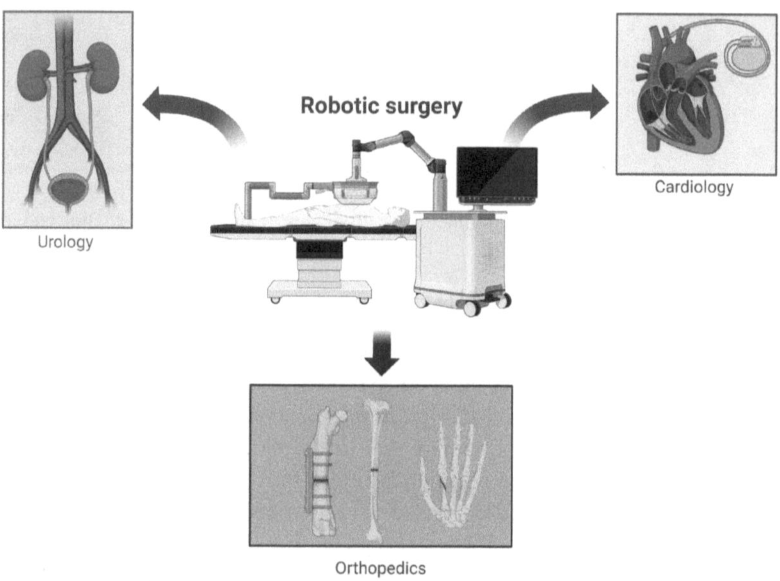

FIGURE 19.3 Schematic diagram for the role of robotics in biomedical science. (Created in https://BioRender.com)

specialties, in orthopedics, urology, and cardiology [22,23], as shown in **Figure 19.3**. These technologies enable a surgeon to manipulate the patient's anatomy in ways that are not possible when using conventional surgery tools. Implementations of robotics in manufacturing workflows allow for faster achievement of goals primarily because they eliminate cases of repeated error common in human operations. Such integration is especially critical in mass production in the biomedical manufacturing industries mainly because precision is critical. In addition, real-time inspection using robots at different production times means that the products will meet regulatory requirements before it is released to the market [24–27].

19.3 SOCIAL ASPECTS OF AMP IN BIOMEDICAL SCIENCES

Social aspects of AMP in biomedical sciences are illustrated in **Figure 19.4**. The detailed discussion is as follows.

19.3.1 Accessibility and Equity

AMPs improve manufacturing costs since they reduce wastages common with conventional manufacturing techniques but allow production to be localized [28,29]. These savings could possibly make existing superior treatment plans within reach for more people across all classes. For instance, 3D printing can be effectively used in areas with restricted access to innovative healthcare products as a result of haulage difficulties [30].

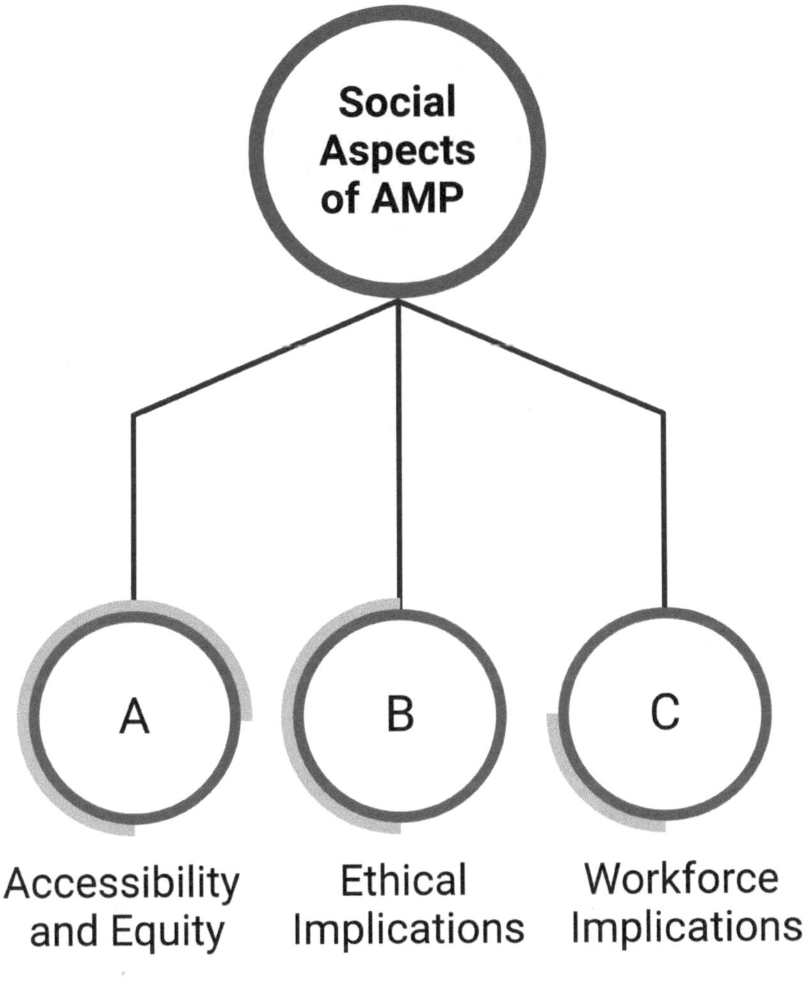

FIGURE 19.4 Social aspects of AMP in biomedical sciences.

As a result, even though developed countries can benefit from AMPs, there are existing regional differences between developed and developing regions for access. Despite this, several developing nations might find it difficult to adopt these technologies after surprisingly fast adoption by already wealthy nations that boast of better improved infrastructural facilities and available funds for technologically related projects. It is important to level the playground to expand appreciations so that it reaches all the population without increasing the gap that is seen in the health sector.

19.3.2 Ethical Implications

It is valuable to address the following ethical concerns regarding the AMPs, which results from the medical uses of bioprinted tissues or genetically modified organisms implemented in the creation of synthetic biology related to tissue engineering [31–33]. They create awareness of the improvements that are required to lessen their negative impacts on human health as well as the impacts of the ecosystem when implemented at a large scale. This means that the utilization of these complex biomaterials in the treatment of diseases entitles the patient to clear information on certain potential dangers and malfunctions of new techniques like bioprinting or genetically modified objects, which emanate from cell-producing organisms [34,35]. As new technologies emerge, existing practices around informed consent must also change to ensure that patients have adequate knowledge of what it is they are consenting to when agreeing to trials or treatments involving these new materials.

19.3.3 Workforce Implications

With increasing automation in the manufacturing processes, issues connected with displacement of workers and changes in demand for skills among the labor force due to robots taking over roles which used to be executed by human beings are other challenges [36,37]. Some workers will end up being locked out of employment chances altogether if they do not possess the education or training needed to effectively transition into the new positions arising from technologization of work. Regarding the evaluation of demands of workforce related to automation trends within the biomedical manufacturing industries that focus on AMPs, educational institutions need to ensure that curricula as well as training programs developed to prepare current workforce to manage new technologies are skills required for management of such changes through delivery systems that are currently in place and those under development globally.

19.4 SOCIAL IMPACT AND ITS OPERATIONAL GUIDELINES/FRAMEWORKS

There is a general agreement that social impacts are significant and should be included in sustainability assessments. However, despite recent progress in this area, there is still a limited understanding of social impact assessment (SIA), particularly concerning its conceptual and theoretical foundations [38]. The definition of "social impact" is not universally agreed upon, which creates challenges in distinguishing social impacts from social changes or broader societal impacts. As a result, some researchers refer to "social impact," while others use "social change" to express similar ideas. Additionally, the term "societal impacts" is often used to describe what essentially social impacts are. The literature presents several varying definitions of social impact, highlighting the complexity of the concept.

19.4.1 Social Impact Operational Guidelines/Frameworks

The United Nations Environment Programme (UNEP) guidelines characterize social impacts as the "outcomes of positive or negative pressures on social endpoints, such as stakeholder well-being" [39–41]. Social impacts are seen as the results of social interactions that occur within the framework of an activity—be it production, consumption, or disposal—and can also emerge from preventive or reinforcing actions taken by stakeholders, such as implementing safety protocols in a facility. Notably, the concept of social impact does not encompass processes of social change. The UNEP Setac Life Cycle Initiative recommends utilizing the social life cycle assessment (S-LCA) methodology to evaluate social impacts across different stages of a product's life cycle [42]. This assessment framework considers five categories of stakeholders: workers/employees, local communities, society at large, consumers (including both end users and other consumers), and actors within the value chain.

19.4.2 Vanclay's Theoretical Framework

Vanclay has laid the theoretical groundwork for social impact assessment (SIA) [43]. He thoroughly examines the challenge of differentiating between social change processes and social impacts. According to Vanclay [44–46], social impacts are "experienced or perceived in both tangible and intangible ways." These impacts can differ significantly depending on the location and the specific project involved, with the importance assigned to each impact varying across different communities and among various groups within a single community. This concept encompasses a wide range of factors that influence individuals directly or indirectly, including their lifestyles, cultural practices, community dynamics, political structures, environmental conditions, health and well-being, personal and property rights, as well as their fears and aspirations.

19.5 SOCIAL IMPACTS OF ADVANCED MANUFACTURING

There is an absence of social impact repositories specifically related to AM technology. This chapter draws upon several categories proposed by Vanclay as a foundational framework [46]. Four categories of social impacts were identified as particularly relevant: (1) health and social well-being, (2) institutional, legal, political, and equity issues, (3) quality of the living environment (livability), and (4) economic and material well-being. Although Vanclay's categories are designed to apply broadly to various topics and do not specifically address AM, these four categories were chosen based on evidence found in the existing AM literature and insights from a recent study. The objective of this research was to identify specific keywords or "pointers" that highlight the social impacts associated with AM technology.

19.5.1 Social Impacts of AM

The data gathered were examined using a color-coding method (refer to Table 19.1) to show the level of agreement among the four respondents about the "direction" of each impact, which was classified as positive, negative, neutral, or mixed. The goal is to demonstrate the relationship between factors identified as "causes" and their resulting outcomes, termed "impacts." The "causes" refer to the distinct features of AM technology that may contribute to understanding the perceived "impact." The subsequent subsections analyze the primary results.

19.5.2 Impacts on Quality of Life

This category encompasses elements like recreational and leisure activities, along with perceptions of the impact of AM on crime and violence. All interviewees expressed that this technology opens up a wide range of leisure activities, emphasizes the do-it-yourself (DIY) approach, and fosters creativity by enabling the creation of objects for cultural expression and educational purposes [48,49]. These insights support other findings identified in the literature review. Furthermore, the ability to utilize AM technology to produce replicas of museum artifacts and create "3D museums" was also mentioned, offering opportunities for social inclusion, particularly for individuals with visual impairments.

19.5.3 Impacts on Institutional and Legal Levels

The interviewees held varying opinions regarding their legal rights. Organizations B and C indicated that they were unaware of any potential impacts, while organizations A and D asserted that there are indeed implications. Organization A argues that the protection of patent rights has a negative effect, as AM allows for the production of multiple copies, which jeopardizes patent security. Conversely, organization D sees this as a positive aspect, highlighting the significance of open-source models where information is freely available to all.

TABLE 19.1
Level of Agreement between Interviewees (Reproduced from Matos et al. [47], under Creative Commons Attribution 4.0)

Colour Code	
Green	All positive (the four respondents agree on a positive impact)
Light Green	Positive + null
Yellow	Positive + negative and/or mixed and/or null (i.e., undefined)
Orange	Negative + null
Red	All negative (the four respondents agree on a negative impact)
Light Gray	All null (the four respondents agree—no impact)

19.5.4 Impacts on Economic and Material Well-Being

The key category, "economic and material well-being," addresses concerns related to disruptions in the local economy, economic growth, community employment rates, and the types of professional status or employment available (as shown in **Table 19.2**). The results reveal that respondents frequently expressed aligned opinions about the impacts within this category, with a largely positive perspective. In fact, more than half of the items are indicated in green (21% + 32%).

19.5.5 Emerging Social Impacts and Factors

Each respondent was asked to identify the most significant social impacts of AM and the factors contributing to them [47]. Several key items emerged from their responses, including customization, which allows individuals to replicate necessary parts or create and print new components as needed. The ease of repair associated with AM also leads to decreased consumerism, encouraging a shift away from purchasing new items. Additionally, the ability to maintain and repair equipment with customized 3D-printed parts may enhance the durability of products, while the adoption of AM technology reduces the necessity for maintaining large inventories. Respondents also highlighted environmental concerns, emphasizing the need to systematically categorize different materials and establish mechanisms for their classification, separation, and recycling. Furthermore, AM technology has notable implications for quality of life, particularly in medical applications where it facilitates the production of prostheses, organs, and dental implants. While there are concerns that AM may lead to job losses among unskilled workers, it can also create opportunities for skilled individuals. The technology can enhance educational processes and learning experiences and can be applied in cultural contexts by rapidly reproducing 3D miniatures for museums and thematic events [50]. So AM technology can promote social inclusion by enabling visually impaired individuals to engage with museums in a more meaningful way.

19.6 ECONOMIC ASPECTS OF AMPS IN BIOMEDICAL SCIENCES

19.6.1 Cost Implications

Figure 19.5 represents a schematic diagram showing the economic aspects of AMPs in biomedical sciences. They make big input to reductions in overall production costs by optimizing material use coupled with efficient workflows where there are huge savings by manufacturers who use these practices than by owners who use the conventional processes that normally create high wastage due to long times required to produce both standard and customized products consistent with the needs of clients/patients. Overall, manufacturing sectors that use advanced manufacturing practices reap from economies of scale whereby the output capacities create more profits for the various sectors that rely on [51]. Long-term benefits which accrue to organizations that have implemented advanced manufacturing technologies include high efficiency and reduced operational costs [52,53]. However, the initial investment needed

TABLE 19.2
Cross Case Analysis (Reproduced from Matos et al. [47], under Creative Commons Attribution 4.0)

	AM Changes	Answers			AM Social Impacts	Answer				
Social Impact Categories	Can AM technology lead to changes in the following factors?	No	Don't know	Yes	What is your perception of the factor effect on:	+ve	–ve	Null	Mixed	Full Assessment (in colors)
Economic and Material Well-being	Adaptation of products' characteristics to the needs/expectations of the community, e.g., making traditional objects/artifacts			ABCD	Disruption with the local economy	ABCD				Green
	Creation/disappearance of small local businesses, e.g., local production models			ABCD		AB			CD	Yellow
	Customization/personalization and creating personalized products			ABCD	Economic prosperity	ABCD				Green
	Reward systems, e.g., compensation by objectives, to guarantee efficiency in production	BCD		A			A	CD		Parrot
	Development of new skills that can be used in new businesses, e.g., digital entrepreneurship			ABCD		ACD			B	Yellow
	Creation/disappearance of jobs, e.g., work at home or new jobs			ABCD	Level of employment in the community				ABCD	Yellow
	Educational curricula, e.g., the teaching of AM technology in technical-vocational education			ABCD	Professional status and employment type	ABCD				Green
	Need to participate in training and professional requalification, e.g., training in new software/hardware			ABCD		ABCD				Green

Function analysis (roles), e.g., new tasks within the product design/production processes	D		ABC	ABC		D		Parrot
Work organization, e.g., changes in workspaces and layouts		C	ABD	ABD				Parrot
More flexible work schedules, e.g., adapting human resource needs to the production cycle	AB		CD	CD		AB		Parrot
Performance assessment system, e.g., introducing management by objectives	BCD		A	A		BCD		Parrot
Responsibility for the tasks performed, e.g., production errors are costly	CD		AB	AB		CD		Parrot
Need of teamwork. Need to join different skills	D		ABC	C		D	AB	Yellow
Need to develop new skills, e.g., the use of the new equipment and software			ABCD	ACD			B	Yellow
New work schemes, e.g., remote work/ work at home	A		BCD	CD		A	B	Yellow
Precarious contracts, e.g., the provision of services and fixed-term contracts based on productive objectives	D		ABC	A		D	BC	Yellow
Turnover, because of the high demand for specialists in AM technology	A		BCD	D		A	BC	Yellow
Resistance to organizational and technological change, e.g., difficulties in implementing new work schemes or changing roles	BCD		A		A	BCD		Orange

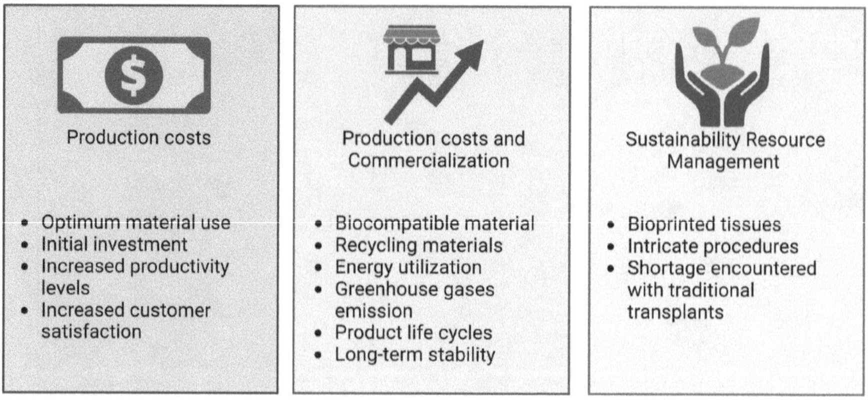

FIGURE 19.5 Economic aspects of AMPs in biomedical sciences.

to procure and maintain necessary equipment/software may be high; organizations, therefore, have to balance the necessary capital outlay against the potential savings in the form of increased productivity levels/increased customer satisfaction due to the ability to meet today's ever-changing demands for customized solutions offered by the marketplace, which is characterized by change-driven.

19.6.2 Market Growth and Commercialization

The commercialization of bioprinted tissues provides fresh market potential as the global demand for organ transplant continues to soar. Companies dedicated to developing a feasible solution addressing shortage encountered with traditional transplant methods stand to gain from growing awareness of the integrity in adopting bioengineered solutions for patients requiring surgeries that entail intricate procedures well known for drawback of mismatched donor/recipient profile and risks associated with the procedure therein [54]. It is therefore profound that startups have critical role advancing innovation within AMP context through introduction of new technologies and business models that disrupt traditional processes in biomedical manufacturing. The flexible organizations seldom restricted norms, such as the big firms adapt venture into new frontiers where breakthroughs can happen, leading change across entire fabrication chain. This can benefit the consumers in the long term and enhance the quality of healthcare worldwide.

19.6.3 Sustainability Resource Management

Finding sustainable raw materials remain difficult in advanced manufacturing processes, especially when demand rises. Biocompatible material is used in medical applications; ensuring there is available environmentally friendly materials is critical to mitigate the negative effects associated with extraction and processing of the conventional materials that leads to depletion of ecosystems and habitats. These ecosystems and habitats are essential for maintaining biodiversity, which also become critical in the long run as the health of the planet is paramount to sustainable efforts required to improve the quality of life of patients [55]. Initiatives in progress within industry are efforts to manage environmental effects of an organization's procedures, such as recycling materials employed in the creation of its products, reducing the amount of energy utilized throughout production processes, the emission of greenhouse gasses in the course of operations, or strategies intended to reduce carbon footprints resulting from all phases of product life cycles which are crucial for guaranteeing the long-term stability of technologies of modern manufacturing.

19.7 CHALLENGES AND FUTURE DIRECTIONS

19.7.1 Regulatory Policy Barriers

While AMPs grow in prominence and momentum, it becomes imperative that regulation catches up to guard against risks that may hinder innovation in the biomedical sector. So a stricter regulatory framework for biomedical devices is required. It is crucial factors in the health sector that understand the regulatory scheme which governs the approval processes as well as the requirements needed for compliance in order to avoid costly delays and setbacks [56,57]. Manufacturers entering into the international markets face problems due to a lack of harmonized global standards. Coordination among regulatory agencies is needed to address problems effectively to guarantee consistency of quality and safety measures worldwide. This simplifies the transition of products across jurisdictions to benefit consumers everywhere who rely on effective, reliable solutions to meet their or others' health care needs.

19.7.2 Constraints, Material Properties, and Scalability

Present-day technological constraints restricting key material properties require constant ongoing research to come up with new material ideal for various biomedical applications [58]; efforts should also be taken to advance the performance attributes of existing material to identify that which is capable of handling the increased pressure being placed on them as they play a crucial role in the advancement of this field and unlock what AMPs offer with regard to transforming the face of global healthcare delivery systems today, characterized by constant change. As such future research endeavors need to be directed at surmounting current technological limitations to discover new uses of sophisticated manufacturing technologies within the biomedical sciences. Interdisciplinary collaboration between engineers, scientists, clinicians is crucial in creating the environment that will lead to the breakthroughs needed to transform the industry and benefit consumers around the world who continue to face a myriad of challenges throughout the continuum of healthcare delivery systems today coping with chronic illnesses and new infectious diseases that demand attention.

19.7.3 Role of Academia, Industry, and Government in Advancing AMPs

The academia, industry stakeholders, and government entities are vital for the advancement of AMPs and the partnerships that facilitate knowledge sharing and funding opportunities, as well as to assess the resources necessary for innovation. Relationships between educational institutions and private sector organizations create an enhanced pipeline of talent for a skilled workforce ready to navigate the complexities that are inherent in the rapid evolution of the landscape and that are characterized by advances in technology that will shape the future delivery of healthcare systems worldwide [28]. International partnerships are crucial in ensuring equitable distribution of advanced manufacturing technologies in different world regions. Collaborative efforts enable addressing disparities and promoting global health equity in the context of fostering environments conducive to sustainable development guiding decisions in all the supply chains involved in the production of medical devices. Therapies intended to enhance the lives of patients face the myriad challenges that encompass chronic illnesses and emergent infectious diseases, which require concerted universal attention as well as knowledge-focused approach to tackle these issues.

19.8 CONCLUSION

AMPs redefine the objectives of biomedical sciences work on the customization ability, enhance the patient's result through evolutionary solutions such as AM, bioprinting automation, robotics, and so on. The economic effect has a direct positive impact on cost, market, and growth and sustains some of the negative effects, and then social results arise concerns related to the access to biomedical sciences and equitable distribution of benefits and risks.

REFERENCES

[1] Kumar K, Zindani D, Davim JP. *Advanced Machining and Manufacturing Processes.* Springer; 2018.

[2] Singh AB, Khandelwal C, Dangayach GS. Revolutionizing healthcare materials: Innovations in processing, advancements, and challenges for enhanced medical device integration and performance. *J Micromanuf.* 2024;25165984241256230.

[3] Yang J, Griffin A, Qiang Z, et al. Organelle-targeted therapies: A comprehensive review on system design for enabling precision oncology. *Signal Transduct Target Ther.* 2022;7:379.

[4] Singh AB. Transforming healthcare: A review of additive manufacturing applications in the healthcare sector. *Eng Proc.* 2024;72:2.

[5] Pathak K, Saikia R, Das A, et al. 3D printing in biomedicine: Advancing personalized care through additive manufacturing. *Explor Med.* 2023;4:1135–67.

[6] Kantaros A, Petrescu FIT, Abdoli H, et al. Additive manufacturing for surgical planning and education: A review. *Appl Sci.* 2024;14:2550.

[7] Jain V, Haider N, Jain K. 3D printing in personalized drug delivery. *Curr Pharm Des.* 2018;24:5062–71.

[8] Singh R, Toseef M, Kumar J, et al. Benefits and challenges in additive manufacturing and its applications. In: Kaushal S, Singh I, Singh S, et al., editors. *Sustainable Advanced Manufacturing and Materials Processing* [Internet]. 1st ed. Boca Raton: CRC Press; 2022. pp. 137–57. Available from: www.taylorfrancis.com/books/9781003269298/chapters/10.1201/9781003269298-8.

[9] Singh J. Sustainability issues in laser-based additive manufacturing. In *Handbook of Laser-Based Sustainable Surface Modification and Manufacturing Techniques*. CRC Press; 2023. pp. 167–89.
[10] Ahmad S, Hashmi AW, Singh J, et al. Innovations in additive manufacturing of shape memory alloys: Alloys, microstructures, treatments, applications. *J Mater Res Technol*. 2024;32:4136–97.
[11] Jegadeesan JT, Baldia M, Basu B. Next-generation personalized cranioplasty treatment. *Acta Biomater*. 2022;154:63–82.
[12] Yan Q, Dong H, Su J, et al. A review of 3D printing technology for medical applications. *Engineering*. 2018;4:729–42.
[13] Sharma V, Singh JP, Hussan K, et al. Machine learning approach for predicting the machining characteristics of additive manufactured ABS material. *Proc Inst Mech Eng Part C J Mech Eng Sci*. 2024;09544062241283330.
[14] Singh JIP, Sharma V, Singh S, et al. Impact of molding temperature, fiber loading and chemical modifications on the physicomechanical, and microstructural morphology properties of woven kenaf Fiber/PLA composites for non-structural applications. *J Nat Fibers*. 2024;21:2326586.
[15] Aljohani W, Ullah MW, Zhang X, et al. Bioprinting and its applications in tissue engineering and regenerative medicine. *Int J Biol Macromol*. 2018;107:261–75.
[16] Murphy SV, Atala A. 3D bioprinting of tissues and organs. *Nat Biotechnol*. 2014;32:773–85.
[17] Mandrycky C, Wang Z, Kim K, et al. 3D bioprinting for engineering complex tissues. *Biotechnol Adv*. 2016;34:422–34.
[18] Bouten CVC, Cheng C, Vermue IM, et al. Cardiovascular tissue engineering and regeneration: A plead for further knowledge convergence. *Tissue Eng Part A*. 2022;28:525–41.
[19] Yadav M, Kumar A, Verma GC. Artificial tissues and organs: Revolutionizing and pioneering the future of medicine and healthcare. In *Additive Manufacturing Biomedical Applications: Recent Trends and Challenges*. Springer; 2024. pp. 105–60.
[20] Bann S, Khan M, Hernandez J, et al. Robotics in surgery. *J Am Coll Surg*. 2003;196:784–95.
[21] Ashrafian H, Clancy O, Grover V, et al. The evolution of robotic surgery: Surgical and anaesthetic aspects. *BJA Br J Anaesth*. 2017;119:i72–i84.
[22] Diana M, Marescaux JJBJ. Robotic surgery. *J Br Surg*. 2015;102:e15–e28.
[23] Reddy K, Gharde P, Tayade H, et al. Advancements in robotic surgery: A comprehensive overview of current utilizations and upcoming frontiers. *Cureus*. 2023;15.
[24] Javaid M, Haleem A, Singh RP, et al. Substantial capabilities of robotics in enhancing industry 4.0 implementation. *Cogn Robot*. 2021;1:58–75.
[25] Bi ZM, Luo C, Miao Z, et al. Safety assurance mechanisms of collaborative robotic systems in manufacturing. *Robot Comput Integr Manuf*. 2021;67:102022.
[26] Liberty JT, Habanabakize E, Adamu PI, et al. Advancing food manufacturing: Leveraging robotic solutions for enhanced quality assurance and traceability across global supply networks. *Trends Food Sci Technol*. 2024;104705.
[27] Borangiu T, Gilbert P, Ivanescu N-A, et al. An implementing framework for holonic manufacturing control with multiple robot-vision stations. *Eng Appl Artif Intell*. 2009;22:505–21.
[28] Ford SLN. Additive manufacturing technology: Potential implications for US manufacturing competitiveness. *J Int'l Com Econ*. 2014;6:40.
[29] Liker JK, Morgan JM. The Toyota way in services: The case of lean product development. *Acad Manag Perspect*. 2006;20:5–20.
[30] Chohan JS, Mittal N, Kumar R, et al. Mechanical strength enhancement of 3D printed acrylonitrile butadiene styrene polymer components using neural network optimization algorithm. *Polymers*. 2020;12(10):2250.

[31] Tripathi S, Dash M, Chakraborty R, et al. Engineering considerations in the design of tissue specific bioink for 3D bioprinting applications. *Biomater Sci.* 2025;13:93–129.
[32] Koutava D. *Printing Life on Demand.* Master Thesis. Tilburg University, Netherlands; 2023. https://arno.uvt.nl/show.cgi?fid=162390
[33] Pushparaj K, Balasubramanian B, Pappuswamy M, et al. Out of box thinking to tangible science: A benchmark history of 3D bio-printing in regenerative medicine and tissues engineering. *Life.* 2023;13:954.
[34] Razavi ZF, Farokhi S, Mahmoudvand G, et al. Stem cells and bio scaffolds for the treatment of cardiovascular diseases: New insights. *Front Cell Dev Biol.* 2024;12:1472103.
[35] Sittadjody S, Criswell T, Jackson JD, et al. Regenerative medicine approaches in bioengineering female reproductive tissues. *Reprod Sci.* 2021;28:1573–95.
[36] Acemoglu D, Restrepo P. Automation and new tasks: How technology displaces and reinstates labor. *J Econ Perspect.* 2019;33:3–30.
[37] West DM. *The Future of Work: Robots, AI, and Automation.* Brookings Institution Press; 2018.
[38] Howitt R. Theoretical foundations. In *New Dir Soc Impact Assess.* Edward Elgar Publishing; 2011.
[39] Di Cesare S, Silveri F, Sala S, et al. Positive impacts in social life cycle assessment: State of the art and the way forward. *Int J Life Cycle Assess.* 2018;23:406–21.
[40] Falcone PM, González García S, Imbert E, et al. Transitioning towards the bio-economy: Assessing the social dimension through a stakeholder lens. *Corp Soc Responsib Environ Manag.* 2019;26:1135–53.
[41] Benoît-Norris C, Vickery-Niederman G, Valdivia S, et al. Introducing the UNEP/SETAC methodological sheets for subcategories of social LCA. *Int J Life Cycle Assess.* 2011;16:682–90.
[42] Hannouf MB, Padilla-Rivera A, Assefa G, et al. Social life cycle assessment (S-LCA) of technology systems at different stages of development. *Int J Life Cycle Assess.* 2024;1–16.
[43] Vanclay F. SIA principles. *Impact Assess Proj Apprais.* 2003;21:5–11.
[44] Becker HA, Vanclay F. *The International Handbook of Social Impact Assessment: Conceptual and Methodological Advances.* Edward Elgar Publishing; 2003.
[45] Vanclay F, Esteves AM. *New Directions in Social Impact Assessment: Conceptual and Methodological Advances.* Edward Elgar Publishing; 2011.
[46] Vanclay F. International principles for social impact assessment. *Impact Assess Proj Apprais.* 2003;21:5–12.
[47] Matos F, Godina R, Jacinto C, et al. Additive manufacturing: Exploring the social changes and impacts. *Sustainability.* 2019;11:3757.
[48] Fauchart E, Bacache-Beauvallet M, Bourreau M, et al. Do-it-yourself or do-it-together: How digital technologies affect creating alone or with others? *Technovation.* 2022;112:102412.
[49] Tanenbaum TJ, Williams AM, Desjardins A, et al. Democratizing technology: Pleasure, utility and expressiveness in DIY and maker practice. In *Proceedings of the SIGCHI Conference on Human Factors in Computing Systems.* ACM Digital Library, New York; 2013. pp. 2603–12.
[50] Li J, Zheng X, Watanabe I, et al. A systematic review of digital transformation technologies in museum exhibition. *Comput Human Behav.* 2024;108407.
[51] Naudé W, Szirmai A. *The Importance of Manufacturing in Economic Development: Past, Present and Future Perspectives*; 2012. https://unu-merit.nl/publications/wppdf/2012/wp2012-041.pdf
[52] Cook JS, Cook LL. Achieving competitive advantages of advanced manufacturing technology. *Benchmarking Qual Manag Technol.* 1994;1:42–63.

[53] Zammuto RF, O'Connor EJ. Gaining advanced manufacturing technologies' benefits: The roles of organization design and culture. *Acad Manag Rev.* 1992;17:701–28.
[54] Akhtar Z Bin, Gupta A Das. Advancements within molecular engineering for regenerative medicine and biomedical applications an investigation analysis towards a computing retrospective. *J Electron Electromed Eng Med Informatics.* 2024;6:54–72.
[55] Tracy AA, Bhatia SK, Ramadurai KW. *Bio-Based Materials as Applicable, Accessible, and Affordable Healthcare Solutions.* Springer; 2018.
[56] Mackey TK, Kuo T-T, Gummadi B, et al. 'Fit-for-purpose?'–challenges and opportunities for applications of blockchain technology in the future of healthcare. *BMC Med.* 2019;17:1–17.
[57] Disease WHON, Cluster MH. *Innovative Care for Chronic Conditions: Building Blocks for Action: Global Report.* World Health Organization; 2002.
[58] Holzapfel BM, Reichert JC, Schantz J-T, et al. How smart do biomaterials need to be? A translational science and clinical point of view. *Adv Drug Deliv Rev.* 2013;65:581–603.

20 Pioneering Biomedical Manufacturing

A Glimpse into Future Trends and Obstacles

Ruchira Srivastava, Ayushi Thakur, and Sunil Verma

CONTENTS

DOI: 10.1201/9781003516064-20

20.1 INTRODUCTION

Manufacturing a variety of medications, biologics, and medical devices for use in healthcare is referred to as biomedical manufacturing. Products that detect, cure, or prevent illnesses and medical disorders are designed, developed, manufactured, and distributed in this industry [1]. Biomedical manufacturing encompasses various disciplines, including engineering, biology, chemistry, and materials science, to create innovative solutions that improve patient care and advance medical science [2]. There is no one accepted definition for biomedical manufacturing. The definition of biomedical manufacturing as the production process is excessively limited of medical gadgets, which makes up only a tiny percentage of the healthcare sector. Biomedical manufacturing must be defined broadly enough to include both present and upcoming healthcare manufacturing research [3]. Biomedical implants are being manufactured more quickly because of a rapidly evolving technology called additive manufacturing (AM). Owing to its customized design, faster manufacture, and lower cost, it presents a large and promising opportunity for the bio-mimicry of necessary complex biological implant properties. Biomedical implants made of metal alloys (AM) have drawn the interest of several medical professionals due to their superior corrosion resistance, enhanced fatigue strength, and ability to be patient-specific, resulting in a quicker recovery compared to amputation [4]. It takes a deep and complete understanding of the method and material to manufacture such biomedical components with comprehensively enhanced qualities interdependent to microstructure, mechanical property, and design constraints using the AM process. The previously mentioned specifics and concerns with AM of magnesium components are highlighted in the current review study [5]. The special qualities of magnesium-based biomaterials—their mechanical strength being comparable to that of bone, their capacity to regulate deterioration, and their bio-absorbable and bio-resorbable properties—make them an obvious choice for the creation of biomedical implants [6]. The research also describes the existing barriers and difficulties that prevent the medical sciences from fully using the benefits presented by advanced manufacturing. These include challenges with manufacturing capacity, post-processing, product quality, range of materials, standards compliance, and maintenance [7]. Among the industries using additive manufacturing technology rapidly are healthcare, aerospace, biomedical, manufacturing, and construction. One example of the technical advancements brought about by the industrial period is the creation of

3D printers. It has been a regular occurrence for a considerable amount of time. The healthcare sector has been using this incredible production technique more and more as time has gone on. The evolution of personalized implants and prostheses, organ printing, tissue engineering, surgery, medicines, and disease modeling have all been studied in contrast to more traditional methods in the field of 3D printing [8]. The work provides a route toward their development by applying strategies for manufacturing optimization, process–structure–property relationships that control performance and alloy composition design in addition with computer-aided structural design tools [9]. AM methods are frequently used to produce components with intricate geometric designs, sometimes to the breaking point. The AM approaches are not yet able to claim their rightful place in biological and medical applications due to several limitations [10].

20.2 GENERAL CHARACTERISTICS OF BIOMEDICAL MANUFACTURING

Biomedical-grade alloy compositions have been developed with great success and are widely accessible; yet these materials still have several drawbacks. This suggests that to develop new, optimized, biocompatible compositions with improved capabilities that are appropriate as candidate materials for biomedical devices, more thorough study is required. This book's primary goal is to discuss biomedical device production issues from both a materials and manufacturing standpoint. The intended features, categorization, and processes for obtaining regulatory authority clearance for these biomedical devices are reviewed in the chapter [11].

The impact of process parameters and AM technique type on surface topography, geometric characteristics, mechanical properties, biocompatibility, and in vitro and in vivo performance of various orthopedic applications is reviewed in this chapter. There have been attempts to point out gaps, offer concepts for new advancements, and highlight the need for standards [12]. **Table 20.1** represents a comparison on the hospital and factory manufacturing utilization. The goal of this comprehensive view of biomedical production is to apply science of manufacturing and engineering to medical treatment and scientific research. The hospital bed is like a fixture, the doctor is like an operator, the surgical equipment is like a machine tool, and so on in the hospital–factory comparison. The tissue/object/patient is similar to a workpiece [13]. This comparison suggests that a wide range of industrial methods and ideas are easily transferable to biological and healthcare settings. Adding value to the manufacturing process is one justification for using a wide elaboration of biomedical manufacturing [14].

Biomedical manufacturing encompasses the production or manufacturing of medical devices, equipment, diagnostics, and pharmaceuticals. The characteristics and needs of this field are shaped by the unique requirements and regulations governing healthcare products. Here are some key characteristics and needs.

20.2.1 Quality Commitment

Biomedical manufacturing requires strict adherence to quality guidelines to guarantee the effectiveness and safety of medical goods. Compliance with regulations such as good manufacturing practices (GMP) is essential to meet quality requirements

TABLE 20.1
Biomedical Manufacturing—Comparison of Hospital and Factory Manufacturing Utilization

S. No.	Medical Prerequisites	Manufacturing Parts and Process
1.	Tissue thermal damage	Workpiece thermal damage
2.	Patient cycle time	Part-to-part cycle time
3.	Hospital	Factory
4.	Patient rooms	Inventory area
5.	Tissue/patient	Workpiece
6.	Doctor	Operator
7.	Waiting room	Loading dock
8.	Surgical instrument	Machine tool
9.	Diagnosis machines	Inspection machines
10.	Sterilization	Cleanliness
11.	Bed	Fixture
12.	Bracelets	In-process tags
13.	Patient scheduling	Production scheduling
14.	Stretcher	Pallet
15.	Preclinical trials	Prototyping

[15]. Medical device manufacturers must carefully follow quality assurance (QA) procedures throughout the production process since they are subject to stringent regulatory frameworks. Even if they are effective, traditional quality assurance (QA) methods can demand significant time and resource commitments, which can lead to difficulties and increased costs [16]. The advent of artificial intelligence (AI) in recent times has brought about a total revolution in quality assurance (QA) techniques across several industries, offering unmatched opportunities for enhanced efficiency, accuracy, and expandability [17]. The strict requirements on the quality level and its replication for medical appliances necessitate the observation of certain features during the establishment of quality systems. A manufacturer must ensure that all hazards associated with using medical devices are eliminated or reduced, primarily through proper design, material selection, and manufacturing processes [18].

20.2.2 Regulatory Adherence

The industry is heavily regulated by agencies such as the FDA (United States), EMA (Europe), and similar bodies worldwide. Companies must navigate complex regulatory frameworks to gain approval for their products [19]. The emergence of new technologies like genomics integration, quantum computing, and AI-driven diagnostics opens up a world of potential and challenges for us as we look to the future. The environment of BioMEMS security must change in parallel, embracing ethical concerns, regulatory compliance, and collaborative initiatives to address emerging threats [20]. Given the changing political and regulatory landscape in the

United States and the public interest in exposing and discouraging dubious research practices, a shared understanding of scientific integrity is crucial and should guide research conduct and reporting as well as regulatory and clinical decision-making. Here, we go over these ideas within the context of biomedical research and point out areas that need more attention [21].

20.2.3 Research and Development (R&D)

Continuous innovation is crucial to developing new medical technologies and improving existing ones. Biomedical manufacturing companies invest heavily in research and development to stay competitive and address unmet medical needs [22]. To define biomedical manufacturing widely and inclusively, the hospital as a factory comparison is investigated. The features and technical requirements of biomedical production are examined. Examples of the wide range of biomedical manufacturing are given, such as the laparoscopic surgery on reducing the heat injury to nerve tissue during surgery and the grinding and cutting of plaque in interventional cardiology [23].

20.2.4 Equipment and Facilities with Specialization

Manufacturing facilities for biomedical products often require specialized equipment and cleanroom environments to maintain sterility and prevent contamination [24]. Multinational corporations' site strategy reorganizes the district's structure and alters its evolutionary pattern. MNCs operate as catalysts, bringing in new capital, concepts, and management techniques as well as opening the district up to outside markets and global technology flows. The Italian Biomedical Valley is a relatively new high-tech area that makes sense in this context [25].

20.2.5 Supply Chain Management (SCM)

Biomedical manufacturing depends on a convoluted international supply network to get basic ingredients, components, and specialized equipment. Effective supply chain management is essential to ensure the availability of high-quality inputs [26]. The manufacturing of medical supplies and their transfer to a distribution center marks the start of the healthcare supply chain. Depending on the product, hospitals can buy products straight from the manufacturer or distributor; alternatively, they can use a group purchasing organization to negotiate a purchase arrangement with the manufacturer on their behalf [27].

20.2.6 Risk Management

Given the critical nature of healthcare products, risk management is a top priority. Companies must identify and mitigate risks throughout the manufacturing process to prevent product defects and ensure patient safety [28]. At the Flinders Medical Centre (FMC), a strategy for prioritizing equipment for replacement has been successfully tested. Device managers throughout FMC have access to software created by Flinders Biomedical Engineering (www.fbe.org.au), which allows them to enter readily established factors related to the probability of a device problem arising and the impact of the problem [29].

20.2.7 Skilled and Trained Workforce

A competent workforce with knowledge of fields including engineering, biochemistry, microbiology, and regulatory affairs is needed for biomedical production. Training and retaining qualified personnel are essential for success in the industry [30]. The manufacturing of vaccines is a labor-intensive, intricate, costly, and highly technical process that necessitates close coordination and cooperation between numerous businesses with various inputs, including glass, active pharmaceutical ingredients, and specializations, as well as supply chains spanning numerous nations. The COVID-19 pandemic showed that there can be frightening and disastrous consequences from disregarding the necessity for a worldwide effort in vaccine production and delivery, particularly when a strong healthcare ecosystem is required to ensure everyone's safety [31].

20.2.8 Traceability, Recognition, and Documentation

Comprehensive documentation and traceability systems are necessary to track materials, components, and processes throughout the manufacturing life cycle. This facilitates compliance with regulatory requirements and enables effective recall management if issues arise [32]. The internal and external viewpoints of traceability are frequently discussed in the literature, as seen in **Figure 20.1**. Internal traceability in this context refers to a product's record-keeping inside a single production process. External traceability, often known as chain traceability, describes the flow between several "traceability partners" of a product. For complete supply chain traceability, both internal and external traceability are required [33].

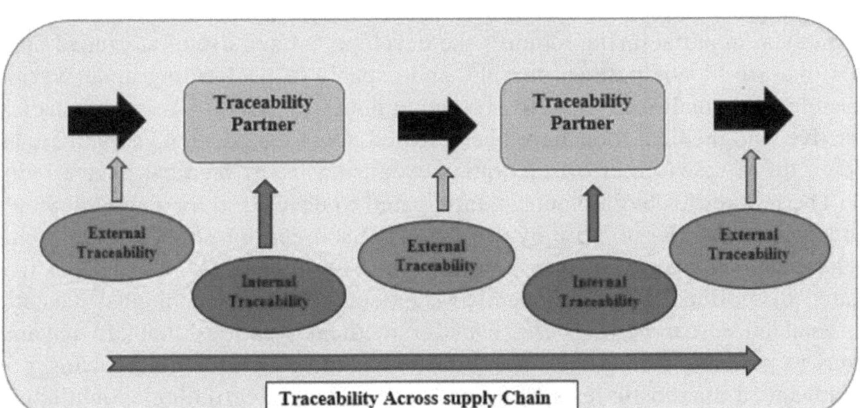

FIGURE 20.1 Illustration of traceability in supply chain.

20.2.9 Continuous and Regular Improvement

Biomedical manufacturing companies must embrace a culture of continuous improvement to optimize processes, reduce costs, and enhance product quality. This involves regularly assessing and refining manufacturing practices [34].

20.2.10 Ethical Considerations

Companies must prioritize ethical principles in their research, development, and manufacturing activities [35]. Ethical issues associated with this topic have been addressed in light of the use and promise of cutting-edge nanoscience techniques in nanomedicine, including targeted medication delivery, tissue engineering, and nano surgery. These ethical issues include research into human embryonic stem cells; treatment using somatic cells as opposed to germ line cells; risk assessment in general; the toxicity, self-assembly, and uncontrollable activity of nanoparticles and nano systems; and the improvement of human capacities [36].

20.3 NEED FOR ENGINEERING IN BIOMEDICAL PRODUCTION

Biomedical manufacturing is an emerging research area that has seen quick expansion within the previous ten years. Biomedical manufacturing is heavily reliant on ethical issues, including patient privacy, informed permission, and responsible use of developing technology (such as gene editing). For the manufacturing community, biomedical manufacturing is an emerging field of study that has grown rapidly in the last ten years. This development trajectory is accompanied by an expanding range of applications for biomedical manufacturing technologies, such as improvements in healthcare service and research speed, cost, quality, safety, and efficiency [37]. Some key points on the engineering needs in biomedical manufacturing are discussed here.

20.3.1 Advanced and Trending Materials

Biomedical manufacturing requires the development and use of advanced materials that are biocompatible, durable, and capable of performing under various physiological conditions [38]. To prolong human life, a wide variety of surgical, assistive, and medical tools have been created. Over the past ten years, there has been a lot of research effort and quick expansion in the medical device industry. The market for bioimplants is anticipated to develop at a compound annual growth rate (CAGR) of 8.6% by 2023. Recent sources state that the bioimplant sector has a valuation of over $100 billion. The integration of concepts from related disciplines including chemistry, bioengineering, and biopharmaceutics has enabled researchers to create better medical solutions that are advantageous to patients. The global medical device market is seeing a growing need for advanced diagnostic tests along with ortho, dental, cardiologic, ophthalmic, and IVD equipment because of things like an elderly population, accidents, and sports-related injuries [39].

20.3.2 Precision Engineering

The manufacturing processes in this field need to be extremely precise due to the small scale of many biomedical devices and the high standards for reliability and safety [40]. The ability to construct complex structures at will is made possible by engineering through multilayered, "top-down" techniques that are reinventing manufacturing processes at several scale levels with atomic accuracy in the age of multidimensional digital printing technology. This calls into question the current understanding of traditional machining methods for non-conventional materials (such as smart-stimuli responsive materials), which present obstacles to bridging the manufacturing process gap with the growing need for quick assembly processes, miniaturized products, and affordable goods anticipated for emerging industries that will supply cutting-edge goods to an expanding number of end users [41].

20.3.3 Quality Control (QC)

Comprehensive quality control procedures are necessary to guarantee the security and effectiveness of biological products. This includes robust testing procedures and adherence to regulatory standards [42]. The present state and technological requirements in process monitoring and control and risk analysis are discussed after an introduction to systems integration, continuous production, and control systems. The following are some important points to remember which are also depicted in **Figure 20.2**. (a) Continuous manufacturing should aim to fulfill all critical quality characteristics (CQAs), not to maintain constant values for all variables; (b) The way a continuous manufacturing process is designed to start and stop can have a big impact on how profitable it is; (c) Residence time distributions can be used to handle the critical issue of material traceability as it moves through the production facility, at least in part; and (d) In the face of dynamics, nonlinearities, uncertainties, disturbances, and restrictions, control systems technologies must guarantee quality [43].

20.3.4 Automation

With the increasing complexity of biomedical products, there is a growing need for automation in manufacturing processes to improve efficiency, accuracy, and scalability. Despite being at the vanguard of scientific research, technical innovation, and clinical translation, the large-scale manufacturing and repeatability of regenerative medicine products are hindered by concerns related to automation, standardization, and monitoring [44]. To overcome these constraints, extensive research is being conducted on new technologies at the hardware (such as automated liquid handling, automated colony-forming unit counting, automated cell expansion bioreactor systems and characterization units, and scalable cell culture plates) and software (such as algorithms and artificial intelligence models mixed with image software and machine learning approaches) levels. Automation, monitoring, and standardization should be included early in the development cycle of cell products to save healthcare costs, improve services and patient care, and bring more comprehensive and effective treatments and treatment processing ideas to the bedside [45].

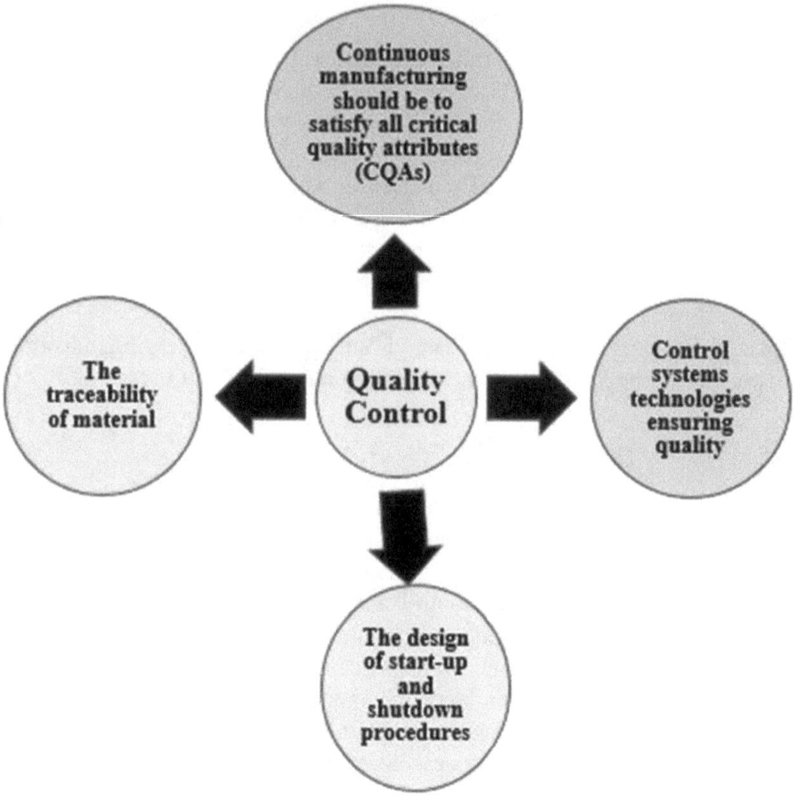
Continuous manufacturing should be to satisfy all critical quality attributes (CQAs)
The traceability of material
Quality Control
Control systems technologies ensuring quality
The design of start-up and shutdown procedures

FIGURE 20.2 Key factors to ensure quality control.

20.3.5 Sustainability

Making biomedical manufacturing processes more sustainable is becoming more and more important. This includes using eco-friendly materials and energy-saving techniques. When studying matter at the nanoscale level, where cooperative behaviors among atomic and molecule assemblies are most effective, nanoscience is a potent tool. Through applications in industries including environmental and materials science, pharmacy, and medicine, its integration into technology is anticipated to bring about novel approaches to enhancing our quality of life. Considering the advancements made in these fields, it's not too soon to consider producing goods based on nanotechnology on a broad scale. However, the effects of a large-scale growth of nanomanufacturing processes have not yet received enough consideration, particularly concerning the effects on the environment [46].

20.3.6 Interdisciplinary Collaboration

Mechanical, electrical, and chemical engineering are just a few of the technical disciplines that are frequently integrated into biomedical manufacturing. This requires effective collaboration and communication among different teams [47]. Nursing innovation and practice are enhanced by interdisciplinary nursing and engineering interactions. These partnerships are still new and in their infancy, nevertheless. In the future, nurses ought to play a bigger role in the demand analysis and design phases of problem-solving in the healthcare industry [48].

20.3.7 Innovation

As the field of biomedical science keeps changing, there is a constant need for innovative engineering solutions to meet new challenges and opportunities. The process of additive manufacturing offers a versatile and economical way to print intricate body components, promote tissue development, and offer individualized fixes for a variety of issues. In areas like tissue engineering, temporal bone dissection, implant design, surgical planning, and medicine distribution, additive manufacturing is essential [49].

These are just some of the many engineering needs in biomedical manufacturing. The specific needs can vary greatly depending on the particular product or application.

20.4 CHALLENGES OF BIOMEDICAL MANUFACTURING

In the realm of biomedical manufacturing, several trends and challenges are likely to shape the industry's trajectory in the future.

20.4.1 Personalized Medicine

The demand for personalized medical treatments tailored to individual patient's genetic makeup and specific needs is expected to increase. Biomedical manufacturing will need to adapt to produce customized medical devices, pharmaceuticals, and therapies efficiently. Tissue engineering, transgenesis, and rapid prototyping have brought about the emergence of spatially complex tissues [50]. A single build that combines a mechanically stable design, a synergistic multicellular organization, and a nutrition delivery mechanism would be the perfect artificial organ. Multi-nozzle rapid prototyping technology, which concurrently and reliably assembles vascular systems, including hierarchical multicellular formations, using automation, makes successful treatment of organ failures conceivable [51].

20.4.2 Cutting-Edge Technologies (Advanced Manufacturing)

Technologies such as 3D printing, nanotechnology, and robotics are revolutionizing biomedical manufacturing processes. These advancements offer the potential for greater precision, customization, and cost-effectiveness in producing medical devices and pharmaceuticals [52]. Improved characterization techniques and testing facilities have contributed to the manufacturing aspects improvement. The industry and consumers place the utmost importance on product quality, particularly when it comes to biomedical devices. The biomedical sector not only preserved and improved the quality of the existing gadgets but also acquired new technologies by using an interdisciplinary strategy. For instance, the technology used to create electrical devices is also employed to create microfluidic devices. Similar technologies are employed in the development of personalized biomedical equipment, such as 3D printing and vapor deposition procedures [53].

20.4.3 Biopharmaceuticals and Biologics

Biopharmaceuticals and biologics, such as gene therapies, cell-based therapies, and monoclonal antibodies, are becoming more and more important. Biomedical manufacturing must address the complexities of producing these advanced therapies at scale while ensuring safety, efficacy, and regulatory compliance [54]. Novel ideas for producing biologics have emerged as a consequence of recent advancements. The industrial transfer of chemical engineering tools, such as process modeling and comprehension, miniaturization/scaled-down equipment for quick process development, advanced process control, creative analytics, mass transfer enhancement, and process integration, is prepared for the adoption of process intensification methods to biologics [55].

20.4.4 Digitalization and Data Integration

Supply chain management, quality assurance, and production efficiency may all be improved by using digital technology and data analytics into biomedical manufacturing operations. However, this integration also brings challenges related to data security, interoperability, and regulatory compliance [56]. Emerging digital technologies with enormous promise to solve global issues and advance development include artificial intelligence, biotechnology, the Internet of Things, data analytics, and digital transformation. Artificial intelligence and machine learning algorithms have the potential to improve resource management, healthcare, education, and transportation through the analysis of vast amounts of data [57].

20.4.5 Sustainability and Green Manufacturing

There is increasing pressure to adopt environmentally sustainable practices in biomedical manufacturing to reduce waste, energy consumption, and environmental impact. This includes exploring eco-friendly materials, optimizing resource utilization, and implementing green manufacturing processes [58]. Global pollution has risen as a result of population growth and greater use of fossil fuels. Large metropolitan centers are home to alarmingly high levels of pollution, which is generally accepted to be the primary cause of chronic and fatal illnesses that annually harm millions of people. The impacts of pollution and its influence on human health are undeniable and widely apparent, even though the relationship between environmental pollution and global warming is questionable [59].

20.4.6 Regulatory Compliance and Quality Assurance

Biomedical manufacturing is subject to strict and complex regulatory requirements to ensure product safety, efficacy, and quality. Keeping pace with evolving regulatory standards and navigating complex global regulatory landscapes pose significant challenges for manufacturers [60].

20.4.7 Supply Chain Resilience and Security

The production of biomedical devices depends on intricate worldwide supply networks for components and raw materials and equipment. Ensuring supply chain resilience, mitigating risks such as disruptions and shortages, and addressing issues of counterfeit and substandard products are critical concerns [61].

20.4.8 Workforce Skills and Training

The evolving nature of biomedical manufacturing requires a highly skilled workforce proficient in advanced technologies, data analytics, regulatory compliance, and quality assurance. Continuous training and professional development initiatives will be essential to meet workforce demands [62].

Addressing these trends and challenges in biomedical manufacturing will require collaboration among industry stakeholders, regulatory agencies, academic institutions, and research organizations to drive innovation, ensure product quality and safety, and ultimately improve patient outcomes.

20.5 EXPLORING THE IMPACT OF ADDITIVE MANUFACTURING ON BIOMEDICAL PRODUCTION

Biomedical production has undergone a transformation thanks to additive manufacturing, commonly related to as 3D printing [63]. It has created new opportunities and is essential to the development of medical technology. **Figure 20.3** shows some important fields where additive manufacturing has a big influence.

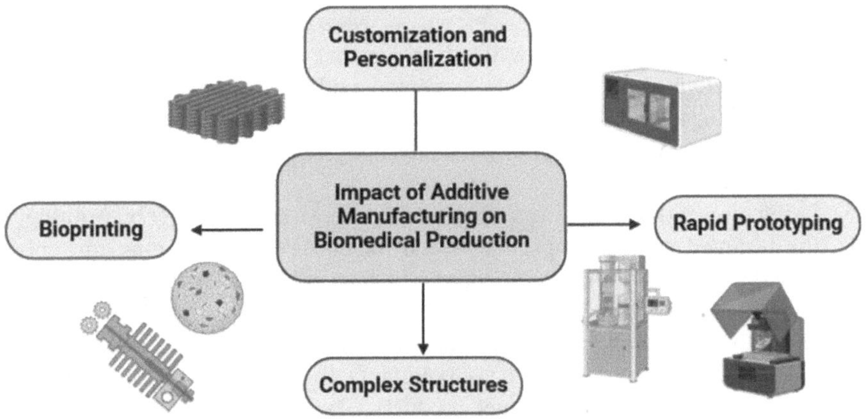

FIGURE 20.3 Impact of additive manufacturing on biomedical production.

- One of the most significant advantages of additive manufacturing is the ability to create customized medical devices. Traditional manufacturing methods often produce standard-sized items, which may not fit every patient perfectly [64]. With additive manufacturing, medical devices such as prosthetics, dental implants, and orthopedic implants can be tailored to the specific needs and anatomy of each patient.
- Complex structures that are hard or impossible to fabricate with conventional manufacturing techniques may now be created, thanks to additive manufacturing. When creating porous scaffolds for tissue engineering, where the scaffold needs to replicate the intricate microstructure of actual tissue, this capacity is very helpful [65].
- Rapid prototyping is made possible by additive manufacturing and is essential for the creation of novel medical equipment. Designers are able to rapidly develop a prototype, test it, make the required adjustments, and then manufacture the finished product [66]. This leads to a significant reduction in the time and cost associated with product development.
- One of the most intriguing applications of additive manufacturing in the field of biomedical manufacturing is bioprinting. This entails creating live tissue for transplantation, such as skin, bone, and cartilage, using 3D printing technology [67].

20.6 3D BIOPRINTING OF THE AIR–LIQUID INTERFACE (ALI) FOR THE ASSESSMENT OF NANOTOXICITY

An innovative method in environmental and biomedical research is the use of 3D bioprinting to produce an artificial material for the air–liquid interface (ALI) for the nanotoxicity evaluation of particulate matter [68], as shown in **Figure 20.4**. Researchers can get a better understanding of the possible health impacts of airborne contaminants and nanoparticles by modeling the interface between lung epithelial cells and inhaled particulate matter. Here's how the process might work.

- Researchers would design a 3D structure that mimics the airway epithelium, where lung cells are in direct contact with air on one side and a liquid medium (usually culture media or a physiological fluid) on the other. This design is crucial for replicating the physiological conditions of the respiratory system [69].
- Using bioprinting techniques, such as extrusion-based or inkjet bioprinting, the designed structure is printed layer by layer. Bio-ink containing lung epithelial cells and supporting materials (such as hydrogels or scaffold materials) is deposited with high precision to create the ALI model [70].
- Once the ALI model is fabricated, it can be exposed to particulate matter samples of interest, such as pollutants from industrial emissions or nanoparticles used in consumer products. The particles are introduced to the air side of the ALI model, allowing them to interact with the lung cells at the air–liquid interface [71].

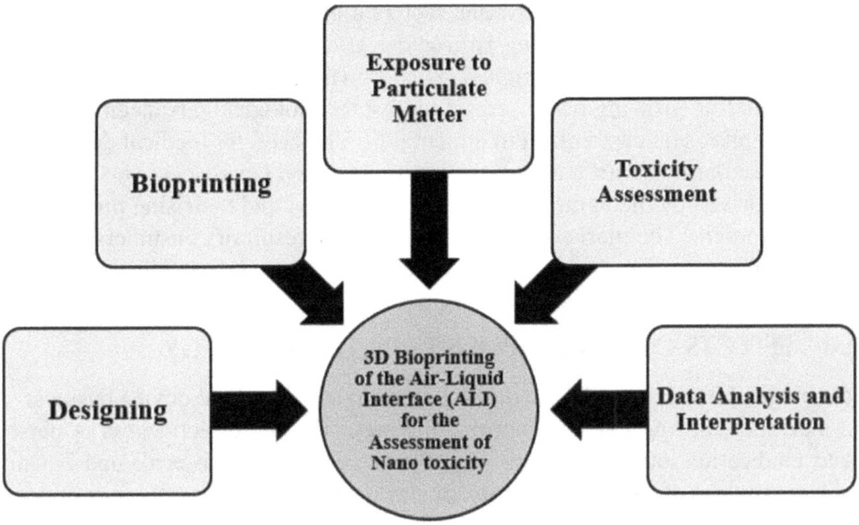

FIGURE 20.4 3D bioprinting of the air-liquid interface (ALI) for the assessment of nanotoxicity.

- Researchers can then assess the toxicological effects of the particulate matter on the lung cells. This includes evaluating cell viability, inflammation, oxidative stress, genotoxicity, and other relevant endpoints using techniques like cell viability assays, cytokine analysis, and gene expression profiling [72].
- Data obtained from the toxicity assessments are analyzed to understand the potential health risks associated with exposure to particulate matter. This information can contribute to regulatory decisions, the development of safer materials, and the design of strategies to mitigate air pollution-related health effects [73]. By utilizing 3D bioprinting to create ALI models, researchers can overcome some of the limitations of traditional 2D cell culture models, which do not accurately represent the complex physiological conditions of the respiratory system. This approach allows for more realistic and predictive toxicity testing, ultimately advancing our understanding of the health impacts of airborne pollutants and nanoparticles [74].

20.7 PROSPECTS AND DEVELOPMENTS FOR THE BIOMEDICAL DEVICE INDUSTRY

This chapter examines the growth factors, emerging trends, and factors that make the medical device manufacturing sector well-positioned for the future. With the market expected to increase from $637 billion in 2024 to around $893 billion by 2029, the medical device manufacturing sector is set for substantial change (Bainbridge EDGE Report, June 2024). Technological developments and rising healthcare needs are the main drivers of this remarkable growth, which makes the industry a desirable place to invest [75]. For stakeholders hoping to take advantage of these opportunities, it is essential to comprehend the motivating factors and new trends. The global market for medical device manufacturing is growing at a compound annual growth rate (CAGR) of 5.8% (Bainbridge Insights). This growth is being fueled by a variety of factors, including growing healthcare expenses, technological advancements, and a growing emphasis on customized treatment [76]. The need for medical devices such as cardiovascular implants, telemedicine equipment, and laparoscopic instruments is also being driven by the aging of the global population and the rising prevalence of chronic disorders. The market is still expanding as a result of consumers' changing treatment choices and increased patient awareness of innovative medical procedures.

20.8 EFFECTS OF DEVELOPMENTS IN TECHNOLOGY

Technological breakthroughs are driving growth in the medical device business. AI and machine learning together increase the precision and effectiveness of personalized medication and diagnostics [77]. By decreasing human error and boosting precision, the use of robots and automation in manufacturing and surgery improves patient outcomes. Additionally, 3D printing technology allows for the customization of implants and prostheses. Faster data transfer and support for the Internet of Medical Things (IoMT) are two ways that 5G technology is transforming the healthcare sector. More interconnected healthcare ecosystems and real-time remote procedures will be made possible by this [78]. Additionally, 5G technology improves the functionality and connection of telehealth equipment, allowing for real-time data transfer and remote treatments. These developments simplify industrial operations, lowering costs and raising production, in addition to improving the precision of diagnostic and therapeutic results.

20.9 CHANGING PREFERENCES OF CONSUMERS

The medical device manufacturing business is appealing for investment and expansion since it provides a wealth of options. The inclination of consumers is moving toward minimally invasive techniques, such as robotic, laparoscopic, and endoscopic technologies, along with gadgets that provide individualized care and remote monitoring [79]. Growing consumer demand for preventive care and continuous health monitoring is driving the popularity of wearable health gadgets, such as fitness trackers and continuous glucose monitors. Furthermore, the market for diagnostic devices, which includes CT and ultrasound scanners, is expanding rapidly. Manufacturers are placing even more focus on quality assurance, which is driving this boom with the integration of AI for improved accuracy. The cardiovascular device market is still growing as a result of the introduction of sophisticated cardiovascular implants like stents and catheters [80].

20.10 HANDLING DIFFICULTIES AND HAZARDS

The medical device manufacturing sector faces several risks and obstacles despite its encouraging growth. Strong cybersecurity measures are essential since the risk of cyberattacks and data breaches rises as devices become increasingly linked [81].

Furthermore, it is still difficult to comply with strict standards, especially in light of the constant revisions to guidelines like the EU MDR and FDA. Significant compliance expenses are associated with these upgrades, which disproportionately affect smaller enterprises. Financial difficulties arise from high R&D expenses and pressure on prices from payers and healthcare providers, which will require striking a balance between innovation and cost-effectiveness [82].

20.11 CONCLUSION

By addressing these characteristics and needs, biomedical manufacturing companies can develop safe, effective, and innovative medical products to improve patient outcomes and advance healthcare globally. These are just a few of the many engineering needs in the field of biomedical manufacturing. The domain is constantly generating, and new technologies and techniques are continually being designed and produced. Additive manufacturing is playing a transformative role in biomedical manufacturing, driving innovation and improving patient care. As technology continues to advance, the impact of additive manufacturing on the biomedical field is expected to grow even further. Technology developments and rising healthcare costs will propel the medical device manufacturing sector's rapid expansion. Patient results and satisfaction are being revolutionized by cutting-edge healthcare technologies like 3D-printed implants and AI-driven diagnostics. Through comprehension of market dynamics, adoption of innovation, and resolution of obstacles, interested parties can leverage prospects in this ever-changing industry. Bainbridge is prepared to assist businesses in managing the disruptive growth of this potential industry, thanks to its expertise in strategy and M&A advising.

REFERENCES

1. Chen, R., Chang, R. C., Tai, B., Huang, Y., Ozdoganlar, B., Li, W., & Shih, A. (2020). Biomedical manufacturing: A review of the emerging research and applications. *Journal of Manufacturing Science and Engineering*, *142*(11), 110807. Chen, Y., Lai, Z., Zhang, X., Fan, Z., He, Q., Tan, C., & Zhang, H. (2020). Phase engineering of nanomaterials. *Nature Reviews Chemistry*, *4*(5), 243–56.
2. Kumar, R., Kumar, M., & Chohan, J. S. (2021). The role of additive manufacturing for biomedical applications: A critical review. *Journal of Manufacturing Processes*, *64*, 828–50.
3. Shahrubudin, N., Koshy, P., Alipal, J., Kadir, M. H. A., & Lee, T. C. (2020). Challenges of 3D printing technology for manufacturing biomedical products: A case study of Malaysian manufacturing firms. *Heliyon*, *6*(4).
4. Vignesh, M., Ranjith Kumar, G., Sathishkumar, M., Manikandan, M., Rajyalakshmi, G., Ramanujam, R., & Arivazhagan, N. (2021). Development of biomedical implants through additive manufacturing: A review. *Journal of Materials Engineering and Performance*, *30*, 4735–44.
5. Allavikutty, R., Gupta, P., Santra, T. S., & Rengaswamy, J. (2021). Additive manufacturing of Mg alloys for biomedical applications: Current status and challenges. *Current Opinion in Biomedical Engineering*, *18*, 100276.
6. Kaushik, V., Kumar, N., & Vignesh, M. (2022). Magnesium role in additive manufacturing of biomedical implants–challenges and opportunities. *Additive Manufacturing*, *55*, 102802.

7. Wazeer, A., Das, A., Sinha, A., Inaba, K., Ziyi, S., & Karmakar, A. (2023). Additive manufacturing in biomedical field: A critical review on fabrication method, materials used, applications, challenges, and future prospects. *Progress in Additive Manufacturing*, *8*(5), 857–89.
8. Francis Luther King, M., Robert Singh, G., Gopichand, A., & Srinivasan, V. (2023). Challenges and perspective of manufacturing techniques in biomedical applications. In *Advanced Materials and Manufacturing Techniques for Biomedical Applications* (pp. 345–81). Wiley.
9. Attar, H., Ehtemam-Haghighi, S., Soro, N., Kent, D., & Dargusch, M. S. (2020). Additive manufacturing of low-cost porous titanium-based composites for biomedical applications: Advantages, challenges and opinion for future development. *Journal of Alloys and Compounds*, *827*, 154263.
10. Koptioug, A., Rännar, L. E., Bäckström, M., & Cronskär, M. (2014, June). Additive manufacturing for medical and biomedical applications: Advances and challenges. In *Materials Science Forum* (Vol. 783, pp. 1286–91). Trans Tech Publications Ltd.
11. Munir, K., Biesiekierski, A., Wen, C., & Li, Y. (2020). Introduction to biomedical manufacturing. In *Metallic Biomaterials Processing and Medical Device Manufacturing* (pp. 3–29). Woodhead Publishing.
12. Singh, S., & Ramakrishna, S. (2017). Biomedical applications of additive manufacturing: Present and future. *Current Opinion in Biomedical Engineering*, *2*, 105–15.
13. Özel, T., Bártolo, P. J., Ceretti, E., Gay, J. D. C., Rodriguez, C. A., & Da Silva, J. V. L. (Eds.). (2016). *Biomedical Devices: Design, Prototyping, and Manufacturing*. John Wiley & Sons.
14. Ciurana, J. (2013). New opportunities and challenges for additive manufacturing to produce biomedical devices. *IFAC Proceedings Volumes*, *46*(24), 283–8.
15. Kim, H., Lin, Y., & Tseng, T. L. B. (2018). A review on quality control in additive manufacturing. *Rapid Prototyping Journal*, *24*(3), 645–69.
16. Khinvasara, T., Ness, S., & Shankar, A. (2024). Leveraging AI for enhanced quality assurance in medical device manufacturing. *Asian Journal of Research in Computer Science*, *17*(6), 13–35.
17. Kuba, J. (2003, May). Quality assurance in production of medical devices. In *26th International Spring Seminar on Electronics Technology: Integrated Management of Electronic Materials Production, 2003* (pp. 141–4). IEEE.
18. Ranebennur, R., Thirumaleshwar, S., Somareddy, H. K., Desai, R., & Sandeep, D. S. (2023). Development of automated quality assurance systems for pharmaceutical manufacturing: A review. *Journal of Coastal Life Medicine*, *11*, 1855–64.
19. Yu, J. R., Navarro, J., Coburn, J. C., Mahadik, B., Molnar, J., Holmes IV, J. H., . . . & Fisher, J. P. (2019). Current and future perspectives on skin tissue engineering: Key features of biomedical research, translational assessment, and clinical application. *Advanced Healthcare Materials*, *8*(5), 1801471.
20. Jaime, F. J., Muñoz, A., Rodríguez-Gómez, F., & Jerez-Calero, A. (2023). Strengthening privacy and data security in biomedical microelectromechanical systems by IoT communication security and protection in smart healthcare. *Sensors*, *23*(21), 8944.
21. Wallach, J. D., Gonsalves, G. S., & Ross, J. S. (2018). Research, regulatory, and clinical decision-making: The importance of scientific integrity. *Journal of Clinical Epidemiology*, *93*, 88–93.
22. Vogt, L., Ruther, F., Salehi, S., & Boccaccini, A. R. (2021). Poly (glycerol sebacate) in biomedical applications—A review of the recent literature. *Advanced Healthcare Materials*, *10*(9), 2002026.
23. Shih, A. J. (2008). Biomedical manufacturing: A new frontier of manufacturing research. *International Manufacturing Science and Engineering Conference*, *130*(2), 021009.

24. González-Henríquez, C. M., Sarabia-Vallejos, M. A., & Rodriguez-Hernandez, J. (2019). Polymers for additive manufacturing and 4D-printing: Materials, methodologies, and biomedical applications. *Progress in Polymer Science*, *94*, 57–116.
25. Biggiero, L. (2002). The location of multinationals in industrial districts: Knowledge transfer in biomedicals. *The Journal of Technology Transfer*, *27*(1), 111–22.
26. Ahmad, A., Banat, F., Alsafar, H., & Hasan, S. W. (2024). An overview of biodegradable poly (lactic acid) production from fermentative lactic acid for biomedical and bioplastic applications. *Biomass Conversion and Biorefinery*, *14*(3), 3057–76.
27. Sakly, H., Said, M., & Tagina, M. (2021). Healthcare supply chain management: Towards 3D MRI aorta model with CPU-GPU parallel architecture for medical manufacture. *Cogent Medicine*, *8*(1), 2012888.
28. Carvalho, M. M. D., & Rabechini Junior, R. (2015). Impact of risk management on project performance: The importance of soft skills. *International Journal of Production Research*, *53*(2), 321–40.
29. Niinomi, M. (Ed.). (2019). *Metals for Biomedical Devices*. Woodhead Publishing.
30. Leal, F., Chis, A. E., Caton, S., González–Vélez, H., García-Gómez, J. M., Durá, M., . . . & Mier, M. (2021). Smart pharmaceutical manufacturing: Ensuring end-to-end traceability and data integrity in medicine production. *Big Data Research*, *24*, 100172.
31. Radon, J., & Pan, G. (2023). Pharma—manufacturing: The unappreciated and overlooked indispensable skill. *Current Opinion in Immunology*, *84*, 102385.
32. Daly, A. C., Riley, L., Segura, T., & Burdick, J. A. (2020). Hydrogel microparticles for biomedical applications. *Nature Reviews Materials*, *5*(1), 20–43.
33. Schuitemaker, R., & Xu, X. (2020). Product traceability in manufacturing: A technical review. *Procedia Cirp*, *93*, 700–5.
34. Andersen, M. L., & Winter, L. M. (2017). Animal models in biological and biomedical research-experimental and ethical concerns. *Anais da Academia Brasileira de Ciências*, *91*, e20170238.
35. Zhang, L. C., & Chen, L. Y. (2019). A review on biomedical titanium alloys: Recent progress and prospect. *Advanced Engineering Materials*, *21*(4), 1801215.
36. Ebbesen, M., & Jensen, T. G. (2006). Nanomedicine: Techniques, potentials, and ethical implications. *BioMed Research International*, *2006*.
37. Ruban, R., Rajashekhar, V. S., Nivedha, B., Mohit, H., Sanjay, M. R., & Siengchin, S. (2022). Role of additive manufacturing in biomedical engineering. In *Innovations in Additive Manufacturing* (pp. 139–57). Cham: Springer International Publishing.
38. Shin, D. G., Kim, T. H., & Kim, D. E. (2017). Review of 4D printing materials and their properties. *International Journal of Precision Engineering and Manufacturing-Green Technology*, *4*, 349–57.
39. Kim, H., Lin, Y., & Tseng, T. L. B. (2018). A review on quality control in additive manufacturing. *Rapid Prototyping Journal*, *24*(3), 645–69.
40. González-Henríquez, C. M., Sarabia-Vallejos, M. A., & Rodriguez-Hernandez, J. (2019). Polymers for additive manufacturing and 4D-printing: Materials, methodologies, and biomedical applications. *Progress in Polymer Science*, *94*, 57–116.
41. Khare, V., Sonkaria, S., Lee, G. Y., Ahn, S. H., & Chu, W. S. (2017). From 3D to 4D printing–design, material and fabrication for multi-functional multi-materials. *International Journal of Precision Engineering and Manufacturing-Green Technology*, *4*, 291–9.
42. Kulkarni, P. G., Paudel, N., Magar, S., Santilli, M. F., Kashyap, S., Baranwal, A. K., . . . & Singh, A. V. (2024). Overcoming challenges and innovations in orthopedic prosthesis design: An interdisciplinary perspective. *Biomedical Materials & Devices*, *2*(1), 58–69.

43. Myerson, A. S., Krumme, M., Nasr, M., Thomas, H., & Braatz, R. D. (2015). Control systems engineering in continuous pharmaceutical manufacturing May 20–21, 2014 continuous manufacturing symposium. *Journal of Pharmaceutical Sciences, 104*(3), 832–9.
44. Prakash, C., Singh, S., Singh, R., Ramakrishna, S., Pabla, B. S., Puri, S., & Uddin, M. S. (Eds.). (2019). *Biomanufacturing* (Vol. 20). Cham, Switzerland: Springer.
45. Doulgkeroglou, M. N., Di Nubila, A., Niessing, B., König, N., Schmitt, R. H., Damen, J., . . . & Zeugolis, D. I. (2020). Automation, monitoring, and standardization of cell product manufacturing. *Frontiers in Bioengineering and Biotechnology, 8*, 811.
46. Szkodny, A. C., & Lee, K. H. (2022). Biopharmaceutical manufacturing: Historical perspectives and future directions. *Annual Review of Chemical and Biomolecular Engineering, 13*, 141–65.
47. Aceto, G., Persico, V., & Pescapé, A. (2020). Industry 4.0 and health: Internet of things, big data, and cloud computing for healthcare 4.0. *Journal of Industrial Information Integration, 18*, 100129.
48. Devarajaiah, D., & Muthumari, C. (2018). Evaluation of power consumption and MRR in WEDM of Ti–6Al–4V alloy and its simultaneous optimization for sustainable production. *Journal of the Brazilian Society of Mechanical Sciences and Engineering, 40*, 1–18.
49. Sastri, V. R. (2021). *Plastics in Medical Devices: Properties, Requirements, and Applications*. William Andrew.
50. Senna, P., Reis, A., Dias, A., Coelho, O., Guimaraes, J., & Eliana, S. (2023). Healthcare supply chain resilience framework: Antecedents, mediators, consequents. *Production Planning & Control, 34*(3), 295–309.
51. Wang, X., Yan, Y., & Zhang, R. (2010). Recent trends and challenges in complex organ manufacturing. *Tissue Engineering Part B: Reviews, 16*(2), 189–97.
52. Singh, S., Ramakrishna, S., & Singh, R. (2017). Material issues in additive manufacturing: A review. *Journal of Manufacturing Processes, 25*, 185–200.
53. Samuel, G. L., Kong, L., Arcot, Y., & Pandit, P. (2022). Principles of advanced manufacturing technologies for biomedical devices. In *Advanced Micro-and Nano-manufacturing Technologies: Applications in Biochemical and Biomedical Engineering* (pp. 361–402). Singapore: Springer.
54. Chhaya, M. P., Poh, P. S., Balmayor, E. R., Van Griensven, M., Schantz, J. T., & Hutmacher, D. W. (2015). Additive manufacturing in biomedical sciences and the need for definitions and norms. *Expert Review of Medical Devices, 12*(5), 537–43.
55. Guzzi, E. A., & Tibbitt, M. W. (2020). Additive manufacturing of precision biomaterials. *Advanced Materials, 32*(13), 1901994.
56. Kumar, A., Mishra, D. K., Upadhyay, L., Srivastava, M., & Pathak, D. K. (2023). Additive manufacturing technologies for on-demand production of personalized goods. In *Laser Applications in Manufacturing* (pp. 120–52). CRC Press.
57. Ashima, R., Haleem, A., Bahl, S., Javaid, M., Mahla, S. K., & Singh, S. (2021). Automation and manufacturing of smart materials in Additive Manufacturing technologies using Internet of Things towards the adoption of Industry 4.0. *Materials Today: Proceedings, 45*, 5081–8.
58. Pathak, K., Saikia, R., Das, A., Das, D., Islam, M. A., Pramanik, P., . . . & Borthakur, B. (2023). 3D printing in biomedicine: Advancing personalized care through additive manufacturing. *Exploration of Medicine, 4*(6), 1135–67.
59. Pathak, K., Saikia, R., Das, A., Das, D., Islam, M. A., Pramanik, P., . . . & Borthakur, B. (2023). 3D printing in biomedicine: Advancing personalized care through additive manufacturing. *Exploration of Medicine, 4*(6), 1135–67.
60. Ozbolat, I. T., Peng, W., & Ozbolat, V. (2016). Application areas of 3D bioprinting. *Drug Discovery Today, 21*(8), 1257–71.

61. Horváth, L., Umehara, Y., Jud, C., Blank, F., Petri-Fink, A., & Rothen-Rutishauser, B. (2015). Engineering an in vitro air-blood barrier by 3D bioprinting. *Scientific Reports*, *5*(1), 7974.
62. Gidwani, M., & Singh, A. V. (2013). Nanoparticle enabled drug delivery across the blood brain barrier: In vivo and in vitro models, opportunities and challenges. *Current Pharmaceutical Biotechnology*, *14*(14), 1201–12.
63. Ochs, M., Nyengaard, J. R., Jung, A., Knudsen, L., Voigt, M., Wahlers, T., . . . & Gundersen, H. J. G. (2004). The number of alveoli in the human lung. *American Journal of Respiratory and Critical Care Medicine*, *169*(1), 120–4.
64. Singh, A. V., Laux, P., Luch, A., Sudrik, C., Wiehr, S., Wild, A. M., . . . & Sitti, M. (2019). Review of emerging concepts in nanotoxicology: Opportunities and challenges for safer nanomaterial design. *Toxicology Mechanisms and Methods*, *29*(5), 378–87.
65. Holgate, S. T. (1999). The epidemic of allergy and asthma. *Nature*, *402*(6760).
66. Zarrabeitia-Bilbao, E., Álvarez-Meaza, I., Río-Belver, R. M., & Garechana-Anacabe, G. (2019). Additive manufacturing technologies for biomedical engineering applications: Research trends and scientific impact. *Profesional de la información/Information Professional*, *28*(2).
67. Harding, A., Pramanik, A., Basak, A. K., Prakash, C., & Shankar, S. (2023). Application of additive manufacturing in the biomedical field-A review. *Annals of 3D Printed Medicine*, 100110.
68. Verboeket, V., Khajavi, S. H., Krikke, H., Salmi, M., & Holmström, J. (2021). Additive manufacturing for localized medical parts production: A case study. *IEEE Access*, *9*, 25818–34.
69. Rehman, M., Yanen, W., Mushtaq, R. T., Ishfaq, K., Zahoor, S., Ahmed, A., . . . & Sultana, J. (2023). Additive manufacturing for biomedical applications: A review on classification, energy consumption, and its appreciable role since COVID-19 pandemic. *Progress in Additive Manufacturing*, *8*(5), 1007–41.
70. Zadpoor, A. A., & Malda, J. (2017). Additive manufacturing of biomaterials, tissues, and organs. *Annals of Biomedical Engineering*, *45*, 1–11.
71. Butt, J. (2020). Exploring the interrelationship between additive manufacturing and Industry 4.0. *Designs*, *4*(2), 13.
72. Velu, R., Calais, T., Jayakumar, A., & Raspall, F. (2019). A comprehensive review on bio-nanomaterials for medical implants and feasibility studies on fabrication of such implants by additive manufacturing technique. *Materials*, *13*(1), 92.
73. Sheoran, A. J., Kumar, H., Arora, P. K., & Moona, G. (2020). Bio-medical applications of additive manufacturing: A review. *Procedia Manufacturing*, *51*, 663–70.
74. Srivastava, R., & Srivastava, V. K. (2020). Changing scenario of manufacturing industries due to Covid 19. *International Journal for Modern Trends in Science and Technology*, *6*(10), 143–6.
75. Bahadur, P. S., Jaiswal, S., Srivastava, R., & Kumar, A. (2021, November). Advanced application of nanotechnology in engineering. In *2021 International Conference on Technological Advancements and Innovations (ICTAI)* (pp. 92–5). IEEE.
76. Srivastava, R., Thakur, A., & Rana, A. (2024). The basic understanding of nano materials: A review. In A. Thakur & A. Kumar (Eds.), *Innovations in Nanomaterials-Based Corrosion Inhibitors* (pp. 1–20). IGI Global. https://doi.org/10.4018/979-8-3693-3088-3.ch001
77. Srivastava, R., Arun, J., & Patel, D. K. (2019). Amalgamating the service quality aspect in supply chain management. In *2019 International Conference on Automation, Computational and Technology Management (ICACTM)* (pp. 63–7). London. https://doi.org/10.1109/ICACTM.2019.8776839

78. Thakur, A., Vates, U. K., & Mishra, S. (2024). Parametric optimization of 3D-printed PLA part using response surface methodology for mechanical properties. *Smart Science, 12*(1), 91–104.
79. Andreoni, G., Barbieri, M., & Colombo, B. (2014). *Developing Biomedical Devices: Design, Innovation and Protection.* Springer International Publishing.
80. Mamo, H. B., Adamiak, M., & Kunwar, A. (2023). 3D printed biomedical devices and their applications: A review on state-of-the-art technologies, existing challenges, and future perspectives. *Journal of the Mechanical Behavior of Biomedical Materials, 143*, 105930.
81. Dobrzański, L. A., Dobrzańska-Danikiewicz, A. D., & Dobrzański, L. B. (2021). Effect of biomedical materials in the Implementation of a long and healthy life policy. *Processes, 9*(5), 865.
82. Sugahara, T. (2023). Challenges and prospects in the medical device industry-heading toward a leading Japanese industry. *The Institute of Comparative Economic Studies Hosei University, 37*, 55–67.

21 Bioimplants Redefined
The Role of Advanced Biomaterials in Load-bearing Solutions

Sahil Kainth and Gaurav Prashar

CONTENTS

21.1 INTRODUCTION

Bioimplants have become a cornerstone of modern medicine, restoring function and improving lives. The need for bioimplants arises from a variety of medical diseases in which native tissues or organs are damaged, defective, or absent, resulting in diminished function or quality of life. Bioimplants are designed to support, restore, or rectify the operational behavior of an injured body part. In medical words, medical implants are equipment, tools, and devices or tissues put within the body or on the surface of the body. Most of the implants are prostheses designed to replace lost/missing body parts, while others administer medication, observe bodily functions and work as support for tissues and organs. Several implants are manufactured out of bones, skin segments, and other bodily parts while many of them are manufactured of ceramics, polymers, metals, and other biomaterials. Implants can either be installed permanently or withdrawn when no longer required. For instance, stents

DOI: 10.1201/9781003516064-21

and hip implants are aimed to be permanent. Bioimplants act as replacements for various body components to repair, preserve, or change wounded tissues and organ function (1).

21.1.1 Need for Bioimplants

Accidents, diseases, and congenital conditions can cause bone fractures, joint degeneration, or missing teeth. Bioimplants provide a way to replace or repair these damaged tissues, restoring functionality and alleviating pain. Bioimplants can go beyond simple repair. In some cases, they can enhance a person's capabilities, such as with joint replacements that allow for a more active lifestyle. The need for implants in the body may arise for an injury, accident, or due to malfunctions of the body parts of tissues such as a fracture due to injury or joints degradation due to some disease. Bioimplants are most commonly used in orthopedics. They include joint replacements, bone plates, and ligaments among other. Medical implants are classed based on many qualities that distinguish them from others in terms of behavior, body acceptance rate, cost, and tribo-corrosive nature (2).

Figure 21.1 describes the classification of bioimplants depending upon their usability in the body. Bioimplants can also be classified depending upon their usage in the body. As some implants in the body function as a structural member of the body, they bear and support heavy loads. Bioimplants are a diverse group of medical devices that are surgically placed into the body to replace, repair, or augment a tissue or organ function. Metals, ceramics, polymers, and even biological tissues are among the materials that can be used to create them. Here's a classification of bioimplants based on their application in the body as shown in **Figure 21.2**.

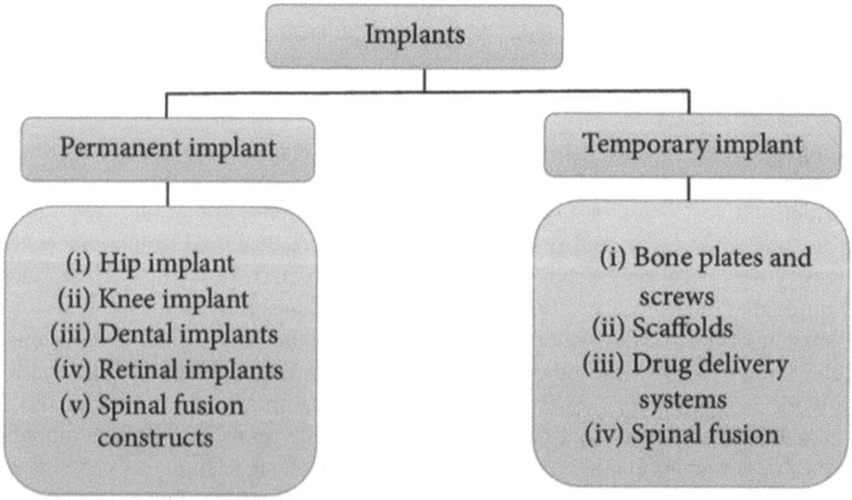

FIGURE 21.1 Classification of bioimplants.

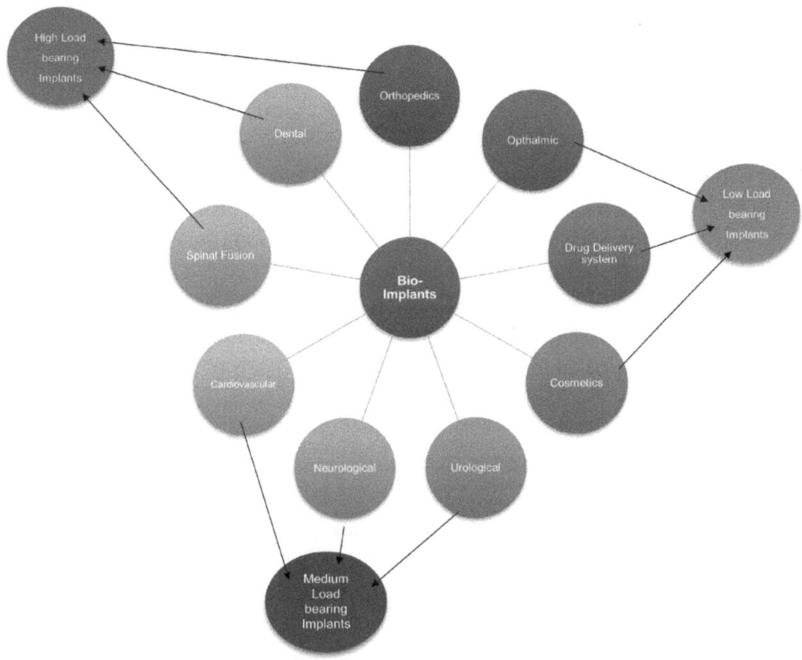

FIGURE 21.2 Classification of implants on the basis of their application and load-bearing capacity.

Once the implant is placed in the body, it will function as an integral part of the body, cooperating with surrounding cells, tissues, and muscles. Implants may be placed permanently or temporarily in the body. In case of temporary implants they are removed from the body when their desired purpose is achieved such as growth of bones or new generation of tissues. While choosing implant material their fundamental characteristics must be considered A bioimplant material ought to have all essential characteristics and shouldn't have any detrimental effects on human anatomy (3).

The structural implants like plates and screws which are placed to support bone fractures, cages, or plates have to undergo severe wear and heavy loads as their primary objective is to provide mechanical strength to the bones, joints, and replaced body parts.

The ideal biomaterial for these implants should be super strong and durable to resist wear and tear. It should also last a long time without breaking down or rusting. Ultimately, the goal is for the implant to become one with the body's bones and minimize any friction, damage, or negative reactions from surrounding tissues (4). As discussed earlier, the function of bioimplants is to serve as an integral part of human body for a long duration. Hence, a good bioimplant must have the following properties:

i) Biocompatibility
ii) High corrosion and wear resistance
iii) Appropriate mechanical properties

iv) 20–50% porosity
v) Good bioactivity for osteointegration (5)

To achieve these properties, various materials like metals and alloys, ceramics, polymers, and various composites have been used in the manufacture of bio implants. The requirement and applicability of the material depend upon the type of implants being placed in the body, the load capacity of the implant, biocompatibility, and cost. With the advancements in materials new advanced biomaterials have been introduced which provide better desired properties in implants (6). This chapter discusses the advancements in bioimplant materials for load-bearing applications.

Multiple implants are employed to replace various parts of the body and prostheses. In addition, other medical implants serve the purpose of diagnosis, monitoring, and provide support for malfunctioning organs or tissues (6). Some implants are constructed of natural materials such as bones, skins, and tissues, while others are made of man-made materials such as ceramics, metals, and plastics (7). There is a continuous improvement in implant materials on a daily basis by incorporating innovative technology at cheap prices (8,9). There are performance factors that are used to select an implant. The parameters are described in **Figure 21.3**.

There are specific features that an implant must demonstrate to be chosen (10). The properties are listed here. It is necessary that a biomaterial has all the primary qualities and does not have a negative impact on human anatomy. The key properties of an implant can be defined as follows.

- *Biocompatibility*: Any material is considered biocompatible when it has no negative influence or toxicity on the environment in which it is used. It should be compatible and friendly with the surrounding tissues and cells.

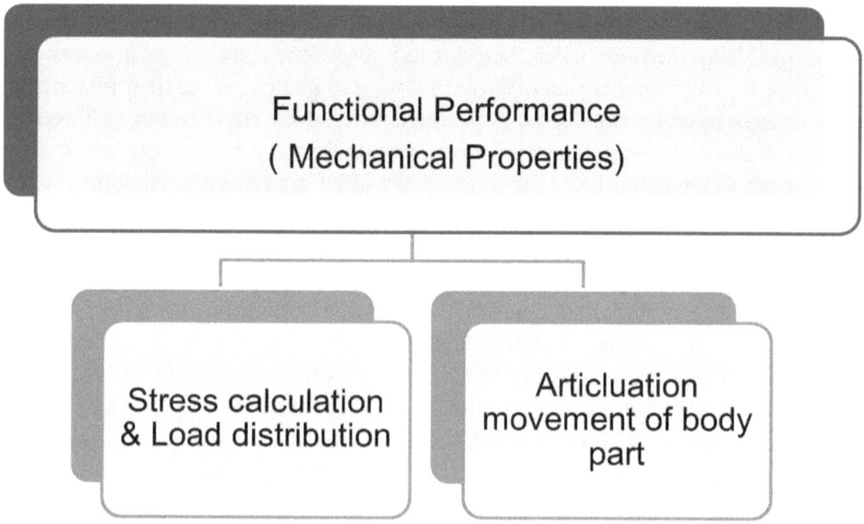

FIGURE 21.3 Performance parameters for selecting implants.

- *Bio tolerant*: If a material is not disapproved by the human body and may easily build a fibrous coating around the bones it is said to be a bio tolerant.
- *Bioinert*: A substance is termed to be bioinert when it has compatibility with its tissues or surface.
- *Bioactive*: Any material is considered bioactive if a material allows other materials to develop around itself and become an integral structure of the parent bone.
- *Osteoconductive Materials*: These allow transplanted bone to merge with normal bone without producing material debris or deformation.
- *Osteoinductive Materials*: These materials can create new bones in the human body. Bioimplants are composed of a range of materials (11).

21.2 SELECTION OF BIOIMPLANTS

Some crucial points are examined while selecting materials for biological purposes (12). Non-toxic materials must be used, and these materials should not cause any type of contamination in the body. Because the human system is extremely reactive to alien materials, wearing them may induce debris buildup, perhaps causing tumors, circulate corroded particles in the body, and healthy tissues are damaged. All these reasons shorten the life of the medical implant (13). Also, economics plays a significant part in the choosing process. Materials that are readily available and take less time to make (14) are also given weightage.

21.2.1 Modulus of Elasticity

The elasticity modulus of natural bone ranges from 10 GPa to 40 GPa. Multiple methods are used to calculate the elasticity modulus of different materials. The elasticity modulus for implant materials should be similar to natural bone. This shielding effect happens when there is non-uniform transfer of load through the bone, and it does not generate enough robustness to withstand against stresses (15). Low load and stress can lead to insufficient thickness of the bone and loss of mass of the bone. Furthermore, the shielding effect can damage the implants by promoting loosening of the implants and various other issues. As a result, implants with low elasticity modulus have the tendency to identically transmit stress as well as load over implant and bone, hence extending an implant's life period. The materials which have low modulus of elasticity are beta-phase titanium alloys (16).

21.2.2 Biocompatibility

Implant materials must be nontoxic, biologically compatible, and shouldn't cause any inflammatory reactions or other medical issues. The interaction between implant material and internal body surroundings material determines the implant's success and lifespan. Other aspects that influence an implant's biocompatibility include immune system reactions and implant degrading qualities. Implant materials are classified as bioresorbable, bioactive, and bio tolerant (17). Bioactive materials are favored because of their high attraction and interaction in the internal conditions of the body. Impulses generated along with responses at the tissue/implant contact determine how well the implant is integrated. Successful implants are biocompatible and bioactive. Some of the concerns associated with the body's responses include thrombosis, which refers to the clotting, blood coagulation, or adherence of blood cells to the implant material, and the formation of a layer of fat or tissues surrounding the implant material (18).

21.2.3 Fatigue Limit

The longevity of an implant is significantly influenced by its fatigue strength and resistance. Bone implants are subject to cyclic loads due to body movements, which may lead to plastic deformation. Stress concentration around manufacturing flaws and material inconsistencies can precipitate implant failure. Bending, torsion, tension, and compression tests are used to determine fatigue strength. Titanium-based alloys are known for their high fatigue resistance (19).

21.2.4 Corrosion/Wear Resistance

Implant materials need to have good wear and corrosion resistivity. The continuous loss of material and corrosion can produce debris along with ions that cause significant consequences resulting in inflammation, toxicity, and allergic contamination. The immune system attacks an implant and releases wear debris, which can have a substantial impact on its lifespan. Furthermore, poor wear resistivity might cause loosening of implant and finally failure (20,21).

21.3 MATERIAL USED FOR BIOIMPLANTS: HISTORY AND PRESENCE

Bioimplants are synthetic medical devices designed and employed to substitute for impaired skeletal components and bolster biological structures. These implants are composed of synthetic materials endowed with biocompatibility and mechanical characteristics that ensure no detrimental effects on tissues, such as appropriate porosity, chemical neutrality, load-bearing capacity, and resilience (22). The fundamental objective of bioimplants is to restore the functionality of compromised human anatomical parts. These implants serve a broad spectrum of duties, including sensory devices for the brain, retina, and cochlea, as well as dental, orthopedics, and cardiovascular applications (23). A variety of these devices, like pacemakers, heart valves, stents, dental crowns, braces, and prosthetic hip and knee joints, are surgically implanted to regulate, monitor, and sustain the operations of damaged organs or tissues. The history of implants can be traced from early Egyptians along with evidences of implants from South American cultures, and following continuous enhancements in the area of materials and medical sciences we have been able to achieve substantial breakthroughs in implantation technology. Improvements in the quality of materials for implants as well as quantity have resulted in this treatment technique highly anticipated, emerging, and widely used in the modern day (24). Dating back to 2500 BC, the Egyptians pioneered the use of gold ligatures to secure damaged teeth. Subsequently, around 500 BC, the Etruscans innovated with gold to create pointed dental structures. This positions gold as one of the earliest materials utilized in engineering, predating the use of bronze, iron, and steel. Gold's unique mechanical qualities, such as its ductility and malleability, made it a metal of choice for early dental implants among various ancient cultures (25). The Phoenicians were particularly adept at crafting gold wires and using carved ivory to correct and stabilize misaligned teeth. The Mayan civilization marked a departure from metal, introducing the use of seashell implants. However, it was the 18th century that heralded a significant advancement in dental implantology, with notable figures like Pierre Fauchard and John Hunter leading successful tooth transplantations. In the early 20th century, specifically 1913, Greenfield utilized a 24-gauge wire made from an iridium-platinum alloy, which was soldered using 24-carat gold. The advent of the Industrial Revolution brought about transformative changes in the manufacturing and design of dental implants, including the introduction of stainless steel wires to address dental deformities (26).

The positive outcomes from these metallic implants paved the way for the use of cobalt and chromium in the creation of subperiosteal implants. These materials were also instrumental in the development of implants with mushroom-shaped designs, which gained popularity during that period (27). Modern implants play an essential role in enhancing human lifespan and quality of life. This technology offers solutions that are not only cost-effective but also resist wear and tear (tribocorrosion). While the concept of implants has roots in ancient civilizations like Egypt, Rome, and Maya (primarily for dental applications), the modern scientific revolution has seen their use expand dramatically. Implantology, the field dedicated to implant development and use, has gained widespread recognition and acceptance within the global medical community (28). Following the advancements in science, the use of implants has seen a significant rise, not just in dentistry, but across all aspects of human anatomy. The field of implantology has developed and gained recognition from the global medical community. As of 2019, approximately 85% of the global population under the age of 40 experienced conditions such as bone defects, fractures, and excessive strain, leading to severe pain and reduced mobility. These conditions have limited their physical activities, often leading to disability. Consequently, the demand for medical implants is on the rise, as they offer a solution for replacing defective bones without causing harm to natural tissues, cells, or the human body as a whole (29).

For load-bearing applications, mechanical performance behavior and biocompatibility of material is a prime factor to classify the material for implant. As research and technological efforts evolved in 21st century the desire for more efficient, optimum, strong, and more durable materials for bioimplants resulted in advanced biomaterials. These materials are easy to manufacture, have greater biocompatibility, high load-bearing capacities, and have positive economic impacts. The developments in materials engineering lead to development of such materials which become significant in the manufacture of bioimplants.

During heavy load-bearing applications when a metallic substance undergoes wear and corrosion, it might induce inflammation in the tissues around the implant location, yielding negative biological responses inside the body. Byproducts generated from metallic materials, such as ions and harmful substances, have the potential to cause severe diseases and increase the dangers connected with the incorporation of metals as implants. As a result, when executing bioimplants, it becomes essential to select the suitable material for the correct applications. Furthermore, the biomaterial's mechanical performance should be equal to the material it replaces. It should be able to sustain intricately variable mechanical load cycles. Teeth, knee joints, and hips are common implantation sites. Choosing a biomaterial considering its physical and mechanical qualities is critical in avoiding implant malfunctions and failures since the body experiences repeated loading cycles over its lifespan. Furthermore, whatever material is used must be simultaneously friendly with the surrounding tissues as well as financially practical. Subsequently, the material should be affordable, efficient, and compatible with the human body. Following these requirements, a variety of materials have been progressed over the last few decades especially biomaterials in biomedical applications. However, meeting all of the desired qualities with a single metallic material remains a challenge. Biomaterials utilized for biological purposes are commonly classified into ceramics, polymers, and metallic systems, as detailed here (30).

21.3.1 Metallic Implants

Because of their biomechanical qualities, metals are a good choice for implant materials. Apart from these features, they are simple to treat because of their smooth surface. Metal implants can be cleaned and sterilized using the standard techniques, making them convenient to utilize. However, following developments in materials and similarly inadequate successive rates with metals (cobalt–chromium stainless steel and gold), these materials have been outdated and have been substituted by newer ones. Metallic implants are suitable for high load-bearing functions due to their excellent mechanical qualities. Some of the attributes of metallic implants are as follows.

Metallic implants have been a mainstay in orthopedic surgery and dentistry for decades, due to their peerless set of traits that make them well-suited for replacing or reinforcing bones and teeth. Figure 21.5 shows the application of metallic implants being used to replace deteriorated hips. Here are some key properties of metallic implants:

- *High Mechanical Strength*: Metals like titanium and stainless steel boast superior strength and stiffness compared to bone. This allows them to withstand significant loads and stresses placed upon bones, particularly in weight-bearing applications like hips and knees.
- *Durability and Wear Resistance*: Metallic implants are built to last for many years within the body. They exhibit excellent wear resistance, minimizing friction and wear debris that could lead to implant loosening or failure.
- *Biocompatibility*: While not perfect, some metals like titanium and certain alloys have good biocompatibility, meaning they are relatively well-tolerated by the body and cause minimal immune response.
- *Osteoconductivity*: Certain metallic implants, particularly those with textured surfaces, promote bone growth on their surface. This osseointegration is vital for long-term stable operation of the implant.

21.3.1.1 Stainless Steel

The most prevalent metallic implant material is surgical-grade stainless steel 316LSS. This grade has a wide spectrum of mechanical, physical, and chemical qualities and costs a reasonable amount due to the readily available materials. Stainless steel has several alloying elements, including Cr, Cu, Mo, Mn, Si, Ni, and C. Its great corrosion resistance comes from the production of a chromium oxide film that prevents oxidation. However, stainless steel can leak metal ions that include Cr, Fe, and Ni, which can be toxic to the humans and can lead to serious medical problems (31). To reduce these harmful consequences, several surface modification techniques are used. Ceramic, polymer, and composite coatings are placed on implants made from metals to avoid any contamination. The polymer PCL approved by FDA is preferred for its biocompatibility and strong mechanical strength. Due of its hydrophobic character, PCL is frequently mixed with hydrophilic polymers to improve cell proliferation and adherence (32). The ability to resist corrosion of SS316L can be improved further by adding Ni to it. However, carbon present in stainless steel can cause oxidation of Cr at grain boundaries, resulting in pitting action or corrosion. Despite these challenges, SS is commonly utilized for biomedical implants and critical operations, such as knee, ankle, and hip replacements. Stainless steel implants offer excellent physical and tribological characteristics while also being compatible with the body's biological systems. Because of metallic leaching concerns, these implants are normally reserved for short-term use (33). Implants can be subjected to both dynamic and static loading conditions when they are placed in the body. Dynamic loading includes the implant's fatigue strength, and fatigue is a common cause of failure. Biological conditions within the human body can cause corrosion and pitting, which significantly reduce implant's fatigue strength. Corrosion is particularly not required since it brings down the implant's fatigue power (34).

21.3.1.2 Co-based Alloys

Co-based alloys are regarded as one of the prominent materials for implant applications. These type of alloys initially appeared in the beginning of the 1900s as hip replacement implant material. Co-based alloys exhibit improved corrosion, mechanical attributes, and wear resistance properties and are mostly employed in bioimplant applications. In vitro studies and in vivo studies indicated that Co-based alloys have superior biological compatibility and also can be used to manufacture surgical implants for the knee, hip, broken bone surfaces, and shoulder (35). Co-Cr-Mo is the widely utilized combination of Co alloys because of its unique mix of ductility, stiffness, and strength. As compared to implants made from other metallic materials, they demonstrate increased density, elastic modulus, and stiffness, this makes it an appropriate material for the implant technique (36). This form of alloy is commonly used for long-term fixation of implant since it maintains its original properties for a long period after implantation. For patients aged 60 and older had a cumulative chance of endurance of 96% after 12 years. These alloys and polyethylene with a high molecular weight are used in prosthetic ankles and knees. These are still not suggested for joint attachments because of their low friction along with tensile strength. Co-based alloys have low frictional qualities, making them unsuitable for joints and bearing surfaces, despite their biocompatibility and corrosion resistance (37).

21.3.1.3 Titanium-based Alloys

Titanium-based alloys are preferred for implants because of their superior strength, resistance to corrosion, passiveness, improved biological compatibility, low density and low modulus. The aviation industry was the first to witness the use of Ti-based alloys because of their high corrosion resistivity. Its high biological compatibility with the bodily conditions made it ideal for bioimplants. The modulus of titanium is substantially low as compared to steel and Co-based implants, favoring its applicability for implantation. Aside from implants, titanium is employed in a variety of medical applications, including synthetic legs, limbs, and wheelchairs. The strength of Ti alloy implants is comparable to that made of stainless steel alloys, but their density is substantially lower. Titanium-based alloys are deployed in manufacturing of hip and knee replacements, dental implants, pacemakers, heart valves, bone screws, and several types of surgical equipment. Ti-based alloys have limitations, such as decreased shear strength, leaving them unsuitable for some medical uses. Furthermore, the high value of coefficient of friction in Ti-based alloys can cause wear debris and may release these particles to the body, resulting in pain and suffering (38).

21.3.1.4 Iron-Chromium-Nickel-based Alloys

Stainless steel alloys are commonly used to make orthopedic and implant devices. Ramus blades, ramus frames, and stabilizer pins are made of iron-based alloys. The alloy is specifically vulnerable to pitting corrosion, as nickel being a key element, it must be used with precaution to preserve its passivated (oxide) surface condition. Their use in allergic people should be avoided. They are corrosion resistant because of their high corrosion potential. If implant made from cobalt, titanium, zirconium, or carbon biomaterials are employed, it may result in the formation of galvanic couple and bio corrosion may occur (39).

21.3.1.5 Titanium-Zirconium Alloy (Straumann Roxolid)

Titanium zirconium alloys containing 13%–17% zirconium (TiZr1317) are exceptional to pure titanium in terms of mechanical performance such as fatigue resistance and tensile strength. Titanium and zirconium do not hinder the development of bone-forming cells, which are needed for implant anchorage. Roxolid, which is 50% durable in terms of strength than pure titanium and fulfills the criteria of dental implantologists, was created by Straumann. The surfaces which are topographically identical to pure titanium implants can be produced by performing sandblasting and by doing acid etching on TiZr1317 having monophasic structure since it has exceptional mechanical qualities. TiZr1317 due to its higher mechanical properties is also used to manufacture implants and implant components which are very thin and can be subjected to heavy loads and wear, considering that the material has to exhibit the same good biocompatibility as pure titanium (40).

21.3.1.6 Mg Alloys

The biodegradable orthopedic implants based on the magnesium alloys eliminate the difficulties related with long duration of implant placement in the human body. Recently, decomposable metallic implants have been studied as biomedical implants. Magnesium (Mg) is the fourth most prevalent ion in the human body and performs a substantial part in biological mechanism. Mg corrodes faster in a chloride-containing anatomical milieu, hence it has developed as a biocompatible and decomposable material for use in implants. Furthermore, magnesium and its alloys have gained significant recognition in the domain of biodegradable alloys because of their prime qualities such as low density, an elastic modulus similar to that of bones, biological compatibility, lightweight, and outstanding mechanical qualities.

When the desired purpose of these implanted components, orthopedics screw and plate, for which they were implanted is fulfilled, the after surgeries done to extract them are painful and pose economic impact on patients. Patients may end up in contacting nosocomial infections as the result of surgeries to remove implants from the body of patient thus delaying the patient's return to a regular lifestyle. These biodegradable metallic implants are helpful in preventing operations done to remove implant components by disintegrating in situ, eliminating the need of after surgery to remove them (41,42).

21.3.2 Polymers-based Implants

Initial attempts for resin implants by using methyl methacrylate were mainly ineffective. However, in 1969, Hodosh proved that polymers are biologically friendly materials. His study on the creation of replica of tooth implants with polymethacrylate led to the concept of polymer-based tooth implants. When natural teeth were replaced, these polymer copies proved to be the most effective at restoring both function alongside look.

Polymers were chosen for several reasons:

- The physical properties of polymers can be easily altered depending upon their applications and specific purpose in the body such as being made porous and softer.
- Polymer-based implants provide a wider range of flexibility for better replication of body part.
- Polymers, unlike metals, do not generate microwaves or electrolytic currents.
- Their fibrous connective tissue attachment is evident.
- Polymers are easier to inspect microscopically than metals.
- They provide a more visually appealing appearance.

Despite these advantages, there are notable disadvantages:

- Poor mechanical characteristics
- Evidences of low adhesiveness to living tissues
- Prone to severe immunologic reactions

The biodegradable implant products are generally made from polymers which may be natural polymers (42) or synthetic polymers (43). Polymers are macromolecular arrangements made up of covalently bound monomers. The repeated arrangement of prevalent monomers from the same group or different group determines whether they belong to homopolymers or copolymers. The source for natural polymers is taken from starch, collagen, hyaluronic acid derivatives, chitosan, silk, and fibrin gels. The limited mechanical strength, uncertain breakdown rate, repellency, and significant physiological activity of these natural-based polymers limit adaptability of their practical applications. The variation of breakdown rate is mostly dependent upon the type of arrangement of polymer chains, whether they are of linear, branched, or cross-linked (44), and crystallinity/amorphous nature. Polymers are flexible due to their glass transition temperature (45); therefore, above-normal body temperature polymers must be biodegradable. Polyglycolic acid (PGA), polylactic acid (PLA), poly-_-hydroxybutyrate (PHB), poly (lactic acid-co-glycolic acid) (PLGA), and poly-"-caprolactone (PCL) are the commonly employed biodegradable polymers (45). Degradable sutures are made from polymers such as PLA, PGA, and poly lactic acid-co-glycolic acid. The first known polymer used for sutures was PLA (47). PLA was made from natural materials like starch and corn. L-PLA (crystalline PLA) is less hostile to hydrolysis than DL-PLA (amorphous PLA).

Other types of polymers which include hyaluronan, collagens, and fibrin glue are also degraded enzymatically through collagenase, hyaluronic acid hydrolase, and plasmin, sequentially. Implants for bone restoration and other load-bearing applications demand high mechanical strength; hence metals and ceramics are favored. However, in some situations, adverse consequences such as corrosion, inflammation, and bone loss are reported. As a result, polymers are being evaluated for bone restoration applications due to their high tensile strength, elastic elasticity, and resistance to corrosion. It is important to remember that as implantation time increases, polymers lose mechanical strength due to degradation/resorbability. Polymers such as PGA, PLA, and PLGA are now routinely used for bone implants. Screws, bone fixation objects, anklebones, patella, and other fixing devices are also used in various applications. Some downsides of these polymers include X-ray transparency, unexplained effects of foreign body interactions, and decreasing mechanical strength with time (46–48).

21.3.3 Ceramic-based Implants

Ceramic implants serve their purpose in a range of applications, including orthopedic and dental implants and many other applications. Ceramic implants interact with the internal environment of the body through physical attachment, fixation, and bone tissue growth within their porous structure. Calcium phosphate, often known as hydroxyapatite (HA), is a frequently employed bioactive ceramic material for implants. Calcium-based ceramic materials have been defined by their calcium-to-phosphate ratio. Hydroxyapatite's bioactivity for implants depends on its ratio. Hydroxyapatite is suitable for non-load-bearing implants and has degradable characteristics. When degradable ceramic implants, such as calcium phosphate, are subjected to water and a specific temperature, they produce HA phase (49). These degradable property of implants are temperature sensitive, which causes problems when fabricating them. Moreover, HA is coated on a variety of metallic implants using surface modification techniques like laser coating and plasma spraying processes. These coatings enhance the underlying material's biocompatibility, improve interfacial characteristics, and prevent deterioration (50–53). HA is used as bone cement material for prosthetic joints. In similar function, additional ceramic materials including SiO_2, P_2O_5, CaO, and Na_2O are employed in comparable applications. Some downsides of these polymers include X-ray transparency, unexplained effects of interaction with foreign bodies, and decreasing mechanical strength with time.

Ceramics are popular for their stress-shielding effects due to their high elastic moduli and high hardness, and slow propagation of crack growth over time, which considerably decrease the dependability of the implants. As well, fabrication, brittleness, and fracture toughness issues limit their application as bioimplants. Ceramics hold the brittleness factor, which prohibits their functionality in terms of load-bearing applications (hip implants). If the difference between mechanical properties of ceramic material used and bone is large, then the bone will not be able to bear the load, thus leading to catastrophic failure of the bone (54). Ceramic composite materials present unmatched qualities compared to single materials. The deficient mechanical properties of monolithic ceramics can be resolved by composite ceramics while declining the drawbacks of each component. The noticeable features of composites, for instance the weight to strength ratio, enable them to be used extensively for the refurbishment of bones and restoration of dental fillings and ligaments. Further, the composites produced through the combination of ceramics which are non-reactive to biological environment of the body and bio active show better bioactivity and mechanical strength (55). Key mentionings are hydroxyapatite and Al_2O_3 composites which show better bone and tissue, good bioactivity, and superior load resistance (56).

21.4 CONCLUSION

The chapter underscores the critical importance of selecting and engineering biomaterials for load-bearing bioimplants. By leveraging the strengths of advanced materials like alloys, ceramics, and polymers, and through meticulous design and surface modification, the feasibility of production is possible for bioimplants that are not only mechanically robust but also highly biocompatible and effective in long-term applications.

- Understanding key characteristics of biomaterials is very crucial which influence their bioactivity. These characteristic properties are critical for selecting the appropriate material for bioimplant applications, particularly in load-bearing scenarios.
- For implants under heavy load-bearing applications such as orthopedic implants, implants used in dental applications, and spinal implants, the materials must possess excellent mechanical strength but also needs to ensure biocompatibility so that they do not react with the body.
- Advanced alloys provided greater flexibility for creation of such implants which can provide specific and stringent requirements for various medical conditions.

- Modern sophisticated biomaterials, namely ceramics, metals, and polymers, have revolutionized the field of bioimplants. These materials have enabled the development of implants that can withstand heavy loads and high strains, particularly in orthopedic applications where they can serve to repair broken or damaged parts of joints and bones.

21.5 FUTURE PERSPECTIVES

The field of improved biomaterials for load-bearing bioimplants is on the verge of substantial achievements. Future biomaterials are projected to have improved mechanical qualities, particularly increased tensile strength and durability against cyclic loading while retaining or enhancing biocompatibility. Material science innovations, such as novel polymer composites and ceramic–metal hybrids, will be critical to comprehending these advances. Smart and sensitive biomaterials will become more common, allowing implants to respond to physiological changes within the body. For example, smart implants could release anti-inflammatory medications when inflammation is detected or modify their mechanical properties in real time to match the surrounding tissues. There will also be an emphasis on biodegradable and bioactive materials that stimulate tissue regeneration and repair, lowering the need for additional procedures and enhancing patient outcomes. Moreover, additive manufacturing techniques like 3D printing will play a pivotal role in manufacturing specific implants depending upon the medical requirements and properties of tissues and bones.

REFERENCES

1. Kaivosoja, E.; Tiainen, V.-M. *Materials used for hip and knee implants.* Helsinki University Central Hospital, Orton Orthopaedic Hospital of the Invalid Foundation, Finland.
2. Awasthi, A.; Saxenam, K.K.; Dwivedi, R.K. An investigation on classification and characterization of bio materials and additive manufacturing techniques for bioimplants. https://doi.org/10.1016/j.matpr.2020.12.176
3. Awasthi, A.; Saxenam, K.K.; Dwivedi, R.K. An investigation on classification and characterization of bio materials and additive manufacturing techniques for bioimplants. https://doi.org/10.1016/j.matpr.2020.12.176
4. Kaivosoja, E.; Tiainen, V.-M. *Materials used for hip and knee implants.* Helsinki University Central Hospital, Orton Orthopaedic Hospital of the Invalid Foundation, Finland.
5. Aliyu, A.A.A.; Abdul-Rani, A.M.; Ginta, T.L.; Prakash, C.; Axinte, E.; Razak, M.A.; Ali, S. A review of additive mixed-electric discharge machining: Current status and future perspectives for surface modification of biomedical implants. *Adv. Mater. Sci. Eng.* 2017; 2017(1): 8723239.
6. Manivasagam, G.; Suwas, S. Biodegradable Mg and Mg based alloys for biomedical implants. *Mater. Sci. Technol.* 2014. https://doi.org/10.1179/1743284713Y.0000000500.
7. Ratner, B.D.; Hoffman, A.S.; Schoen, F.J.; Lemons, J. E. *Biomaterials science: An introduction to materials in medicine.* Academic Press Elsevier. 2004.
8. Luthringer, T.A.; Vigdorchik, J.M. A preoperative workup of a 'hip-spine' total hip arthroplasty patient: A simplified approach to a complex problem. *J. Arthroplasty.* 2019. https://doi.org/10.1016/j.arth.2019.01.012.

9. Zwawi, M. Recent advances in bio-medical implants; Mechanical properties, surface modifications and applications. https://doi.org/10.1088/2631-8695/ac8ae2
10. Sharma, K.; Saxena, K.K.; Shukla, M. Effect of multiple stone-wales and vacancy defects on the mechanical behavior of carbon nanotubes using molecular dynamics. 2012. https://doi.org/10.1016/j.proeng.2012.06.390.
11. Zwawi, M. Recent advances in bio-medical implants; Mechanical properties, surface modifications and applications. https://doi.org/10.1088/2631-8695/ac8ae2
12. Kang, C.W.; Fang, F.Z. State of the art of bioimplants manufacturing: Part II, *Adv. Manuf.* 2018. https://doi.org/10.1007/s40436-018-0218-9.
13. Advincula, M.C.; Petersen, D.; Rahemtulla, F.; Advincula, R.; Lemons, J.E. Surface analysis and biocorrosion properties of nanostructured surface sol-gel coatings on Ti6Al4V titanium alloy implants. *J. Biomed. Mater. Res.-Part B Appl. Biomater.* 2007. https://doi.org/10.1002/jbm.b.30575.
14. Özkurt, Z.; Kazazoğlu, E. Zirconia dental implants: A literature review. *J. Oral Implantol.* 2011. https://doi.org/10.1563/AAID-JOI-D-09-00079.
15. Teo, A.J.T.; Mishra, A.; Park, I.; Kim, Y.J.; Park, W.T.; Yoon, Y.J. Polymeric biomaterials for medical implants and devices, *ACS Biomater. Sci. Eng.* 2016. https://doi.org/10.1021/acsbiomaterials.5b00429.
16. Witte, F. The history of biodegradable magnesium implants: A review. *Acta Biomater.* 2010. https://doi.org/10.1016/j.actbio.2010.02.028.
17. Radovic. M.; Lara-Curzio, E.; Riester, L. Comparison of different experimental techniques for determination of elastic properties of solids. *Mater. Sci. Eng. A.* 2004; 368: 56–70.
18. Mohammed, M.T.; Khan, Z.A.; Siddiquee, A.N. Beta titanium alloys: The lowest elastic modulus for biomedical applications: A review. *Int. J. Chem. Mol. Nucl. Mater. Met. Eng.* 2014; 8: 726.
19. Chen, Q.; Thouas, G.A. Metallic implant biomaterials. *Mater. Sci. Eng. R Rep.* 2015; 87: 1–57.
20. Mecenas, P.; Espinosa, D.G.; Cardoso, P.C.; Normando, D. Stainless steel or titanium mini-implants? A systematic review. *Angle Orthod.* 2020; 90: 587–97.
21. Khosravi, F.; Nouri Khorasani, S.; Khalili, S.; Esmaeely Neisiany, R.; Rezvani Ghomi, E.; Ejeian, F.; Das, O.; Nasr-Esfahani, M.H. Development of a highly proliferated bilayer coating on 316L stainless steel implants. *Polymers.* 2020; 12: 1022
22. Sidambe, A.T. Biocompatibility of advanced manufactured titanium implants—A review. *Materials.* 2014; 7: 8168–88.
23. Ibrahim, M.Z.; Sarhan, A.A.; Yusuf, F.; Hamdi, M. Biomedical materials and techniques to improve the tribological, mechanical and biomedical properties of orthopedic implants–A review article. *J. Alloys Compd.* 2017; 714: 636–67.
24. Saini, M. Implant biomaterials: A comprehensive review. *World J. Clin. Cases.* 2015. https://doi.org/10.12998/wjcc.v3.i1.52.
25. Ratner, B.D.; Hoffman, A.S.; Schoen, F.J.; Lemons, J.E. *Biomaterials science: An introduction to materials in medicine.* Academic Press Elsevier. 2004.
26. Saini, M.; Singh, Y.; Arora, P.; Arora, V.; Jain, K. Implant biomaterials: A comprehensive review. *World J. Clin. Cases.* 2015; 3(1): 52–7.
27. Awasthi, A.; Saxenam, K.K.; Dwivedi, R.K. An investigation on classification and characterization of bio materials and additive manufacturing techniques for bioimplants. https://doi.org/10.1016/j.matpr.2020.12.176
28. Kargozar, S.; Ramakrishna, S.; Mozafari, M. Chemistry of biomaterials: Future prospects. *Curr. Opin. Biomed. Eng.* 2019. https://doi.org/10.1016/j.cobme.2019.07.003
29. Mohammed, M.T.; Khan, Z.A.; Siddiquee, A.N. Beta titanium alloys: The lowest elastic modulus for biomedical applications: A review surface modifications through FSP view project machining view project. *Int. J. Chem. Nucl. Metall. Mater. Eng.* 2014; 8(8): 726–31.

30. Park, G.E.; Webster, T.J. A review of nanotechnology for the development of better orthopedic implants. *J. Biomed. Nanotechnol.* 2006. https://doi.org/10.1166/jbn.2005.003
31. Saini, M.; Singh, Y; Arora, P.; Arora, V.; Jain, K. Implant biomaterials: A comprehensive review. *World J. Clin. Cases.* 2015; 3(1): 52–7.
32. Geetha, M.; Singh, A.K.; Asokamani, R.; Gogia, A.K. Ti based biomaterials, the ultimate choice for orthopaedic implants–A review. *Prog. Mater. Sci.* 2009; 54: 397–425.
33. Kamachimudali, U.; Sridhar, T.M.; Raj, B. Corrosion of bio implants. *Sadhana.* 2003; 28: 601–37.
34. Patnaik, L.; Maity, S.R.; Kumar, S. Status of nickel free stainless steel in biomedical field: A review of last 10 years and what else can be done. *Mater. Today Proc.* 2020; 26: 638–43.
35. Mahmoudi Hashemi, P.; Borhani, E.; Nourbakhsh, M.S. A review on nanostructured stainless steel implants for biomedical application. *Nanomedicine J.* 2016; 3: 202–16.
36. Amirtharaj Mosas, K.K.; Chandrasekar, A.R.; Dasan, A.; Pakseresht, A.; Galusek, D. Recent advancements in materials and coatings for biomedical implants. *Gels.* 2022; 8: 323. https://doi.org/10.3390/gels8050323
37. Yu, W.; Li, X.; Ma, X.; Xu, X. Biomechanical analysis of inclined and cantilever design with different implant framework materials in mandibular complete-arch implant restorations. *J. Prosthet. Dent.* 2022; 127(5): 783–e1.
38. González-Mora, V.A.; Hoffmann, M.; Stroosnijder, R.; Espinar, E.; Llamas, J.M.; Fernández-Fairén, M.; Gil, F.J. Influence of different cocrmo counterfaces on wear in UHMWPE for artificial joints. *J. Biomed. Sci. Eng.* 2011; 4: 375–82.
39. Sidambe, A.T. Biocompatibility of advanced manufactured titanium implants—A review. *Materials.* 2014; 7: 8168–88.
40. Saini, M.; Singh, Y.; Arora, P.; Arora, V.; Jain, K. Implant biomaterials: A comprehensive review. *World J. Clin. Cases.* 2015; 3(1): 52–7.
41. Chiapasco, M.; Casentini, P.; Zaniboni, M.; Corsi, E.; Anello, T. Titanium-zirconium alloy narrow-diameter implants (Straumann Roxolid(®)) for the rehabilitation of horizontally deficient edentulous ridges: Prospective study on 18 consecutive patients. *Clin. Oral Implants Res.* 2012; 23: 1136–41. PMID: 22092806. https://doi.org/10.1111/j.1600-0501.2011.02296.x
42. Amukarimi, S.; Mozafari, M. Biodegradable magnesium-based biomaterials: An overview of challenges and opportunities. *Med. Comm.* 2021; 2: 123.
43. Tsakiris, V.; Tardei, C.; Clicinschi, F.M. Biodegradable Mg alloys for orthopedic implants—A review. *J. Magnes. Alloy.* 2021; 9: 1884–1905.
44. Gunatillake, P.A.; Adhikari R. Biodegradable synthetic polymers for tissue engineering. *Eur. Cell Mater.* 2003; 5: 01–16. https://doi.org/10.22203/eCM.v005a01.
45. He, S.; Yaszemski, M.J.; Yasko, A.W.; Engel, P.S.; Mikos, A.G. Injectable biodegradable polymer composites based on poly (propylene fumarate) crosslinked with poly (ethylene glycol)-dimethacrylate. *Biomaterials.* 2000; 21: 2389–94.
46. Lodge, T.P.; McLeish, T.C. Self-concentrations and effective glass transition temperatures in polymer blends. *Macromolecules.* 2000; 33: 5278–84
47. Singh, J. Sustainability issues in laser-based additive manufacturing. In *Handbook of laser-based sustainable surface modification and manufacturing technologies.* CRC Press. 2023. pp. 167–89.
48. Witte, F.; Hort, N.; Vogt, C.; Cohen, S.; Kainer, K.U.; Willumeit, R.; Feyerabend, F. Degradable biomaterials based on magnesium corrosion. *Curr. Opin. Solid State Mater. Sci.* 2008; 12: 63–72.
49. Cappiello, M.; Luongo, R.; Di Iorio, D.; Bugea, C.; Cocchetto, R.; Celletti, R. Evaluation of peri-implant bone loss around platform-switched implants. *Int. J. Periodontics Restor. Dent.* 2008; 28: 347–55.

50. Yedida, V.V.S.; Vasudev, H. A review on the development of thermal barrier coatings by using thermal spray techniques. *Mater. Today Proc.* 2022; 50: 1458–64.
51. Prashar, G.; Vasudev, H. A review on the influence of process parameters and heat treatment on the corrosion performance of Ni-based thermal spray coatings. *Surf. Rev. Lett.* 2022; 29: 2230001.
52. Prashar, G.; Vasudev, H.; Surface topology analysis of plasma sprayed Inconel625-Al2O3 composite coating. *Mater. Today Proc. [Internet].* 2022; 50: 607–11. Available from: https://linkinghub.elsevier.com/retrieve/pii/S221478532102109X.
53. Majji, B.G.R.; Vasudev, H.; Bansal, A. A review on the oxidation and wear behavior of the thermally sprayed high-entropy alloys. *Mater. Today Proc.* 2022; 50: 1447–51.
54. Andreiotelli, M.; Wenz, H.J.; Kohal, R.-J. Are ceramic implants a viable alternative to titanium implants? A systematic literature review. *Clin. Oral Implants Res.* 2009; 20: 32–47.
55. Ridzwan, M.I.Z.; Shuib, S.; Hassan, A.Y.; Shokri, A.A.; Mohammad Ibrahim, M.N. Problem of stress shielding and improvement to the hip implant designs: A review. *J. Med. Sci.* 2007; 7: 460–7.
56. Fiorillo, L.; Cicciù, M.; Tozum, T.F.; Saccucci, M.; Orlando, C.; Romano, G.L.; D'amico, C.; Cervino, G. Endosseous dental implant materials and clinical outcomes of different alloys: A systematic review. *Materials.* 2022; 15: 1979.

22 Advancing Surface Quality in Metal Additive Manufacturing

The Role of Magnetorheological Finishing

Manoj Kumar and Manpreet Singh

CONTENTS

22.1 INTRODUCTION

The technique known as additive manufacturing or 3D printing has changed the face of manufacturing in the last couple of decades [1–4]. This new technology dates back to the 1980s, when Chuck Hull pioneered stereolithography, a technique that enables

 DOI: 10.1201/9781003516064-22

manufacturing of prototype product through layering by successively printing cross-sectional layers of ultraviolet cure of material [5–8]. Since then AM has come a long way for what it is now comprising a variety of technology and material and spread in a number of industrial applications. Basically, AM is every technique that involves bonding materials to form objects from 3D model data, layer by layer rather than from cutting or etching away material [5]. It is possible to fabricate structures of various shapes and patterns that are hardly practicable with other techniques [6–8]. The common starting point for the AM process is a 3D computer-aided design model or a CAD that is processed by specific software to section the model into thin layers [9]. These layers act as a map or/and templates for the AM machine, where layers of material are deposited or solidified. The kind of materials to be used also varies with the different AM technologies where they can include plastics and/or metals and even ceramics and biological materials [10].

Several necessary AM technologies have appeared and developed in the course of several years. One of the most common techniques is fused deposition modeling (FDM) that extrudes thermoplastic, relatively inexpensive and not very complicated to use. Selective laser sintering (SLS) and (selective laser melting) (SLM)—differ in that layers of powder materials are sintered or melted with the help of lasers to make strong, functional parts. Stereolithography (SLA) and digital light processing (DLP) use the photopolymers that undergo polymerization in the presence of light to form very accurate models from liquid resins [11–15]. There are various reasons that have led to the adoption of AM, some of them being following the various benefits that come with the new technology over the conventional means. The first one is what one might call the unparalleled design freedom [16]. AM facilitates the development of intricate internal structures, networks, and natural shapes which are almost impracticable or would require humongous capital to build when employing conventional technologies. This capability has been used to achieve great strides in areas like aerospace, where one can have strong yet exceptionally light components that can be designed and manufactured having the best topology [17]. Third, AM helps to avoid expensively equipped large batch production and high tools costs for single, unique pieces. It has been especially revolutionary in such manufacturing sectors as the medical ones, as custom-made implants and prosthetics for individuals can be produced. Further, AM has tremendously reduced the product development time due to incorporation of the tool called rapid prototyping, whereby the designers and engineers are able to produce many patterns and test their efficiencies [18]. The impact of AM on the environment is also quite viable as well. By accumulating the object in structure on the layer by layer basis, AM reduces material waste as compared to the subtraction strategies [19–21]. In addition, it is pointed out that on-demand manufacturing of products and in particular manufacturing of parts and components near the point of usage can minimize transport costs and thus, carbon footprint [22]. However, these are not the only issues AM faces as we will discuss in the rest of the chapter. Some of them include, the material limitations, slow production rates for the large volume production, and mechanical properties which have limited its applicability in the past [23]. Nevertheless, current research studies are constantly working toward overcoming these restrictions that help to unravel the opportunities of using AM in different fields. There are also predictions of the growth of influence of AM technology in the future as it develops in the industry and society. From providing a basis for new forms of mass customization to changing the scope of supply networks through demand-based production, AM is being one of the key technologies for the future manufacturing industry. Arguably, the future developments of AM will be enhanced with the integration of other similar technologies like artificial intelligence, robotics, and the Internet of Things [23–26].

22.1.1 Overview of Magnetorheological Finishing

Magnetorheological Finishing (MRF) is one of the state-of-the-art polishing techniques that have been receiving much attention for the last few years, especially for the fine finishing of the precision molds [27]. **Figure 22.1** shows the schematic diagram of the turning-type MR finishing experimental setup on the standard conventional lathe machine which helps to perform the MR finishing. This new method utilizes the characteristics of magnetorheological (MR) fluids in producing a manageable and very accurate polishing tool. The main part of the MRF is a smart material—the magnetorheological fluid, including micron-sized particles of magnetically soft materials dispersed in a carrier liquid such as water or oil [28–30]. These particles, usually carbonyl iron particles, are combined with abrasives and stabilizing agents. The main features of MR fluids are their capability to respond to alteration of rheological characteristics and do it reversibly and quickly upon exposure to a magnetic field. This means that when there is no applied magnetic field, the MR fluid works like the ordinary fluid. Nevertheless, when placed in a magnetic field, the

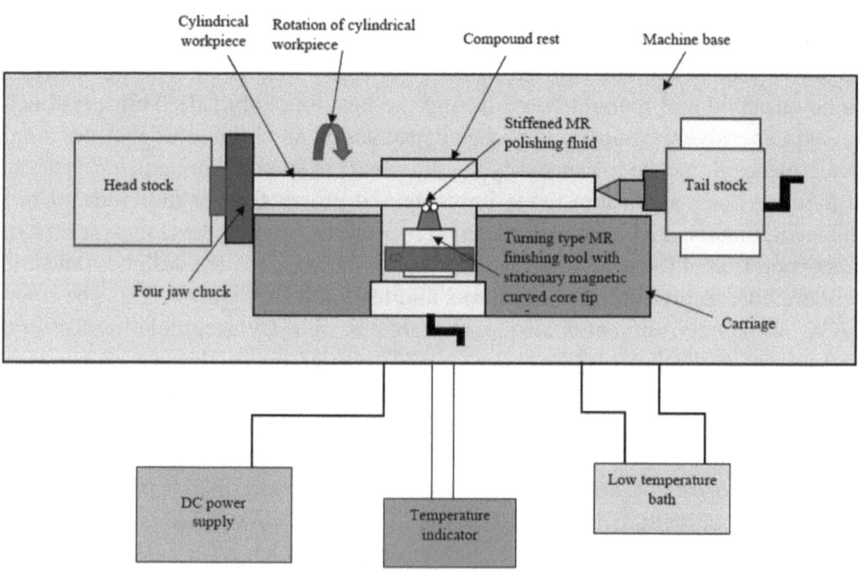

FIGURE 22.1 Schematic diagram of the turning-type MR finishing experimental setup on the standard conventional lathe machine. (Created by authors)

suspended particles in real plasma respond to the field and chain up along the field lines. This alignment substantially enhances the increase in the shear viscosity and yield stress of the fluid and seems to transform the fluid to a semi solid material. It is observed that the strength of this transformation can be changed as per one's requirement through the variation in the strength of the magnetic field [31–34]. In the MRF process, this controllable stiffening of the fluid is used to design the tool to precisely polish [35]. A standard setup of MRF comprises a wheel that is partially immersed in an MR fluid containment. The wheel, in its motion, presents a ribbon of the MR fluid toward the polishing zone of the workpiece. In this area, a large magnetic field is used, and this makes the fluid turn into a compliant-polishing tool [36–40]. The stiffened fluid ribbon comes into contact with the workpiece which needs to be polished. The abrasive particles in the fluid, that is, the cutting tool, will now be fixed in place, and as the magnetic field envelops the workpiece, material will be cut on the microscopic level. The polishing action is very specific and selective thus allowing the developer to remove material in the specific part of the surface that needs to be shaped [37]. MRF has significant and unique advantages, and one of that is its ability to fine finish intricate and free form surfaces. It adapts to the complex shapes of the workpiece, allowing uniform pressure regardless of the shape of the workpiece. Due to this, MRF is especially appropriate in the finishing of optical elements, precision molds, and intricate aerospace components. Thus, in an MRF it becomes possible to achieve very fine control over the material removal rate [38].

These are the magnetic field, the distance from the wheel to the working piece, wheel speed, and MR fluid type. The level of control is such that material removal is possible on a nanometer scale for the attainment of substrates having very low roughness with measurements in sub-nanometer range. The last important dimension, which can be isolated in the structure of MRF, is regarding its determinism. While other methods of polishing are appreciable as they might involve the use of expert operators, MRF has the capability of being simulated to a near accuracy. This makes it easy to predict how much material is being removed and the final surface finish, which means that the process can be fully automated to deliver excellent reproducibility. The MRF is also beneficial in terms of providing the surface finish [3, 31]. The process causes lower subsurface damage and residual stresses as compared to the conventional abrasives polishing. This is especially useful in applications that demand polished surfaces for operations, such as in the manufacturing of optical components or high-precision mechanical parts. Thus, all in all, MRF has depicted appreciable competencies in learning, but some challenges have been identified as well. Disadvantages of the MR fluids are that the fluids and equipment are costly, especially for small uses, and the systems may also be somewhat complicated [41–44].

Also, controlling the stability of MR fluids for several weeks/months and handling the issue of fluid disposal are continual research topics. Nevertheless, due to the specific features that become possible through its use, MRF is used in a variety of highly accurate industries [45]. MRF is used in the semiconductor industry where silicon wafer and other components are polished [46]. The aerospace and defense industries also use MRF for the finishing of such critical components that have very demanding surface finish specifications. New applications and improvements

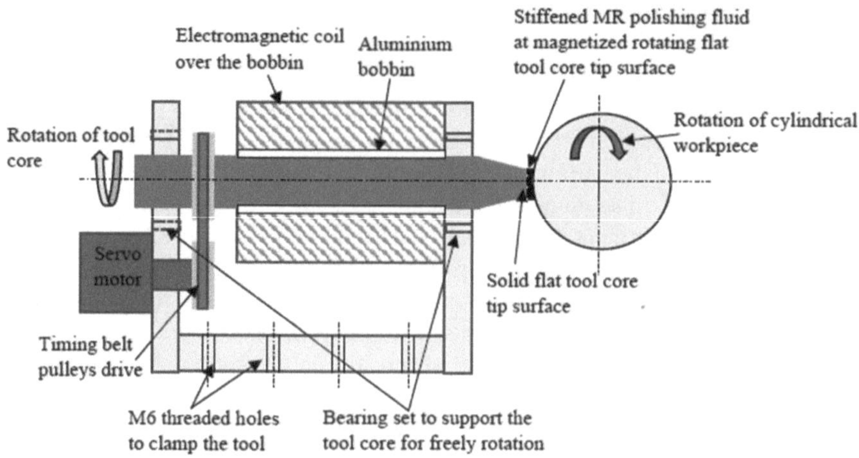

FIGURE 22.2 A rotating flat tool core tip surface in the present improved magnetorheological (MR) finishing process to fine finish the external surface of the cylindrical workpieces. (Created by authors)

have continued to appear on the research front as work on MRF goes on [33–37]. **Figure 22.2** depicts the rotating flat tool core tip surface in the present improved magnetorheological (MR) finishing process to fine finish the external surface of the cylindrical workpieces.

22.1.2 Scope and Objectives of the Chapter

This chapter seeks to give a systematic evaluation of the relationship between AM and MRF while also concentrating on the function of MRF as a post-processing method for AM products. Being two very active research areas, this chapter aims at providing a step toward an organized knowledge as well as focusing on recent developments in the fields and future trends for research in the areas. The primary objective of this chapter is to assess the effectiveness and potential of MRF in addressing one of the key challenges in AM: on the other hand, decreasing the surface roughness increases the surface finish. AM has changed the way components are manufactured due to the ability to produce complex geometries and customized parts; however, the process of building up a component layer by layer produces surface defects such as stair-step effects, partially melted particles, and support structure residues. This surface roughness can affect functionality, appearance, and dimensional tolerances of the final product in AM. In this chapter, an attempt will be made to investigate the use of MRF to AM parts to understand its suitability to the surface quality problems currently facing the AM industry. The chapter starts with discussing the main surface features characteristic of diverse AM processes in terms of their surface characteristics. It will be discussed how the material properties, process parameters, and the geometry of the part can affect surface quality in various categories of AM techniques. This analysis will form a basic comprehension of the surface finish issue particular to AM to precede the introduction of MRF as a solution. In this chapter, the basics of MRF as well as the method of its operation, influence of crucial parameters, and characteristics of MR fluids are described. We will explore how each of these aspects of MRF can be adapted to the AM parts such as complexity, geometrical aspect, and material aspect. Finally, a great part of this chapter is allocated to outline the case studies and experimental findings of the application of MRF to AM parts. By scrutinizing papers in aerospace, medical, and precision engineering industries, we will be able to produce a holistic qualitative assessment on the efficiency of the proposed MRF system. This section will present a quantitative analysis on how the surface roughness has been improved, how the dimensions have been accurately developed and the mechanical properties affected. Apart from the assessment of strengths, this chapter will also discuss the weakness and shortcomings of applying MRF on AM parts. **Table 22.1** represents the challenges in MRF for AM parts and potential solutions. The target is to make a SWOT analysis regarding the applicability of MRF in an industrial, large-scale setting when evaluating the economic sanity of the proposed technology and equipment in terms of their cost, processing time and efficiency, and other facilities. The chapter will also position MRF in the larger category of post-processing methods for applications in AM. Finally, we will seek to explain how MRF can be benefited from other works done in the same finishing field, including abrasive flow machining and chemical as well as laser polishing. MRF can then be shown to have a number of benefits that are not realized when alternative techniques are adopted, before going through cases where MRF may not be the best solution.

Future directions of this chapter will be to discuss possible trends and development in the subject area. We will further talk about existing and planned research work in the areas like characteristic MR fluid for specific AM materials, the combination of MRF with AM processes for finish during manufacturing, and MRF integrated with other processes. The implications of these trends to the extension of AM in the continuation of precision applications will also be assessed. Environmental concerns as well as safety issues will also be included in this reviewing. In the next step, MRF's sustainability in regard to conventional finishing approaches will be compared in terms of material input, waste production, and energy demand. Measures used in the handling of MR fluids and explanation on how to operate MRF equipment will be covered, giving users a broad outlook on the technology.

TABLE 22.1
Challenges in MRF for AM Parts and Potential Solutions

Challenge	Impact	Potential Solution
MR Fluid Stability	Inconsistent finishing	Advanced formulations, continuous circulation
Process Control	Variable results	AI-driven adaptive control, in-situ monitoring
Cost	Limited adoption	Process optimization, longer-lasting fluids
Complex Geometries	Difficult to access all surfaces	Multi-axis systems, specialized fluid delivery
Material Compatibility	Limited applicability	Custom fluid formulations for different materials

22.2 COMMON AM TECHNOLOGIES

AM is known as the process that includes many technologies, which are different from one another, have specific features, strengths, and weaknesses. It is important to know these typical technologies applied in AM to comprehend the distinctions in surface roughness which such methods create and which demand further treatment.

Fused deposition modeling (FDM), also known as fused filament fabrication (FFF) is one of the most familiar and easily available forms of AM. In FDM, a thermoplastic filament is melted by heating it to its melting point and extruding it through a nozzle on to a build plate [21]. In X and Y directions, the nozzle dispenses material in a desired manner to fabricate each layer. When one layer is built, the build platform descends and/or the nozzle ascends to commence work on the subsequent layer. FDM is said to be relatively inexpensive to use, very accessible, and there are many materials that can be used such as ABS, PLA, nylon, and different composites [46, 47]. However, it often produces parts with visible layer lines and may require support structures for overhanging features.

Stereolithography (SLA) is one of the oldest AM technologies and is renowned for its ability to produce parts with high resolution and smooth surfaces. **Figure 22.3** represents the product development cycle. SLA uses a vat of liquid photopolymer resin and a UV laser to selectively cure and solidify the resin layer by layer [48, 49]. The laser traces the cross-section of each layer on the surface of the liquid resin, causing it to harden [50]. After each layer, the build platform lowers slightly, allowing fresh resin to flow over the previous layer. SLA can produce parts with very fine details and smooth surfaces, making it popular for applications requiring high aesthetic quality or intricate features [51]. Digital light processing (DLP) is similar to SLA but uses a digital projector screen to flash a single image of each layer at once. This can make the process faster than SLA for some geometries [52]. Like SLA, DLP produces parts with high resolution and smooth surfaces, but it can be limited in build size due to the projector's resolution.

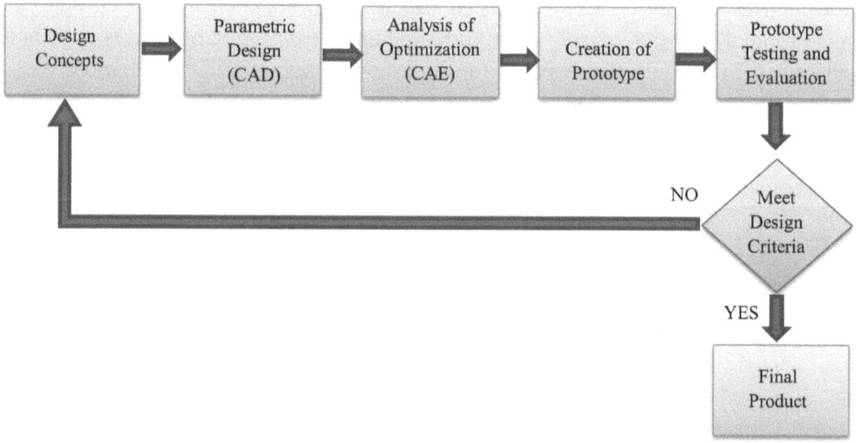

FIGURE 22.3 Product development cycle. (Created by authors)

Selective laser sintering (SLS) uses a high-power laser to sinter powdered materials, typically nylon or other thermoplastics. The laser selectively fuses the powder particles in the shape of each cross-section [53–56]. After each layer, a roller spreads a new layer of powder over the build area. SLS does not require support structures as the unsintered powder supports the part during the build. This allows for complex geometries and nested parts. SLS parts often have a slightly grainy surface finish due to the powder particles.

Selective laser melting (SLM) and direct metal laser sintering (DMLS) are similar to SLS but are used for metal powders. These processes fully melt the metal particles, creating dense, strong parts. They are widely used in aerospace, automotive, and medical industries for producing complex metal components [57–61]. The surface finish of SLM and DMLS parts can be rough and may require significant post-processing. Electron beam melting (EBM) is another metal AM technology that uses an electron beam instead of a laser to melt metal powder. EBM operates in a vacuum and at high temperatures, which can result in parts with less residual stress compared to SLM. However, the surface finish is often rougher than SLM parts. Binder jetting deposits a liquid binding agent onto a bed of powder material. The binder holds the powder particles together like a glue stick and fixes them to one another to create each layer. Following the construction of the build, the part might be sintered in a bid to enhance its sturdiness. In binder jetting, it is possible to use metal, ceramic, and polymer materials as well as some of the combinations of them. It tends to have shorter build times, but it creates parts with lower density and strength compared to other metal AM processes [62]. Casting can be likened to material jetting where droplets of a build material are dispensed and cured or solidified. Compared with existing conventional technologies, this technology can fabricate multi-material and multi-color parts with high accuracy. It can be often applied to prototype making and creating actual models [63].

DED is a 3D EUR made with a nozzle attached to a robotic manipulator that applies melted material on a surface to solidify it. This in the form of either metal wire or metal powder is fused as it is deposited by laser, electron beam, or plasma arc. Some of the typical applications of DED include repairing of worn-out parts, addition of material to the parts to increase their thickness as well as the manufacturing of hybrid components [64–69]. All these technologies possess advantages and disadvantages in relation to the available materials, construction rates, aspects of strength, precision, and surface quality. The surface texture of the produced parts and the need for its further correction as well as the intensity of the work in this area will be depending on the type of AM technology used.

22.2.1 Surface Characteristics of AM Parts

Styling parameters are the direct function of the AM technique used and have a direct relation to the functioning, looks, and efficiency of the part being made. In general, knowing these characteristics is essential for selecting the further processing methods and assessing whether the final parts correspond to the required characteristics [70].

Layer Lines and Stair-Stepping Effect: AM parts may exhibit the layer lines as a type of surface features due to the layer build-up method used in the process [71]. This is especially seen in some technologies like FDM for the reason that successive layers are clearly distinguishable. The layer lines give the appearance of steps especially on the inclined or curved structures; this is because it is hard to achieve smoothness in layering structures. The degree of this influence, the layer thickness, and the angle to the build direction have an impact on this behavior [72–75]. Higher incidence rates are more likely to exhibit stair-stepping more significantly.

Surface Roughness: The surface roughness of AM parts can vary widely depending on the technology and process parameters used. FDM parts often have relatively high surface roughness due to the visible layer lines and the rounded profile of extruded filaments. SLA and DLP typically produce smoother surfaces, but the layer lines can still be visible under close inspection. SLS parts have a characteristic grainy texture due to the partially sintered powder particles adhering to the surface [76]. Metal AM processes like SLM and EBM often result in rough surfaces due to partially melted powder particles and the formation of small spherical protrusions known as balling. **Table 22.2** represents the common AM technologies and their surface characteristics.

Support Structure Remnants: Many AM technologies require support structures to build overhanging features. After removal, these supports can leave marks or rough patches on the part surface. In FDM, support removal can sometimes damage the part surface. For resin-based technologies like SLA, support removal points are usually smaller but can still be visible and affect surface smoothness [77–82].

Warping and Curling: Thermal stresses during the build process can cause parts to warp or curl, especially in processes involving high temperatures like FDM and SLM. This can result in dimensional inaccuracies and surface deformations, particularly at the corners and edges.

Porosity: Some AM processes, particularly those involving powder bed fusion, can result in parts with internal and surface porosity. This can affect not only the surface finish but also the mechanical properties and fluid tightness of the part.

Texture and Orientation Effects: The surface texture of AM parts can vary depending on the orientation of the surface relative to the build direction. Surfaces parallel to the build platform often have different characteristics compared to that perpendicular or at an angle to it. In FDM, for example, top surfaces may have a different texture compared to side walls due to the different ways material is deposited [83].

Material-specific Effects: Different materials can result in varying surface characteristics even when using the same AM technology. For instance, some materials may be more prone to warping or may produce smoother surfaces due to better flow characteristics.

TABLE 22.2
Common AM Technologies and their Surface Characteristics

AM Technology	Typical Surface Roughness (Ra)	Common Surface Defects
FDM	5–20 μm	Layer lines, stair-stepping
SLA	1–5 μm	Support marks, resin residue
SLS	5–15 μm	Powder adhesion, porosity
SLM	5–20 μm	Partially melted particles, balling
EBM	20–35 μm	Powder sintering, surface waviness

Resolution Limitations: The minimum feature size and surface detail that can be accurately produced are limited by the resolution of the AM process. This can result in the loss of fine surface details or the rounding of sharp edges.

Surface Defects: Various defects can occur on the surface of AM parts.

22.2.2 Need for Post-processing

The unique surface characteristics of additively manufactured parts, as discussed in the previous section, often necessitate post-processing to achieve the desired final properties. The need for post-processing in AM is driven by various factors, including functional requirements, aesthetic considerations, and industry standards [84–89].

Dimensional Accuracy: While AM technologies have improved significantly in terms of accuracy, many applications require tighter tolerances than what can be achieved directly from the AM process [90]. Post-processing techniques such as machining or polishing can help achieve the required dimensional accuracy, especially for mating surfaces or critical dimensions.

Surface Finish Improvement: One of the primary reasons for post-processing is to improve surface finish. The layer lines, stair-stepping effect, and other surface irregularities characteristic of AM parts are often unacceptable for final use. Industries such as aerospace, automotive, and medical devices often require smooth surfaces for functional or aesthetic reasons [91]. Techniques like sanding, polishing, and chemical treatments can significantly reduce surface roughness.

22.2.2.1 Removal of Support Structures

Many AM processes require support structures to build overhanging features. These supports need to be removed after the build, and the areas where supports were attached often require additional finishing smoothing out any remaining marks or roughness [92]. For instance, heat treatment can help to reduce the internal stresses caused by AM of metal parts and enhance their strength and fatigue characteristics. Hot isostatic pressing or HIP can bring improvements in the density and mechanical properties of a part since it is effective against the presence of porosity in the metal.

Surface Sealing: In cases where the fluid tightness or pressure containment is necessary at the surface of the AM parts, post-processing might be required, in this case to seal the surface of the AM parts. This is particularly relevant for parts manufactured by PBF process that could contain surface porosity after the build process [93].

22.2.2.2 Improving Aesthetic Appeal

In many consumer as well as design applications of parts, the aesthetic appearances of the parts are very important. Surface finishes produced from painting, coating, or polishing can easily improve on the appearance of AM parts.

Meeting Industry Standards: There are so many industries that have set standards on surface finish, material properties, and part performance. It is often required to post-process the AM parts to meet these requirements and pass the certification test for utilizing the product in aerospace and medicine fields.

Functional Surface Modification: According to Chuang and Wu, post-processing can be employed to change the surface properties for the intended functions [94]. This may comprise raising hardness by case carburizing, improving wear and tear resistance through the application of coatings or improving the degree of slipperiness for the moving parts of the metal merchandise.

22.2.2.3 Removing Residual Powder or Resin

The PBF process and resin-based processes generally involve the use of a spare material that can stick to the part surface or become trapped inside the part. The final processes include powder removal, washing, and curing since all unused material must be eliminated.

Stress Relief: The stratification manner of constructing parts in AM can lead to application of residual stresses in parts [95]. Stresses developed during these post-processing heat treatments can alleviate these stresses and possibly prevent warpage or dimensional changes.

22.2.2.4 Improving Fatigue Performance

Stress concentrators are the surface roughness and pores which might be present in as-built AM parts. Stress concentrators also affect the fatigue life of component. There are treatments to the surface like shot peening or polishing that could further enhance the surface finish and introduce beneficial compressive stresses that would effectively contribute to the enhancement of fatigue properties [96].

Biocompatibility: In medical applications, post-processing may be necessary to ensure the biocompatibility of implants or medical devices. This could involve surface treatments to promote cell adhesion or prevent bacterial growth.

22.2.2.5 Enhancing Optical Properties

For AM parts used in optical applications, post-processing is often critical to achieve the required surface finish and optical clarity. This might involve polishing to a mirror finish or applying coatings to modify reflectivity or transmission properties.

22.2.2.6 Removing Chemical Contaminants

Inherent to some form of AM processes is that they can deposit a chemical residue on the outer surface of the parts. These contaminants are required to be cleaned post-processing, and the procedure is more critical for parts that are used in such applications as medical devices or high-purity chemical processing.

22.2.2.7 Assembling Multi-Part Constructions

For huge parts, complicated parts that need to be built as individual parts because of the size of the build platform and other factors such as build direction, there requires additional processing to integrate the whole part.

22.2.2.8 Tailoring Surface Texture

As it has been indicated that AM can create some roughness on the surface, post-processing provides the best control regarding roughness. This can be crucial in cases where an application needs to exhibit certain friction coefficient or when it is needed to nurture or hinder the growth of certain types of cells in the biomedical field.

22.2.2.9 Color and Texture Matching

In areas where AM parts are required to interface with other elements, the final surface finish is often attained through painting, dyeing, or texturing. The AM process may leave defects such as pores in the final product; post-processing allows the defects to be filled in or the features to be repaired. The degree and kind of post-processing required will vary with respect to the type of AM technology used, the material applied, and the geometry of the part as well as the intended use that the final part will have. Occasionally, simple post-processing treatments would be all that is needed for the part, whereas at other times complex multiple-step post-processing treatments may be needed to obtain the desired part characteristics [97–103]. However, on this note, it can be seen that the need for post-processing is regarded as a disadvantage of AM technologies since it turns out to be time-consuming and expensive in the production process. Therefore, there is further enhancement in finding ways and means of minimizing the extent of post-processing. These are the enhancement of function of AM resolution and surface finish and the creation of new material practices with improved as-built features as well as the fusion of AM with conventional manufacturing technologies [104]. Still, it is recognized that post-processing is often necessary in various applications even as AM technologies improve steadily. It makes it possible to adjust the properties of additively manufactured parts and guarantee that the components will meet specific demands of different industries. Therefore, post-processing techniques' characterization and optimization serve as critical factors when it comes to AM technology deployment. Post-processing of AM parts is still an area of research and development focus for improving the manufacturing practice, as the current technological methods for depositing materials for post-processing AM constructions are costly and resource-ineffective [105–110]. Technologies like MRF are promising to solve the requirements that are specific to finishing of AM parts and particularly those with complex shapes. With these technologies getting developed, they have potential to bring immeasurable change in the functionalities and scope of AM in different sectors.

22.3 FUNDAMENTALS OF MAGNETORHEOLOGICAL FINISHING

Magnetorheological finishing (MRF) is another of the modern polishing technologies that are based on the properties of magnetorheological (MR) fluids with the view of attaining a very high degree of surface accuracy [111].

The working principle of MRF is therefore rooted in the aspect of the controllable alteration of rheological characteristics of MR fluids in the presence of a magnetic field. **Figure 22.4** shows the experimental setup of rotary rectangular core magnetorheological finishing process. The core of the MRF process is a magnetic fluid which is a suspension of micron dimensions particles, magnetic soft material, usually carbonyl iron in a fluid base which may be a liquid. In the cases when no magnetic field is applied, this fluid has characteristics of a Newtonian fluid characterized by low

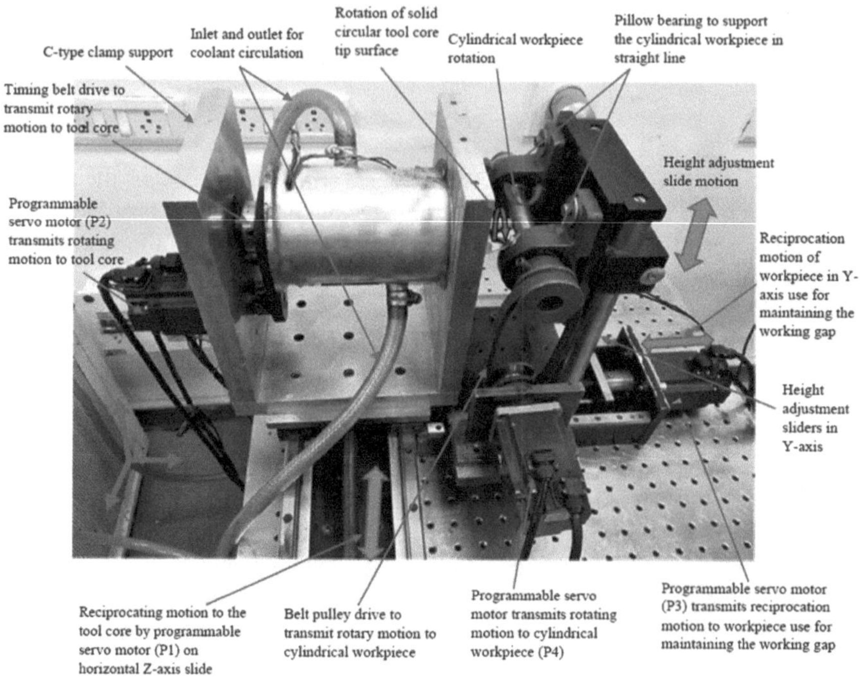

FIGURE 22.4 Experimental setup of rotary rectangular core magnetorheological finishing process. (Created by authors)

viscosity [112]. When exposed to the magnetic field, all the particles are oriented in an aligned manner along the vector field, giving a cylindrical arrangement-like structure. Simple shear strains of such types of MR fluids align the particles, and this greatly augments their viscosity and yield stress which in effect turns the fluid into a gel-like substance [113–117]. Fundamentally, the MRF system comprises a wheel that is partially immersed in a containing bath of the MR fluid. During a rotation of the wheel, the mouth of the ribbon that contains the fluid is transported to the polishing section. Here a strong magnetic field is used, which makes the fluid turn into a compliant polishing tool there [118]. This flexible fluid ribbon is stiffened, and the workpiece that has to be polished is made to come into contact with it. The polishing action in MRF is a two-step operation using either mechanical means or chemical treatments. The stiffened MR fluid, which has become a flexible abrasive tool, matches with the surface of the workpiece [119]. The solid particles in the fluid, being anchored firmly by the magnetic force, act on the surface of the workpiece and resultantly exert a shearing action which takes off a very thin layer of material at a time.

This material removal is very selective and can be controlled so that structures at different places are shaped as needed. **Figures 22.5 (a–c)** show the mechanism of material removal during the interaction of active abrasive particle with roughness peaks to finish the cylindrical workpiece surface. MRF has the

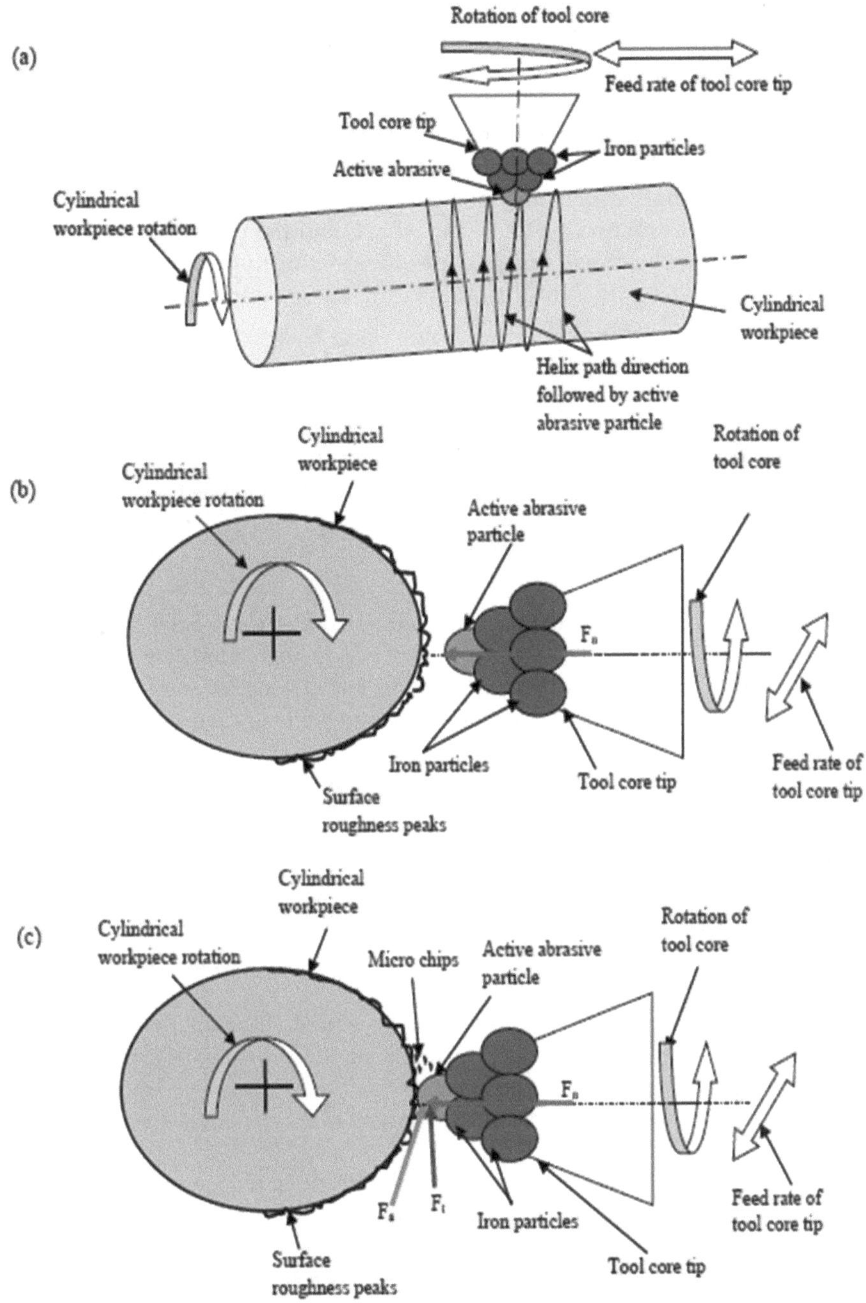

FIGURE 22.5 Mechanism of material removal: (a) Helical path of the active abrasive over the external surface of the cylindrical workpiece, (b) Force acting on abrasive particle before interaction with roughness peaks, and (c) Forces acting during the interaction of active abrasive particle with roughness peaks to finish the cylindrical workpiece surface. (Created by authors)

capacity of finishing high-precision and free form surface which is one of the major strengths of this finish. In this case, the fluid ribbon which is employed can easily wrap itself along the surface geometries without varying the amount of polishing pressure that is exerted on it. And this makes MRF especially appropriate for the finishing of optics, precision molds, and other intricate aerospace components. In MRF, material removal can be easily and accurately set by just regulating the strength of the magnetic field, the distance between the workpiece and the wheel, the rotation speed of the wheel, and the type of MR fluid. Such level of control is beneficial and provides the possibility to remove material in scales of nanometers, which results in the ultra-smooth surfaces with the roughness of values in sub-nanometers [120].

22.3.1 MR Fluid Composition and Properties

The composition and properties of the MR fluid are crucial to the effectiveness of the MRF process. A typical MR fluid used in finishing applications consists of several key components.

22.3.1.1 Magnetic Particles

These are usually carbonyl iron particles with sizes ranging from 1 micrometer to 10 micrometers. The particles are magnetically soft, meaning they can be easily magnetized and demagnetized. The size, shape, and concentration of these particles significantly influence the fluid's response to magnetic fields and its polishing capabilities [121].

22.3.1.2 Abrasive Particles

These are non-magnetic particles added to enhance the material removal rate. Common abrasives include cerium oxide, diamond, or aluminum oxide. The choice of abrasive depends on the workpiece material and the desired surface finish [122].

22.3.1.3 Carrier Fluid

This is typically water- or oil-based. The carrier fluid suspends the magnetic and abrasive particles and also acts as a coolant during the polishing process.

22.3.2 Stabilizers and Additives

Various additives are included to prevent particle settling, reduce wear, and enhance the overall stability and performance of the fluid [123–127]. **Table 22.3** represents the MR fluid composition. The properties of MR fluids are complex and can be tailored for specific applications. Key properties include the following.

22.3.2.1 Magnetorheological Effect

This is the fluid's ability to change its rheological properties in response to a magnetic field. The strength of this effect determines how quickly and effectively the fluid can stiffen to form a polishing tool [123].

TABLE 22.3
MR Fluid Composition

Component	Typical Percentage	Function
Magnetic Particles	20–40%	Provide magnetorheological effect
Abrasive Particles	5–20%	Material removal
Carrier Fluid	40–70%	Suspend particles, provide lubrication
Additives	1–5%	Improve stability, modify viscosity

22.3.2.2 Yield Stress

In the presence of a magnetic field, MR fluids exhibit a yield stress, which is the minimum stress required to initiate flow. This property is crucial for maintaining the shape of the polishing ribbon.

22.3.2.3 Viscosity

The fluid's viscosity changes dramatically with the application of a magnetic field. Understanding and controlling this change is essential for precise material removal [128–131].

22.3.2.4 Stability

MR fluids must remain stable over time, resisting particle settling and maintaining consistent properties throughout the polishing process [130].

22.3.2.5 Thermal Properties

As the polishing process generates heat, the thermal stability of the MR fluid is important for maintaining consistent performance.

22.3.3 Process Parameters and their Effects

The effectiveness of MRF is governed by several key process parameters, each of which can significantly influence the final surface quality and material removal rate.

22.3.3.1 Magnetic Field Strength

This is perhaps the most critical parameter in MRF. The strength of the magnetic field determines the stiffness of the MR fluid ribbon. A stronger field generally results in higher material removal rates but may also increase the risk of surface damage if not properly controlled [132].

22.3.3.2 Wheel Speed

The rotation speed of the wheel affects how the MR fluid is delivered to the polishing zone. Higher speeds can increase material removal rates but may also lead to fluid splashing and reduced control [133].

22.3.3.3 Gap between Wheel and Workpiece

This gap, often referred to as the "working gap," influences the pressure applied by the MR fluid on the workpiece surface. A smaller gap typically leads to higher removal rates but requires more precise control to avoid damage [134].

22.3.3.4 Fluid Flow Rate

The rate at which fresh MR fluid is supplied to the polishing zone affects the consistency of the polishing process and the removal of debris.

22.3.3.5 Workpiece Feed Rate

In systems where the workpiece moves relative to the polishing wheel, the feed rate affects the dwell time of any given area under the polishing spot.

22.3.3.6 MR Fluid Composition

The specific proportions of the magnetic particles, the abrasives, and the carrier fluid can be varied to achieve the best results on different types of materials and the end product that is required.

22.3.3.7 Temperature

When the MR fluid and the workpiece are heated, they might enhance the viscosity of the fluid and the mode of material removal.

22.3.3.8 Polishing Time

The two polish parameters are the total amount of material removed and the final surface quality, which depend on the polishing time. The combined effect of these parameters at a certain degree may significantly affect the surface finish. For instance, an increase in magnetic field can also enable the enhancement of a larger working gap or higher wheel speed though the MRR remains constant [135]. **Table 22.4** represents the MRF process parameters and their effects.

Likewise, alterations in the composition of the fluid may require that the other parameters be tweaked to get good outcomes. The control of these parameters is important within the context of achieving the appropriate surface finish and in maintaining stable machining conditions. Parameters that show variability generally are regulated in complex and real-time style constantly via state-of-art MRF systems [136].

TABLE 22.4
MRF Process Parameters and their Effects

Parameter	Effect on Surface Finish	Effect on Material Removal Rate
Magnetic Field Strength	Increases with strength	Increases with strength
Wheel Speed	Improves with higher speed (up to a limit)	Increases with speed
Gap Distance	Improves with smaller gap	Increases with smaller gap
Polishing Time	Improves with longer time	Increases with time
MR Fluid Viscosity	Improves with higher viscosity	Decreases with higher viscosity

22.4 POST-PROCESSING FOR AM PARTS

22.4.1 Versatility for Complicated Shapes

Another very profound benefit of MRF for AM parts is that it is highly versatile particularly with regard to free-form surface finishes. Free-form shapes are the key strength of AM technologies, especially because some of them cannot be produced using conventional methods [121]. However, this means that while finishing a workpiece one is presented with several problems concerning traditional finishing methods. Because of its several characteristics, MRF is especially suitable to face such threats [123]. Thus, the capability of MRF to adapt to different applications is couched in the composition of the magnetorheological fluid. When invaded by the magnetic field the fluid transforms into a soft polishing tool able to make contact with the various surface irregularities. This conformability enables MRF to apply equal pressure on the complicated curves and planes, holes and recesses, outer contours, and other intricate edges [137–140]. As for the surface angles of AM parts, MRF can adapt to them and does not require repositioning or tools of high specificity. This is especially helpful for applications that require polishing of components with organic forms or members with topology-optimized designs, which are frequently found in AM but difficult with conventional polishing techniques. Among all these aspects, MRF's capability of post-processing the internal features is highly effective for AM parts. In many AM designs, designers provide internal channels, lattice structures, or honeycomb to reduce the weight or for some functional requirements. These internal features are, as a rule, inaccessible to the traditional polishing instruments. MRF, however, can be adapted to polish these internal surfaces by using specialized delivery systems or by temporarily filling the part with MR fluid and applying a magnetic field to activate polishing in specific areas. The non-contact nature of MRF (as the actual polishing is done by the fluid, not a solid tool) also makes it suitable for delicate or thin-walled structures often found in AM parts [141]. This reduces the risk of deformation or damage during the finishing process. Furthermore, MRF can be easily automated and integrated with computer-controlled systems. This allows for precise control over the polishing process across complex geometries, ensuring consistent material removal and surface finish even on parts with varying feature sizes and orientations [142].

22.4.2 Material Compatibility

MRF demonstrates broad material compatibility, making it suitable for finishing a wide range of AM parts. However, the effectiveness and specific process parameters can vary depending on the material being polished. Here's an overview of MRF compatibility with common AM materials.

- *Metals*: MRF is highly effective on most metals used in AM, including titanium alloys, stainless steels, aluminum alloys, and nickel-based superalloys. For these materials, MRF can achieve extremely smooth surfaces with roughness values in the nanometer range. The process is particularly valuable for high-performance alloys used in aerospace and medical applications, where surface quality is critical [143].

- *Ceramics*: AM-produced ceramics, such as alumina or zirconia, can also be effectively polished using MRF. The process is particularly useful for ceramic parts with complex geometries, such as custom dental implants or intricate industrial components. MRF can achieve the high-quality surface finish required for these applications without the risk of chipping or cracking associated with mechanical polishing methods [144].
- *Polymers*: While less common, MRF can be adapted for use with certain polymer materials produced by AM. However, care must be taken to prevent chemical interactions between the MR fluid and the polymer surface. For some thermoplastics, the process parameters may need to be adjusted to avoid thermal deformation.
- *Composites*: For composite materials produced through AM, such as carbon fiber-reinforced plastics, MRF can be effective but may require careful optimization. The heterogeneous nature of composites can lead to differential polishing rates between the matrix and reinforcement materials [145].
- *Glass and Optical Materials*: Although not typically produced by AM, it's worth noting that MRF is highly effective on glass and optical materials. This capability could become relevant, as AM technologies for transparent materials continue to develop.

When applying MRF to AM parts, several material-specific considerations must be taken into account:

a) *Hardness and Abrasion Resistance*: The composition of the MR fluid, particularly the choice of abrasive particles, may need to be adjusted based on the hardness of the AM material.
b) *Chemical Compatibility*: The carrier fluid and additives in the MR fluid must be chemically compatible with the AM material to avoid unwanted reactions or degradation.
c) *Thermal Sensitivity*: For materials with low melting points or glass transition temperatures, the heat generated during MRF must be carefully managed.
d) *Surface Porosity*: Some AM processes can produce parts with surface porosity. The MRF process may need to be optimized to effectively polish these surfaces without excessive fluid penetration into the pores.
e) *Residual Stress*: AM parts may have residual stresses from the building process. MRF parameters should be chosen to avoid exacerbating these stresses or causing deformation.

22.4.3 Surface Roughness Improvement

One of the primary objectives of applying MRF to AM parts is to improve surface roughness. AM technologies, while capable of producing complex geometries, often result in parts with surface irregularities such as stair-stepping effects, partially melted particles, or support structure remnants [146]. MRF has demonstrated significant capabilities in reducing these surface imperfections and achieving high-quality finishes [147–152].

The effectiveness of MRF in improving surface roughness can be quite remarkable. Studies have shown that MRF can reduce the surface roughness of AM parts from initial values of several micrometers (μm) to final values in the nanometer (nm) range. For example, metal AM parts with initial surface roughness (Ra) values of 5–10 μm can be polished to achieve Ra values of 10–50 nm or even lower. The level of improvement in surface roughness depends on several factors:

a) *Initial Surface Condition*: The starting surface roughness and the nature of surface irregularities (e.g., layer lines, partially melted particles) influence the polishing time and the final achievable smoothness.
b) *Material Properties*: Different materials respond differently to MRF. Generally, harder materials can achieve lower final roughness values but may require longer polishing times.
c) *Process Parameters*: The magnetic field strength, polishing time, MR fluid composition, and other parameters can be optimized to achieve the desired surface finish.
d) *Geometry*: While MRF is adaptable to complex geometries, very intricate features or deep recesses may be more challenging to polish to the same level of smoothness as more accessible surfaces.

MRF is particularly effective at reducing the layer lines and stair-stepping effects common in AM parts. These periodic surface structures can be smoothed out uniformly across the part surface, resulting in a more isotropic surface texture. This is advantageous for applications where consistent surface properties are required in all directions. **Table 22.5** represents the surface roughness improvement by MRF for different AM materials.

For PBF processes, which often result in partially melted particles adhering to the surface, MRF can effectively remove these particles and smooth out the underlying surface. This is necessary for those forms of parts where surface finish is a critical parameter, for instance, in medical devices or certified mechanical parts. It is worth mentioning that mean roughness will be not only low, but also other parameters of the roughness profile such as the skewness and kurtosis will be improved at the same time while using MRF. This means that the surface produced is more even and functionally superior to the value indicated by the Ra value.

TABLE 22.5
Surface Roughness Improvement by MRF for Different AM Materials

Material	Initial Ra (μm)	Final Ra (μm)	Improvement Factor
Ti-6Al-4V	15	0.1	150x
AlSi10Mg	10	0.2	50x
316L Stainless	8	0.05	160x
Inconel 718	12	0.08	150x
CoCr	5	0.02	250x

22.4.4 Dimensional Accuracy Enhancement

Dimensional accuracy of AM technologies has progressed with time, but most of the applications demand a higher degree of accuracy than what can be offered without post-processing. This way, MRF can also help increase the dimensional stability of the AM parts and, as a result, meet higher standards for precision applications. The ability of MRF to enhance dimensional accuracy stems from several key characteristics of the process.

a) *Controlled Material Removal*: MRF enables very close to ideal control of the material removal process. Using such factors as magnetic field strength, polishing time, and type of fluid, one can reduce the material at the nanometer level. The real level of control allows for achieving very small part dimensions and meeting quite stringent tolerances.
b) *Uniform Processing*: In contrast to some of the other traditional finishing processes, which might remove the material in a more aggressive manner from the edges or the protrusion, MRF might prove to be better at removing the appropriate amount of material evenly over the whole of a part's surface. This supports the general geometry to be kept stable constant while at the same time giving the surface a polished finish.
c) *Non-Contact Nature*: MRF does not place significant pressure on a surface as the polishing is not done by a solid tool, and this minimizes the probability of deformation or over polishing hence affecting dimensional stability.
d) *Adaptive Processing*: Complex MRF systems can include the measurements done during the manufacturing process and the feedback control system. This helps the user to follow the removal of material and control the process parameters to achieve the required dimensions accurately. The enhancement of dimensional accuracy through MRF can be particularly beneficial for AM parts in several ways.
e) *Correction of AM Process Variations*: When it comes to aspects such as thermal distortion or shrinkage, it is possible for AM processes to cause slight changes in the dimensions. MRF can be utilized for correction of these variations, thus getting the parts into the desired specification.
f) *Achieving Tight Tolerances*: In those fields where applications demand very small tolerances, such as the mechanical components or the optical parts, MRF can enhance the corresponding dimensions up to the desired tolerance levels.
g) *Improving Mating Surfaces*: MRF may be applied in assemblies that require connection with other components on the AM parts, for adjustment of the fit and performance.
h) *Enhancing Geometric Accuracy*: Dependent on the build, AM may allow high detail features but certain regions must engage a high degree of tolerance (e.g., inlets/outlets, bearing surfaces). It is found that MRF can selectively enhance the accuracy of these significant features.
i) *Compensating for Support Removal Effects*: In AM, the elimination of supports sometimes causes an impact on shells neighboring to the structure

formed. This is where MRF can fit in and help restore the parts to their correct dimensional accuracy. It's, however, very pertinent that MRF can greatly improve the dimensional accuracy, but its application is best done where small corrections in the material removal are required. However, the process is most effective when AM parts are made near to finish size, and a slight finish is provided by the MRF. Therefore, the improvement of the surface roughness and dimensional accuracy makes MRF an effective solution in the post-processing of the AM parts. It allows for the manufacturing of parts with both finishes of the surface and dimensions that are required in high-performance applications. This capability thus helps to increase adoption of AM in aerospace components and parts, medical devices, and instruments to mention but a few, where surface finish and accurate dimensions are very crucial.

22.5 CASE STUDIES AND APPLICATIONS

22.5.1 Aerospace Components

The aerospace industry has already benefited from AM technologies a lot because of their potential to create strong yet lightweight structures and to significantly decrease the number of parts in the assembly. However, the surface finish and dimensional tolerances of certain parts used in aerospace require applications of higher sophistication of post-processing, such as MRF. Some of the case studies clearly depict the extent to which MRF has improved the AM aerospace parts.

There is an example of using hybrid coatings on the titanium alloy (Ti-6Al-4V) turbine blades fabricated with SLM that has been mentioned earlier. In the case study, the as-built blades measured a surface roughness (Ra) of approximately 15 μm, and layer lines were clearly visible as was the partially melted particles that had bonded to the blade surface. In conventional finishing techniques there was a problem of polishing the geometry of the airfoil in a uniform manner while maintaining the thinness of the trailing edge. MRF was carried out using an in-house built fluid delivery system with the capability of reaching every part of the blade. In addition to the optimization of the parameters such as magnetic field strength and time of polishing, the Ra surface roughness was brought down to 0.1 μm at all the regions of the blade. Most importantly, the key aerodynamic profiles were held to within ±10 μm on critical dimensions, required to manufacture abrasive efficient turbomachinery. Another case study focused on lightweight structural components for satellite applications. These parts, produced using EBM of aluminum alloys, featured intricate lattice structures designed for optimal strength-to-weight ratio. The as-built parts had rough surfaces with Ra values around 20–30 μm, which could potentially impact the mechanical properties and thermal performance of the structures. MRF was employed using a specially formulated MR fluid compatible with aluminum alloys. The process successfully reduced the surface roughness to Ra 0.5 μm without damaging the delicate lattice structures. Post-finishing analysis showed a 15% improvement in fatigue life and enhanced thermal conductivity due to the smoother surface finish.

In the realm of spacecraft propulsion, MRF has been applied to AM-produced rocket engine components. A case study on inconel fuel injector nozzles highlighted the importance of surface finish for fluid dynamics and combustion efficiency. The AM process allowed for the creation of complex internal flow passages but left surface roughness that could disrupt fuel atomization. MRF was used to polish both external and internal surfaces, reducing roughness from Ra 10 μm to Ra 0.05 μm. Flow testing of the finished components showed a 5% increase in spray uniformity and improved combustion efficiency.

These aerospace case studies demonstrate the capability of MRF to address the unique challenges posed by AM components in high-performance applications. The ability to achieve excellent surface finish while maintaining tight dimensional tolerances on complex geometries positions MRF as a key enabler for the broader adoption of AM in the aerospace sector.

22.5.2 Medical Implants

The medical field has embraced AM for its ability to produce patient-specific implants and complex biomedical devices. However, the surface quality of these components is crucial for biocompatibility, wear resistance, and functionality. MRF has shown promising results in finishing various types of medical implants produced by AM. A significant case study involved the finishing of titanium dental implants produced via direct metal laser sintering (DMLS). The as-built implants had a rough surface (Ra ~10 μm) with partially melted particles, which could potentially lead to poor osseointegration and increased risk of infection. MRF was applied using a biocompatible MR fluid formulation. The process reduced the surface roughness to Ra 0.2 μm on the implant body while maintaining the micro-roughness on the bone-interfacing surfaces, which is beneficial for cell adhesion. In vitro testing showed improved fibroblast attachment and proliferation on the MRF-finished surfaces compared to conventionally polished implants.

Another compelling application of MRF in the medical field is the finishing of cobalt-chromium knee implants manufactured using EBM. These implants require exceptionally smooth articulating surfaces to minimize wear and extend the implant's lifespan. In this case study, MRF was used to polish the complex, free-form surfaces of the femoral component. The process reduced surface roughness from Ra 5 μm to Ra 0.02 μm, achieving a mirror-like finish. Wear testing demonstrated a 30% reduction in particulate generation compared to conventionally manufactured and polished implants.

MRF has also been applied to AM-produced titanium spinal implants featuring porous structures for bone ingrowth. The challenge here was to selectively polish certain surfaces while preserving the intentional porosity of others. A masked MRF process was developed, allowing precise control over which areas were polished. The smooth surfaces achieved Ra values of 0.1 μm, while the porous regions maintained their original structure. Post-processing analysis showed improved cell viability on the polished surfaces and unimpeded bone growth in the porous regions. In the field of cardiovascular implants, a case study on AM-produced nitinol stents highlighted MRF's ability to polish extremely delicate structures. The stents, with strut thicknesses of less than 100 μm, required smooth surfaces to prevent thrombosis. MRF, using a specially designed fixture and low-viscosity MR fluid, successfully reduced surface roughness from Ra 3 μm to Ra 0.05 μm without deforming the stent structure.

In vitro flow studies have shown reduced platelet adhesion on the MRF-finished stents compared to as-built samples. These medical case studies underscore the versatility of MRF in addressing the diverse surface finishing requirements of AM-produced implants. The ability to achieve high-quality finishes on complex, biocompatible materials while preserving critical features positions MRF as a valuable tool in the production of next-generation medical devices.

22.5.3 Optical Elements

While not typically associated with AM, the production of optical elements through advanced manufacturing techniques is an emerging field where MRF has shown significant promise. This includes both traditional optical materials finished after AM-assisted fabrication and novel AM-produced optically functional components.

A noteworthy case study involved the finishing of free-form optics produced through a hybrid manufacturing process. The base shape was created using precision AM of a polymer substrate, which was then coated with optical glass using chemical vapor deposition. The resulting surface, while close to the desired form, had irregularities and mid-spatial frequency errors that affected optical performance. MRF was applied to correct these errors and achieve the required surface quality. The process reduced the surface form error from 5 μm PV (Peak-to-Valley) to 50 nm PV and surface roughness from Ra 20 nm to Ra 1 nm. The finished optic met the stringent specifications for use in a high-resolution imaging system. Another case study focused on AM-produced metal mirrors for space-based telescopes. These lightweight mirrors, made from aluminum alloys using selective laser melting (SLM), required exceptional surface quality for optical performance. The as-built surfaces had roughness values of Ra 5 μm and significant form errors due to residual stresses in the AM process. MRF was employed in a two-stage process: first, to correct the overall form error and then to achieve the final surface finish. The process reduced form error from 50 μm PV to 100 nm PV and surface roughness to Ra 2 nm. The finished mirrors met the specifications for visible and near-infrared astronomy applications.

In the field of integrated photonics, MRF has been applied to AM-produced waveguides and optical couplers. A case study on polymer-based optical waveguides produced via multi-photon polymerization demonstrated MRF's ability to reduce sidewall roughness, a critical factor in minimizing optical losses. The MRF process, using a specially formulated low-viscosity MR fluid, reduced sidewall roughness from Ra 100 nm to Ra 5 nm, resulting in a 50% reduction in propagation losses. Thus, these case studies of optical applications demonstrate that MRF confirms a very high surface quality needed for optical elements. The information enables the process to generate accurate corrective actions based on form errors and surface roughness to apply in making next-generation optical components that have geometries created by next-generation AM technology.

22.5.4 Tooling and Molds

One of the industries that have embraced AM is the tooling and mold making due to the complexity of the molds and dies required. But, typically, the surface quality of the fabricated AM tools is not up to the mark in comparison to the required surface finish of molded parts. MRF has been proven to be quite helpful for the improvement of the surface finish of the AM-generated tooling. A major application incorporated the roughing and finishing of injection mold inserts manufactured by DMLS of tool steel. The mold surfaces were as-built, and the roughness of the surface was in the Ra 10 μm range, and layer lines were also visible which would appear on the molded part. The finished molds delivered consistent and smooth surface quality of the parts, and hence there was little requirement for subsequent finishing of the molded parts. Also, the realization of smoother mold surface provided easy removal of the part and improved the service life of molds due to minimum wear. The fourth case describes the application of AM in manufacturing the extrusion dies for polymer processing. These dies were made out of high-performance alloys materials, and these new dies had internal mazes which were designed to allow even distribution of the material. The built surfaces of the internal environment had roughness values of Ra 15 μm, which led to a variation in the flow rate and hence the quality of manufactured products. It was necessary to create a specialized MRF setup for improved finishing of the internal channels to attain roughness of Ra 0. 2 μm. The cooperation of MRF and the FAMD found out that there was a 20% enhancement in flow characteristics and pressure drop for the MRF-finished dies as compared to as-built dies. **Table 22.6** represents the MRF applications in different industries.

In the field of sheet metal forming, a case study on AM-produced hydroforming dies highlighted MRF's ability to enhance both surface finish and dimensional accuracy. The dies, produced via EBM of titanium alloys, required a smooth surface to prevent marking of the formed parts and precise dimensions to ensure part accuracy. MRF was used to reduce surface roughness from Ra 25 μm to Ra 0.05 μm while also correcting form errors introduced during the AM process. The finished dies produced parts with improved surface quality and tighter dimensional tolerances compared to conventionally manufactured dies. These case studies in tooling and mold applications

TABLE 22.6
MRF Applications in Different Industries

Industry	Typical Components	Key Requirements	MRF Advantages
Aerospace	Turbine blades, structural components	High surface quality, fatigue resistance	Uniform finishing, stress control
Medical	Implants, prosthetics	Biocompatibility, complex geometries	Smooth surfaces, controlled texture
Optics	Free-form mirrors, waveguides	Sub-nanometer finish, form accuracy	Ultra-smooth surfaces, figure correction
Tooling	Injection molds, Extrusion dies	Wear resistance, uniform channels	Smooth internal features, extended tool life

demonstrate MRF's capability to bridge the gap between the geometric freedom offered by AM and the surface quality requirements of high-performance tooling. **Table 22.7** represents the recent advancements in MRF technology. The ability to achieve excellent surface finish on complex geometries, including internal features, positions MRF as a key enabler for the broader adoption of AM in the tooling industry.

The integration of MR finishing with AM processes themselves is an exciting possibility. Concepts such as in-situ MR finishing during the AM build process, or layer-by-layer finishing for large AM parts, are being explored. **Table 22.8** represents the comparison of MRF with other finishing techniques for AM parts. These approaches could potentially address surface quality issues as they arise during the build rather than as a separate post-processing step. Another promising direction is the development of multi-stage hybrid finishing systems. These would combine several finishing techniques in a single setup, with MR finishing as one of the stages.

A system might be designed to first carry out abrasive flow machining in an upstream stage for bulk material removal and then execute MR finishing process to attain final surface quality, all through a single automated cycle. **Table 22.9**

TABLE 22.7
Recent Advancements in MRF Technology

Advancement	Description	Potential Impact
Hybrid Techniques	Combining MRF with other processes (e.g., ultrasonic, electrochemical)	Enhanced material removal, broader material compatibility
Smart Fluids	MR fluids with embedded sensing capabilities	Improved process control, real-time monitoring
In-situ Metrology	Integration of advanced measurement techniques	Closed-loop control, consistent results
AI-driven Control	Machine learning algorithms for process optimization	Adaptive finishing, improved efficiency
Multi-functional Fluids	Fluids that polish and impart surface properties	Enhanced functionality, reduced processing steps

TABLE 22.8
Comparison of MRF with Other Finishing Techniques for AM Parts

Technique	Surface Finish Capability (Ra)	Geometry Adaptability	Material Removal Control
MRF	0.01–0.5 μm	Excellent	Excellent
Abrasive Flow	0.05–1 μm	Good	Moderate
Chemical Polish	0.1–2 μm	Excellent	Poor
Laser Polish	0.1–5 μm	Good	Moderate
Hand Polish	0.1–1 μm	Poor	Poor

TABLE 22.9
Environmental and Safety Considerations of MRF

Aspect	Consideration	Mitigation Strategy
Waste Management	Disposal of used MR fluids	Recycling systems, biodegradable formulations
Energy Consumption	High power requirements for electromagnets	Energy-efficient designs, optimized process duration
Operator Safety	Exposure to magnetic fields and chemicals	Enclosed systems, personal protective equipment
Noise	Potential high-frequency noise from equipment	Sound insulation, low-noise component design
Material Efficiency	Potential for overprocessing	Precision control systems, optimized material removal

represents the environmental and safety considerations of MRF. In their continued refinement, these hybrid techniques are poised to expand the reach of MR finishing and ensure that it remains a valuable weapon in overcoming this unique set of challenges related specifically to AM part finishing.

22.6 CONCLUSION

In practice, integration of MRF with AM represents the first step toward addressing some long-standing factory-floor surface quality challenges associated with AM processes. Through this chapter, the impressive capability presented by MRF in delivering superior surface finish and shape precision achievable on complex parts is established across diverse market sectors (from aerospace to medical implants). Despite many challenges associated with MR fluid stability, process control, and cost-effectiveness, further research into hybrid techniques [23], smart fluids [13], and in-situ monitoring systems has continued to broaden the capabilities of MRF. The combination of AM's geometric flexibility with MRF precision finishing could expand the use-case scenarios for AM in high-performance industries. With the continuing evolution of these technologies, we can look forward to more integrated use of MRF in AM workflows that may one day materialize at the level of in situ processes itself, enabling new vistas in bespoke design and part performance. As a result of the unresolved issues, AM combined with MRF is an important approach to implement in practice for producing excellent precision parts and add more research activity since it promises at this stage high dimensional accuracy into complex shapes.

REFERENCES

1. Abdel-Aal, H. A. (2003). On the interdependence between kinetics of friction-released thermal energy and the transition in wear mechanisms during sliding of metallic pairs. *Wear*, 254(9), 884–900.

2. Agrawal, A., & Pandithevan, P. (2021). A review on surface finishing of additively manufactured metal parts. *Materials Today: Proceedings*, 44, 4748–53.
3. Ahuir-Torres, J. I., Arenas, M. A., Perrie, W., & de Damborenea, J. (2018). Influence of laser parameters in surface texturing of Ti6Al4V and AA2024-T3 alloys. *Optics and Lasers in Engineering*, 103, 100–9.
4. Altan, T., & Lilly, B. (2005). Manufacturing of dies and molds. *CIRP Annals*, 54(2), 675–99.
5. Arun, K., Sabarish, R., & Madhavan, N. (2020). Surface modification of additively manufactured parts using magnetic abrasive finishing process. *Materials Today: Proceedings*, 27, 1691–5.
6. Astakhov, V. P. (2010). Surface integrity–definition and importance in functional performance. In *Surface Integrity in Machining* (pp. 1–35). London: Springer.
7. Attaran, M. (2017). The rise of 3-D printing: The advantages of additive manufacturing over traditional manufacturing. *Business Horizons*, 60(5), 677–88.
8. Babu, P. D., & Venkateswara Rao, P. (2020). A review on magneto rheological fluid (MRF) finishing process. *Materials Today: Proceedings*, 27, 1752–7.
9. Bai, Y., & Williams, C. B. (2015). An exploration of binder jetting of copper. *Rapid Prototyping Journal*, 21(2), 177–85.
10. Barletta, M., & Tagliaferri, V. (2006). Development of an abrasive flow machining (AFM) cell for the deburring of aerospace components. *International Journal of Machine Tools and Manufacture*, 46(14), 1937–44.
11. Barton, K. L., & Rampersad, G. (2017). The impact of additive manufacturing on the aerospace industry. *Journal of Manufacturing Technology Management*, 28(1), 75–94.
12. Berman, B. (2012). 3-D printing: The new industrial revolution. *Business Horizons*, 55(2), 155–62.
13. Bhattacharya, M., & Blawat, M. (2020). Additive manufacturing of metals: Current state and future scope. *Journal of Manufacturing Processes*, 56, 1353–77.
14. Bhushan, B. (2000). *Modern Tribology Handbook, Two Volume Set*. CRC Press.
15. Boschetto, A., & Bottini, L. (2016). Surface improvement of fused deposition modeling parts by barrel finishing. *Rapid Prototyping Journal*, 22(1), 145–56.
16. Bourell, D., Kruth, J. P., Leu, M., Levy, G., Rosen, D., Beese, A. M., & Clare, A. (2017). Materials for additive manufacturing. *CIRP Annals*, 66(2), 659–81.
17. Brinksmeier, E., Riemer, O., & Gessenharter, A. (2006). Finishing of structured surfaces by abrasive polishing. *Precision Engineering*, 30(3), 325–36.
18. Calignano, F., Manfredi, D., Ambrosio, E. P., Biamino, S., Lombardi, M., Atzeni, E., & Fino, P. (2017). Overview on additive manufacturing technologies. *Proceedings of the IEEE*, 105(4), 593–612.
19. Cattano, C., Nikou, T., & Klotz, L. (2011). Teaching systems thinking and biomimicry to civil engineering students. *Journal of Professional Issues in Engineering Education and Practice*, 137(4), 176–82.
20. Chandra, H., Allen, S. W., Oberloier, S. W., Bihari, N., Gwamuri, J., & Pearce, J. M. (2017). Open-source automated mapping four-point probe. *Materials*, 10(2), 110.
21. Chen, M., Zheng, K., Xie, Y., & Liu, X. (2018). Finishing of additively manufactured metal parts by abrasive flow machining. *The International Journal of Advanced Manufacturing Technology*, 96(5), 2075–83.
22. Chen, X., & Hutchinson, J. W. (2004). Herringbone buckling patterns of compressed thin films on compliant substrates. *Journal of Applied Mechanics*, 71(5), 597–603.
23. Cheng, J., & Yang, S. (2009). Development of a magnetorheological abrasive flow machining process. *Journal of Materials Processing Technology*, 209(9), 4367–73.

24. Choi, J. W., & Kim, H. C. (2015). 3D printing technologies–A review. *Journal of the Korean Society of Manufacturing Technology Engineers*, 24(3), 311–7.
25. Chun, D. M., Davaasuren, G., Ahn, S. H., & Lee, C. S. (2014). Abrasive flow polishing of micro-components fabricated by selective laser melting. *International Journal of Precision Engineering and Manufacturing*, 15(9), 1801–07.
26. Cortina, M., Arrizubieta, J. I., Calleja, A., Ukar, E., & Alberdi, A. (2018). Case study to illustrate the potential of conformal cooling channels for hot stamping dies manufactured using hybrid process of Laser Metal Deposition (LMD) and milling. *Metals*, 8(2), 102.
27. Li, C., Wang, J., Huang, X., & Luo, J. (2020). Mechanism and modeling of magneto-rheological polishing on hard-brittle materials. *The International Journal of Advanced Manufacturing Technology*, 109(5), 1491–503.
28. Choi, H. S., & Jeon, B. G. (2020). Parametric optimization of magnetorheological finishing process using response surface methodology. *International Journal of Precision Engineering and Manufacturing*, 21(5), 819–30.
29. Nagaraj, B. K., Raji, A. K., & Prabhakaran, P. (2020). Empirical modeling and optimization of magneto-rheological finishing process parameters for surface quality improvement of aluminum alloy. *Materials Today: Proceedings*, 33, 1305–09.
30. Han, X., Li, H., Zhu, H., & Zeng, W. (2020). Influence of abrasive particle size and content on surface roughness and material removal rate in magnetorheological finishing. *The International Journal of Advanced Manufacturing Technology*, 107(11), 4919–30.
31. Babu, P. D., & Rao, P. V. (2020). Enhancement of surface quality of DMLS Ti6Al4V components using magnetorheological abrasive flow finishing. *Materials Today: Proceedings*, 27, 1752–57.
32. Arun, K., Sabarish, R., & Madhavan, N. (2020). Surface modification of additively manufactured parts using magnetic abrasive finishing process. *Materials Today: Proceedings*, 27, 1691–95.
33. Mishra, R., Jain, V. K., & Munjal, A. (2020). Experimental investigations and modeling of surface roughness in magnetorheological abrasive flow finishing. *The International Journal of Advanced Manufacturing Technology*, 106(11), 4927–43.
34. Sharma, A., Jain, V. K., & Ramkumar, J. (2019). Magnetorheological fluid-based finishing process for enhancement of surface quality of additively manufactured parts. *Precision Engineering*, 60, 290–307.
35. Jain, V. K., & Sidpara, A. (2019). A review on magnetorheological abrasive flow finishing. *Materials and Manufacturing Processes*, 34(5), 481–502.
36. Kumar, S., Jha, S., & Jain, V. K. (2019). Experimental investigations and modeling of surface roughness in magneto-rheological abrasive flow finishing. *The International Journal of Advanced Manufacturing Technology*, 101(1), 969–87.
37. Jha, S., Jain, V. K., & Rajurkar, K. P. (2018). Modeling and optimization of surface roughness in magnetorheological abrasive flow finishing (MRAFF) process. *The International Journal of Advanced Manufacturing Technology*, 97(5), 2453–70.
38. Singh, D. K., Jain, V. K., & Raghuram, V. (2017). Experimental investigations and modeling in magnetorheological abrasive flow finishing (MRAFF) process. *The International Journal of Advanced Manufacturing Technology*, 89(5), 2485–501.
39. Sidpara, A., & Jain, V. K. (2017). Experimental investigations into the behavior of magnetorheological fluid and finishing of silicon wafer. *Materials and Manufacturing Processes*, 32(13), 1568–75.
40. Sidpara, A., & Jain, V. K. (2016). Experimental investigations and modeling of forces in magnetorheological fluid-based finishing process. *The International Journal of Advanced Manufacturing Technology*, 84(1), 433–46.

41. Sidpara, A., & Jain, V. K. (2015). Theoretical analysis and experimental investigation in nanofinishing of silicon wafer. *The International Journal of Advanced Manufacturing Technology*, 76(1), 83–94.
42. Sidpara, A., & Jain, V. K. (2012). Nano-level finish on single crystal silicon substrate by magnetorheological finishing process. *Precision Engineering*, 36(2), 291–9.
43. Sidpara, A., Das, M., & Jain, V. K. (2011). Experimental investigations into the surface roughness and flow stability in the magnetorheological fluid-based finishing process. *Proceedings of the Institution of Mechanical Engineers, Part B: Journal of Engineering Manufacture*, 225(10), 1785–98.
44. Jha, S., & Jain, V. K. (2011). Modeling and simulation of surface roughness in magnetorheological abrasive flow finishing (MRAFF) process. *The International Journal of Advanced Manufacturing Technology*, 55(5), 612–28.
45. Jha, S., & Jain, V. K. (2007). Investigations on surface properties in magnetorheological abrasive flow finishing (MRAFF) process. *Materials and Manufacturing Processes*, 22(4), 463–7.
46. Danforth, S. C. (2019). On the future of additive manufacturing. *Journal of Materials Science*, 54(6), 4147–68.
47. Jha, S., & Jain, V. K. (2004). Design and development of the magnetorheological abrasive flow finishing (MRAFF) process. *The International Journal of Advanced Manufacturing Technology*, 26(11), 1471–78.
48. Das, S., Wohlert, M., Beaman, J. J., & Bourell, D. L. (1998). Producing metal parts with selective laser sintering/hot isostatic pressing. *JOM*, 50(12), 17–20.
49. Dehoff, R. R., Kirka, M. M., Sames, W. J., Bilheux, H., Tremsin, A. S., Lowe, L. E., & Babu, S. S. (2015). Site specific control of crystallographic grain orientation through electron beam additive manufacturing. *Materials Science and Technology*, 31(8), 931–8.
50. Ding, D., Pan, Z., Cuiuri, D., & Li, H. (2015). Wire-feed additive manufacturing of metal components: Technologies, developments and future interests. *The International Journal of Advanced Manufacturing Technology*, 81(1–4), 465–81.
51. Doubrovski, E. L., Tsai, E. Y., Dikovsky, D., Geraedts, J. M., Herr, H., & Oxman, N. (2015). Voxel-based fabrication through material property mapping: A design method for bitmap printing. *Computer-Aided Design*, 60, 3–13.
52. Duflou, J. R., Sutherland, J. W., Dornfeld, D., Herrmann, C., Jeswiet, J., Kara, S., . . . & Kellens, K. (2012). Towards energy and resource efficient manufacturing: A processes and systems approach. *CIRP Annals*, 61(2), 587–609.
53. Dutta, B., & Froes, F. H. (2017). The additive manufacturing (AM) of titanium alloys. *Metal Powder Report*, 72(2), 96–106.
54. Emmelmann, C., Scheinemann, P., Munsch, M., & Seyda, V. (2011). Laser additive manufacturing of modified implant surfaces with osseointegrative characteristics. *Physics Procedia*, 12, 375–84.
55. Everton, S. K., Hirsch, M., Stravroulakis, P., Leach, R. K., & Clare, A. T. (2016). Review of in-situ process monitoring and in-situ metrology for metal additive manufacturing. *Materials & Design*, 95, 431–45.
56. Farina, I., Fabbrocino, F., Carpentieri, G., Modano, M., Amendola, A., Goodall, R., . . . & Fraternali, F. (2016). On the reinforcement of cement mortars through 3D printed polymeric and metallic fibers. *Composites Part B: Engineering*, 90, 76–85.
57. Feygin, M., Shkolnik, A., Diamond, M. N., & Dvorskiy, E. (1998). *Laminated object manufacturing system*. U.S. Patent No. 5,730,817. Washington, DC: U.S. Patent and Trademark Office.
58. Frazier, W. E. (2014). Metal additive manufacturing: A review. *Journal of Materials Engineering and Performance*, 23(6), 1917–28.

59. Gao, W., Zhang, Y., Ramanujan, D., Ramani, K., Chen, Y., Williams, C. B., . . . & Zavattieri, P. D. (2015). The status, challenges, and future of additive manufacturing in engineering. *Computer-Aided Design*, 69, 65–89.
60. Gibson, I., Rosen, D. W., & Stucker, B. (2014). *Additive Manufacturing Technologies* (Vol. 17). New York: Springer.
61. Gokuldoss, P. K., Kolla, S., & Eckert, J. (2017). Additive manufacturing processes: Selective laser melting, electron beam melting and binder jetting—Selection guidelines. *Materials*, 10(6), 672.
62. Gu, D. D., Meiners, W., Wissenbach, K., & Poprawe, R. (2012). Laser additive manufacturing of metallic components: Materials, processes and mechanisms. *International Materials Reviews*, 57(3), 133–64.
63. Gupta, K., & Laubscher, R. F. (2017). Sustainable machining of titanium alloys: A critical review. *Proceedings of the Institution of Mechanical Engineers, Part B: Journal of Engineering Manufacture*, 231(14), 2543–60.
64. Herzog, D., Seyda, V., Wycisk, E., & Emmelmann, C. (2016). Additive manufacturing of metals. *Acta Materialia*, 117, 371–92.
65. Huang, Y., Leu, M. C., Mazumder, J., & Donmez, A. (2015). Additive manufacturing: Current state, future potential, gaps and needs, and recommendations. *Journal of Manufacturing Science and Engineering*, 137(1), 014001.
66. Jacobs, P. F. (1992). *Rapid Prototyping & Manufacturing: Fundamentals of Stereolithography*. Society of Manufacturing Engineers.
67. Jain, V. K., & Adsul, S. G. (2000). Experimental investigations into abrasive flow machining (AFM). *International Journal of Machine Tools and Manufacture*, 40(7), 1003–21.
68. Jha, S., & Jain, V. K. (2004). Design and development of the magnetorheological abrasive flow finishing (MRAFF) process. *International Journal of Machine Tools and Manufacture*, 44(10), 1019–29.
69. Jiang, X. J., & Whitehouse, D. J. (2012). Technological shifts in surface metrology. *CIRP Annals*, 61(2), 815–36.
70. Karunakaran, K. P., Bernard, A., Suryakumar, S., Dembinski, L., & Taillandier, G. (2012). Rapid manufacturing of metallic objects. *Rapid Prototyping Journal*, 18(4), 264–80.
71. Kaynak, Y., & Kitay, O. (2018). Porosity, surface quality, microhardness and microstructure of selective laser melted 316L stainless steel resulting from finish machining. *Journal of Manufacturing and Materials Processing*, 2(2), 36.
72. Kellens, K., Baumers, M., Gutowski, T. G., Flanagan, W., Lifset, R., & Duflou, J. R. (2017). Environmental dimensions of additive manufacturing: Mapping application domains and their environmental implications. *Journal of Industrial Ecology*, 21(S1), S49–68.
73. Khoo, Z. X., Teoh, J. E. M., Liu, Y., Chua, C. K., Yang, S., An, J., . . . & Yeong, W. Y. (2015). 3D printing of smart materials: A review on recent progresses in 4D printing. *Virtual and Physical Prototyping*, 10(3), 103–22.
74. Klocke, F., & Kuchle, A. (2011). *Manufacturing Processes 1: Cutting*. Springer Science & Business Media.
75. Korner, C. (2016). Additive manufacturing of metallic components by selective electron beam melting—A review. *International Materials Reviews*, 61(5), 361–77.
76. Kruth, J. P., Leu, M. C., & Nakagawa, T. (1998). Progress in additive manufacturing and rapid prototyping. *CIRP Annals*, 47(2), 525–40.
77. Kumar, S., & Kruth, J. P. (2010). Composites by rapid prototyping technology. *Materials & Design*, 31(2), 850–6.
78. Leary, M., Merli, L., Torti, F., Mazur, M., & Brandt, M. (2014). Optimal topology for additive manufacture: A method for enabling additive manufacture of support-free optimal structures. *Materials & Design*, 63, 678–90.

79. Lee, J. Y., An, J., & Chua, C. K. (2017). Fundamentals and applications of 3D printing for novel materials. *Applied Materials Today*, 7, 120–33.
80. Leong, K. F., Cheah, C. M., & Chua, C. K. (2003). Solid freeform fabrication of three-dimensional scaffolds for engineering replacement tissues and organs. *Biomaterials*, 24(13), 2363–78.
81. Li, N., Huang, S., Zhang, G., Qin, R., Liu, W., Xiong, H., & Blackburn, J. (2019). Progress in additive manufacturing on new materials: A review. *Journal of Materials Science & Technology*, 35(2), 242–69.
82. Liu, R., Wang, Z., Sparks, T., Liou, F., & Newkirk, J. (2017). Aerospace applications of laser additive manufacturing. In *Laser Additive Manufacturing* (pp. 351–71). Woodhead Publishing.
83. Loh, G. H., Pei, E., Harrison, D., & Monzón, M. D. (2018). An overview of functionally graded additive manufacturing. *Additive Manufacturing*, 23, 34–44.
84. Mahmood, M. A., & Popescu, A. C. (2017). Laser-assisted additive manufacturing processes: A review. *Lasers in Manufacturing and Materials Processing*, 4(3), 155–92.
85. Manfredi, D., Calignano, F., Krishnan, M., Canali, R., Ambrosio, E. P., & Atzeni, E. (2013). From powders to dense metal parts: Characterization of a commercial AlSiMg alloy processed through direct metal laser sintering. *Materials*, 6(3), 856–69.
86. Mellor, S., Hao, L., & Zhang, D. (2014). Additive manufacturing: A framework for implementation. *International Journal of Production Economics*, 149, 194–201.
87. Merklein, M., Junker, D., Schaub, A., & Neubauer, F. (2016). Hybrid additive manufacturing technologies—An analysis regarding potentials and applications. *Physics Procedia*, 83, 549–59.
88. Mohammadian, N., Turenne, S., & Brailovski, V. (2018). Surface finish control of additively-manufactured Inconel 625 components using combined chemical-abrasive flow polishing. *Journal of Materials Processing Technology*, 252, 728–38.
89. Mori, K., Maeno, T., & Nakagawa, Y. (2014). Dieless forming of carbon fibre reinforced plastic parts using 3D printer. *Procedia Engineering*, 81, 1595–600.
90. Mourtzis, D., Doukas, M., & Bernidaki, D. (2014). Simulation in manufacturing: Review and challenges. *Procedia CIRP*, 25, 213–29.
91. Murr, L. E., Gaytan, S. M., Ramirez, D. A., Martinez, E., Hernandez, J., Amato, K. N., ... & Wicker, R. B. (2012). Metal fabrication by additive manufacturing using laser and electron beam melting technologies. *Journal of Materials Science & Technology*, 28(1), 1–14.
92. Muthu, S. S., & Savalani, M. M. (Eds.). (2016). *Handbook of Sustainability in Additive Manufacturing*. Springer.
93. Ngo, T. D., Kashani, A., Imbalzano, G., Nguyen, K. T., & Hui, D. (2018). Additive manufacturing (3D printing): A review of materials, methods, applications and challenges. *Composites Part B: Engineering*, 143, 172–96.
94. Nickels, L. (2015). AM and aerospace: An ideal combination. *Metal Powder Report*, 70(6), 300–3.
95. Ning, F., Cong, W., Qiu, J., Wei, J., & Wang, S. (2015). Additive manufacturing of carbon fiber reinforced thermoplastic composites using fused deposition modeling. *Composites Part B: Engineering*, 80, 369–78.
96. Olakanmi, E. O., Cochrane, R. F., & Dalgarno, K. W. (2015). A review on selective laser sintering/melting (SLS/SLM) of aluminium alloy powders: Processing, microstructure, and properties. *Progress in Materials Science*, 74, 401–77.
97. Palanivel, S., Nelaturu, P., Glass, B., & Mishra, R. S. (2015). Friction stir additive manufacturing for high structural performance through microstructural control in an Mg based WE43 alloy. *Materials & Design*, 65, 934–52.

98. Park, J., Tari, M. J., & Hahn, H. T. (2000). Characterization of the laminated object manufacturing (LOM) process. *Rapid Prototyping Journal*, 6(1), 36–50.
99. Singh, M., Singh, A., & Singh, A. K. (2019). Nanofinishing of external cylindrical surface of C60 steel using rotating core-based magnetorheological finishing process. In *Advances in Unconventional Machining and Composites: Proceedings of AIMTDR 2018* (pp. 53–66). Singapore: Springer Singapore.
100. Petrovic, V., Vicente Haro Gonzalez, J., Jordá Ferrando, O., Delgado Gordillo, J., Ramón Blasco Puchades, J., & Portolés Griñan, L. (2011). Additive layered manufacturing: Sectors of industrial application shown through case studies. *International Journal of Production Research*, 49(4), 1061–79.
101. Singh, M., & Singh, A. K. (2021). Magnetorheological finishing of variable diametric external surface of the tapered cylindrical workpieces for functionality improvement. *Journal of Manufacturing Processes*, 61, 153–72.
102. Singh, M., & Singh, A. K. (2021). Magnetorheological finishing of copper cylindrical roller for its improved performance in printing machine. *Proceedings of the Institution of Mechanical Engineers, Part E: Journal of Process Mechanical Engineering*, 235(1), 103–15.
103. Pham, D. T., & Gault, R. S. (1998). A comparison of rapid prototyping technologies. *International Journal of Machine Tools and Manufacture*, 38(10–11), 1257–87.
104. Singh, M., & Singh, A. K. (2018, June). Parametric optimization for nano-finishing of the external cylindrical surfaces using rotating core magnetorheological finishing process. In *International Manufacturing Science and Engineering Conference* (Vol. 51388, p. V004T03A006). American Society of Mechanical Engineers.
105. Qi, Q., Pagani, L., Scott, P. J., & Jiang, X. (2020). A categorical framework for formalising knowledge in additive manufacturing. *Procedia CIRP*, 75, 87–91.
106. Qian, Y. P., Huang, J. H., Zhang, H. O., & Wang, G. L. (2008). Direct laser fabrication of nickel alloy samples. *International Journal of Machine Tools and Manufacture*, 48(2), 237–43.
107. Raghavan, N., Dehoff, R., Pannala, S., Simunovic, S., Kirka, M., Turner, J., & Babu, S. S. (2016). Numerical modeling of heat-transfer and the influence of process parameters on tailoring the grain morphology of IN718 in electron beam additive manufacturing. *Acta Materialia*, 112, 303–14.
108. Rajan, K., Deshpande, A. P., & Narasimhan, K. (2010). Effect of heat treatment on the magnetic and magnetorheological properties of magnetite nanoparticles in magnetorheological fluids. *Journal of Magnetism and Magnetic Materials*, 322(18), 2685–8.
109. Ramu, M., Prabhu Raja, V., & Thyla, P. R. (2013). Establishment of structural similarities and evaluation of solid freeform fabrication processes. *International Journal of Advanced Manufacturing Technology*, 65(5–8), 1049–59.
110. Reeves, P. (2017). Additive manufacturing–A supply chain wide response. *European Journal of Operational Research*, 258(1), 296–307.
111. Rejeski, D., Zhao, F., & Huang, Y. (2018). Research needs and recommendations on environmental implications of additive manufacturing. *Additive Manufacturing*, 19, 21–8.
112. Singh, M., & Singh, A. K. (2019). Magnetorheological finishing of micro-punches for enhanced performance of micro-extrusion process. *Materials and Manufacturing Processes*, 34(14), 1646–57.
113. Rombouts, M., Kruth, J. P., Froyen, L., & Mercelis, P. (2006). Fundamentals of selective laser melting of alloyed steel powders. *CIRP Annals*, 55(1), 187–92.
114. Sames, W. J., List, F. A., Pannala, S., Dehoff, R. R., & Babu, S. S. (2016). The metallurgy and processing science of metal additive manufacturing. *International Materials Reviews*, 61(5), 315–60.

115. Singh, M., & Singh, A. K. (2020). Magnetorheological finishing of grooved drum surface and its performance analysis in winding process. *The International Journal of Advanced Manufacturing Technology*, 106, 2921–37.
116. Sánchez-Salinas, A., Blanco-Villalobos, C., Neto, J. C., Greer, A. L., Vogiatzis, P., & Jiménez, J. A. (2019). On the role of Nb and Ti on microsegregation and microstructure selection in laser-melted Inconel 718. *Metallurgical and Materials Transactions A*, 50(6), 2859–72.
117. Santecchia, E., Hamouda, A. M. S., Musharavati, F., Zalnezhad, E., Cabibbo, M., El Mehtedi, M., & Spigarelli, S. (2016). A review on fatigue life prediction methods for metals. *Advances in Materials Science and Engineering*, 2016.
118. Santos, E. C., Shiomi, M., Osakada, K., & Laoui, T. (2006). Rapid manufacturing of metal components by laser forming. *International Journal of Machine Tools and Manufacture*, 46(12–13), 1459–68.
119. Schmidt, M., Merklein, M., Bourell, D., Dimitrov, D., Hausotte, T., Wegener, K., . . . & Levy, G. N. (2017). Laser based additive manufacturing in industry and academia. *CIRP Annals*, 66(2), 561–83.
120. Seifi, M., Salem, A., Beuth, J., Harrysson, O., & Lewandowski, J. J. (2016). Overview of materials qualification needs for metal additive manufacturing. *JOM*, 68(3), 747–64.
121. Seyda, V., Kaufmann, N., & Emmelmann, C. (2012). Investigation of aging processes of Ti-6Al-4 V powder material in laser melting. *Physics Procedia*, 39, 425–31.
122. Shapiro, A. A., Borgonia, J. P., Chen, Q. N., Dillon, R. P., McEnerney, B., Polit-Casillas, R., & Soloway, L. (2016). Additive manufacturing for aerospace flight applications. *Journal of Spacecraft and Rockets*, 53(5), 952–9.
123. Shishkovsky, I., Yadroitsev, I., Bertrand, P., & Smurov, I. (2007). Alumina–zirconium ceramics synthesis by selective laser sintering/melting. *Applied Surface Science*, 254(4), 966–70.
124. Singh, M., Singh, A., & Singh, A. K. (2018). A rotating core-based magnetorheological nano-finishing process for external cylindrical surfaces. *Materials and Manufacturing Processes*, 33(11), 1160–8.
125. Sing, S. L., An, J., Yeong, W. Y., & Wiria, F. E. (2016). Laser and electron-beam powder-bed additive manufacturing of metallic implants: A review on processes, materials and designs. *Journal of Orthopaedic Research*, 34(3), 369–85.
126. Singh, S., Ramakrishna, S., & Singh, R. (2017). Material issues in additive manufacturing: A review. *Journal of Manufacturing Processes*, 25, 185–200.
127. Slotwinski, J. A., Garboczi, E. J., Stutzman, P. E., Ferraris, C. F., Watson, S. S., & Peltz, M. A. (2014). Characterization of metal powders used for additive manufacturing. *Journal of Research of the National Institute of Standards and Technology*, 119, 460.
128. Song, B., Dong, S., Zhang, B., Liao, H., & Coddet, C. (2012). Effects of processing parameters on microstructure and mechanical property of selective laser melted Ti6Al4V. *Materials & Design*, 35, 120–5.
129. Strano, G., Hao, L., Everson, R. M., & Evans, K. E. (2013). Surface roughness analysis, modelling and prediction in selective laser melting. *Journal of Materials Processing Technology*, 213(4), 589–97.
130. Sun, J., Yang, Y., & Wang, D. (2013). Parametric optimization of selective laser melting for forming Ti6Al4V samples by Taguchi method. *Optics & Laser Technology*, 49, 118–24.
131. Taminger, K. M., & Hafley, R. A. (2003). Electron beam freeform fabrication: A rapid metal deposition process. In *Proceedings of the 3rd Annual Automotive Composites Conference* (pp. 9–10).

132. Tan, X., Kok, Y., Tan, Y. J., Descoins, M., Mangelinck, D., Tor, S. B., . . . & Chua, C. K. (2015). Graded microstructure and mechanical properties of additive manufactured Ti–6Al–4V via electron beam melting. *Acta Materialia*, 97, 1–16.
133. Thijs, L., Verhaeghe, F., Craeghs, T., Van Humbeeck, J., & Kruth, J. P. (2010). A study of the microstructural evolution during selective laser melting of Ti–6Al–4V. *Acta Materialia*, 58(9), 3303–12.
134. Thompson, M. K., Moroni, G., Vaneker, T., Fadel, G., Campbell, R. I., Gibson, I., . . . & Martina, F. (2016). Design for additive manufacturing: Trends, opportunities, considerations, and constraints. *CIRP Annals*, 65(2), 737–60.
135. Töppel, T., Müller, B., Hoeren, K. P., & Witt, G. (2016). Eigenspannungen und Verzug bei additiver Fertigung durch Strahlschmelzen. *Schweissen und Schneiden*, 68(4), 176–86.
136. Trevisan, F., Calignano, F., Lorusso, M., Pakkanen, J., Aversa, A., Ambrosio, E. P., . . . & Fino, P. (2017). On the selective laser melting (SLM) of the AlSi10Mg alloy: Process, microstructure, and mechanical properties. *Materials*, 10(1), 76.
137. Vaezi, M., Seitz, H., & Yang, S. (2013). A review on 3D micro-additive manufacturing technologies. *The International Journal of Advanced Manufacturing Technology*, 67(5–8), 1721–54.
138. Valente, E. H., Nadimpalli, V. K., Andersen, O., Christiansen, T. L., & Somers, M. A. (2019). Effect of moisture content in MIM feedstock on the sintering behavior of stainless steel components. *Powder Technology*, 343, 68–72.
139. Van Bael, S., Kerckhofs, G., Moesen, M., Pyka, G., Schrooten, J., & Kruth, J. P. (2011). Micro-CT-based improvement of geometrical and mechanical controllability of selective laser melted Ti6Al4V porous structures. *Materials Science and Engineering: A*, 528(24), 7423–31.
140. Singh, M., & Singh, A. K. (2019). Performance investigation of magnetorheological finishing of rolls surface in cold rolling process. *Journal of Manufacturing Processes*, 41, 315–29.
141. Singh, M., & Singh, A. K. (2019). Improved magnetorheological finishing process with rectangular core tip for external cylindrical surfaces. *Materials and Manufacturing Processes*, 34(9), 1049–61.
142. Singh, M., & Singh, A. K. (2020). Theoretical investigations into magnetorheological finishing of external cylindrical surfaces for improved performance. *Proceedings of the Institution of Mechanical Engineers, Part C: Journal of Mechanical Engineering Science*, 234(24), 4872–92.
143. Vayre, B., Vignat, F., & Villeneuve, F. (2012). Metallic additive manufacturing: State-of-the-art review and prospects. *Mechanics & Industry*, 13(2), 89–96.
144. Venuvinod, P. K., & Ma, W. (2004). *Rapid Prototyping: Laser-Based And Other Technologies*. Springer Science & Business Media.
145. Wang, F., Williams, S., Colegrove, P., & Antonysamy, A. A. (2013). Microstructure and mechanical properties of wire and arc additive manufactured Ti-6Al-4V. *Metallurgical and Materials Transactions A*, 44(2), 968–77.
146. Wang, X., Gong, X., & Chou, K. (2015). Review on powder-bed laser additive manufacturing of inconel 718 parts. *Proceedings of the Institution of Mechanical Engineers, Part B: Journal of Engineering Manufacture*, 231(11), 1890–903.
147. Weller, C., Kleer, R., & Piller, F. T. (2015). Economic implications of 3D printing: Market structure models in light of additive manufacturing revisited. *International Journal of Production Economics*, 164, 43–56.
148. Williams, S. W., Martina, F., Addison, A. C., Ding, J., Pardal, G., & Colegrove, P. (2016). Wire+ arc additive manufacturing. *Materials Science and Technology*, 32(7), 641–47.

149. Wong, K. V., & Hernandez, A. (2012). A review of additive manufacturing. *ISRN Mechanical Engineering*, 2012.
150. Wu, A. S., Brown, D. W., Kumar, M., Gallegos, G. F., & King, W. E. (2014). An experimental investigation into additive manufacturing-induced residual stresses in 316L stainless steel. *Metallurgical and Materials Transactions A*, 45(13), 6260–70.
151. Yadroitsev, I., Krakhmalev, P., & Yadroitsava, I. (2015). Selective laser melting of Ti6Al4V alloy for biomedical applications: Temperature monitoring and microstructural evolution. *Journal of Alloys and Compounds*, 583, 404–9.
152. Yang, L., Hsu, K., Baughman, B., Godfrey, D., Medina, F., Menon, M., & Wiener, S. (2017). *Additive Manufacturing of Metals: The Technology, Materials, Design and Production*. Springer.
153. Singh, A. K., Kumar, S., & Singh, V. P. (2014). Optimization of parameters using conductive powder in dielectric for EDM of super Co 605 with multiple quality characteristics. *Materials and Manufacturing Processes*, 29(3), 267–73.
154. Sankhyan, A., & Pawar, P. K. (2013). Metformin loaded non-ionic surfactant vesicles: Optimization of formulation, effect of process variables and characterization. *DARU Journal of Pharmaceutical Sciences*, 21, 1–8.

23 Regulating Pyrimethamine Resistance in Malaria via Virtual Screening Techniques based on the PubChem Derivatives

Anish Kumar, Aeimy Mary Jose, Karuna Khajuria, and Anshika Mahajan

CONTENTS

23.1 INTRODUCTION

Malaria is a disease which is caused by the malarial parasite which falls under the species Plasmodium. Malaria is by far a very deadly disease that affects other people through the malaria parasite, which is believed to be found in the infected female Anopheles. Even though malarial diseases are deadly these can be prevented as well as it is curable. Malaria mainly affects the kidney as well as the liver, or it can even cause the spleen to be ruptured. Having malaria causes red blood cells to decrease that supply oxygen to the tissues in our body. As compared to other infectious diseases, malaria

DOI: 10.1201/9781003516064-23

possess a much greater effect on the world [1]. The data collected from the World Health Organization WHO reveals that there is 247 million new cases of malaria in the year 2021 all over the world, out of that the African region has 95% of cases, and the death rate was 96% in which 80% of the death is of children below the age of 5 years. There are five main parasite species of which two are of immense danger to humans, *P. falciparum* and *P. vivax*. The early stages of symptoms are fever, headache, and cold which occur within 10–15 days of infection, and in case it is left undetected it causes severe ailment or even be the cause of death of a person [2].

P. falciparum was identified to be the most prevalent species of parasite to be living in some areas of Asia, Africa, and Latin America which is credited for the massive increase in malaria cases, for which various drugs or medicines have been developed to curb and eradicate malarial parasite. *P. falciparum* has a higher malaria mortality rate than *P. vivax* although the latter has more dangerous and fatal malarial contagion [3]. Pyrimethamine is an anti-parasitic used in the management of malaria and as a prophylactic agent against malaria. The sporozoite which gets in to the human being through the bite migrates to the liver, and when the mosquito bites an infected person the parasite will again enter [4]. From the observation, there was an increase in the development of resistance as opposed to pyrimethamine was caused by various mutations that occur in the genes. Comparing the development of pyrimethamine resistance with resistance to other drugs, it is necessary to have an anti-malarial drug to treat the pyrimethamine resistance. Newer generation medicines are used by the people of the world extensively due to which there is a lot of concern about the availability of the medicines and the side effects which are associated with these medicines [5]. The key information regarding the mechanism of drug resistance is of utmost importance to the advancement of the therapeutic sector. Resistance to pyrimethamine is attributed to changes in genes for which our body is unable to respond to the drug. Malaria is also preventable and also curable, but if the parasite is not treated it multiplies within 48 hours and also leads to death caused by malaria. Due to several mutations in the malarial parasite, they have become resistant to antimalarial drugs which reduces the productiveness of the malarial treatment. Several steps are taken for the better treatment of malarial parasite; first, proper diagnosis is done; proper and correct doses of drugs are to be used on time, and this is because the incomplete dosage would lead to the failure of the treatment [6]. The development of the anti-malarial drugs for pyrimethamine resistance is achieved with the help of virtual screening technique such as Molinspiration and OSIRIS program. The analysis is done with PubChem database, and it is later inspected with Lipinski's rule of five. Molecular docking is done in which the computational reconstruction of ligand–receptor interaction/protein–protein interaction occurs. The OSIRIS software is used to ascertain from the main molecules whether or not they exhibit toxicity, drug-likeness, clogP, and other physico-chemical properties of the drugs. PubChem database offers free and easily available data, allowing the users to compare as well as to examine and to collect any biological tests [7–8]. The causative agent of malaria is coccidian parasitic protozoan subclass; this mostly affects the red blood cells, and there are some other organisms such as small insects and few mites which transmit malaria to mammals including humans and other animals. The sporozoite is transferred through the saliva of mosquitoes into the bloodstream from where it infiltrates the liver where it divides, and then it is passed back into the bloodstream [8]. There has been an increase in the malarial drug resistance, and the rate of mortality is higher, so it is essential to recognize and acknowledge the malarial drug resistance, improving the techniques which are used to detect the resistance in the drugs. There are various antimicrobial drugs utilized against malaria such as co-trimoxazole, ketolides, thiopeptides, quinolones, tigecycline, and others [9]. It has already been long understood that computer techniques including virtual screening (VS) can be incredibly helpful in speeding up and decreasing the cost of drug design. In accordance with the literature evidence, authors claimed that VS methods provided qualitative predictions between active and inactive compounds efficiently. Research has also shown that VS may also be used to develop new drugs to fight pyrimethamine resistance in malaria. Moreover, the search for new medications has become more and more important due to the trends toward and increase in patient numbers. Today, the molecular docking method allows cutting the time to search for the necessary molecules and effective studying of several compounds in reference to the given target [10–11]. Pharmacological tools are useful to fast forward the evaluation of the molecule in question to determine the suitability of the compound as a drug candidate. After passing through the screening process the drug candidate can be tested in vitro and in vivo models and in various phases of clinical trials before getting to the market. Using the molecular docking tool known as Seamdock in parallel with the advanced screening tools which include Molinspiration and OSIRIS property explorer, a pharmacological replacement to pyrimethamine-resistant malaria was determined in this investigation [12]. The software, web servers, and technique used in this study are outlined in the flowchart shown in **Figure 23.1**.

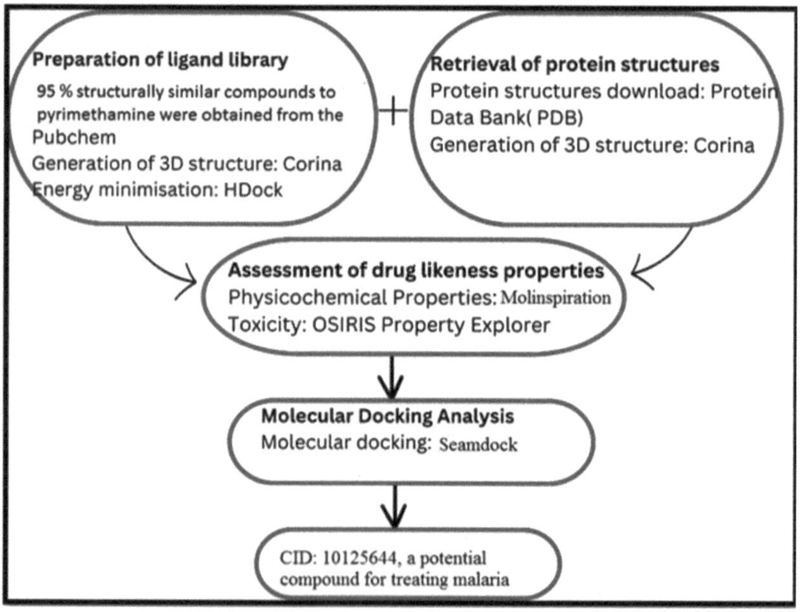

FIGURE 23.1 Flowchart of methodology, software, and web servers used in this study.

23.2 MATERIALS AND METHODS

23.2.1 Dataset

The native structure and the mutant structure at amino acid level are taken from Protein Data Bank [PDB] for performing the analysis in the 3D structure [13]. Pyrimethamine chemical name: 5–(4-chlorophenyl)-6-ethyl-2,4-dimethylpyrimidin; Chemical formula: $C_{12}H_{13}C_{1}N_{4}$. The PDB codes are 2BL9 and 2BLC, both for native and the mutant structures (which is pyrimethamine resistant) as shown in **Figure 23.2**. From the PubChem database which provides information on various compounds including their biological activities, safety, toxicity, and physical properties, we obtained the SMILES string of the lead compounds used in this study. The PubChem database, a comprehensive database containing information on numerous compounds including their biological activity, safety, toxicity, and physical qualities, is where we received the SMILES string of lead compounds used in our study. Every compound in PubChem is assigned a unique CID, and regardless of the type of information one wants, the CID number is used to retrieve it. We used the SMILES string in the CORINA 3D structure generator to generate 3D structure of lead compounds to allow for further study (**Figure 23.3**). A free web application called CORINA is

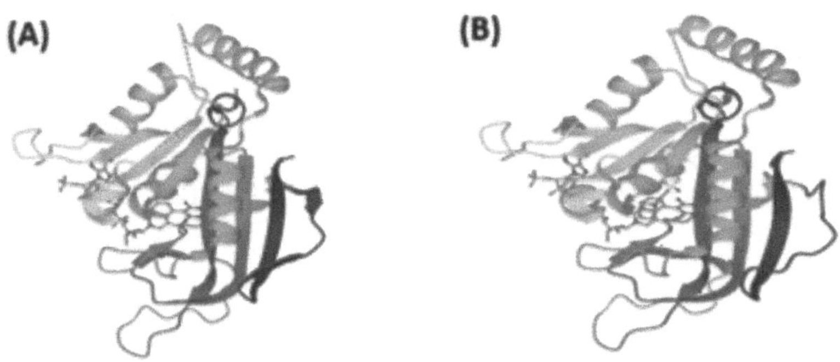

FIGURE 23.2 Protein structure obtained from PDB (A) Native structure 2BL9 (B) Mutant structure 2BLC.

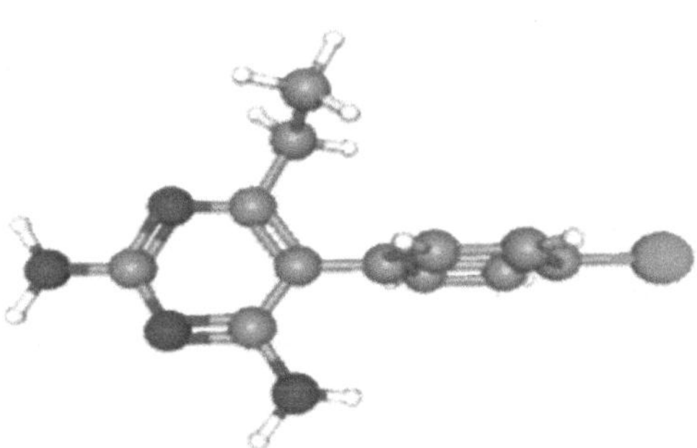

FIGURE 23.3 3D structure of pyrimethamine.

a must to build the 3D structures of many different compounds and is used when seeking a medicinal compound [14]. This provides a fast, high-quality molecular structure that is useful for analyzing numerous lead compounds and in the long run useful for developing new drugs [15].

23.2.2 Manufacturing Techniques

Virtual screening (VS) is a computational technique which is used in screening and discovery of drugs. With the help of computer tools present in the laboratory we can automatically screen large libraries. It is more accurate, and the cost is less due to which VS is an important part of the discovery of drugs [16]. The virtual screening technique using PubChem database with pyrimethamine as the query was utilized. According to statistics, PubChem database holds about 27 million unique chemical substances for which compound ID (CID) is derived from about 70 million substance deposition (SID) [17]. PubChem database which is publicly accessible is a golden opportunity for scientists to perform VS technique. Several hits are acquired from PubChem database, which in return are further examined with the help of molecular docking.

One of the discoveries enabled by this technique is venetoclax, a BCL-2 antagonist which is prescribed for the management of hematological cancers and CLL. Small molecules selective for BCL-2 were identified using computational tools and led to the development of venetoclax, a targeted therapy for CLL [18–19]. Dasatinib, a tyrosine kinase inhibitor for CML was identified through the VS technique. Discovery of dasatinib, a tyrosine kinase inhibitor used to treat chronic myeloid leukemia (CML), was also made possible by computational techniques, particularly VS. Additionally, targeted therapy for CML, known as dasatinib, was created through applying these methods to search for small molecules that potentially may block the BCR-ABL kinase [20].

23.2.3 ADME and Toxicity

Regarding the molecular properties of the lead compounds, Lipinski's rule of five was applied to determine the bioavailability of the lead compounds, As it is known, Lipinski formulated the rule of five, which is, in fact, four main molecular properties put together in an ensemble called the rule of five [21]. These are as follows logP (partition coefficient), hydrogen bond donors and acceptors in the molecule, and molecular weight (MW) are the factors resulting in the rule of five. It has been noted that around 51% of drugs provided by FDA complies with Lipinski's rule of five [22]. According to this rule, a molecular weight less than or equal to equal to 500 Daltons, log P less than 5, and hydrogen bond donors not more than 5 and hydrogen bond acceptors not more than 10, as well as Van der Waals bumps polar surface must be below 120 $Å^2$[23]. All the different physiochemical properties of lead molecules in the study are determined by using Molinspiration program [24].

Toxicity is the next characteristics used to determine if the lead compounds are toxic or not, which in return is responsible for the failure of most of the lead compounds. The clogP value is calculated with the help of Molinspiration techniques [25]. Tumorigenicity, mutagenicity, and reproductive effects of the lead compounds are the parameters which are used when trying to determine toxicity. For the lead compounds, the toxicity is determined by utilizing OSIRIS program. While the OSIRIS program allows us to analyze the lead compounds drug-likeness and drug score, there is 5,300 substructure fragments formed by 3,300 traded drug and 15,000 compounds indicate the absolute list of all the available fragments associated with drug-likeness. Drug-likeness, log S, clog P, molecular weight, and risk of toxicity are important preclusion and used to decide whether a chemical fragment belongs to a drug or not is a drug score. The danger levels of various drug molecules can be readily identified by using the color-coded approach. Red highlights high-risk drug features, while green highlights safe pharmaceuticals [26–27].

23.2.4 Molecular Docking

Estimation of how the target proteins or receptors or ligands will interact is an essential component of virtual screening called docking. The main procedure of docking is to predict the orientation and interactions between ligand and the protein's binding site [28]. Furthermore, the biological activity of the screened lead compounds is crucial to give royalty to the study of docking, first of all, the SMILES string is used to build the 3D structure of the lead compounds. Following this, through the Seamdock server the server docking was executed. Estimation of the activity of target proteins, or receptors, or ligands, is an imperative step in VS, which is called docking. Predicting the position and orientation of the ligands within the binding site of the protein is the major objective of docking [28]. It can be used in cooperation with partners from all over the world or, leaving aside the installation of the software and command lines in Unix, in a class specific to docking techniques or receptor–ligand interactions [29]. Planned enhancements include more docking engines, better protonation control, and choice of one or more scoring functions. Studies of the binding of pyrimethamine and the lead compounds are explained by means of 2BL9 and 2BLC; these are the native and the mutated protein structures [30].

23.3 RESULTS AND DISCUSSION

23.3.1 Virtual Screening Techniques

The study was done by using compounds which are similar to pyrimethamine from the PubChem database and pyrimethamine was opted as the query molecule. On the base of the aim, the virtual screening parameters differ but the protocol is similar [31]. Ninety-five percent similarity cutoff was stained for the analysis, as a result 60 compounds were obtained, which are used for further study. For understanding bioavailability of the pyrimethamine and its lead compounds Molinspiration program (**Figure 23.4**) is used. The properties of pyrimethamine are calculated by Molinspiration program, and it will be used in designing the library to screen the lead compound using computational techniques [32]. **Table 23.1** shows the results; it indicates that four compounds, CID:330711, CID:53345306, CID:21689899, CID:5797178. Out of these, all four compounds demonstrated one violation of Lipinski's rule of five, The remaining 56 compounds showed zero violations, and hence, the bioavailability of these 56 compounds is significantly more. These hits have been further classified based on the number of rotatable bonds, which should

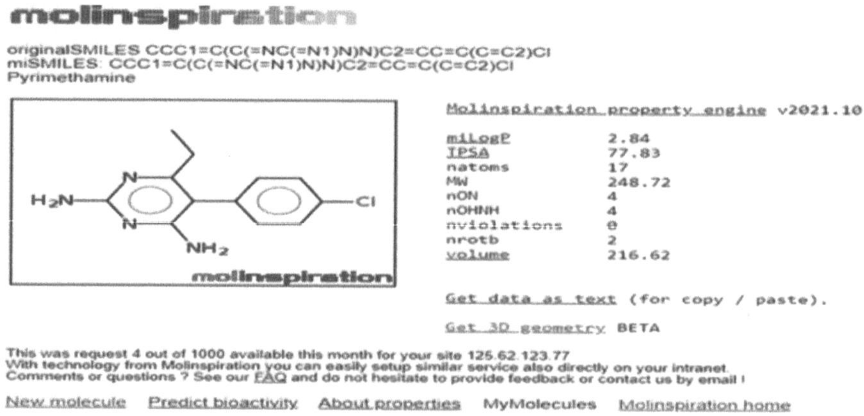

FIGURE 23.4 Molecular properties of pyrimethamine calculated using the Molinspiration program.

TABLE 23.1
Calculations of Molecular Properties of Pyrimethamine and Lead Compound using Molinspiration

S. No.	Compound	miLogP	TPSA	MW	nON	nOHNH	nviolation	Volume
1.	Pyrimethamine	2.84	77.83	248.72	4	4	0	216.62
2.	CID:24466	2.87	77.83	269.13	4	4	0	213.35
3.	CID:93114	2.16	77.83	214.27	4	4	0	203.08
4.	CID:29142	3.44	77.83	283.16	4	4	0	230.15
5.	CID:9881905	4.23	77.83	270.38	4	4	0	270.29
6.	CID:9860692	3.13	77.83	287.12	4	4	0	218.52
7.	CID:343098	3.81	127.58	289.73	7	4	0	241.51
8.	CID:240802	2.51	51.81	205.65	3	2	0	171.96
9.	CID:134621	2.43	77.83	248.72	4	4	0	216.62
10.	CID:134531	2.26	77.83	234.69	4	4	0	199.81
11.	CID:72565	1.58	77.83	200.25	4	4	0	186.28
12.	CID:13926968	2.24	77.83	234.69	4	4	0	199.81
13.	CID:12293991	4.06	51.81	281.78	3	2	0	243.37
14.	CID:1156921	3.23	51.81	233.76	3	2	0	205.33
15.	CID:10060600	2.81	77.83	248.72	4	4	0	216.62
16.	CID:6365291	2.84	77.83	248.72	4	4	0	216.62
17.	CID:3154202	3.62	51.81	267.15	3	2	0	218.86
18.	CID:2777563	1.99	77.83	220.66	4	4	0	183.25
19.	CID:516689	1.75	77.83	214.27	4	4	0	203.08
20.	CID:341268	2.72	93.43	318.81	6	4	0	285.78
21.	CID:332598	3.53	105.80	319.80	7	4	0	281.62
22.	CID:330711	2.25	103.85	263.73	5	6	1	227.90

TABLE 23.1 *(Continued)*
Calculations of Molecular Properties of Pyrimethamine and Lead Compound using Molinspiration

S. No.	Compound	miLogP	TPSA	MW	nON	nOHNH	nviolation	Volume
23.	CID:309512	3.18	77.83	288.66	4	4	0	214.55
24.	CID:125330	3.79	127.58	289.73	7	4	0	241.51
25.	CID:92135840	2.84	77.83	248.72	4	4	0	216.62
26.	CID:58089417	3.98	25.78	272.66	2	0	0	208.53
27.	CID:53345306	1.47	17	249.71	5	6	1	211.34
28.	CID:53345189	3.90	77.83	276.77	4	4	0	250.22
29.	CID:44532049	2.01	77.83	214.27	4	4	0	202.84
30.	CID:25099455	3.32	77.83	262.74	4	4	0	233.20
31.	CID:23423608	3.58	77.83	276.77	4	4	0	250.00
32.	CID:23423607	3.34	77.83	262.74	4	4	0	233.42
33.	CID:21689932	3.48	77.83	303.58	4	4	0	226.88
34.	CID:21689899	2.28	103.85	284.15	5	6	1	224.64
35.	CID:18549177	2.48	77.83	369.13	4	4	0	213.35
36.	CID:14810438	2.61	51.81	219.68	3	2	0	188.53
37.	CID:13377422	2.88	51.81	219.68	3	2	0	188.53
38.	CID:11132208	−1.44	105.98	275.72	6	4	0	231.96
39.	CID:10125644	3.42	77.83	310.79	4	4	0	271.46
40.	CID:9974420	4.76	77.83	338.84	4	4	0	305.07
41.	CID:5797178	5.24	77.83	371.27	4	4	1	312.42
42.	CID:3331411	−1.44	105.98	275.72	6	4	0	231.96
43.	CID:3013252	3.05	76.20	303.80	5	3	0	274.35
44.	CID:3013250	3.03	76.20	303.80	5	3	0	274.35
45.	CID:894261	3.48	52.81	272.74	4	0	0	240.24
46.	CID:796128	2.79	25.78	204.66	2	0	0	177.24
47.	CID:456236	3.90	105.80	333.83	7	4	0	298.43
48.	CID:353605	3.81	127.58	289.73	7	4	0	241.51
49.	CID:343992	2.33	118.12	404.90	8	2	0	314.83
50.	CID:309506	2.25	101.62	259.70	5	4	0	216.91
51.	CID:134975	2.64	77.83	228.30	4	4	0	219.67
52.	CID:134622	4.40	77.83	290.80	4	4	0	267.02
53.	CID:134265	2.66	77.83	228.30	4	4	0	219.88
54.	CID:163242788	3.40	51.81	251.69	3	2	0	210.02
55.	CID:155553964	3.88	51.81	273.77	3	2	0	244.92
56.	CID:154722295	2.96	25.78	222.65	2	0	0	182.17
57.	CID:153919816	2.17	77.83	256.64	4	4	0	193.12
58.	CID:153867667	3.28	51.81	258.08	3	2	0	190.43
59.	CID:150093118	4.49	77.83	363.22	4	4	0	289.96
60.	CID:146266628	3.05	51.81	237.66	3	2	0	193.46

be less than ten to pass the oral bioavailability criterion. **Table 23.2** shows the final results; it is visible that all the 60 compounds which are selected by the ADME study has enough number of rotatable bonds <10, due to which these compounds are used as the lead compounds [33]. Toxicity is an important concern which is taken into consideration for the compounds before it is selected.

23.3.2 Toxicity Analysis

Toxicology testing is an important part in discovering new drugs as well as helps to improve the currently available drugs for therapeutic purpose. In the course of the drug development process, in early phases, it is a common experience that compounds

TABLE 23.2
Details of Number of Rotatable Bonds

S. No.	Compound	nrotb	S. no	Compound	nrotb
1.	Pyrimethamine	2	31	CID:23423608	3
2.	CID:24466	1	32	CID:23423607	3
3.	CID:93114	2	33	CID:21689932	1
4.	CID:29142	2	34	CID:21689899	1
5.	CID:9881905	6	35	CID:18549177	1
6.	CID:9860692	2	36	CID:14810438	1
7.	CID:343098	3	37	CID:13377422	1
8.	CID:240802	1	38	CID:11132208	2
9.	CID:134621	2	39	CID:10125644	3
10.	CID:134531	1	40	CID:9974420	5
11.	CID:72565	1	41	CID:5797178	4
12.	CID:13926968	1	42	CID:3331411	2
13.	CID:12293991	2	43	CID:3013252	5
14.	CID:1156921	2	44	CID:3013250	5
15.	CID:10060600	2	45	CID:894261	3
16.	CID:6365291	2	46	CID:796128	1
17.	CID:3154202	2	47	CID:456236	5
18.	CID:2777563	1	48	CID:353605	3
19.	CID:516689	2	49	CID:343992	6
20.	CID:341268	4	50	CID:309506	2
21.	CID:332598	4	51	CID:134975	2
22.	CID:330711	2	52	CID:134622	5
23.	CID:309512	2	53	CID:134265	3
24.	CID:125330	3	54	CID:163242788	1
25.	CID:92135840	2	55	CID:155553964	1
26.	CID:58089417	2	56	CID:154722295	1
27.	CID:53345306	2	57	CID:153919816	1
28.	CID:53345189	4	58	CID:153867667	1
29.	CID:44532049	1	59	CID:150093118	3
30.	CID:25099455	2	60	CID:146266628	1

are washed out because of the problems which are arising out of their pharmacokinetics as well as their toxicity [34]. The issues were conveyed in the recent works with the help of OSIRIS property explorer. Various criteria such as the clogP value and logS value are used to examine the pharmacokinetic properties of the lead compound [35]. The results obtained when all the lead compounds were subjected to OSIRIS property explorer program are shown in **Table 23.3**. Since the hydrophilicity is determined by the clogP value, the compound that has a high logP value will have minimum hydrophilicity, which leads to poor absorptiveness as well as permeability of the lead compound [36]. The value of logP of the lead compound is below 5 so that there is a better chance of getting absorbed properly. The value of logP was determined for all the 57 compounds using the parameters set as given in the **Table 23.1**. It is observed that the solubility affects the absorption as well as the distribution properties of the compounds; if a drug is having low absorption, then it is due to low solubility. The solubility unit is logS measured in mol/L. Around more than 80% of the drugs which are present in the market have logP value more than −4 [37].

23.3.3 Drug-Likeness

Drug-likeness is an important feature because drug-like molecules exhibit absorption, distribution, metabolism, excretion, and toxicity (ADMET) [38]. Drug-likeness of pyrimethamine and other virtually screened compounds is determined by using the OSIRIS program (**Figure 23.5**). According to the present study, drug-likeness of all the 57 lead compounds was within acceptable ranges; drug-likeness in a molecule could be evaluated if the molecule has the potentiality to become a drug in terms of its bioavailability [39].

23.3.4 Drug Score and Toxicity

The lead 57 compounds are put through the test for mutagenicity and tumorigenicity. From the statistics in the **Table 23.3**, it is realized that 20 compounds are non-tumorigenic as well as non-mutagenic. CID:24466, CID:93114, CID:29142, CID:9881905, CID:343098, CID:13453, CID:72565, CID:13926968, CID:10060600, CID:6365291, CID:341268, CID:332598, CID:330711, CID:309512, CID:92135840, CID:53345306, CID:53345189, CID:44532049, CID:25099455, CID:23423608, CID:23423607, CID:21689932, CID:21689899, CID:18549177, CID:11132208, CID:9974420, CID:5797178, CID:456236, CID:353605, CID:343992, CID:309506, CID:134975, CID:134622, CID:134265, CID:153919816, CID:150093118—these compounds were exhibiting mutagenic and/or tumorigenic properties and did not qualify the OSIRIS program (as seen in **Table 23.3**). The drug score [DS] of the lead compounds were also analyzed and comparison was also made with pyrimethamine. Quiz parameters included drug-likeness, miLogP, logS, toxicity prospects of a molecule, and molecular weight. The DS is helpful criterion to know whether or not the particular compound complies with all the requirements for approval of the drug. The lead compounds when compared to pyrimethamine showed moderate to outstanding DS value. From our dataset, 16 compounds were found to have DS similar to pyrimethamine, and about eight compounds—CID:134621, CID:3154202, CID:2777563, CID:14810438, CID:14810438, CID:3013252, CID:3013250, and

TABLE 23.3
Toxicity Risks and Physiochemical Properties of Pyrimethamine and Virtual Compounds Predicted by OSIRIS Property Explorer.

S. No.	Compound ID	Mutagenic	Tumorigenic	Reproductive Effective	cLogP	Solubility	Drug Likeness	Drug Score
1.	Pyrimethamine	Yes	Yes	Yes	2.54	−4.91	−.24	0.11
2.	CID:24466	Yes	No	Yes	2.73	−5.49	−.96	0.15
3	CID:93114	Yes	Yes	Yes	1.94	−4.17	−2.01	0.13
4.	CID:29142	Yes	Yes	Yes	3.15	−5.65	−1.24	0.11
5.	CID:9881905	No	No	Yes	3.75	−5.25	−16.86	0.19
6.	CID:343098	Yes	Yes	Yes	2.81	−5.61	−1.31	0.11
7.	CID:240802	No	No	No	2.24	−3.24	−1.52	0.52
8.	CID:134621	No	No	No	2.28	−4.38	0.51	0.63
9.	CID:134531	No	No	Yes	2.13	−4.75	0.07	0.34
10.	CID:72565	No	No	Yes	1.52	−4.01	−1.72	0.29
11.	CID:13926968	No	No	Yes	2.13	−4.75	−1.75	0.26
12.	CID:12293991	No	No	No	3.89	−5.25	0.17	0.47
13.	CID:1156921	No	No	No	2.87	−4.31	−0.24	0.56
14.	CID:10060600	Yes	Yes	No	2.54	−4.91	−2.03	0.11
15.	CID:6365291	Yes	Yes	Yes	2.54	−4.91	−0.24	0.11
16.	CID:3154202	No	No	No	3.31	−4.27	0.51	0.61
17.	CID:2777563	No	No	No	1.82	−4.07	0.18	0.64
18.	CID:516689	No	No	No	1.68	−3.64	−1.51	0.51
19.	CID:341268	Yes	Yes	Yes	1.87	−4.77	1.91	0.12
20.	CID:332598	Yes	Yes	Yes	3.18	−5.08	−3.67	0.07
21.	CID:330711	Yes	Yes	Yes	1.86	−4.98	−3.33	0.08
22.	CID:309512	No	No	Yes	2.63	−5.18	−7.01	0.2
23.	CID:92135840	Yes	Yes	Yes	2.54	−4.91	−0.24	0.11
24.	CID:58089417	No	No	No	3.59	−3.63	−8.77	0.39
25.	CID:53345306	No	No	Yes	0.79	−4.37	−0.06	0.36
26.	CID:53345189	No	No	Yes	3.45	−5.45	−5.58	0.18
27.	CID:44532049	No	No	Yes	1.86	−4.36	−2.1	0.27
28.	CID:25099455	No	No	Yes	2.97	−5.28	−0.26	0.28

29.	CID:23423608	No	No	Yes	3.21	−5.34	−0.2	0.28
30.	CID:23423607	No	No	Yes	3.0	−5.18	2.31	0.22
31.	CID:21689932	Yes	Yes	Yes	3.34	−6.22	−1.39	0.1
32.	CID:21689899	No	No	Yes	2.05	−5.56	−1.39	0.23
33.	CID:18549177	No	No	Yes	2.73	−5.49	−0.64	0.26
34.	CID:14810438	No	No	No	2.54	−3.84	0.07	0.63
35.	CID:13377422	No	No	No	2.59	−3.58	−1.57	0.5
36.	CID:11132208	Yes	Yes	Yes	2.3	−5.58	−3.7	0.09
37.	CID:10125644	No	No	No	2.77	−5.83	−0.04	0.44
38.	CID:9974420	No	No	Yes	4.44	−6.31	−5.5	0.14
39.	CID:5797178	No	No	Yes	4.92	−7.18	−1.78	0.13
40.	CID:3013252	No	No	No	2.92	−4.45	0.85	0.63
41.	CID:3013250	No	No	No	2.92	−4.45	1.83	0.69
42.	CID:894261	No	No	No	2.85	−4.05	1.19	0.7
43.	CID:796128	No	No	No	2.78	−2.52	−1.58	0.53
44.	CID:456236	Yes	Yes	Yes	3.58	−5.38	−2.67	0.07
45.	CID:353605	Yes	Yes	Yes	2.81	−5.61	−1.62	0.1
46.	CID:343992	No	No	Yes	1.99	−6.93	2.6	0.28
47.	CID:309506	No	No	Yes	1.79	−5.06	−7.22	0.21
48.	CID:134975	No	No	Yes	2.36	−4.54	−1.91	0.26
49.	CID:134622	No	No	Yes	3.9	−5.72	−10.0	0.17
50.	CID:134265	No	No	Yes	2.39	−4.44	−4.03	0.24
51.	CID:163242788	No	No	No	3.03	−4.24	−1.82	0.26
52.	CID:155553964	No	No	No	4.03	−4.96	−2.31	0.34
53.	CID:154722295	No	No	No	3.14	−3.59	−1.21	0.51
54.	CID:153919816	No	No	Yes	2.02	−4.7	−3.56	0.31
55.	CID:153867667	No	No	No	3.08	−4.55	−1.16	0.46
56.	CID:150093118	No	Yes	Yes	3.53	−5.61	0.21	0.16
57.	CID:146266628	No	No	No	2.69	−3.89	−1.83	0.47

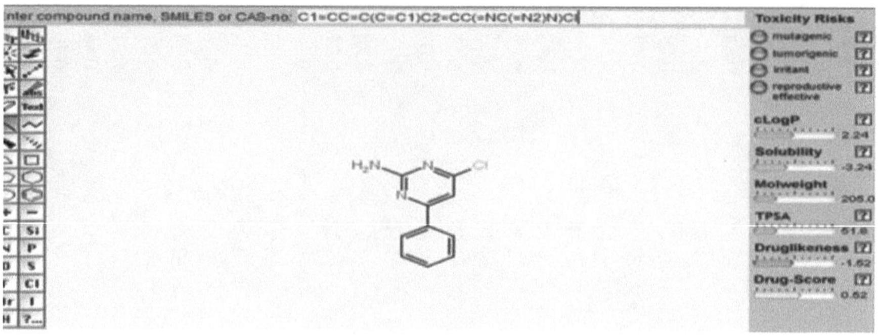

FIGURE 23.5 OSIRIS property explorer displaying drug-likeness of CID:10125644.

CID:894261—have shown a DS of 0.6 and more. Thus, with the 57 lead compounds the study was further continued.

23.3.5 Molecular Docking

When selecting patterns in the development of new drug, it is recommended to go through a docking phase in in silico studies. Molecular docking is a technique which is most commonly used for the discovery of drugs with the help of silico structures. We are able to make compounds which are useful in the therapeutic section if the chemical structure is unknown molecular interaction of a ligand and target [40–41]. The intended structure of the targeted molecule is gained beforehand, and these can be taken from a protein data bank (PDB) and for the 3D structure, ab initio is used and ligand uses PubChem. Molecular docking was invented in the year 1980 and is one of the most acknowledged technologies in computer-aided drug design and supports for prediction of binding site and fast screening of large molecules at low cost, and enhancement in rate of drugs is revealing itself as a dominant tool used globally for drug discovery [42]. This is a theoretical method that can be employed to describe the protein–ligand interaction. The interaction can forecast the strength of the proteins receptor and the binding site allowing for the structure-based drug design (SBDD) [43–44]. Originally employed for molecular recognition, the latest enhancement and advancement in technology enable its use for other main purposes such as recognition of toxicity, drug redesign, characterization, and target pharmacology [45–46]. All the substances were therefore automated docked with the 2BL9 and 2BLC proteins in the Seamdock server. Out of all the compounds in the dataset, the docking score is highest for CID:10125644. **Table 23.4** shows that the native-type docked complex has a docking score of −8.9 kcal/mol. As with the wild-type enzyme, docking studies of the mutant-type docked complex revealed a −9.0 kcal/mol docking score (**Figure 23.6**). The data indicates that CID:10125644 has a higher binding affinity for both the native and mutant forms than does pyrimethamine compared to other compounds. CID:10125644 exhibited superior pharmacokinetic and pharmacodynamic qualities (**Figure 23.7**). CID:10125644 pertain to 5-(Aminomethyl)-6–(4-chlorophenyl)-2-phenylpyrimidin-4-amine derivatives. To our notice, data generated from experimental studies suggests that it also has the ability to treat malaria [47–48].

TABLE 23.4
Docking Score of the Pyrimethamine and Lead Compound obtained from PubChem Database against the Target Structure

		Score (Kcal/mol)	
S. No.	**Compound ID**	**2BL9**	**2BLC**
1.	Pyrimethamine	–7.2	–7.4
2.	CID:894261	–7.6	–7.7
3.	CID:134621	–7.2	–7.6
4.	CID:12293991	–8.8	–8.7
5.	CID:1156921	–8.7	–8.7
6.	CID:3154202	–7.3	–7.6
7.	CID:2777563	–7.0	–6.9
8.	CID:516689	–7.3	–7.5
9.	CID:58089417	–7.7	–7.9
10.	CID:14810438	–6.9	–7.0
11.	CID:13377422	–6.8	–7.0
12.	**CID:10125644**	**–8.9**	**–9.0**
13.	CID:3013252	–8.7	–8.7
14.	CID:3013250	–8.8	–8.5
15.	CID:240802	–6.7	–7.0
16.	CID:796128	–6.7	–6.8
17.	CID:163242788	–7.4	–7.7
18.	CID:155553964	–8.3	–8.6
19.	CID:154722295	–6.9	–7.0
20.	CID:146266628	–7.4	–7.3

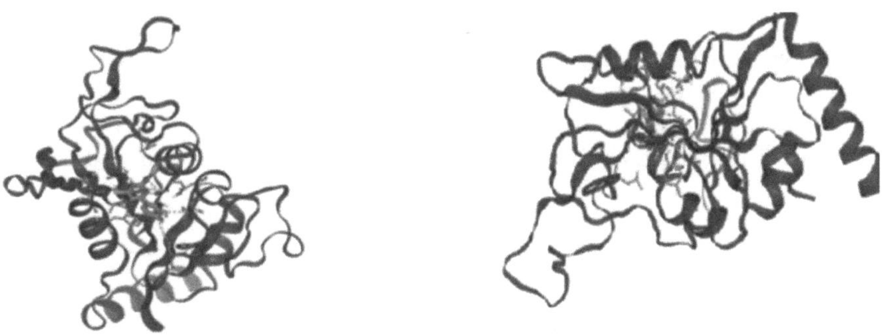

FIGURE 23.6 (a) Native and (b) Mutant with CID: docking result obtained from Seamdock.

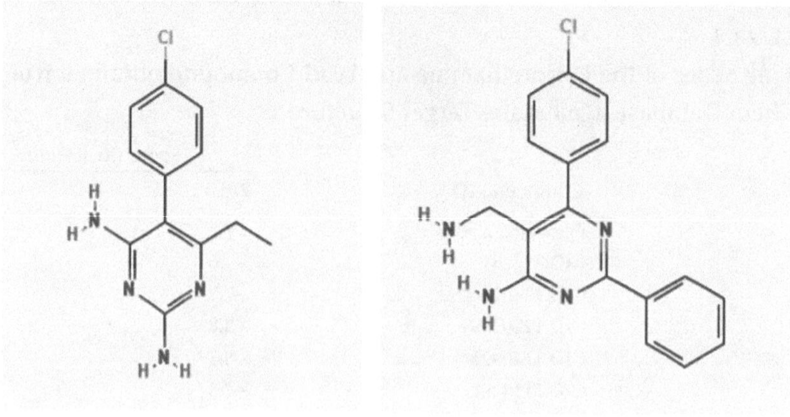

FIGURE 23.7 Structural comparison between (A) pyrimethamine and (B) CID:10125644.

23.4 CONCLUSION

The objective of this chapter was to analyze and identify a possible drug candidate which may replace pyrimethamine. As mentioned earlier, this work was able to address this problem by following VS methods. Out of the 60 analyzed compounds, 56 compounds that conform to Lipinski's rule of five were selected for further study, and 20 compounds were selected for molecular docking study. Among these compounds, conducting toxicity and pharmacokinetics tests on the compound CID:10125644, it was categorized to be more drug-like and therefore will be a much more effective malarial drug in future. Out of all the chemicals collected for the investigation, CID:10125644 reveals that it has the highest binding affinity among the native- and mutant-type malaria among all the lead compounds retrieved from the PubChem database undergoing a docking study. This means that the 5-(Aminomethyl)-6–(4-chlorophenyl)-2-phenylpyrimidin-4-amine derivates have a high propensity to substitute the role played by pyrimethamine in the treatment of malaria. The results obtained in this study align well with the previous experimental study. It is also important to note that the assessed conclusions are in good positive correlation with previous experimental attempts. However, one must not fail to agree that the information presented here assists in encouraging for PB-resistant malaria treatments, whereas did not effective in other terms in curing malaria treatments. This could be further supported by using more number of in vitro and in vivo analyses.

ACKNOWLEDGMENTS

The authors would like to express their gratitude to LPU for their support during the project work and completion of this study.

CONFLICT OF INTEREST

The authors have no conflicts of interest to report.

REFERENCES

1. Garcia, LS. Malaria. *Clinics in Laboratory Medicine.* 2010, 30(1), 93–129. https://doi.org/10.1016/j.cll.2009.10.001
2. Talapko, J.; Škrlec, I.; Alebić, T.; Jukić, M.; Včev, A. Malaria: The past and the present. *Microorganisms.* 2019, 7(6), 179. https://doi.org/10.3390/microorganisms7060179
3. Heidari, A.; Keshavarz, H. The drug resistance of plasmodium falciparum and P. Vivax in Iran: A review article. *Iranian Journal of Parasitology.* 2021, 16(2), 173. https://doi.org/10.18502/ijpa.v16i2.6265
4. Garrido-Cardenas, JA.; Cebrián-Carmona, J.; González-Cerón, L.; Manzano-Agugliaro, F.; Mesa-Valle, C. Analysis of global research on malaria and Plasmodium vivax. *International Journal of Environmental Research and Public Health.* 2019, 16(11), 1928. https://doi.org/10.3390/ijerph16111928
5. McCombie, SC. Treatment seeking for malaria: A review of recent research. *Social Science & Medicine.* 1996, 43(6), 933–45. https://doi.org/10.1016/0277–9536(95)00446–7
6. Bruxvoort, K.; Goodma, C.; Kachur, SP.; Schellenberg, D. How patients take malaria treatment: A systematic review of the literature on adherence to antimalarial drugs. *PLoS ONE.* 2014, 9(1), e84555. https://doi.org/10.1371/journal.pone.0084555
7. Wang, Y.; Xiao, J.; Suzek, TO.; Zhang, J.; Wang, J.; Zhou, Z.; Han, L.; Karapetyan, K.; Dracheva, S.; Shoemaker, BA.; Bolton, E. PubChem's BioAssay database. *Nucleic Acids Research.* 2012, 40(D1), D400–12. https://doi.org/10.1093/nar/gkr1132
8. Aravind, L.; Iyer, LM.; Wellems, TE.; Miller, LH. Plasmodium biology: Genomic gleanings. *Cell.* 2003, 115(7), 771–85. https://doi.org/10.1016/S0092–8674(03)01023–7
9. Gaillard, T.; Madamet, M.; Tsombeng, FF.; Dormoi, J.; Pradines, B. Antibiotics in malaria therapy: Which antibiotics except tetracyclines and macrolides may be used against malaria. *Malaria Journal.* 2016, 15, 1–0. https://doi.org/10.1186/s12936-016-1613-y
10. Kumar, A.; Shanthi, V.; Ramanathan, K. Computational investigation and experimental validation of crizotinib resistance conferred by C1156Y mutant anaplastic lymphoma kinase. *Molecular Informatics.* 2015 Feb, 34(2–3), 105–14. https://doi.org/10.1002/minf.201400070. Epub 2015 Jan 30. PMID: 27490033.
11. Kumar, A.; Ramanathan, K. Analyzing resistance pattern of non-small cell lung cancer to crizotinib using molecular dynamic approaches. *Indian Journal of Biochemistry and Biophysics.* 2015 Feb, 52(1), 23–8. PMID: 26040108.
12. Murail, S.; de Vries, SJ.; Rey, J.; Moroy, G.; Tufféry, P. SeamDock: An interactive and collaborative online docking resource to assist small compound molecular docking. *Frontiers in Molecular Biosciences.* 2021 Sep, 17(8), 716466. https://doi.org/10.3389/fmolb.2021.716466. PMID: 34604303; PMCID: PMC8484321.
13. Berman, HM.; Westbrook, J.; Feng, Z.; Gilliland, G.; Bhat, TN.; Weissig, H.; Shindyalov, IN.; Bourne, PE. The protein data bank. *Nucleic Acids Research.* 2000, 28(1), 235–42. https://doi.org/10.1093/nar/28.1.235
14. Kim, S. Getting the most out of PubChem for virtual screening. *Expert Opinion on Drug Discovery.* 2016, 11(9), 843–55.
15. Sadowski, J.; Schwab, CH.; Gasteiger, J. *3D structure generator.* Thesis, UC Irvine Donald Bren School of Information and Computer Sciences, California, 2003.
16. Feldman, HJ.; Snyder, KA.; Ticoll, A.; Pintilie, G.; Hogue, CW. A complete small molecule dataset from the protein data bank. *FEBS Letters.* 2006, 580(6), 1649–53. https://doi.org/10.1016/j.febslet.2006.02.003
17. Lin, Y.; Zhang, Y.; Wang, D.; Yang, B.; Shen, Y-Q. Computer especially AI-assisted drug virtual screening and design in traditional Chinese medicine. *Phytomedicine.* 2022 Dec, 107, 154481.

18. Da Silva Rocha, SFL.; Olanda, CG.; Fokoue, HH.; Sant'Anna, CMR. Virtual screening techniques in drug discovery: Review and recent applications. *Current Topics in Medicinal Chemistry*. 2019, 19(19), 1751–67.
19. Pan, R.; Hogdal, L.; Benito, J. Selective BCL-2 inhibition by ABT-199 causes on-target cell death in acute myeloid leukemia. *Cancer Discovery*. 2014, 4(3), 362–75.
20. Schindler, T.; Bornmann, W.; Pellicena, P.; Miller, W T. Structural mechanism for STI-571 inhibition of abelson tyrosine kinase. *Science*. 2000, 289(5486), 1938–42.
21. Lipinski, CA.; Lombardo, F.; Dominy, BW.; Feeney, PJ. Experimental and computational approaches to estimate solubility and permeability in drug discovery and development settings. *Advanced Drug Delivery Reviews*. 2012, 64, 4–17. https://doi.org/10.1016/j.addr.2012.09.019
22. Zhang, MQ.; Wilkinson, B. Drug discovery beyond the 'rule-of-five'. *Current Opinion in Biotechnology*. 2007, 18(6), 478–88. https://doi.org/10.1016/j.copbio.2007.10.005
23. Muegge, I. Selection criteria for drug-like compounds. *Medicinal Research Reviews*. 2003, 23(3), 302–21. https://doi.org/10.1002/med.10041
24. Kilic, B.; Gulcan, HO.; Aksakal, F.; Ercetin, T.; Oruklu, N.; Bagriacik, EU.; Dogruer, DS. Design and synthesis of some new carboxamide and propanamide derivatives bearing phenylpyridazine as a core ring and the investigation of their inhibitory potential on in-vitro acetylcholinesterase and butyrylcholinesterase. *Bioorganic Chemistry*. 2018, 79, 235–49. https://doi.org/10.1016/j.bioorg.2018.05.006
25. Mabkhot, YN.; Alatibi, F.; El-Sayed, NN.; Al-Showiman, S.; Kheder, NA.; Wadood, A.; Rauf, A.; Bawazeer, S.; Hadda, TB. Antimicrobial activity of some novel armed thiophene derivatives and petra/osiris/molinspiration (POM) analyses. *Molecules*. 2016, 21(2), 222. https://doi.org/10.3390/molecules21020222
26. Kumar, A.; Ramanathan, K. Exploring the structural and functional impact of the ALK F1174L mutation using bioinformatics approach. *Journal of Molecular Modeling*. 2014 Jul, 20(7), 2324. https://doi.org/10.1007/s00894-014-2324-3. Epub 2014 Jun 21. PMID: 24952065.
27. Wang, A.; Durrant, JD. Open-source browser-based tools for structure-based computer-aided drug discovery. *Molecules*. 2022 Jul 20, 27(14), 4623. https://doi.org/10.3390/molecules27144623. PMID: 35889494; PMCID: PMC9319651.
28. Morris, GM.; Lim-Wilby, M. Molecular docking. *Molecular Modeling of Proteins*. 2008, 365–82. https://doi.org/10.1007/978-1-59745-177-2-19
29. Kontoyianni, M. Docking and virtual screening in drug discovery. *Proteomics for Drug Discovery: Methods and Protocols*. 2017, 255–66. https://doi.org/10.1007/978-1-4939-7201-2-18
30. Dorgham, K.; Murail, S.; Tuffery, P.; Savier, E.; Bravo, J.; Rebollo, A. Binding and kinetic analysis of human protein phosphatase PP2A interactions with caspase 9 protein and the interfering peptide C9h. *Pharmaceutics*. 2022 Sep 27, 14(10), 2055. https://doi.org/10.3390/pharmaceutics14102055. PMID: 36297489; PMCID: PMC9609871.
31. López-Vallejo, F.; Caulfield, T.; Martínez-Mayorga, K.; A Giulianotti, M.; Nefzi, A.; A Houghten, R.; L Medina-Franco, J. Integrating virtual screening and combinatorial chemistry for accelerated drug discovery. *Combinatorial Chemistry & High Throughput Screening*. 2011, 14(6), 475–87. https://doi.org/10.2174/138620711795767866
32. Oprea, TI. Property distribution of drug-related chemical databases. *Journal of Computer-Aided Molecular Design*. 2000, 14, 251–64. https://doi.org/10.1023/a:1008130001697
33. Bugrim, A.; Nikolskaya, T.; Nikolsky, Y. Early prediction of drug metabolism and toxicity: Systems biology approach and modeling. *Drug Discovery Today*. 2004, Feb, 9(3), 127–35. https://doi.org/10.1016/S1359–6446(03)02971–4
34. Kumar, A.; Shanthi, V.; Ramanathan, K. Discovery of potential ALK inhibitors by virtual screening approach. *3 Biotech*. 2016, 6, 1–2. https://doi.org/10.1007/s13205-015-0336-z

35. Coltescu, AR.; Butnariu, M.; Sarac, I. The importance of solubility for new drug molecules. *Biomedical and Pharmacology Journal.* 2020, 13(2), 577–83. https://doi.org/10.13005/bpj/1920
36. Pradhan, M.; Kumar, A. Managing rifampicin resistance in tuberculosis utilizing virtual screening techniques. *Plant Archives.* 2022, 22(2). ISSN 0972–5210. https://doi.org/10.51470/PLANTARCHIVES.2022.v22.no.2.004
37. Ferreira, LL.; Andricopulo, AD. ADMET modeling approaches in drug discovery. *Drug Discovery Today.* 2019, 24(5), 1157–65. https://doi.org/10.1016/j.drudis.2019.03.015
38. Daina, A.; Michielin, O.; Zoete, V. SwissADME: A free web tool to evaluate pharmacokinetics, drug-likeness and medicinal chemistry friendliness of small molecules. *Scientific Reports.* 2017, 7(1), 42717. https://doi.org/10.1038/srep42717
39. Pinzi, L.; Rastelli, G. Molecular docking: Shifting paradigms in drug discovery. *International Journal of Molecular Sciences.* 2019, 20(18), 4331. https://doi.org/10.3390/ijms20184331
40. Vilar, S.; Costanzi, S. Application of Monte Carlo-based receptor ensemble docking to virtual screening for GPCR ligands. *Methods in Enzymology.* 2013, 522, 263–78. https://doi.org/10.1016/B978-0-12-407865-9.00014
41. Stanzione, F.; Giangreco, I.; Cole, JC. Use of molecular docking computational tools in drug discovery. *Progress in Medicinal Chemistry.* 2021, 60, 273–343. https://doi.org/10.1016/bs.pmch.2021.01.004
42. Burger, A.; Abraham, DJ. *Burger's medicinal chemistry and drug discovery.* 2003. https://doi.org/10.1002/0471266949
43. Ferreira, LG.; Dos Santos, RN.; Oliva, G.; Andricopulo, AD. Molecular docking and structure-based drug design strategies. *Molecules.* 2015, 20(7), 13384–421. https://doi.org/10.3390/molecules200713384
44. Dai, W.; Zhan, B.; Jiang, XM.; Su, H.; Li, J.; Zhao, Y.; Xie, X.; Jin, Z.; Peng, J.; Liu, F.; Li, C. Structure based design of antiviral drug candidates targeting the SARS-CoV-2 main protease. *Science.* 2020, 368(6497), 1331–5. https://doi.org/10.1126/science.abb4489
45. Kumar, A.; Mahajan, A.; Khajuria, K.; Singh, M.; Singh, M. Management of Gefitinib resistance in lung cancer utilizing virtual screening techniques. In *AIP Conference Proceedings.* 2024 Feb, 2986(1). AIP Publishing.
46. Kumar, A.; Shanthi, V.; Ramanathan, K. Discovery of potential ALK inhibitors by virtual screening approach. *3 Biotech.* 2016, 6, 1–12.
47. Singh, K.; Kaur, H.; Chibale, K.; Balzarini, J. Synthesis of 4-aminoquinoline-pyrimidine hybrids as potent antimalarials and their mode of action studies. *European Journal of Medicinal Chemistry.* 2013 Aug, 66, 314–23. https://doi.org/10.1016/j.ejmech.2013.05.046.
48. Cieplik, J.; Pluta, J.; Bryndal, I.; Lis, T. Two polymorphic forms of N-(4-chlorophenyl)-5-[(4-chlorophenyl)aminomethyl]-6-methyl-2-phenylpyrimidin-4-amine. *Acta Crystallogr C.* 2006 May, 62(Pt 5), o259–61. https://doi.org/10.1107/S0108270106010390. Epub 2006 Apr 13. PMID: 16679597.

24 On-Process Capability Analysis of Novel Cerclage Strip for Health Monitoring of Comminuted Fracture in Canines

Gurwinder Singh, Rupinder Singh, Minhaz Husain, and Amrinderpal Singh

CONTENTS

24.1 INTRODUCTION

Three-dimensional (3D) printing, which is also known as additive manufacturing (AM), involves the creation of 3D objects by depositing material layer by layer through a computer and utilizing digital models or electronic data sources. Various industries, including automotive electronics, aerospace, food, and construction, utilize AM technologies for their production needs (Kamran and Saxena, 2016). A common AM technique called MEX involves extruding thermoplastic filaments layer by layer to produce 3D objects. MEX has been increasingly popular in the biomedical industry because of its affordability and adaptability. It is used to create anatomical models, prosthetics, surgical instruments, and a variety of medical devices. MEX makes it possible to customize medical implants to fit the unique anatomy of each patient, improving results and patient satisfaction. Various types of biocompatible polymer materials are used in the biomedical field i.e. ABS, PLA, PEEK, PETG, TPU, and many more (Singh et al., 2020). Polylactic acid (PLA) is a biodegradable and bioactive thermoplastic. PLA is widely utilized as a 3D printing filament,

 DOI: 10.1201/9781003516064-24

packaging material, and medical implants. PLA offers good mechanical properties, including high stiffness and strength, allowing it to provide structural support during the healing process while gradually being absorbed by the body (Van den Eynde and Van Puyvelde, 2018). In the field of biomedical applications, PLA exhibits great potential, especially for biomedical implants. Over time, PLA implants dissolve naturally within the body, removing the need for subsequent surgeries. The use of PLA in 3D printing makes it possible to create implants that are precisely tailored to each patient's anatomy. PLA's versatility continues to revolutionize medical treatments, providing safer and more effective solutions for patients in need, from scaffolds for tissue engineering to bone fixation devices (Jamshidian et al., 2010). PLA is rapidly being also used in bone sensing capabilities within biomedical implants. PLA-based sensors provide real-time monitoring of bone biomechanics, revealing important information about load distribution, stress levels, and healing progression. These sensors allow healthcare providers to evaluate implant effectiveness, detect early indicators of problems, and adjust rehabilitation programs to each patient's specific needs (Singh et al., 2022). There are a few examples such as Tesse et al. (2019) outlined a PLA with sunflower seed shells (SSS)-based sensor for human health applications, Benaissa et al., (2023) reported a versatile conformal patch antenna embedded within ingestible boluses for animal health monitoring applications and a miniaturized microstrip patch antenna used for the biomedical applications i.e. breast cancer, brain tumor, and blood glucose monitoring (Shamim et al., 2021). In this study, the process capability of the MEX-fabricated prototype sensor was determined as a novel cerclage strip for health monitoring of comminuted fracture in the canine.

Long bone fractures are common in canine orthopedics, typically caused by normal pressures and unanticipated trauma. Non-physiological forces observed in accidents, gunshots, or falls may increase the physiological pressures inherent in normal activity. In extreme cases where these forces surpass the bone's capability, they directly impact the bone, resulting in fracture (Bidari et al., 2023). The tibia fractures in dogs are very common. Severe trauma is the most common reason for tibial fractures. The tibia may undergo multiple, spiral, greenstick, and comminuted fractures, among other types of fractures. One of the most frequent fractures in dogs is the comminuted fracture (Harasen, 2003). Adult dogs experience the majority of comminuted fractures, which are frequently caused by mature bone's increased brittleness and decreased ability to tolerate external stresses. Orthopedic surgeons face difficulties in treating comminuted fractures that penetrate the articular cartilage because of the intricate nature of the condition. Jain et al. (2016) and Presnell (1979) outlined detecting fractures in dogs using radiography and treatment of comminuted fractures using Kirchner wires and screws. However, long-term insertion of sharp-edged screws and wires inside the body can lead to tissue damage, discomfort, and irritation. A minimally invasive repair fracture (MIRF) technique was used to treat canine comminuted fractures. This technique reduces the possibility of soft tissue injury and speeds up recovery. However, relying entirely on fluoroscopic guidance raises the risk of implant malposition, which leads to inadequate stability (Beale and McCally, 2020). Dogs with comminuted fractures were found to have a higher risk of major implant failures or surgical site infections, as well as delays or malfunctions in the healing process of their fractured bones. Marshall et al. (2022)

and Johnson et al. (1996) reported type II external fixator was used to treat comminuted tibia fractures and promote healing at the site of injury in dogs. Sensors are devices developed to monitor and identify physical characteristics of the surroundings and then convert the information into electrical signals for reporting or analysis. They are essential for real-time data collecting and well-informed decision-making in a variety of industries, including healthcare, automotive, environmental monitoring, and industrial applications. With the ability to provide real-time information on physiological indicators and overall health, sensors play a crucial role in animal health monitoring parameters like heart rate, temperature, and activity level. These types of sensors help to detect health problems early on and provide important information for veterinarian care (Weston et al., 2021). There are a few examples of such types of sensors. Windolf et al. (2022) outlined a fracture monitor implantable data logger sensor for assessing the condition of bone repair by continuously tracking the implant load applications. Carmona et al. (2020) outlined an affordable, compact, battery-powered data acquisition system, ease of use, and advanced external fixator for monitoring bone regeneration in lower limbs. McGilvray et al. (2015) reported mechanical and electrical implants designed to track and evaluate the body's repair of bone fractures during diagnosis and following surgical procedures. These sensors give real-time data that can help with postoperative outcome prediction and healing progress diagnosis. Tan et al. (2017) outlined intelligent bone plates based on magnetostriction material allowing real-time monitoring of bone plate strain and assessment of patients' fracture healing status. Malizos et al. (2006) outlined a telemedicine system that employs ultrasonic monitoring to accelerate bone fracture healing. In this system, a transducer has been implanted near the site of fracture for transosseous wave propagation. So, in this study, a novel cerclage strip sensor was fabricated through MEX with 80% infill density for online health monitoring of comminuted fractures in canines. Furthermore, for health monitoring purposes, the process capability of the MEX-fabricated prototype sensor was also determined.

24.2 METHODOLOGY

Figure 24.1 shows the adopted methodology for this study. The novel cerclage strip sensor (as per Indian patent 202411005905 TEMP/E-1/6817/2024-DEL) was designed in ANSYS electronics software with 80% infill density. The sensor was designed on the microstrip patch antenna concept (MPA). The sensor was designed

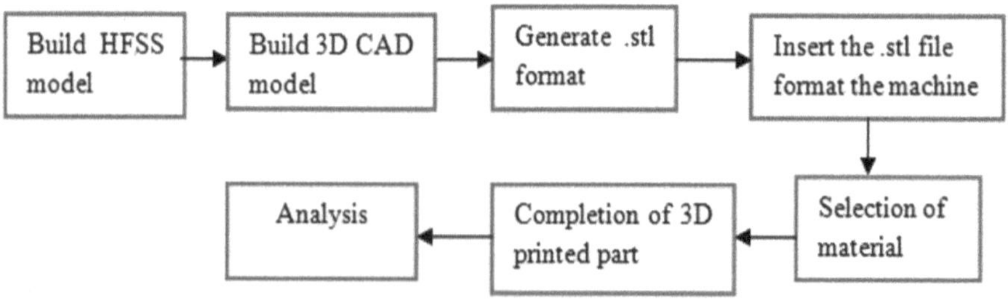

FIGURE 24.1 Adopted methodology.

with a 50 impedance and 2.45GHz operating frequency to assure sensing capability. The sensor consists of three parts i.e. patch, substrate, and ground. Biocompatibility is taken into account when selecting materials for each part. After the simulation of the sensor, the 3D CAD models were generated using SOLIDWORKS software and conversion of CAD files in standard triangular language (.stl) format for printing purposes. The substrate was made of PLA. PLA is a biocompatible polymer with high strength, making it suitable for load-bearing applications. The substrate was fabricated using the MEX. The silver conductive ink was used for the ground and patch. Silver ink is biocompatible which is safe for implant application and provides excellent electrical conductivity, allowing for efficient transmission of electrical signals within the sensor. Additionally, silver ink is deposited in exact patterns and thin layers, allowing the fabrication of flexible sensors ideal for implantation.

24.3 RESULTS

MPA comprises, non-conductive (substrate) and conductive (ground and patch) layers, much like a sandwich. Generally, Cu alloy is used to make the conducting parts, while for precise geometric dimensions 3D printing is used to create the non-conductive parts. The length, width, and height of the substrate (non-conducting part) were 49.59 × 61.71 × 2, and for conducting parts (patch and ground), the length, width, and height were 37.53 × 43.34 × 0.08 and 49.59 × 56.21 × 0.08. The dielectric constant and loss tangent were used at 2.125 and 0.0038. **Figure 24.2** shows the actual design of the sensor. Equations 24.1–24.6 were used for calculations of dimensions of MPA based on per reported literature (Yadav et al., 2017). The width (W) of the patch is given by:

$$W = \frac{C}{2f_r}\sqrt{2/\left(\varepsilon_r + 1\right)} \tag{24.1}$$

To determine the fringe factor (ΔL), the effective dielectric constant (ε_{eff}) needs to be calculated i.e.

$$\varepsilon_{eff} = \left[\frac{\left(\varepsilon_r + 1\right)}{2}\right] + \left[\left(\frac{\left(\varepsilon_r - 1\right)}{2}\right)\left(1 + 12\frac{h}{w}\right)^{-0.5}\right] \tag{24.2}$$

$$\Delta L = 0.42h\left[\frac{\left(\varepsilon_{eff} + 0.3\right)\left(\frac{w}{h} + 0.264\right)}{\left(\varepsilon_{eff} - 0.258\right)\left(\frac{w}{h} + 0.8\right)}\right] \tag{24.3}$$

The length (L) of the patch is given by:

$$L = \frac{1}{2f_r\sqrt{\left(\varepsilon_{eff}\varepsilon_o\mu_o\right)}} - 2\Delta L \tag{24.4}$$

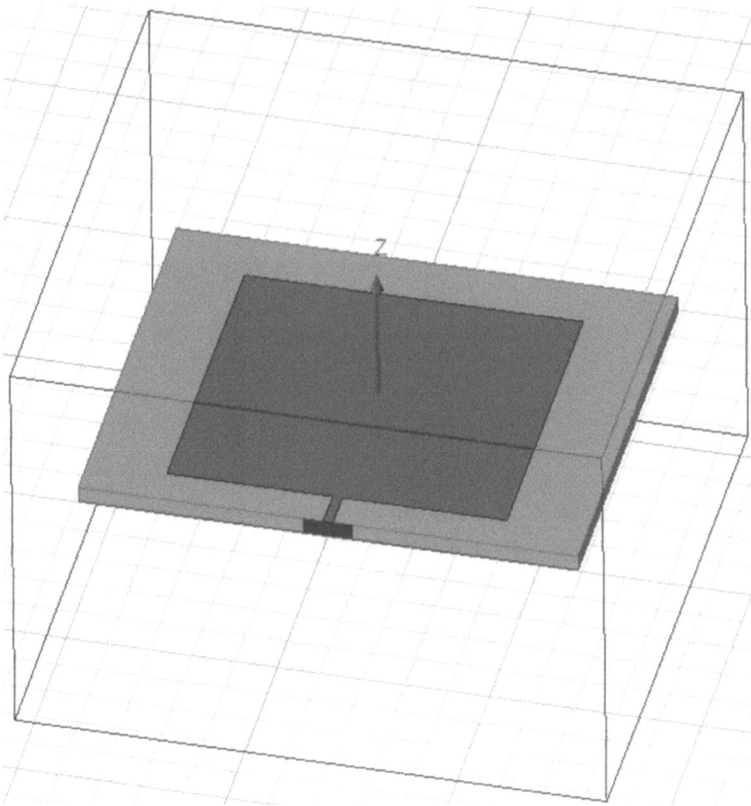

FIGURE 24.2 Actual design of MPA.

The dimensions of the substrate were given by following equations:

$$W_s = W + 6 \tag{24.5}$$

$$L_s = L + 6h \tag{24.6}$$

To check the dimensional stability of the novel cerclage strip sensor, the process capability analysis was performed with the help of process capability wizard software. The process capability wizard software is utilized to assess the manufacturing process involved in the fabrication of sensors operating on industrial, scientific, and medical (ISM) bands. Using the relevant data regarding the resonating frequency of the sensor at 80% infill density, the software helps to analyze the process capability to consistently fabricate the sensor. After the simulation on ANSYS electronics software, the vector network analyzer (VNA) was performed for the prediction of different resonating frequencies of the sensor at 80% infill density. **Table 24.1** shows the resonating frequencies of the sensor.

Based on **Table 24.1**, **Figure 24.3** indicates the summary of the process capability data. The Cp value of 1.98 demonstrates that the process spread is small in comparison to the tolerance, while the Cpk value of 1.35 demonstrates that the process

TABLE 24.1
Different Resonating Frequencies of the Sensor

S. No.	Target Resonate Frequency (GHz)	VNA Observations
1.	2.45	2.60
2.	2.45	2.62
3.	2.45	2.63
4.	2.45	2.61
5.	2.45	2.64
6.	2.45	2.65

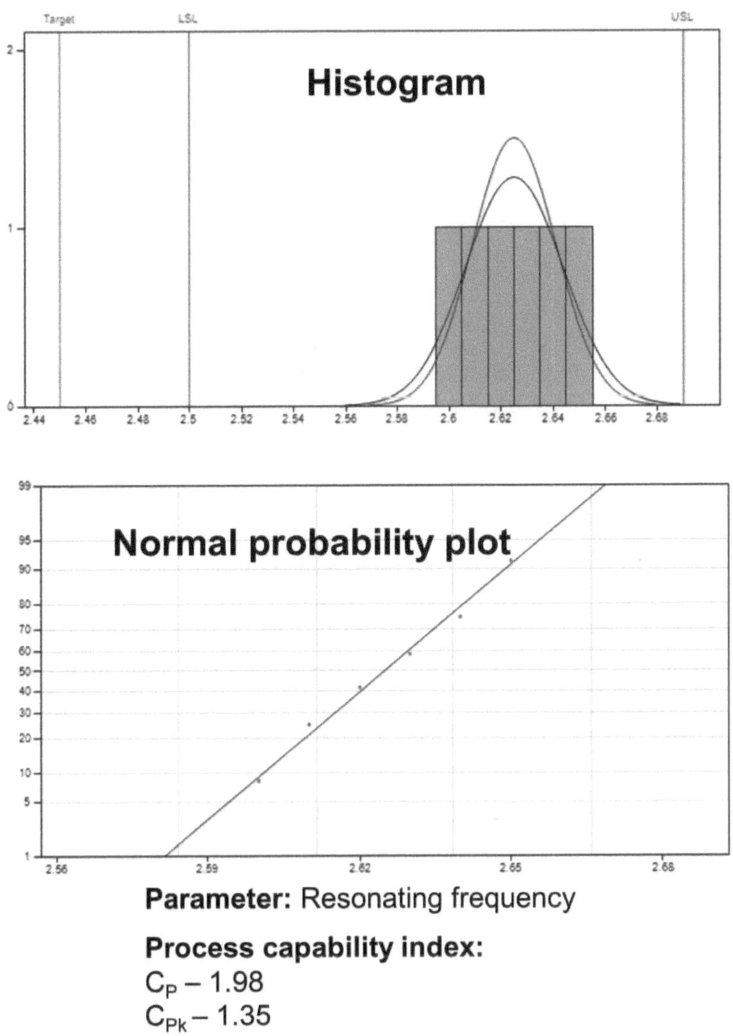

FIGURE 24.3 Summary of process capability data.

was capable of meeting specification limits and ensures the resonance frequencies fall within desired ranges with low variation. This indicates the capability and reliability of resonating frequencies within the designed frequency range, ensuring the suitability of a novel cerclage strip sensor for online health monitoring of comminuted fractures in canines at the ISM band. These findings highlight the fabrication process's dependability and quality, guaranteeing that fabricated sensors meet the demanding quality standards and execute reliably in their intended roles.

24.4 CONCLUSION

In this chapter, the process capability of MEX-fabricated novel cerclage strip sensor for online health monitoring of comminuted fractures in canines was discussed. After fabrication, VNA was conducted on the sensor. The Cp and Cpk values were calculated based on resonating frequency of the sensor, and the values were observed to be greater than 1.3. Hence, the process is statistically controlled and may be used for batch production.

ACKNOWLEDGMENT

The authors are thankful to NITTTR Chandigarh for the lab facility and technical support.

REFERENCES

Beale B, McCally R, 2020. Minimally invasive fracture repair of the tibia and fibula. *Veterinary Clinics: Small Animal Practice*, 50(1):183–206.

Benaissa S, Nikolayev D, Vermeeren G, Deprez K, Goethals J, Sonck B, Tuyttens FA, Martens L, Plets D, Joseph W, 2023. Design and experimental validation of a multiband conformal patch antenna for animal ingestible bolus applications. *IEEE Transactions on Antennas and Propagation*, 71(8):6365–77.

Bidari K, Jahangirbasha D, Dilipkumr D, Bhagavantappa B, 2023. Incidence of long bone fractures in dogs a retrospective study (2016–2021). *Journal of Pharmaceutical Innovation*, 12:531–4.

Blázquez-Carmona P, Sanchez-Raya M, Mora-Macías J, Gómez-Galán JA, Domínguez J, Reina-Romo E, 2020. Real-time wireless platform for in vivo monitoring of bone regeneration. *Sensors*, 20(16):4591.

Harasen G, 2003. Common long bone fracture in small animal practice—Part 2. *The Canadian Veterinary Journal*, 44(6):503.

Indian patent No. 202411005905 TEMP/E-1/6817/2024-DEL. *3D printed smart cerclage strip for medicinal monitoring of comminuted fracture in canine.*

Jain R, Parihar AS, Kamble S, Parihar YS, Ganguly S, 2016. Multiple fractures in tibia bone of dog: A case study. *International Journal*, 2(1):83.

Jamshidian M, Tehrany EA, Imran M, Jacquot M, Desobry S, 2010. Polylactic acid: Production, applications, nanocomposites, and release studies. *Comprehensive Reviews in Food Science and Food Safety*, 9(5):552–71.

Johnson AL, Seitz SE, Smith CW, Johnson JM, Schaeffer DJ, 1996. Closed reduction and type-II external fixation of comminuted fractures of the radius and tibia in dogs: 23 cases (1990–1994). *Journal of the American Veterinary Medical Association*, 209(8):1445–8.

Kamran M, Saxena A, 2016. A comprehensive study on 3D printing technology. *MIT International Journal of Mechanical Engineering*, 6(2):63–9.

Malizos KN, Papachristos AA, Protopappas VC, Fotiadis DI, 2006. Transosseous application of low-intensity ultrasound for the enhancement and monitoring of fracture healing process in a sheep osteotomy model. *Bone*, 38(4):530–9.

Marshall WG, Filliquist B, Tzimtzimis E, Fracka A, Miquel J, Garcia J, Fontana MD, 2022. Delayed union, non-union, and mal-union in 442 dogs. *Veterinary Surgery*, 51(7):1087–95.

McGilvray KC, Unal E, Troyer KL, Santoni BG, Palmer RH, Easley JT, Demir HV, Puttlitz CM, 2015. Implantable microelectromechanical sensors for diagnostic monitoring and post-surgical prediction of bone fracture healing. *Journal of Orthopaedic Research*, 33(10):1439–46.

Presnell KR, 1979. Surgical repair of a comminuted distal femoral fracture in a dog. *The Canadian Veterinary Journal*, 20(7):196.

Shamim SM, Uddin MS, Hasan MR, Samad M, 2021. Design and implementation of miniaturized wideband microstrip patch antenna for high-speed terahertz applications. *Journal of Computational Electronics*, 20:604–10.

Singh R, Barwar A, Kumar A, 2022. Investigations on primary and secondary recycling of PLA and its composite for biomedical and sensing applications. *Journal of The Institution of Engineers (India) Series C*, 103(4):821–36.

Singh S, Singh G, Prakash C, Ramakrishna S, 2020. Current status and future directions of fused filament fabrication. *Journal of Manufacturing Processes*, 55:288–306.

Tan Y, Hu J, Ren L, Zhu J, Yang J, Liu D, 2017. A passive and wireless sensor for bone plate strain monitoring. *Sensors*, 17(11):2635.

Tesser A, Alemaryeen A, Lewis J, Alshami A, Haghshenas M, Noghanian S, 2019. Synthesis and use of bio-based dielectric substrate for implanted radio frequency antennas. *IEEE Access*, 7:123268–79.

Van den Eynde M, Van Puyvelde P, 2018. 3D printing of poly (lactic acid). *Industrial Applications of Poly (lactic acid)*, 139–58.

Weston M, Geng S, Chandrawati R, 2021. Food sensors: Challenges and opportunities. *Advanced Materials Technologies*, 6(5):2001242.

Windolf M, Varjas V, Gehweiler D, Schwyn R, Arens D, Constant C, Zeiter S, Richards RG, Ernst M, 2022. Continuous implant load monitoring to assess bone healing status—evidence from animal testing. *Medicine*, 58(7):858.

Yadav MB, Singh B, Melkeri VS, 2017. Design of rectangular microstrip patch antenna with DGS at 2.45 GHz. In *2017 International Conference of Electronics, Communication and Aerospace Technology (ICECA)*, 1, 367–70.

25 Lab-based 3D-printed Wearable Sweat Sensor for Online Health Monitoring

Sanjeev Kumar, Rupinder Singh, and Amrinderpal Singh

CONTENTS

25.1 INTRODUCTION

To keep the human body at a healthy temperature and preserve homeostasis, sweat must be produced and evaporated from the skin's surface (Lim et al., 2008). High sweat losses are common among endurance athletes because they often work and compete in challenging environments. Research suggests that dehydration-induced loss of 2–7% body weight might have a major negative impact on exercise performance (Hawkins et al., 2010). In some circumstances, particularly during extended and intense activity, sweat losses may be enough to result in severe water/electrolyte imbalances (Baker, 2017), which can lead to the danger of more severe medical effects, such as heat stroke, if dehydration is prolonged (Maughan et al., 2015). Eccrine gland activity causes sweat, and the pace at which it evaporates is determined by the quantity secreted by each gland (Kondo et al., 2001). The number of eccrine glands varies from around 1.6 million to 4 million, and they are irregularly distributed across the skin. The densities of 600–700 glands/cm^2 are found in the palms of hands and the soles of feet, while the densities of less than one-third of the human body are found in other areas, such as the forehead (181 glands/cm^2) and the forearm (108 glands/cm^2) (Robinson and Robinson, 1954). Perspiration is composed of 99% water and 1% electrolytes, namely potassium, sodium, and chloride (Salvo et al., 2018). Sweat testing can be conducted using whole-body techniques or localized to a specific anatomical site. In this research, a prototype has been designed for the wearable sensor

 DOI: 10.1201/9781003516064-25

(forearm band) to measure the sweat rate in that localized area. Numerous industries are being impacted by wearable technology, including entertainment, leisure, safety, and medicine (Lymberis and De Rossi, 2004; Kumar et al., 2023a). E-textiles, or textile electronics combined, give textile products "smart" capabilities, which boost the wearable technology market (Kumar et al., 2022). Technical domains, including aerospace, biomedicine, electronics, and many more, have shown promise for the use of 3D printing (Husain et al., 2023a, 2023b) (builds items by stacking them one after another) (Singh et al., 2020). Researchers have investigated the use of FFF in the printing of PET and LDPE substrates for microstrip patch antennas (MPA) (Singh et al., 2022a; Singh et al., 2002b). An antenna is an essential component of wearable communication systems and needs to be flexible, compliant, lightweight, and low profile, among other requirements (Kumar et al., 2023b). Since MPA are mostly hard PCB-based, the results are uncomfortable and impractical apparel for a user for wearable applications (Kumar et al., 2023c). Scalable systems for printed electronics have been developed recently using inkjet and screen-printing processes that optimize liquid phase inks for high efficiency, stability, low cost, and zero waste materials (Tran et al., 2018). Even though inkjet printing has garnered a lot of interest from the scientific community, it has limitations, including poor ink stability, nozzle clogging, and surface restrictions since printing on rough textile surfaces can be challenging (Ibanez et al., 2021). The most common and straightforward type of traditional printing is screen printing, which is also the fastest, most affordable, versatile, and flexible (Karim et al., 2019). In screen printing, ink is transferred to a surface using a stencil design using a squeegee and a mesh screen made of silk or nylon. By adjusting the squeegee's form, pressure, speed, and snap-off distance, the print quality may be enhanced (Zhong et al., 2019). Complete electrical circuits may be produced flat, cheaply, and with great reproducibility, thanks to conductive printing. The largest obstacle to conductive printing on textiles, nevertheless, is the substrate itself since the weft and warp strands are woven together. A textile structure is typically somewhat rough and contains discernible dips. This type of surface structure is highly unsuitable for direct conductive printing on textiles because of the uneven ink dispersion over the surface. It is therefore impossible to achieve suitable connection and acceptable conductivity (Whittow et al., 2014a, 2014b). Thus, for conductive printing to be successful, the cloth surface must be smoothed and made uniform. To overcome the cloth's flaws and porosity, a thick interface layer can be printed on it. An intermediate polyurethane-based dielectric layer can be used in the interface layer technique to cover a material's surface profile and make it fairly smooth and flat (Whittow et al., 2014a). To make textile-based antennas, conductive textiles are usually attached to thick woven materials, which are not good candidates for wearable applications because of their roughness. Therefore, to build e-textile antennas without altering the feel of the fabric, a demonstration of screen printing on 3D printed thermoplastic polyurethane (TPU) films—which have already been printed on woven fabric—has been presented (Kumar et al., 2023d, 2023e). Researchers have successfully designed the wearable MPA resonating at 2.44 GHz with an SAR value of 1.383 W/kg, well within the permissible limits of 1.6W/kg as per the IEEE standard. To fabricate this MPA, recycled primary (1°) TPU was successfully printed on the cotton lycra fabric using FFF followed by screen printing of silver ink successfully on the TPU substrate (Kumar et al., 2023c). HFSS was used to build and simulate the MPA, and wearable conformability was achieved by bending the MPA at various cylinder radii (Kumar et al., 2023c). It is difficult to measure sweat rate, and as of now, there is no method for doing so outside of controlled laboratories when a subject is being trained or going about their regular business (Coyle et al., 2009). The iodine starch technique has also been used in which iodine powder is sprayed over the skin resulting in a change of powder's color into dark purple when it comes into touch with sweat. However, this technique is limited only to determining whether perspiration is present (Sato et al., 1988). Further wearable technology has also been used because of the shrinking of electrical equipment, but it was dependent on the measurement of skin impedance, though, and this can be influenced by artifacts from the electrodes (Lymberis and De Rossi, 2004; Massie et al., 2000). Other common methods consist of weighing patches placed on the subject's skin before and after exercise (Casa et al., 2000).

The present study is the extension to previously reported work (Kumar et al., 2023f), where the authors have printed TPU on the cotton lycra fabric, and silver ink has been screen printed on the TPU as a microstrip patch antenna resonating at 2.45 GHz, and SAR value has been simulated as 1.383 W/kg well within the permissible limits of 1.6 W/kg as per the IEEE standard, making this sensor safe for wearable applications, whereas conformability of the TPU+fabric-based sensor has also been explored by the author in previous research (Kumar et al., 2023f). In this study, the authors have fabricated a prototype for a sweat rate sensor as a forearm band that will be exposed to sweat (in the form of saline water) resulting in a change of the resonating frequency (showing 4D capabilities) which can be observed for online health monitoring.

25.2 METHODOLOGY

The methodology used for this work is shown in **Figure 25.1**. Given their great elasticity and flexibility, the recycled (1°) TPU granules with an MFI of 29.758 g/10min (ASTM D 1238) and 85 A shore hardness were chosen. The CLWF (lycra and cotton yarns on the weft and warp side respectively) was chosen to be comfortable for the user. In previous work, Kumar et al. (2023c) have reported the optimized printing settings as shown in **Table 25.1** for printing TPU on cotton lycra fabric. TPU filament (diameter~1.75±0.05 mm) was fabricated on a single screw extruder (SSE) (170°C temperature and 7 rpm). Additionally, the 60 × 54 × 0.65 mm TPU substrates were printed using FFF on fabric.

Further, the silver ink (ElectraPolymers ED3000) was screen printed for a ring (13.50 mm, 12.55 mm, and 14.55 mm as mean, inner, and outer ring radius respectively) feed lines (1.91 mm width, 10.82 mm length, 0.90 mm coupling gap), and ground of the ring resonator, onto TPU layer using TWS screen printer through a screen with 61/64 polyester mesh. The ring resonator was then tested on the VNA for dielectric properties, and the effect of loading and loading was also explored by applying a tensioning load of 25 N on the printed sample, but there wasn't any change in the results (**Table 25.2**). So this suggested that the MPA can be used as an armband because there is no effect on the performance by any force.

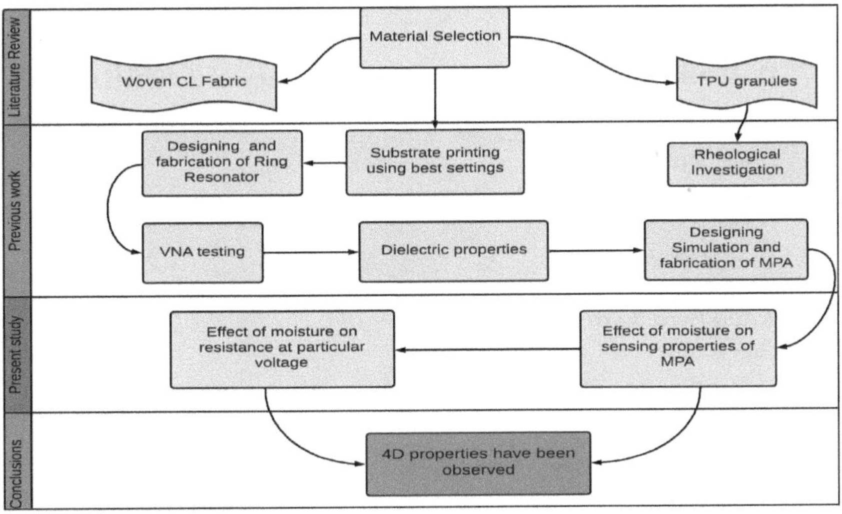

FIGURE 25.1 Methodology used.

TABLE 25.1
Optimized Printing Settings

Nozzle Temperature	Bed Temperature	Printing Speed	Infill Density
225°C	60°C	18 mm/sec	60%

TABLE 25.2
RF and Dielectric Properties of Substrate

Cycles	RF (GHz)	ε_r	Insertion Loss (dB)
Cycle 1	2.86	1.74	–86
Cycle 2	2.86	1.74	–86

Dimensions of MPA have been calculated and the design was then simulated using the HFSS for a resonating frequency of 2.45 GHz. Additionally, employing HFSS, the SAR analysis was carried out on 1 g of human tissue at a resonance frequency of 2.45 GHz. The greatest SAR value for the silver-based MPA that was recorded was 1.383 W/kg, which is well within the IEEE standard's allowable limits of 1.6 W/kg. So this suggested that the MPA can be used as an armband, and there is no effect of any force on the performance of the MPA.

In the paper, the author has expanded on earlier research by employing a TWS screen printer (printing speed 70 mm/sec, 6 layers, squeezing pressure 5 bar, curing

TABLE 25.3
Dimensions of MPA for Resonating Frequency of 2.45 GHz

Dimensions	Value (mm)
Length of Patch (Lp)	34
Width of Patch (Wp)	40
Length of Substrate (Ls)	52
Width of Substrate (Ws)	58
Substrate Thickness (Hs)	0.85
Coaxial Probe (X-axis)	11
Coaxial Probe (Y axis)	2.2

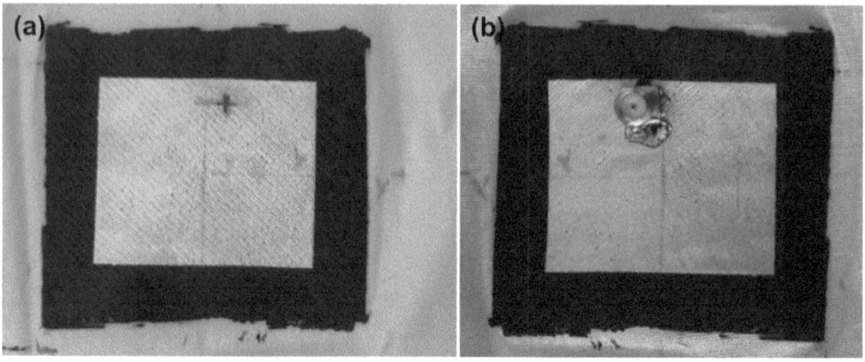

FIGURE 25.2 (a) Patch screen printed and (b) SMA connector soldered.

at 100°C for 15 minutes) to print a patch of silver ink on TPU (printed on CL woven cloth) through a screen made of 61/64 polyester mesh, followed by an oven curing. The printed patch has the dimensions of MPA calculated for a resonating frequency of 2.45 GHz (Table 25.3) as shown in **Figure 25.2**. Further, the author has explored the capabilities of a sensor under the effect of moisture (0.5 mL and 1mL saline water analogs to the sweat of the user) in terms of RF characterization (using VNA) and VR characteristics using a source meter.

25.3 RESULTS AND DISCUSSION

As shown in **Figure 25.3**, the MPA was assessed for RF characteristics on the VNA in a dry condition before being exposed to 0.5 mL of saline water and an additional 0.5 mL of saline water on its back to investigate the effects of sweating (saline water). It was observed that the exposure to moisture has affected the resonating frequency, describing the 4D characteristics of the MPA sensor (**Table 25.4** and **Figure 25.4**).

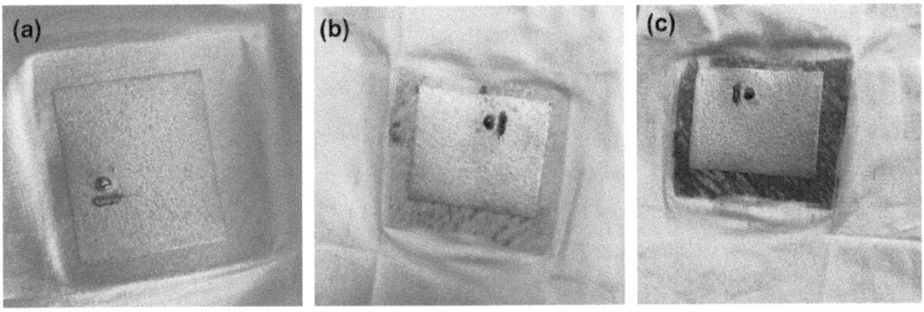

FIGURE 25.3 Back of the sensor (a) without any saline water exposure, (b) 0.5 mL saline water exposure and (c) 1 mL saline water exposure.

TABLE 25.4
Resonating Frequency of the MPA at Different Conditions

Moisture Exposure (mL)	Resonating Frequency (GHz)	Reflection loss (dB)
No Exposure (0)	2.48	−13.57
0.5	2.4	−12.74
1	2.36	−11.70

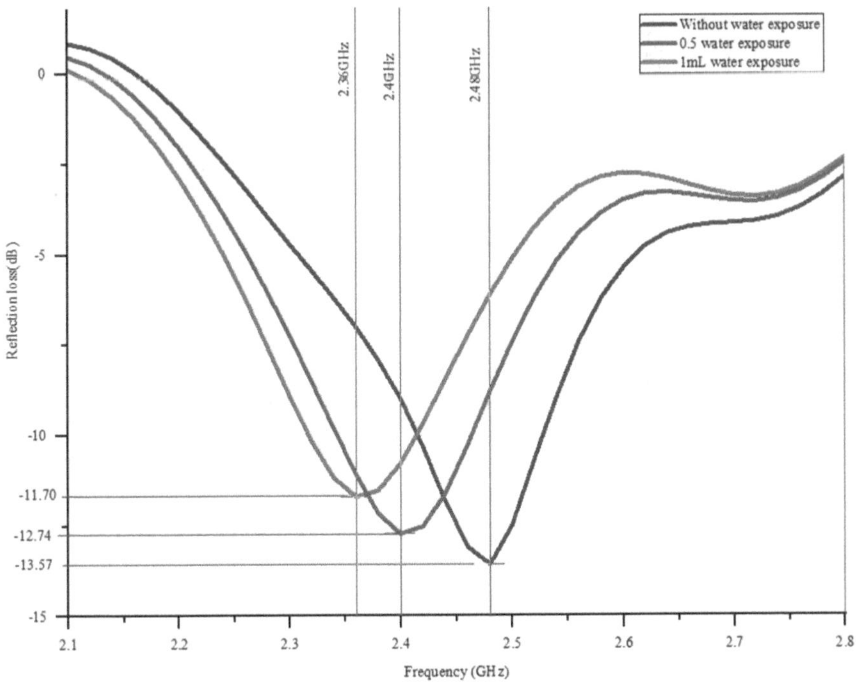

FIGURE 25.4 Resonating frequency at different conditions.

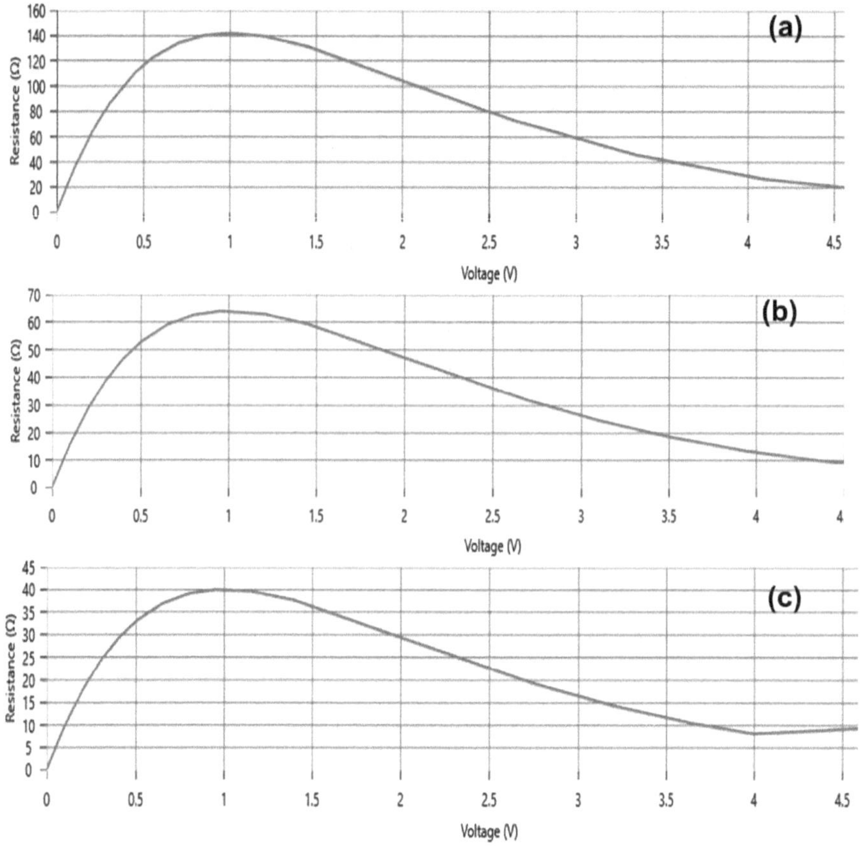

FIGURE 25.5 VR characteristics (a) without water exposure, (b) 0.5 mL water exposure, and (c) 1mL water exposure.

Further to support these results, VR (voltage-resistance) characteristics of the MPA sensor were observed under the same conditions (**Figure 25.5**) which show a change in resistance from 140 Ω (with no water exposure), 65 Ω (0.5 mL water exposure) and 40 Ω (1 mL water exposure). It may be observed that the exposure to water has affected the characteristics of the sensor in terms of resonating frequency and resistance at a particular voltage. So the proposed sensor has shown 4D characteristics and can be used as an armband to detect the sweat rate of a person during exercise or training as required.

25.4 CONCLUSION

The MPA was fabricated by screen printing silver ink on recycled (1°) TPU (printed by FFF) on CL fabric. The 4D characteristics of the MPA were tested on VNA which shows the change in resonating frequency when exposed to the saline water (sweat). So the proposed sensor can be used to detect the sweat rate when the user wears it as a forearm band.

ACKNOWLEDGMENTS

The authors are thankful to Panjab University, Chandigarh, and NITTTR Chandigarh for the lab facility and technical support.

REFERENCES

Baker, L. B. 2017. Sweating rate and sweat sodium concentration in athletes: A review of methodology and intra/interindividual variability. *Sports Medicine*, *47*, 111–28.

Casa, D. J., Armstrong, L. E., Hillman, S. K., Montain, S. J., Reiff, R. V., Rich, B. S., . . . & Stone, J. A. 2000. National athletic trainers' association position statement: Fluid replacement for athletes. *Journal of Athletic Training*, *35*(2), 212.

Coyle, S., Morris, D., Lau, K. T., Diamond, D., Taccini, N., Costanzo, D., . . . & Luprano, J. 2009. Textile sensors to measure sweat pH and sweat-rate during exercise. In *2009 3rd International Conference on Pervasive Computing Technologies for Healthcare* (pp. 1–6). IEEE.

Hawkins, C., Andrews, I., Aston, T., Beyer, T., Cairns, J., & Hansford, B. 2010. Multidisciplinary approach to nutritional problems. *Nutrition and the Cancer Patient*, 237.

Husain, M., Singh, R., & Pabla, B. S. 2023a. On digital twinning of fused filament fabrication for tensile properties of polyvinylidene fluoride composites-based functional prototypes. *Journal of Thermoplastic Composite Materials*. https://doi.org/10.1177/08927057231211221.

Husain, M., Singh, R., Pabla, B. S. 2023b. Investigating the torsional characteristics of 3D printed polyvinylidene fluoride composite. *Journal of Thermoplastic Composite Materials*. https://doi.org/10.1177/08927057231216746.

Ibanez Labiano, I., Arslan, D., Ozden Yenigun, E., Asadi, A., Cebeci, H., & Alomainy, A. 2021. Screen printing carbon nanotubes textiles antennas for smart wearables. *Sensors*, *21*(14), 4934.

Karim, N., Afroj, S., Tan, S., Novoselov, K. S., & Yeates, S. G. 2019. All inkjet-printed graphene-silver composite ink on textiles for highly conductive wearable electronics applications. *Scientific Reports*, *9*(1), 8035.

Kondo, N., Shibasaki, M., Aoki, K., Koga, S., Inoue, Y., & Crandall, C. G. 2001. Function of human eccrine sweat glands during dynamic exercise and passive heat stress. *Journal of Applied Physiology*, *90*(5), 1877–81.

Kumar, S., Singh, R., Singh, A. P., Stanley, J., & Wei, Y. 2023a. On comparison of sensing capabilities of three-dimensional printed wearable sensors. *Proceedings of the Institution of Mechanical Engineers, Part L: Journal of Materials: Design and Applications*. https://doi.org/10.1177/14644207231198708.

Kumar, S., Singh, R., Singh, A. P., & Wei, Y. 2022. Case study for the development of a hybrid composite structure of thermosetting and thermoplastics. In *Additive Manufacturing for Plastic Recycling* (pp. 141–57). CRC Press.

Kumar, S., Singh, R., Singh, A. P., & Wei, Y. 2023b. Fabrication of conformal antenna by 3D printing of recycled thermoplastic polyurethane on fabric. *Materials Today: Proceedings*.

Kumar, S., Singh, R., Singh, A. P., & Wei, Y. 2023c. Flexible and wearable patch antenna using additive manufacturing for modern wireless applications. In *3D Printing of Sensors, Actuators, and Antennas for Low-Cost Product Manufacturing* (pp. 107–22). CRC Press.

Kumar, S., Singh, R., Singh, A. P., & Wei, Y. 2023d. On 3D printing of thermoplastic polyurethane over woven fabric for wearable sensors. *Advances in Materials and Processing Technologies*, 1–10.

Kumar, S., Singh, R., Singh, A. P., & Wei, Y. 2023e. Three-dimensional printed thermoplastic polyurethane on fabric as wearable smart sensors. *Proceedings of the Institution of Mechanical Engineers, Part L: Journal of Materials: Design and Applications*, *237*(7), 1678–92.

Kumar, V., Singh, R., Ahuja, I. S., & Kumar, S. 2023f. 4D printed smart sensor, actuators, and antennas. In *3D Printing of Sensors, Actuators, and Antennas for Low-Cost Product Manufacturing* (pp. 123–36). CRC Press.

Lim, C. L., Byrne, C., & Lee, J. K. 2008. Human thermoregulation and measurement of body temperature in exercise and clinical settings. *Annals Academy of Medicine Singapore*, *37*(4), 347.

Lymberis, A., & De Rossi, D. E. (Eds.). 2004. *Wearable Ehealth Systems For Personalised Health Management: State of the Art and Future Challenges*. Amsterdam: IOS Press.

Massie, J., Gaskin, K., Asperen, P. V., & Wilcken, B. 2000. Sweat testing following newborn screening for cystic fibrosis. *Pediatric Pulmonology*, *29*(6), 452–6.

Maughan, R. J., Watson, P., & Shirreffs, S. M. 2015. Implications of active lifestyles and environmental factors for water needs and consequences of failure to meet those needs. *Nutrition Reviews*, *73*(suppl_2), 130–40.

Robinson, S., & Robinson, A. H. 1954. Chemical composition of sweat. *Physiological Reviews*, *34*(2), 202–20.

Salvo, P., Pingitore, A., Barbini, A., & Di Francesco, F. 2018. A wearable sweat rate sensor to monitor the athletes' performance during training. *Science & Sports*, *33*(2), e51–e58.

Sato, K. T., Richardson, A., Timm, D. E., & Sato, K. 1988. One-step iodine starch method for direct visualization of sweating. *The American Journal of the Medical Sciences*, *295*(6), 528–31.

Singh, R., Kumar, S., Singh, A. P., & Wei, Y. 2022a. On comparison of recycled LDPE and LDPE–bakelite composite based 3D printed patch antenna. *Proceedings of the Institution of Mechanical Engineers, Part L: Journal of Materials: Design and Applications*, *236*(4), 842–56.

Singh, R., Singh, B. P., Singh, A. P., Kumar, S., & Wei, Y. 2022b. Effect of infill density on the performance of recycled PET-based 3D printed microstrip antenna. *National Academy Science Letters*, *45*(6), 525–9.

Singh, T., Kumar, S., & Sehgal, S. 2020. 3D printing of engineering materials: A state of the art review. *Materials Today: Proceedings*, *28*, 1927–31.

Tran, T. S., Dutta, N. K., & Choudhury, N. R. 2018. Graphene inks for printed flexible electronics: Graphene dispersions, ink formulations, printing techniques and applications. *Advances in Colloid and Interface Science*, *261*, 41–61.

Whittow, W. G., Chauraya, A., Vardaxoglou, J. C., Li, Y., Torah, R., Yang, K., . . . & Tudor, J. 2014a. Inkjet-printed microstrip patch antennas realized on textile for wearable applications. *IEEE Antennas and Wireless Propagation Letters*, *13*, 71–4.

Whittow, W. G., Li, Y., Torah, R., Yang, K., Beeby, S., & Tudor, J. 2014b. Printed frequency selective surfaces on textiles. *Electronics Letters*, *50*(13), 916–7.

Zhong, Z. W., Tang, R. W. L., Chen, S. H., & Shan, X. C. 2019. A study of screen printing of stretchable circuits on polyurethane substrates. *Microsystem Technologies*, *25*, 339–50.

26 Ethnopharmacological, Phytochemical, and Toxicological Characteristics of *Dactylorhiza hatagirea*

A Synoptic Overview

Baburam Pokhrel, Saurabh Singh, Narendra Kumar Pandey, Bimlesh Kumar, Anand Kumar Chaudhary, Saumya Das, Rupa Mazumder, Avijit Mazumder, Shruti Sharma, Kardam Joshi, Dhara Patel, and Dileep Singh Baghel

CONTENTS

26.1 INTRODUCTION

Dactylorhiza hatagirea (*D. hatagirea*) is a terrestrial orchid from temperate regions to high mountains. **Figure 26.1** shows the *D. hatagirea* plant and its shoot tuber and roots. The careless harvesting of this plant from the wild and its excellent decorative

DOI: 10.1201/9781003516064-26

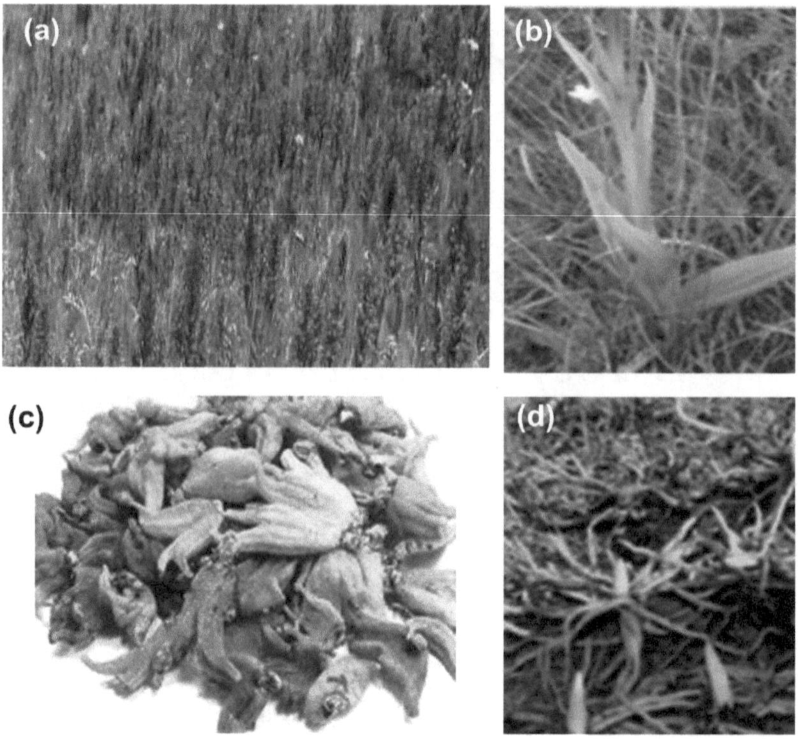

FIGURE 26.1 *D. hatagirea* plant and its shoot tuber and roots.

and medicinal properties have made it rare to find it in its natural habitat [1]. It needs mycorrhizal fungal interaction to germinate. Its natural dissemination is limited. Due to lacuna in research and careless harvesting of this medicinal herb from its natural habitat, it now comes under the endangered species. But due to commercial and medicinal value of the plant, now we have top priority to promote the cultivation which helps to remove it from endangered species category [2, 3]. So with the use of agro-technological advantage, the intensive research, multiplication, reintroduction and commercial cultivation should be promoted [4, 5]. Since the plant has been prized for its biochemical contents, the modern biotechnologies have been used for research. Part used—tuberous root; is round to oval in shape, dull-white to pale yellow in color, slightly wrinkled or smooth, waxy, and hard. Moreover, the tubers resemble the shape of the human hand [6, 7].

This medicinal orchid is enriched with dactylorhin, which has highly therapeutic potential for treating illnesses and maladies [6, 7]. Dactylorhin, known for its aphrodisiac qualities, also has neuro-stimulation, antimicrobial, nutritive, and immunomodulatory properties. The tuber root of this plant has been studied for anti-pyretic, neuro-pharmacological, anti-inflammatory, anti-cancerous, and other effects because of its significant importance for clinical research and drug recovery. This herb has been widely employed in evaluation and ethno-pharmacological uses to validate its efficiency in combating various ailments in global health problems. Recent studies have summarized the botanical, taxonomical, chemical, and ethnopharmacological information of *D. hatagirea* [5, 8–11].

26.2 METHODOLOGY

In this synoptic overview, we refer to the available literature from *Ayurvedic* classical texts, technical reports (published), and scientific databases (online), such as Scopus, Google Scholar, PubMed, Science Direct, EMBASE, and WOS, to investigate its indigenous medicinal practices, plant-based chemical composition, pharmacology, and bio-medicinal implementations. We used listed keywords: "*Dactylorhiza hatagirea*", "*Orchis hatagirea*", "*Orchis latifolia*", "*Salampunja*", "*Munjataka*", "*Hatajiri*", "*Panja*", "*Hatta Haddi*", "*Panchule*", "terrestrial orchid", "phytochemistry", "*Pravahika* (dysentery)", "*Atisara* (diarrhoea)", "*Jwara* (fever)", "*kasa* (cough)", "*Ajirna* (indigestion or upset stomach)", "*Vrana* (wounds)", "*Agnidagdha* (burns)", "*Khanda Bhagna* or *Asthi Bhagna* (fractures)", "*Medhya* (nervine tonic)", and "*Vajikarana or Vrishya chikitsa* (aphrodisiac)". The literature search was done till May 2022 and searches were restricted to the English language only.

26.3 BOTANICAL ASPECTS OF *DACTYLORHIZA HATAGIREA*

Table 26.1 summarizes the scientific classification of *Dactylorhiza hatagirea*. The detailed description is given as follows.

- *Habitat and distribution status*: *D. hatagirea* (Orchidaceae) is found in elevation of 2500–5000 meters from the sea level with temperature ranges (15–18^{0}C), and moist meadow type soils favor the proper growth of the plant. This plant is propagated by seeds and cuttings of sprouting tubers. This is Nepal's native Himalayan region plant and nearly endemic. It is also found in India, Pakistan, Afghanistan, Tibet, and Bhutan.
- *Leaves*: Leaves are 5–6, with sheathing base and obtuse at apex. The base has sub opposite arrangement with linear lanceolate to oblong cluster.
- *Flowers*: Flowers range in color from pink to purple and have six perianth segments. The innermost segment includes a big pink labellum that serves as a pollinator resting cushion. The flower undergoes 180-degree resupination, which places the labellum perpendicular to the ovary. It contains two dark green pollinaria within the anther cap. The zygomorphic flowers are grouped in tall, spike-like inflorescences, and flowering occurs from June through August.
- *Fruits*: Fruits are loculicidal capsules that release very small seeds as immature embryos at globular stage.
- *Tubers*: The tuber of this plant resembles the shape of fingers which gave its Nepali name *Panchaule*. The tuberous root of this plant is 3–7 fingered, slightly flattened, palmately lobed, creamish in color and measures around 3.5 cm in length. The penduncle usually has a length of around 27–41 cm and width of 6.7 cm [1, 2, 12, 13].

TABLE 26.1
Scientific Classification of *Dactylorhiza hatagirea*

S. No.	Class	Scientific classification
1.	Kingdom	Plantae (Plants)
2.	Subkingdom	Tracheobionta (Vascular plants)
3.	Infrakingdom	Streptophyta (land plants)
4.	Division	Magnoliophyta
5.	Phylum	Tracheophyta
6.	Class	Liliopsida
7.	Order	Orchidales, Asparagales
8.	Family	Orchidaceae
9.	Subfamily	Orchidoideae
10.	Genus	Dactylorhiza Neck. ex Neviski
11.	Species	*D. hatagirea* (D. Don) Soó
12.	Ayurvedic name	Salampunja
13.	Unani name	Buzidan, Salab Misri
14.	Hindi name	Salampanja
15.	Sanskrit name	Salam pamisri, salep
16.	English name	Himalayan Marsh Orchid
17.	Trade name	Salampanja
18.	Parts used	Tubers, roots

26.4 PHYTOCHEMICALS FOUND IN *DACTYLORHIZA HATAGIREA*

D. hatagirea contains carbohydrates, flavonoids, glycosides, steroids, tannins, proteins, alkaloids, and saponins. The secondary metabolites contained by *D. hatagirea* are Dactylorhin A, B, C, D, E with chemical formula—$C_{40}H_{56}O_{22}$, $C_{40}H_{56}O_{23}$, $C_{14}H_{24}O_{10}$, $C_{27}H_{40}O_{17}$, $C_{27}H_{40}O_{16}$ respectively (shown in **Figure 26.2**), Dactylose A, B (**Figure 26.3**) with chemical formula $C_{12}H_{16}O_6$, Indole (alkaloid) (**Figure 26.4a**)—C_8H_7N, 1,4-Naphthoquinone (**Figure 26.4b**)—$C_{10}H_6O_2$, Phytonadione/Phylloquinone (**Figure 26.4c**)—$C_{31}H_{46}O_2$, Pyrocatechol/Catechol (**Figure 26.4d**)—$C_6H_6O_2$, Glucomannan (**Figure 26.4e**)—$C_{24}H_{42}O_{21}$, Resveratrol (**Figure 26.4f**)—$C_{14}H_{12}O_3$, Ascorbic Acid (**Figure 26.4g**)—$C_6H_8O_6$, and Cyclamin (Saponin) (**Figure 26.4h**)—$C_{58}H_{94}O_{27}$ [14–16]. Table 26.2 summarizes the ethnopharmacological uses of *Dactylorhiza hatagirea*.

26.5 PHARMACOLOGICAL ACTIVITY OF *D. HATAGIREA*

26.5.1 Aphrodisiac Activity

It has been observed that the lyophilized water-based extract of roots may prevent and enhance the efficiency of sexual organs and also improve sexual performance and behavior. There is also significant evidence that the extract enhances sexual behavior and spermatogenesis activity in male albino rats [23].

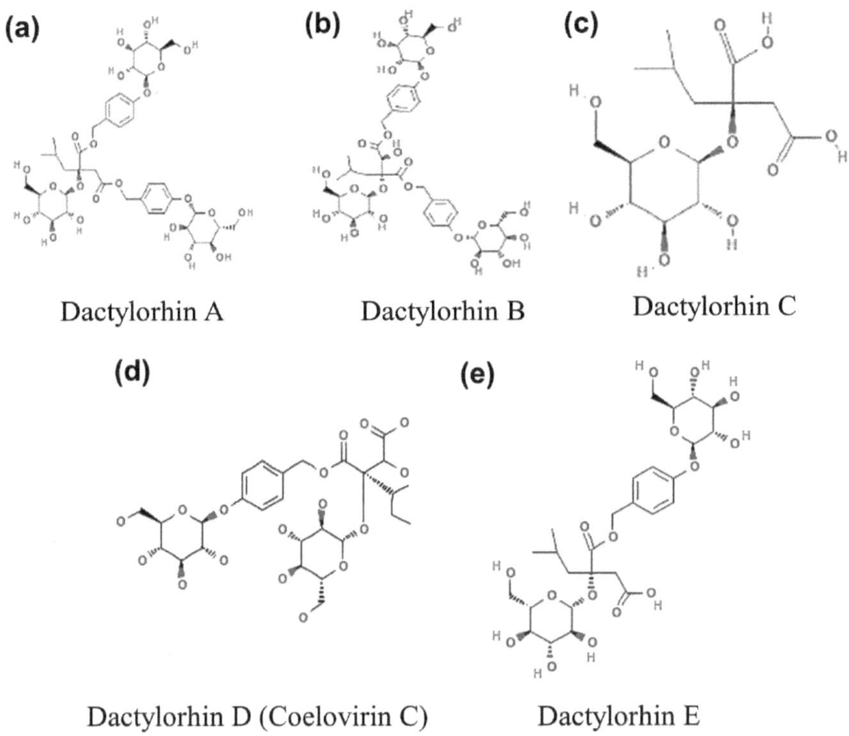

FIGURE 26.2 Chemical structure of Dactylorhin A, B, C, D, E.

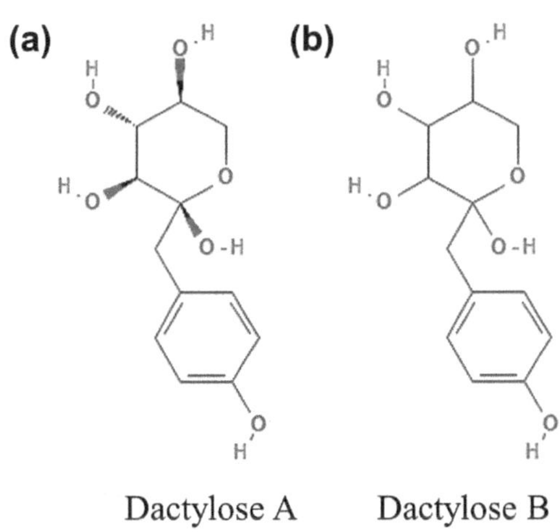

FIGURE 26.3 Chemical structure of Dactylose A and B.

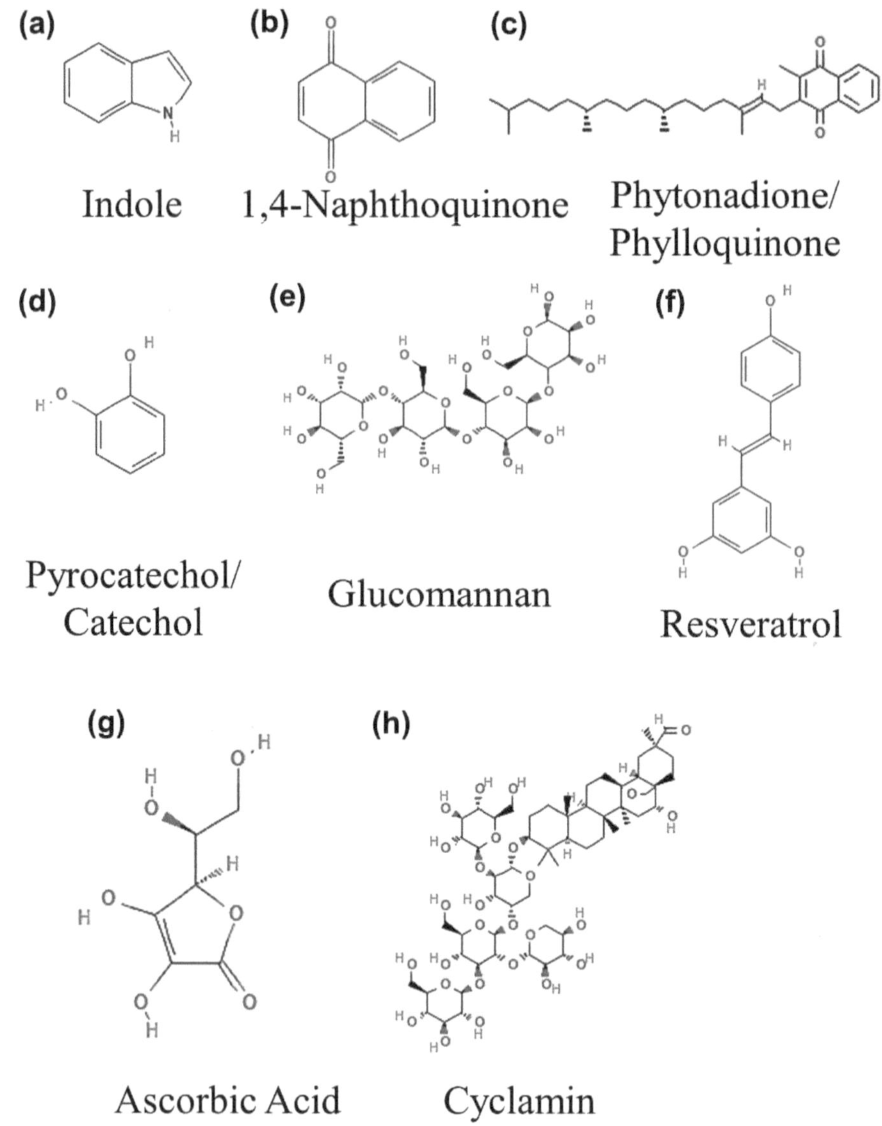

FIGURE 26.4 Chemical structure of (a) Indole, (b) 1,4-Naphthoquinone, (c) Phytonadione/Phylloquinone, (d) Pyrocatechol/Catechol, (e) Glucomannan, (f) Resveratrol, (g) Ascorbic Acid, and (h) Cyclamin.

It has been reported that the water-based extract can enhance penile erection. Further, the herbs help in enhancing reproductive function in Wistar strain male albino rats, established by measuring sperm count, seminal fructose levels in vivo, and nitric oxide release in vitro [32].

TABLE 26.2
Ethnopharmacological Uses of *Dactylorhiza hatagirea*

Sr. No.	Therapeutic Uses	Part of Plant	Territory	Way of Application	Reference
1.	Disorders of lungs	Leaves and tubers	Republic of India and Federal Democratic Republic of Nepal	• Tuber decoction mixed with hot water • Boil plant part in water and inhale the fumes	[5, 17–19]
2.	Improvement of disorders of nervous system	Leaves and tubers		• Decoction	[19–21]
3.	Disorders of digestive system	Underground stems or roots		• Decoction • Together with other therapeutic herbs, a fine powder is taken with milk or water	[20–22]
4.	Erectile dysfunction	Underground stems or roots		• To improve sexual activity, extract prepared from root is taken after dinner	[22, 23]
5.	As a nutrient	Root		• 1 teaspoon of fine powder boiled in milk	[6, 9, 11, 24]
6.	Various clinical conditions related to headache, recovery from developed wound, and dermatological disorders	Underground stems or roots		• Fine powder mixed with turmeric, and used for topical applications • Fine powder uses in wounds to control bleeding • Mustard oil is combined with a fine powder and applied on wounds	[20, 25, 26]
7.	Disorders of nephron	Underground stems or roots	Republic of India	• Not specified	[17, 27, 28]
8.	Useful in clinical conditions, including backache, bone fractures, fever, weakness, general debility, and milk production in lactating mothers	Underground stems or roots and leaves	Republic of India, Federal Democratic Republic of Nepal and Islamic Republic of Pakistan	• Mustard oil is combined with a fine powder of drug for topical applications • Decoction taken after meals	[18, 20, 29–31]

26.5.2 Antibacterial Activity

It has been reported that the ethanolic extracts of the root has resistance against all Gram-positive and Gram-negative bacteria [33].

26.5.3 Antioxidant Activity

It has been reported that the ethanolic extracts of the root has antioxidant properties [33].

26.5.4 Antidiabetic Activity

It is well reported that hydro-alcoholic extracts exhibited antihyperglycemic activity when compared with standard drug glibenclamide [8], and methanolic extract of leaves has potential antidiabetic activity [34].

26.5.5 Antipyretic Activity

According to findings, Wistar rats with pyrexia produced by Brewer's yeast have demonstrated possible antipyretic action when exposed to hydro-alcoholic extract [35].

26.5.6 Neuropharmacological Activity

It has been found that when thiopental sodium was used to induce hypnosis in Swiss albino male mice, the hydro-alcoholic extracts of *D. hatagirea* roots exhibited notable neuropharmacological effects [10].

26.6 CONCLUSION

D. hatagirea is an effective medicinal herb with significant ethnopharmacological value. We will work to prioritize and encourage its cultivation, research, and conservation among the general public, as it has been identified as an endangered plant. It might be a good idea to propagate this medicinal plant in large quantities by adopting in vitro techniques because of its broad variety of therapeutic effects, which include adaptogenic, anti-inflammatory, analgesic, antioxidant, and immunomodulatory effects. More study is required to understand its pharmacokinetics, ideal dosage, and toxicological effects before it can be used in a wide range of therapeutic applications.

REFERENCES

1. Magar, M.M., et al., Dactylorhizahatagirea: A critical issue for research and development in Nepal. *Nepal Journal of Science and Technology*, 2020. **19**(1): pp. 26–38.
2. Warghat, A.R., et al., Population genetic structure and conservation of small fragmented locations of Dactylorhiza hatagirea in Ladakh region of India. *Scientia Horticulturae*, 2013. **164**: pp. 448–54.
3. Khadka, C., et al., Ecological status and diversity indices of Panchaule (Dactylorhiza hatagirea) and its associates in Lete village of Mustang district, Nepal. *Banko Janakari*, 2016. **26**(1): pp. 45–52.

4. Subedi, A., et al., Collection and trade of wild-harvested orchids in Nepal. *Journal of Ethnobiology and Ethnomedicine*, 2013. **9**(1): pp. 1–10.
5. Pant, S. and T. Rinchen, Dactylorhiza hatagirea: A high value medicinal orchid. *Journal of Medicinal Plants Research*, 2012. **6**(19): pp. 3522–24.
6. Singh, L., et al., Process optimization and bioactive compounds quantification from Dactylorhiza hatagirea tuber for alleviating glycemic and oxidative stress. *Journal of Applied Research on Medicinal and Aromatic Plants*, 2022. **26**: p. 100352.
7. Singh, L., et al., Population status, threats, and conservation options of the orchid Dactylorhiza hatagirea in Indian Western Himalaya. *Regional Environmental Change*, 2021. **21**(2): pp. 1–16.
8. Choukarya, R., A. Choursia, and J. Rathi, In vivo and in vitro antidiabetic activity of hydroalcoholic extract of Dactylorhiza hatagirea roots: An evaluation of possible phytoconstituents. *Journal of Drug Delivery and Therapeutics*, 2019. **9**(6-s): pp. 76–81.
9. Sharma, S., P.K. Jain, and G. Parkhe, Extraction, phytochemical screening and anti-inflammatory activity of hydro-ethanolic extract of roots of Dactylorhiza hatagirea. *Journal of Drug Delivery and Therapeutics*, 2020. **10**(3-s): pp. 86–90.
10. Sirohi, B. and R. Sagar, Effect of hydroalcoholic extract of Dactylorhiza hatagirea roots & lavandula stoechas flower on thiopental sodium induced hypnosis in mice. *Journal of Drug Delivery and Therapeutics*, 2019. **9**(4-s): pp. 414–7.
11. Bhattarai, P., et al., Ecology and conservation status of threatened orchid Dactylorhiza hatagirea (D. Don) Soo in Manaslu conservation area, central Nepal. *American Journal of Plant Sciences*, 2014. **5**(23): p. 3483.
12. Warghat, A., et al. Exploring morphological diversity in Dactylorhiza hatagirea (d. don) in the cold arid desert of Ladakh. Souvenir. In *National Conference on Seabuckthorn and Environment: High Altitude Perspectives* (Sept 25–27, 2009). 2009.
13. Kunwar, R.M., et al., Distribution and habitat modeling of Dactylorhiza hatagirea (D. Don) Soo, Paris polyphylla Sm. and Taxus species in Nepal Himalaya. *Journal of Applied Research on Medicinal and Aromatic Plants*, 2021. **20**: p. 100274.
14. Haruhisa Kizu, E.-i.K., Tsuyoshi Tomimori, Studies on nepalese crude drugs. XXVI. Chemical constituents of Panch Aunle, the roots of Dactylorhiza hatagirea D. Don. *Chemical and Pharmaceutical Bulletin*, 1999. **47**(11): pp. 1618–25.
15. Dhiman, N., et al., De novo transcriptome provides insights into the growth behaviour and resveratrol and trans-stilbenes biosynthesis in Dactylorhiza hatagirea-An endangered alpine terrestrial orchid of western Himalaya. *Scientific Reports*, 2019. **9**(1): pp. 1–13.
16. NCBI Data Sources. https://pubchem.ncbi.nlm.nih.gov/sources/ (accessed January 2025).
17. Murugan, M.P., et al., Phytofoods of Nubra valley, Ladakh-the cold desert. *Indian Journal of Traditional Knowledge*, 2010. **9**(2): pp. 303–8.
18. Balkrishna, A., et al., Astavarga plants-threatened medicinal herbs of the North-West Himalaya. *International Journal of Medicinal and Aromatic Plants*, 2012. **2**(4): pp. 661–76.
19. Khajuria, A.K., G. Kumar, and N. Bisht, Diversity with ethnomedicinal notes on Orchids: A case study of Nagdev forest range, Pauri Garhwal, Uttarakhand, India. *Journal of Medicinal Plants*, 2017. **5**(1): pp. 171–4.
20. Uprety, Y., et al., Indigenous use and bio-efficacy of medicinal plants in the Rasuwa district, Central Nepal. *Journal of Ethnobiology and Ethnomedicine*, 2010. **6**(1): pp. 1–10.
21. Arora, M., A. Mahajan, and J.K. Sembi, A review on phytochemical and pharmacological potential of family Orchidaceae. *International Research Journal of Pharmacy*, 2017. **8**(10): pp. 9–24.
22. Tsering, J., et al., Medicinal orchids of Arunachal Pradesh: A review. *Bulletin of Arunachal Forest Research*, 2017. **32**(1&2): pp. 1–16.

23. Thakur, M. and V. Dixit, Aphrodisiac activity of Dactylorhiza hatagirea (D. Don) Soo in male albino rats. *Evidence-Based Complementary and Alternative Medicine*, 2007. **4**(S1): pp. 29–31.
24. Wani, I.A., et al., Dactylorhiza hatagirea (D. Don) Soo: A critically endangered perennial orchid from the North-West Himalayas. *Plants*, 2020. **9**(12): p. 1644.
25. Bhatt, D., et al., Folk herbal remedies for skin care in Kumaun Himalaya. *Journal of Non-Timber Forest Products*, 2012. **19**: pp. 309–12.
26. Hamilton, A.C. and E.A. Radford, *Identification and conservation of important plant areas for medicinal plants in the Himalaya: Project and workshop report.* Ethnobotanical Society of Nepal, 2009.
27. Kunwar, R.M., et al., Ethnomedicine in Himalaya: A case study from Dolpa, Humla, Jumla and Mustang districts of Nepal. *Journal of Ethnobiology and Ethnomedicine*, 2006. **2**(1): p. 1–6.
28. Ballabh, B., et al., Traditional medicinal plants of cold desert Ladakh—used against kidney and urinary disorders. *Journal of Ethnopharmacology*, 2008. **118**(2): pp. 331–9.
29. People, D., S. Sharma, and H. Sood, Optimization of liquid MS medium for enriching biomass of Dactylorhiza hatagirea. *National Academy of Agricultural Science*, 2016. **34**(5): pp. 1271–76.
30. Giri, D. and S. Tamta, A general account on traditional medicinal uses of Dactylorhiza hatagirea (D. Don) Soo. *New York Science Journal*, 2010. **3**(2): pp. 78–9.
31. Rawat, V.S. and J.S. Jalal, Sustainable utilization of medicinal plants by local community of Uttarkashi district of Garhwal, Himalaya, India. *European Journal of Medicinal Plants*, 2011. **1**(2): p. 18.
32. Thakur, M., et al., Improvement of penile erection, sperm count and seminal fructose levels in vivo and nitric oxide release in vitro by ayurvedic herbs. *Andrologia*, 2011. **43**(4): pp. 273–7.
33. Kumar, R., R. Badere, and S.B. Singh, Antibacterial and antioxidant activities of ethanol extracts from trans Himalayan medicinal plants. *Pharmacognosy Journal*, 2010. **2**(17): pp. 66–9.
34. Alsawalha, M., et al., Anti-diabetic activities of Dactylorhiza hatagirea leaf extract in 3T3-L1 cell line model. *Pharmacognosy Magazine*, 2019. **15**(64): p. 212.
35. Sirohi, B. and R. Sagar, Antipyretic activity of hydroalcoholic extract of Dactylorhiza hatagirea roots & lavandula stoechas flowers on Brewer's yeast induced pyrexia in Wistar rats. *Journal of Drug Delivery and Therapeutics*, 2019. **9**(4-A): pp. 701–4.

Index

I

L

M

N

Kolibri 360 GmbH
Ferdinand-Jühlke-Straße 7
99095 Erfurt, Deutschland
produktsicherheit@kolibri360.de